Emergency Medicine

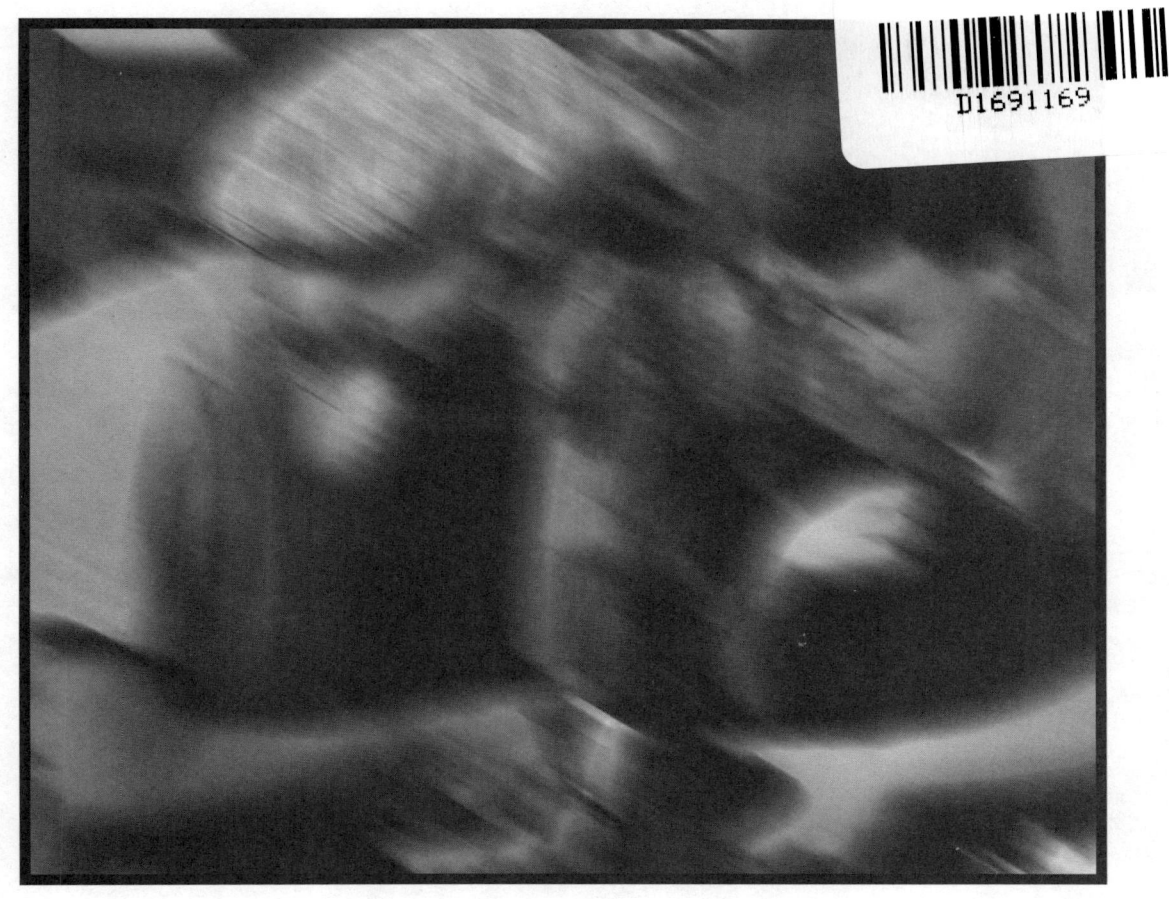

in Small Animal Practice

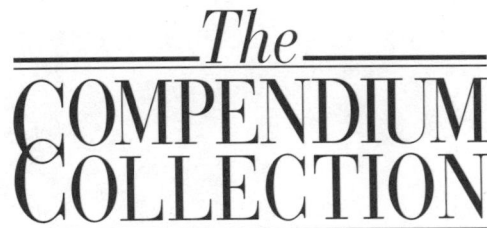

The
COMPENDIUM
COLLECTION

Published by Veterinary Learning Systems
Trenton, New Jersey

Copyright © 1997
Veterinary Learning Systems
All Rights Reserved.
Printed in U.S.A.

ISBN 1-884254-24-1

PREFACE

During veterinary school and then afterwards in private practice, I always looked forward to the next edition of the *Compendium*. The publications often were timely and provided comprehensive and practical clinical information about common conditions in small animal patients. Being veterinary students and not having much money, my former roommate and I split a subscription to the *Compendium*. When we graduated, there was quite an argument as to who would get the journals that we had received. We both recognized their value for clinical practice. The solution is the Compendium Collection series, which consolidates articles pertaining to a group of related topics and makes for easy access off the bookshelf.

Rapid information access is key during an emergency situation. For the second time, VLS Books has assembled a collection of manuscripts on emergency conditions, providing the practitioner with a practical and easy-to-use book. **Emergency Medicine in Small Animal Practice** covers a variety of topics common to veterinary emergency medicine. The articles have been written by clinicians who, because they take a special interest in the various topics, are able to offer the reader a thorough review of each subject. Many of the authors have graciously updated their manuscripts to give the latest information on these issues. Although not comprehensive, this group of manuscripts covers many of the major topics encountered in veterinary emergency medicine, including cardiac failure, shock, trauma, toxicology, seizures, respiratory emergencies, thermal emergencies, acute renal failure, acute gastroenteritis, and radiographic assessment of emergency conditions, to name just a few. Not comprehensive, but certainly extensive!

I think that the reader will find this collection a useful addition to the practice library. My greatest hope is that it is used so much that it becomes worn out. I guess this wish is a double-edged sword: If the book is used so much, then a lot of dogs and cats will have presented with serious conditions; at the same time, a lot of them likely will have been saved. If you have the same passion that I have for veterinary emergency medicine, I am sure you will enjoy this edition. If veterinary emergencies make you uneasy, you likely will enjoy this edition even more.

Finally, to my former roommate and good friend who fought so heartily for his portion of the journals when we graduated, I now have my own collection on emergency medicine.... Get your own!

Kenneth J. Drobatz, DVM
Diplomate, ACVIM and ACVECC
Director, Emergency Service
The Veterinary Hospital of
the University of Pennsylvania
Philadelphia, Pennsylvania

CONTENTS

CARDIAC EMERGENCIES

7 **Endogenous and Exogenous Nitric Oxide Donors**
Gerard J. Rubin

12 **Feline Hypertrophic Cardiomyopathy**
Terry L. Medinger and David S. Bruyette

22 **Heart Failure**
Walter E. Weirich

29 **Feline Aortic Thromboembolism**
James A. Flanders

TRAUMA

40 **Pharmaceutical Treatment of Acute Spinal Cord Trauma**
E. Meintjes, Giselle Hosgood, and Joanna Daniloff

48 **Emergency Management of Traumatic Pulmonary Contusions**
Susan G. Hackner

56 **Feline High-Rise Syndrome**
Amy S. Kapatkin and David T. Matthiesen

63 **Principles of Head Trauma Management in Dogs and Cats—Parts I and II**
Curtis W. Dewey, Steven C. Budsberg, and John E. Oliver, Jr.

84 **Coxofemoral Luxations in Dogs**
Steven M. Fox

93 **Diagnosis of Soft Tissue Injuries Associated with Pelvic Fractures**
Frank J.M. Verstraete and Nic E. Lambrechts

102 **Urethral Trauma and Principles of Urethral Surgery**
Lawrence W. Anson

SHOCK

110 **Shock**
Joseph Taboada, Johnny D. Hoskins, and Rhea V. Morgan

120 **Shock Syndrome in Cats**
Susan L. Ford and Michael Schaer

127 **Use of Hypertonic Saline Solutions in Hypovolemic Shock**
Derek S. Duval

131 **Acute Hemorrhage: A Hematologic Emergency in Dogs**
Mitchell A. Crystal and Susan M. Cotter

139 **An Introduction to Reperfusion Injury**
Mark C. Rochat

147 **Intraosseous Infusion of Fluids and Therapeutics**
Cynthia M. Otto, Geraldine McCall Kaufman, and Dennis T. Crowe, Jr.

TOXICOLOGY

154 **Pyrethrin and Pyrethroid Insecticide Intoxication in Cats**
Ted Whittem

159 **4-Methylpyrazole: An Antidote for Ethylene Glycol Intoxication in Dogs**
Lotfi El Bahri

163 **Management of Cholecalciferol Rodenticide Toxicity**
Marcia Carothers and Dennis Chew

167 **Pathophysiology of Snake Envenomization and Evaluation of Treatments—Parts I-IV**
Stormy Hudelson and Paul Hudelson

190 **Mushroom Poisoning**
Ronald B. Wilson and John A. Holladay

SEIZURE-RELATED DISORDERS

193 **Managing Epileptic Dogs**
William B. Thomas

200 **Seizure Disorders in Companion Animals**
J. E. Oliver, Jr. Update by Stacey A. Sullivan

OPHTHALMIC EMERGENCIES

211 **Assessment and Management of the Ophthalmic Emergency in Cats and Dogs**
Steven M. Roberts

RESPIRATORY EMERGENCIES

227 **Respiratory Emergencies**
Joseph Taboada, Johnny D. Hoskins, and Rhea V. Morgan

248 **Flail Chest: Pathophysiology, Treatment, and Prognosis**
Mark Anderson, John T. Payne, F. A. Mann, and Gheorghe M. Constantinescu

THERMAL EMERGENCIES

259 **Heatstroke in Dogs**
Steven A. Holloway

265 **Hypothermia in Dogs and Cats**
Nishi Dhupa

272 **Fluid and Electrolyte Metabolism During Heat Stress**
Martin J. Fettman

PAIN MANAGEMENT

278 **The Veterinarian's Responsibility: Assessing and Managing Acute Pain in Dogs and Cats. Parts I & II.**
Janna M. Johnson

SELECTED MEDICAL EMERGENCIES

290 **Life-Threatening Bacterial Infection**
Elizabeth M. Hardie

303 **Diagnosis and Symptomatic Therapy of Acute Gastroenteritis**
Albert E. Jergens

311 **Acute Renal Failure. Part I. Risk Factors, Prevention, and Strategies for Protection**
India F. Lane, Gregory F. Grauer, and Martin J. Fettman

324 **Acute Renal Failure. Part II. Diagnosis, Management, and Prognosis**
India F. Lane, Gregory F. Grauer, and Martin J. Fettman

RADIOLOGY OF SELECTED EMERGENCY CONDITIONS

336 **Radiology of Acute Abdominal Disorders in the Dog and Cat: Parts I & II**
Lawrence J. Kleine

352 **Radiologic Aspects of Thoracic Trauma in the Dog and Cat: Parts I & II**
Lawrence J. Kleine

362 **INDEX**

Endogenous and Exogenous Nitric Oxide Donors*

From the *Therapeutics in Practice* series

Gerard J. Rubin, DVM
Diplomate, ACVIM (Cardiology and Internal Medicine)
Animal Internal Medicine Clinic
Dallas, Texas

A survey of scientific material written from 1992 to 1995 revealed that almost 6000 articles on nitric oxide (NO) and the endothelium-derived relaxing factor (EDRF) have been published. The quantity of articles seems considerable for a small molecule whose major claim to fame before 1980 was as an environmental pollutant from the exhaust of cars, thus contributing to the formation of acid rain and destruction of the ozone layer.[1] Endothelium-derived relaxing factor is believed to be nitric oxide or a very similar substance, and much of the literature uses the terms interchangeably. Thus, for the purpose of this presentation, any reference to nitric oxide should be interpreted as also referring to endothelium-derived relaxing factor and vice versa.

Although endogenous nitrovasodilators have been used pharmacologically for more than 100 years, the mechanism of their action was unknown until 1980. Nitrates were better known for their action as fertilizers and in the manufacturing of bombs. The discovery of the importance of nitric oxide in vascular, neural, phagocytic, and a myriad of other functions opened a vast unexplored realm of pathophysiology and pharmacology.

The Endothelium

The vascular endothelium, previously believed to be no more than a cellular lining with a barrier role[2] of maintaining the internal integrity of blood vessels, is now known to be a prodigious manufacturer of vasoactive chemicals. The endothelium exhibits all the characteristics of an endocrine gland.[1] The vasorelaxants produced are the endothelium-derived relaxing factor, endothelium-derived hyperpolarizing factor (EDHF), prostacyclin, and C-type natriuretic peptide (CNP) (Table One). Vasoconstrictors produced are endothelin-1,[3] other endothelins, endothelium-derived contracting factors (ED-CFs), thromboxane-A_2, and free radicals.[4] Most relaxants are inhibitors of growth, and most constrictors are stimulators of growth.[2] In response to some stimuli, the endothelium produces growth factors that, combined with platelet and macrophage growth factors, are responsible for vascular remodeling.

The endothelium-derived relaxing factor is produced in the cytoplasm of vascular endothelial cells, neurovascular cells of the central nervous system,[5] vascular smooth muscle cells, myocardium,[6] endocardium, macrophages, and possibly most of the cells of the body.[7,8] The factor is probably a complex that liberates nitric oxide and may contain a thiol.[9] The major substrate is the amino acid L-arginine found in cellular cytoplasm. The dioxygenase enzyme nitric oxide synthase (NOS) on stimulation catalyzes oxidation of L-arginine, thereby producing nitric oxide and L-citrulline.[10]

Citrulline also is produced from glutamine via glutamate and ornithine in the intestinal epithelial cells and is transported by the bloodstream to the kidneys. Citrulline is converted to arginine in the proximal tubules and made available for nitric

> **KEY POINTS**
> - Endothelium-derived relaxing factor is probably a complex that liberates nitric oxide or a very similar substance.
> - Some nonendothelial agents, such as exogenous nitrovasodilators, can mimic the effects of endothelium-derived relaxing factor.
> - Nitrovasodilators have many beneficial effects as treatment for canine and feline patients with congestive heart failure and no known incompatibility with other common cardiovascular drugs.
> - Dietary deficiency of arginine may be a contributory cause of hypertension and thrombosis in cats.

---

*This column is derived from an in-depth study that includes extensive referencing. A copy of the study, along with the references, is available from the author on request.

TABLE ONE
Comparison of Endothelium-Derived Relaxing Factor (EDRF) and Prostacyclin[21]

Characteristic	EDRF	Prostacyclin
Source	L-arginine	Arachidonic acid
Pathway	Nitric oxide synthase	Cyclooxygenase
Mechanism of action	↑ Cyclic guanine monophosphate	↑ Cyclic adenosine monophosphate
Half-life	Approximately 6 seconds	Approximately 30 seconds
Inhibitors	Oxyhemoglobin, methylene blue	Aspirin and other nonsteroidal antiinflammatory drugs
Stimulus for release	Acetylcholine, calcium ionophore A23187, wall stress, thromboxane A_2, serotonin, thrombin	Acetylcholine, calcium ionophore A23187, wall stress, thrombin, hypoxia
Catabolism	Superoxide radicals	Hydrolysis

oxide synthesis in other tissue. Citrulline also is converted to arginine in endothelial cells and macrophages.[11] The L-citrulline is recycled back to L-arginine by incorporation of one nitrogen from NH_3.[12] Cats cannot produce arginine in sufficient quantities from ornithine or citrulline and therefore require large amounts in the diet.[13,14]

Nitric oxide synthase occurs in two major forms, constitutive and inducible NOS (iNOS), and in three major isoforms. Inducible NOS, also referred to as isoform II, requires induction by immunologic stimulation.[1] Constitutive nitric oxide synthases (cNOSs), isoform I and III, are present under normal physiologic or constitutional conditions, thus the designation constitutive. Isoform I is produced in neurovascular endothelial cells.[5] Isoform III is produced in cardiovascular endothelial cells, endocardium, and myocardium.

The following formula helps to explain the process:

$$\text{L-arginine} + \text{NOS} = \text{EDRF} + \text{L-citrulline}$$

Inhibitors of Nitric Oxide Synthase

Nitric oxide synthase is inhibited by L-arginine analogues[7] (i.e., N^G-monomethyl-L-arginine, N^G-nitro-L-arginine methyl ester, and N-iminoethyl-L-ornithine (Table Two). This inhibition can be overcome by the addition of L-arginine but not D-arginine.[15] These inhibitory agents have been used to define the effects of nitric oxide by blocking nitric oxide production and observing the results. Examples are:

- Induction of an endothelium-dependent constriction of rabbit aortic rings.[16]
- Inhibition of endothelium-dependent relaxation induced by acetylcholine and other relaxant substances.[16]
- Vascular smooth muscle constriction by acetylcholine.[17]
- Increased blood pressure accompanied by decrease in the glomerular filtration rate.[18]
- Induction of dose-related coronary vasoconstriction.[19]

Inducible nitric oxide synthase is also inhibited by glucocorticoid. L-canavanine inhibits nitric oxide synthase in macrophages but not in endothelial cells, platelets, and the brain.[20] Aminoguanidine can be a selective inhibitor of inducible nitric oxide synthase.[21] N-iminoethyl-L-ornithine is a selective inhibitor of nitric oxide synthase in neutrophils.[22]

Nitrovasodilators

Nonendothelial agents that mimic the effects of EDRF are exogenous nitrovasodilators, atrial natriuretic factor,[23] bovine retractor penis inhibitory factor, prostacyclin,[14] and β-adrenergic agonists (Table Three).

The pharmacologic and biochemical effects of endothelium-dependent vasodilators and nitrovasodilators[24] are almost the same.[25] Nitrovasodilators function by releasing nitric oxide independent of L-arginine and nitric oxide synthase. Three groups of drugs are considered to be nitrovasodilators.

The first group is compounds that contain a nitrate ester bond ($R-O-NO_2$). Some of the drugs belonging to the nitrate ester group are isosorbide dinitrate (ISDN), isosorbide-5-mononitrate (IS-5-MN), pentaerythritol tetranitrate, and mannitol hexanitrate.

The second group is nitrocompounds, which have a carbogen-nitrogen bond ($R-C-NO_2$). Belonging to this group is nitroglycerin (chemical name: glyceryl trinitrate).

The third group is nitric-oxide–containing compounds, such as nitroprusside and molsidomine. Nitroprusside and molsidomine can release nitric oxide spontaneously, while other compounds require prior interaction with a thiol, such as cysteine.[25]

Organic nitrates (ISDN, IS-5-MN, and nitroglycerin) are initially converted to nitric acid (HNO_3) intracellularly and subsequently to s-nitrosothiol (SNO) by the addition of a sulfhydryl (SH) group. The s-nitrosothiols and nitric oxide activate soluble guanylate cyclase (GC), which increases cyclic guanine monophosphate (cGMP). Removal of endogenous nitric oxide production or the endothelium enhances the sensitivity of the vasculature to exogenous nitrates and catecholamines,[26] possibly because of the up-regulation of soluble guanylate cyclase.[27] Nitrovasodilators have greater action on coronary arteries than on peripheral arteries, and veins are more sensitive than arteries. The latter effect may be attributable to arteries producing more endogenous nitric oxide than veins do.[28] It has also been found that veins are more subject to developing tolerance to nitrovasodilators than are arteries.[29] Of the three major nitrovasodilators, nitroglycerin is more potent than ISDN, which is more potent than IS-5-MN.[30]

Following are two formulas explaining the process:

Organic nitrates → HNO_3 + SH → SNO

EDRF [SNO or NO] → ↑ GC → ↑ cGMP → ↓ CA^{++} → ↓ contraction

Nitrovasodilators have many beneficial effects in a patient with congestive heart failure.[31] They produce venous dilation and increase venous capacitance, thereby increasing peripheral pooling of blood.[32] The result reduces left- and right-sided ventricular end-diastolic pressure and end-diastolic volume, thereby unloading the heart and reducing myocardial oxygen consumption. The dilation of coronary arteries also leads to an increase of oxygen supply to the heart. Afterload reduction by arterial dilation, reduction of arterial impedance, and increased arterial compliance boost stroke volume and therefore cardiac output. As a result, wall stress is decreased and oxygen consumption is reduced. Nitrovasodilators exert a relaxing effect on the ventricular myocardium by increasing compliance and allowing diastolic filling at a lower filling pressure without affecting systolic function.[33]

Nitrovasodilators have no known incompatibility with other commonly used cardiovascular drugs and may be used with them, some synergistically. Chronic nitrate therapy is believed to improve the hemodynamic benefits of angiotensin-converting enzyme inhibitors.[34]

In Veterans Administration Cooperative Vasodilator–Heart Failure Trials,[35] a combination of hydralazine and nitrates was shown to have a favorable effect on survival when com-

TABLE TWO
Comparison of Forms of Nitric Oxide Synthase

Constitutive	Inducible
Cytosolic	Cytosolic
NADPH[a] dependent	NADPH[a] dependent
Requires tetrahydrobiopterin	Requires tetrahydrobiopterin
Dioxygenase	Dioxygenase
L-arginine analogues inhibit	L-arginine analogues inhibit
Ca^{++} and/or calmodulin dependent	Ca^{++} independent
Picomoles of nitric oxide released	Nanomoles of nitric oxide released
Short-lasting release	Long-lasting release
Unaffected by glucocorticoids	Inhibited by glucocorticoids
Isoform I and III	Isoform II

[a]Nicotinamide adenine dinucleotide phosphate.

TABLE THREE
Comparison of Endothelium-Derived Relaxing Factor (EDRF) and Nitrovasodilators[22]

Nitrovasodilator	EDRF
Stimulates cGMP	Stimulates cGMP
Exogenously administered	Endogenously released
Prolonged circulatory effect	Transient circulatory effect
Increased activity in coronary disease	Decreased activity in coronary artery disease
Systemically active	Locally active
Inhibits smooth muscle growth	Inhibits smooth muscle growth
Inhibits myocyte growth	Inhibits myocyte growth
Tolerance may develop	No tolerance demonstrated

pared with a placebo. A study of the effect of drugs on ventriculoarterial coupling showed that nitrates delayed the peripheral wave reflection and improved the mechanical efficiency of the left ventricle while hydralazine increased the characteristic impedance and shortened wave reflection, thus decreasing the mechanical efficiency of the heart.[36] It is conceivable that trials using nitrates without hydralazine might result in a more favorable response.

Some available forms of nitrovasodilators follow[37]:

- Amyl nitrite is used by inhalation mainly for diagnostic purposes.
  Nitroglycerin is available as a sublingual tablet, oral sustained-release tablet, 2% ointment, transdermal paste, and intravenous solution.
- Nitroprusside is available for intravenous use only.
- Isosorbide dinitrate is available as a sublingual tablet, chewable tablet, tablets of various sizes, oral spray, ointment, and intravenous solution.
- Pentaerythritol tetranitrate is available as a sublingual tablet.
- Erythrityl tetranitrate is available as a sublingual tablet and an oral tablet.
- Molsidomine is a syndonimine that releases nitric oxide without requiring the presence of a thiol group and is less inclined to cause tolerance.[8] Molsidomine is given orally but at this time is not available in the United States.
- Nicorandil is a nicotinamide nitrate that has a dual cellular mechanism as a potassium channel activator and a nitric oxide contributor. Nicorandil acts by dilating large coronary arteries and as a preload and afterload reducer. It causes less tolerance than do the nitrates.[38] Nicorandil is given orally but at this time is not available in the United States.

Use in Veterinary Medicine

I have used nitrates for almost 50 years in clinical practice, originally at the suggestion of another practitioner, Dr. Arthur Trayford, to treat old dog cough (by prescribing mannitol hexanitrate) and subsequently for various forms of diagnosed heart disease. The old dog cough was probably caused by pulmonary edema or mitral regurgitation.

Although reports of the use of nitrovasodilators in veterinary medicine[39–41] have been relatively sparse, a number of pathologic conditions may be improved by their use. Congestive heart failure, especially that attributable to mitral regurgitation, fits this category.

Early studies[42] of dogs have shown that intramural coronary arterial lesions, myocardial necrosis, and myocardial fibrosis (mostly attributable to ischemia) are common findings. Dogs with heart failure are at high risk for developing valvular endocardiosis, arterial lesions, and infarcts, which might be avoided with early treatment using nitrovasodilators. The vasoconstrictor effects of congestive heart failure also might be reversed. Inoperable congenital cardiac conditions, such as septal defects, patent ductus arteriosus with right- to left-sided shunts, aortic stenosis, and valvular dysplasia, may benefit from the use of nitrovasodilators. Hypertrophic cardiomyopathy may be aided by the use of nitrovasodilators, but dilatory cardiomyopathy may not. Dogs with heartworm disease not only have pulmonary hypertension but have endothelial damage as well. It has been demonstrated that factors in serum from heartworm-diseased dogs intefered with endothelium-dependent relaxation. This decreased relaxation is corrected by addition of nitroglycerin.[43] These patients may profit by adding nitrovasodilators to the treatment regimen.

Cats are subject to hypertension as well as to cerebrovascular and caudal aortic thrombosis. Nitrovasodilators may be beneficial in these animals. Cats have a high dietary requirement for arginine because they cannot produce sufficient quantities from ornithine or citrulline.[13,14] Dietary deficiency of arginine may possibly be a contributory cause of the hypertension and thrombosis diagnosed in cats.

I have used nitrovasodilators without observing adverse effects in animals receiving cardioglycosides, diuretics, β-adrenergic blockers, calcium blockers, and angiotensin-converting enzyme inhibitors. The dose of isosorbide dinitrate used is from ¼ to 1 mg/kg twice daily in dogs and cats. The dose of 2% nitroglycerin ointment is from ¼ to 1 inch rubbed into hairless parts of the body (inner thigh or inner ear pinna) twice daily. Although the benefits described here have been anecdotal, the results warrant further trials.

The following trial groups are recommended for a thorough pharmacologic study of animals with congestive heart failure:

- Conventional therapy (i.e., digoxin and/or furosemide)
- Conventional therapy plus angiotensin-converting enzyme inhibitors
- Conventional therapy plus nitrovasodilators
- Conventional therapy plus angiotensin-converting enzyme inhibitors and nitrovasodilators
- Nitrovasodilators and/or angiotensin-converting enzyme inhibitors without conventional therapy.

Conclusion

"The nitrates have not been included in most of the trials carried out in recent years, not because they have been found to be ineffective in the syndrome, but because they are generic drugs without adequate profit margin."[44]

"Because nitrates are very old drugs and are no longer patented, it is unlikely that the pharmaceutical industry will be motivated to fund large placebo-controlled trials of nitrate therapy."[45]

Endogenous and exogenous nitrovasodilators have been studied in detail, and there is little doubt of the efficacy of nitrovasodilators in treating cases of congestive heart failure.[46] The issues that remain to be solved are the best method of use and the extent of nitric oxide toxicity under certain conditions.

References

1. Anggard E: Nitric oxide: Mediator, murderer, and medicine.

Lancet 343:1199–1206, 1994.
2. Schiffrin E: The endothelium and control of blood vessel function in health and disease. *Clin Invest Med* 17:602–620, 1994.
3. Teerlink JR, Loffler B-M, Hess P, et al: Role of endothelin in the maintenance of blood pressure in conscious rats with chronic heart failure: Acute effects of the endothelin receptor antagonist Ro 47-0203 (bosentan). *Circulation* 90:2510–2518, 1994.
4. Anderson TJ, Meredith IT, Ganz P, et al: Nitric oxide and nitrovasodilators: Similarities, differences and potential interactions. *J Am Coll Cardiol* 24:555–566, 1994.
5. Klimaschewski L, Kummer W, Mayer B, et al: Nitric oxide synthase in cardiac nerve fibers and neurons of rat and guinea-pig hearts. *Circ Res* 71:1533–1537, 1992.
6. Bailligand J, Kelly RA, Marsden PA, et al: Control of cardiac muscle cell function by an endogenous nitric oxide signaling system. *Proc Natl Acad Sci USA* 90:347–351, 1993.
7. Moncada S, Palmer RMJ, Higgs EA: Nitric oxide: Physiology, pathophysiology, and pharmacology. *Pharmacol Rev* 43:109–141, 1991.
8. Warren JB, Pons F, Brady AJB: Nitric oxide biology: Implications for cardiovascular therapeutics. *Cardiovasc Res* 28:25–30, 1994.
9. Stamler JS, Loh E, Roddy M-A, et al: Nitric oxide regulates basal systemic and pulmonary vascular resistance in healthy humans. *Circulation* 89:2035–2040, 1994.
10. Palmer R, Ashton D, Moncada S: Vascular endothelial cells synthesize nitric oxide from L-arginine. *Nature* 333:664–665, 1988.
11. Mills CD: Molecular basis of "suppressor" macrophages. *J Immunol* 146:2719–2723, 1991.
12. Hecker M, Sessa WC, Harris HJ, et al: The metabolism of L-arginine and its significance for the biosynthesis of endothelium-derived relaxing factor: Cultured endothelial cells recycle L-citrulline to L-arginine. *Proc Natl Acad Sci USA* 87:8612–8616, 1990.
13. Hodgkins EM, Franks P: Nutritional requirements of the sick cat, in August JR (ed): *Consultations in Feline Internal Medicine*. Philadelphia, WB Saunders Co, 1991, p 26.
14. Brewer NR: Nutrition of the cat. *JAVMA* 180:1179–1182, 1982.
15. Katusic ZS: Role of nitric oxide signal transduction pathway in regulation of vascular tone. *Int Angiol* 11:14–19, 1992.
16. Palmer R, Rees DD, Ashton D, et al: L-arginine is the physiological precursor for the formation of nitric oxide in endothelium-dependent relaxation. *Biochem Biophys Res Comm* 153:1251–1256, 1988.
17. Amezcua JL, Palmer RMJ, deSouza BM, et al: Nitric oxide synthesized from L-arginine regulates vascular tone in the coronary circulation of the rabbit. *Br J Pharmacol* 97:1119–1124, 1989.
18. Tolins J, Palmer RMJ, Moncada S, et al: Role of endothelium-derived relaxing factor in regulation of renal hemodynamic responses. *Am J Physiol* 258:H655–H662, 1990.
19. Chu A, Lin C-C, Chambers DE, et al: Effects of inhibition of nitric oxide formation on basal tone and endothelium-dependent responses of the coronary arteries in awake dogs. *J Clin Invest* 87:1964–1968, 1991.
20. Iyengar R, Stuehr DJ, Marletta MA: Macrophages synthesis of nitrite, nitrate and N-nitrosamines: Precursors and role of the respiratory burst. *Proc Natl Acad Sci USA* 84:6369–6373, 1987.
21. Ignarro LJ: Biological actions and properties of endothelium-derived nitric oxide formed and released from artery and vein. *Circ Res* 65:1–21, 1989.
22. Mellion BT, Ignarro LJ, Ohlstein EH, et al: Evidence for the inhibitory role of guanosine 3'5'-monophosphate in ADP-induced human platelet aggregation in the presence of nitric oxide and related vasodilation. *Blood* 57:946–955, 1981.
23. Black LS, Monroe WE, Lee JC, et al: Atrial natriuretic peptide. *Compend Contin Educ Pract Vet* 16:717–729, 1994.
24. Katsuki S, Arnold W, Mittal CK, et al: Stimulation of guanylate cyclase by sodium nitroprusside, nitroglycerin and nitric oxide in various tissue preparations and comparison to the effects of sodium azide and hydroxylamine. *J Cyclic Nucleotide Res* 3:23–35, 1977.
25. Torfgard KE, Ahler J: Mechanisms of nitrates. *Cardiovasc Drugs Ther* 8:701–717, 1994.
26. Dinnerman JL, Lawson DL, Metha JL: Interactions between nitroglycerin and endothelium in vascular smooth muscle relaxation. *Am J Physiol* 260:H698–H701, 1991.
27. Moncada S, Rees DD, Schulz R, et al: Development and the mechanism of a specific supersensitivity to nitrovasodilators after inhibition of vascular nitric oxide synthesis in vivo. *Proc Natl Acad Sci USA* 88:2166–2170, 1991.
28. Miwa K, Toda N: The regional differences of relaxations induced by various vasodilators in isolated dog coronary and mesenteric arteries. *Jpn J Pharmacol* 38:313–330, 1985.
29. Ghio S, de Servi S, Perotti R, et al: Different susceptibility to the development of nitroglycerin tolerance in the arterial and venous circulation in humans: Effects of N-acetylcysteine administration. *Circulation* 86:798–802, 1992.
30. Toyoda J, Hisayama T, Takayanagi I: Nitro compounds (isosorbide dinitrate, 5-isosorbide mononitrate and glyceryl trinitrate) on the femoral vein and femoral artery. *Gen Pharmacol* 17:89–91, 1986.
31. Cohn JN: Role of nitrates in congestive heart failure. *Am J Cardiol* 60:39H–43H, 1984.
32. Schwarz M, Katz SD, Demopoulos L, et al: Enhancement of endothelium-dependent vasodilation by low-dose nitroglycerin in patients with congestive heart failure. *Circulation* 89:1609–1614, 1994.
33. Paulus WJ, Vantrimpont PJ, Shah AM: Acute effects of nitric oxide on left ventricular relaxation and diastolic distensibility in humans. Assessment by sodium nitroprusside infusion. *Circulation* 89:2070–2078, 1994.
34. Schulz R, Triggle CR: Role of NO in vascular smooth muscle and cardiac muscle function. *TiPS* 15:254–259, 1994.
35. Cohn JN, Archibald DG, Ziesche S, et al: Effect of vasodilator therapy on mortality in chronic congestive heart failure: Results of a Veterans Administration cooperative study. *N Engl J Med* 314:1547–1552, 1986.
36. de Morais HA: Understanding ventriculo-arterial coupling. *Proc 13th Annu Meet ACVIM Forum*:281–284, 1995.
37. Thadani U, Opie LH: Nitrates, in Opie LH (ed): *Drugs for the Heart*. Philadelphia, WB Saunders Co, 1995, pp 31–48.
38. Gross GJ, Auchampach JA, Maruyama M, et al: Cardioprotective effects of nicorandil. *J Cardiovasc Pharmacol* 20(Suppl)3:S22–S28, 1992.
39. Hamlin RL: New ideas in the management of heart failure in dogs. *JAVMA* 171:114–118, 1977.
40. Rubin GJ: Acquired valvular disease, in Morgan RV (ed): *Handbook of Small Animal Practice*, ed 2. New York, Churchill Livingstone, 1992, pp 102–103.
41. Rubin GJ: Chronic atrial-ventricular valvular insufficiency. *Proc Acad Vet Cardiol* 2:49, 1991.
42. Jonsson L: Coronary arterial lesions and myocardial infarcts in the dog. *Acta Vet Scand* 38(Suppl):69, 1972.
43. Lamb VL, Williams JF, Kaiser L: Effect of serum from dogs infected with *Dirofilaria immitis* on endothelium-dependent relations on rat aorta in vitro. *Am J Vet Res* 54:2056-2059, 1993.
44. Cohn JN: Mechanisms of action and efficacy of nitrates in heart failure. *Am J Cardiol* 70:88B–92B, 1992.
45. Abrams J: Nitrates and nitrate tolerance in congestive heart failure. *Coronary Artery Dis* 4:27–36, 1993.
46. Cohn JN: Role of nitrates in congestive heart failure. *Am J Cardiol* 60:39H–43H, 1984.

Feline Hypertrophic Cardiomyopathy

KEY FACTS

- Hypertrophic cardiomyopathy is a disorder characterized by left ventricular hypertrophy, without dilation, occurring in the absence of coexisting cardiac or systemic disease.
- A hypertrophic and nondilated left ventricular wall is the characteristic gross morphologic feature and probably the principal determinant of many clinical features of the disease.
- The proposed pathophysiology of hypertrophic cardiomyopathy is believed to be multifactorial, involving dynamic left ventricular outflow obstruction, ventricular diastolic dysfunction, and myocardial ischemia.
- Clinical manifestations of hypertrophic cardiomyopathy may be typical of cardiac disease. For example, acute dyspnea and detection of abnormal lung sounds (crackles and rales) often are present on thoracic auscultation, thereby indicating pulmonary edema.
- Treatment of feline hypertrophic cardiomyopathy is extrapolated from treatments used for human hypertrophic cardiomyopathy; treatment of the disorder in humans has centered around β-adrenergic-blocking drugs since the mid 1960s.

Pet Practice & Small Animal Medical Referral Center,
Franklin Park, Illinois
Terry L. Medinger, DVM

Overland Park, Kansas
Davis S. Bruyette, DVM

HYPERTROPHIC cardiomyopathy is a disorder characterized by massive left ventricular hypertrophy, without dilation, occurring in the absence of coexisting cardiac or systemic disease.[1] In humans, this disorder has undergone extensive investigation in the areas of morphology, pathophysiology, and disease progression since its recognition during the late 1950s.[2] While increased understanding has emerged from these investigative efforts, the intrinsic complexities of this disorder continue to create uncertainty and debate. Although it is not as well characterized, the disease in cats evidently bears many similarities to the disease that affects humans.[3-7]

CAUSE

Since the reformulation of commercial cat foods in 1987, incidence of dilated cardiomyopathy associated with taurine deficiency has decreased dramatically.[8] Hypertrophic cardiomyopathy (HCM) has now become the most commonly recognized primary feline myocardial disease. Studies in humans have demonstrated the presence of familial transmission with an autosomal dominant mode of inheritance in some cases; however, as a result of wide variability in the degree of expression of the disease, many familial cases may not be detected and all patients may in fact inherit the disease.[9,10] Echocardiographic studies have shown that approximately 33% of first-degree relatives (i.e., parents, siblings, children) of human patients with hypertrophic cardiomyopathy have evidence of the disease. In addition, hypertrophic features in some individuals may not be apparent in early childhood and a single normal echocardiogram in a child does not rule out the presence of the disease in families with a history of hypertrophic cardiomyopathy.[11]

Additional evidence obtained through studies in dogs and humans suggests that hypertrophic cardiomyopathy may be a genetically determined catecholamine disorder affecting embryologic development of the heart. The characteristic histologic abnormality associated with hypertrophic cardiomyopathy is a disordered arrangement of myofibrils resembling those fibers found in the heart of an early embryo or in a more primitive species, such as salamanders.[12] Experimentally, the infusion of norepinephrine (at rates below those required to produce hypertension) or nerve growth factor (a glycoprotein that promotes nerve growth and cardiac adrenergic innervation) produces ventricular hypertrophy in dogs, resulting in gross, histologic changes

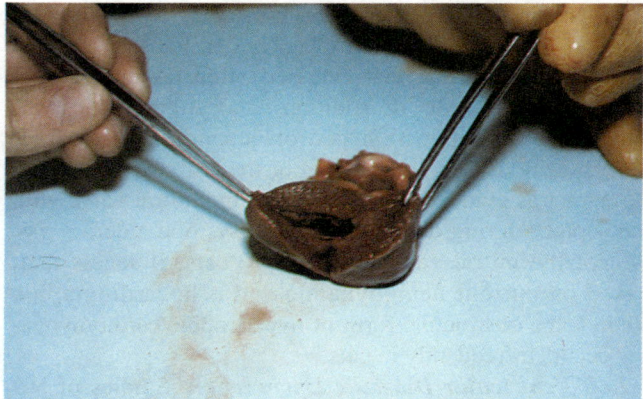

Figure 1—Heart of a five-year-old neutered cat with hypertrophic cardiomyopathy. The left ventricular wall is grossly thickened.

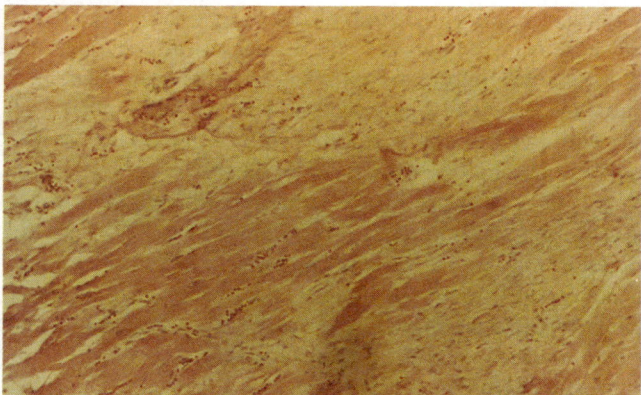

Figure 2—Histologic specimen of a hypertrophic heart from a seven-year-old spayed cat reveals myofibril disorganization and interstitial fibrosis. (H&E, ×40)

similar to those found in cases of hypertrophic cardiomyopathy.[13,14] In addition, in humans several clinical conditions associated with catecholamine dysfunction (including pheochromocytoma, primary hypertension, and neurofibromatosis) often result in hypertrophic cardiomyopathy.[10] Despite what is known about hypertrophic cardiomyopathy, the question of genetic predisposition in cats is currently unresolved as a result of the lack of controlled breeding studies.

ANOTHER speculation is that hypertrophic cardiomyopathy is a disorder of myocardial calcium metabolism.[15] Studies of hereditary hypertrophic cardiomyopathy in Syrian hamsters have shown that myocardial calcium content is increased and that development of cardiomyopathy can be prevented by administration of the calcium channel blocker verapamil.[16] Other possible causes include (1) abnormal compensatory hypertrophy resulting from myocardial ischemia or fibrosis and (2) a primary collagen abnormality with secondary ventricular hypertrophy.[17–19] In cats, excessive basal serum concentrations of growth hormone (acromegaly) result in arthropathy, weight gain, diabetes mellitus, and organomegaly, including a hypertrophic form of cardiomyopathy.[20–23] Recently, however, a cat was described with hypertrophic heart disease and an elevated serum growth hormone concentration without the presence of diabetes mellitus.[24] The role of growth hormone in the pathogenesis of hypertrophic cardiomyopathy in cats is currently under investigation. It is likely that hypertrophic cardiomyopathy is not a single disease but rather a group of causatively different disorders manifesting similar pathologic changes.

GROSS MORPHOLOGY

A hypertrophic, nondilated left ventricular wall is the characteristic gross morphologic feature and probably the principal determinant of many clinical features of the disease[25] (Figure 1). The capacity of the left ventricle is normal to diminished; consequently, increased left ventricular size results exclusively from increased thickness of the ventricular wall.[25] Hypertrophic cardiomyopathy is characterized as symmetric or asymmetric, depending on the ratio of the thickness of the ventricular septum to the ventricular free wall. In humans, 95% of patients experience greater thickening of the ventricular septum than of the free wall (ratio 1.3:1 or greater).

OTHER gross findings include mural endocardial plaque along the outflow tract and thickening of the mitral valve with enlargement of the left atria.[4,10,25] Similar morphologic findings have been described in cats, although the incidence of symmetric hypertrophy versus asymmetric hypertrophy differs between studies.[3,4,6,7] A recent echocardiographic study of cats with hypertrophic cardiomyopathy revealed marked heterogeneity of left ventricular hypertrophy.[26] Three categories of hypertrophy (type 1 = symmetric, type 2 = asymmetric septal, type 3 = asymmetric free wall) were identified and occurred with equal frequency. The clinical significance of the type of hypertrophy is discussed in the pathophysiologic mechanisms section.

HISTOLOGIC ANATOMY

Characteristic histologic findings in cats include myocardial hypertrophy and interstitial fibrosis.[3,4] Myocytes in the ventricular septum and left ventricular free wall are hypertrophied and often arranged in a disorganized pattern, with adjacent cells forming oblique or perpendicular angles to each other.[3,4,6,7] Degeneration, interstitial fibrosis, and chondroid metaplasia may be present focally or diffusely in the endocardium, conduction system, or myocardium[3,4] (Figure 2). These lesions closely resemble the lesions found in human patients with hypertrophic cardiomyopathy and consist of cardiac myofibril disorganization, myocardial scarring, and abnormalities of the small intramural coronary arteries.[27] Small intramural coronary arteries with thickened walls and frequently narrowed lumens are seen in 50% of cats with hypertrophic cardiomyopathy.[3] In humans, abnormal intramural arteries are more frequently observed within or near the margin of a sizable area of fibrosis than in regions of myocardium with little if any fibrosis.[17,27] This association may imply a causal relation between occurrence of abnormal intramural arteries and fibrosis and suggests that a form of small vessel disease may produce or contribute to the myocardial ischemia and necrosis observed in some feline patients.

PATHOPHYSIOLOGIC MECHANISMS

The proposed pathophysiology of hypertrophic cardiomyopathy is believed to be multifactorial, involving dynamic left ventricular outflow obstruction, ventricular diastolic dysfunction, and myocardial ischemia.

Left Ventricular Outflow Obstruction. Hemodynamic studies in both human and feline patients supply supporting evidence for the existence of an obstructive and an unobstructive form of hypertrophic cardiomyopathy.[4,5,10,11,27,28] The obstructive form (which occurs in approximately 25% of human patients) is believed to result from displacement of the mitral valve into the aortic outflow tract during early systole, thereby impeding left ventricular outflow. As a consequence of ventricular hypertrophy, the left ventricular outflow tract is narrowed, which subsequently increases the velocity of blood traveling through this area (Venturi effect). Resultant turbulence in the area of the outflow tract increasingly pulls the mitral valve in an anterior direction causing it to encroach on and ultimately mechanically impede left ventricular ejection.[10,27] This obstruction results in markedly elevated systolic intraventricular pressures, which increase myocardial wall stress and oxygen demand. In humans, it is also believed that displacement of the mitral valve during systole predisposes to mitral regurgitation, a common finding in patients with outflow obstruction.[10,27,29] The degree of mitral regurgitation is proportional to the magnitude of anterior motion of the mitral valve and geometric deformation of the left ventricle. The presence of outflow obstruction with mitral regurgitation represents an unfavorable situation for the left ventricle, as this combination further reduces forward flow and increases mean left atrial pressure resulting in atrial dilation.

THE CLINICAL significance of outflow obstruction in humans with hypertrophic cardiomyopathy is controversial. There evidently is no correlation between left ventricular pressure gradients and symptoms or prognosis.[10,27] Hemodynamic studies have failed to reveal an outflow gradient in most cats with hypertrophic cardiomyopathy, although mid-ventricular gradients have been detected.[4,5] A recent study of 12 cats with hypertrophic cardiomyopathy that had undergone left ventricular catheterization failed to reveal any outflow gradient.[30] In addition, echocardiographic evaluation of eight cats with hypertrophic cardiomyopathy, although demonstrating narrowing of the left ventricular outflow tract as evidenced by contact of the mitral valve with the septum during diastole, revealed systolic anterior motion of the mitral valve in only two cats. It seems that, based on current hemodynamic and echocardiographic studies, the obstructive form of hypertrophic cardiomyopathy occurs infrequently in cats.

Left Ventricular Diastolic Dysfunction. Studies of left ventricular diastolic function in human and feline hypertrophic cardiomyopathy patients have recognized the major hemodynamic abnormality as interference with normal diastolic filling.[4,5,27,31] This occurrence has been recognized in both forms of hypertrophic cardiomyopathy. One contributing factor is decreased distensibility or compliance of the myocardium.[4,5,10,31] The muscle rigidity reflects abnormalities in the intrinsic elastic properties of the myocardium, which may be secondary to increased muscle mass, myocardial fibrosis, or the disordered arrangement of myofibrils characteristic of hypertrophic cardiomyopathy. Hemodynamically, left ventricular diastolic dysfunction in patients with hypertrophic cardiomyopathy is characterized by an elevation in end-diastolic pressure despite a normal or reduced end-diastolic volume.[4,5,27,29]

ANOTHER contributing factor to left ventricular dysfunction is abnormal myocardial relaxation manifested by a prolonged relaxation period and a reduced rate of decline in left ventricular pressure. The mechanisms responsible for myocardial contraction and relaxation are now understood in terms of the central role of calcium as an activator of the contractile process. The relaxation phase is a complex, energy-consuming process by which cytosolic calcium ions are sequestered in the sarcoplasmic reticulum. This occurrence subsequently lowers intracellular calcium concentrations in the region of the myofibrillar contractile proteins and restores these contractile proteins to their relaxed state.[32] The rate of calcium removal from the cytosol determines the rate at which wall tension falls during isovolumetric contraction. Several abnormalities present in patients with hypertrophic cardiomyopathy may interfere with the energy-dependent systems responsible for relaxation. These include abnormalities in left ventricular end-systolic pressure and volume, afterload, wall stress, and ischemia.[27]

The role of abnormal myocardial relaxation and its effect on diastolic function can be evaluated by determining the relaxation half-time. The relaxation half-time is determined directly from the left ventricular pressure (LVP) tracing. The $t_{1/2}$ describes the rate of decline between the time of the maximum rate of left ventricular pressure decline (which marks the beginning of isovolumetric relaxation) and the time at which left ventricular pressure has decreased to half of its value at the beginning of contraction. An increased $t_{1/2}$, as compared with clinically normal controls, has been demonstrated in cats with hypertrophic cardiomyopathy.[33] In addition, $t_{1/2}$ evidently was more accurate in indicating diastolic function when compared with the left ventricular end-diastolic pressure in the same groups of cats.

Myocardial Ischemia. Chest pain, one of the most common symptoms in human patients with hypertrophic cardiomyopathy, is believed to result from regional myocardial ischemia.[34] Mechanisms responsible for the ischemia, although not clearly documented, include diminished capillary density with respect to greatly increased left ventricular mass, the presence of abnormally narrowed small intramural coronary arteries, and systolic compression of large intramyocardial coronary arteries producing functional increases in coronary vascular resistance.[34] Similar capillary abnormalities have been reported in cats.[3,4,6,7] The presence of myocardial ischemia may exacerbate the high left ventricular filling pressures that in turn may cause further ischemia.

SYSTEMIC THROMBOEMBOLISM

Systemic arterial thromboembolism occurs when a thrombus breaks free from its site of origin in the left ventricle and enters peripheral circulation. This occurs in approximately 50% of cats with hypertrophic cardiomyopathy.[35] The pathogenesis of thrombus formation involves a combination of three factors: local vessel or tissue injury, circulatory abnormalities, and altered blood coagulability.[36,37]

Tissue Injury. Abnormal vascular turbulence can damage atrial and ventricular endothelial surfaces exposing endocardial collagen, a potent inducer of platelet adhesion and aggregation and activator of the extrinsic clotting cascade. Activated platelets release adenosine diphosphate, serotonin, and the prostaglandin thromboxane A_2 (TXA_2), all of which promote additional platelet aggregation as well as vasoconstriction. Fibrin, the end product of the coagulation cascade, polymerizes within the platelet aggregate to produce an organized thrombus that adheres to the vascular wall.

Circulatory Abnormalities. Circulatory abnormalities within cardiac chambers may occur, thereby predisposing the chambers to thrombus formation. Left atrial and auricular enlargement, secondary to mitral regurgitation or elevated end-diastolic pressure, results in areas prone to circulatory stasis. Sluggish blood flow in such areas allows activated coagulation factors to accumulate, thereby increasing potential for thrombus formation.[38] Platelet hyperactivity resulting from abnormal circulatory patterns can also be a predisposing factor to thrombus formation. Increased vascular turbulence caused by enlarged papillary muscles, mitral regurgitation, or fibrotic intraventricular lesions can cause activation of platelets, thereby promoting platelet aggregation.[4,39–41] In addition, damage to the platelet membrane exposes phospholipoproteins, thereby providing a site for accumulation and potentiation of clotting factors.[40]

Altered Blood Coagulability. Platelet reactivity is directly related to the size and volume of the cell as well as the cell's storage capacity for serotonin, a vasoactive platelet-aggregating substance.[42,43] Feline platelets are significantly larger than are the platelets of most species, including platelets of humans and dogs[42,44]; consequently, the storage capacity for serotonin is large. In addition, feline platelets tend to be much more responsive to serotonin-induced aggregation than are the platelets of other species,[42,43,45] thereby placing cats in a constant state of increased coagulability as evidenced by spontaneous in vitro aggregation of its platelets.[36,42] This occurrence may explain the frequent occurrence of thromboembolic disease in cats.

CLINICAL MANIFESTATIONS AND DIAGNOSIS

Clinical manifestations of hypertrophic cardiomyopathy may be typical of cardiac disease. Acute dyspnea and the detection of abnormal lung sounds (crackles and rales) on thoracic auscultation are often present, thereby indicating pulmonary edema. If pericardial or pleural effusion is present, heart and lung sounds may be muffled. Arrhythmia may be detected on cardiac auscultation and simultaneous evaluation for pulse deficits by palpation of the femoral artery. Palpation of the femoral artery also may reveal a weak pulse if cardiac output is severely compromised. A cardiac murmur also may be discerned by auscultation. Conversely, signs of thromboembolism may dominate the clinical picture. Presenting signs vary with the location of the embolus, but the most common presentation is hindlimb paresis or paralysis resulting from embolization of the aortic trifurcation (Figure 3); however, forelimb paresis and pain after brachial artery embolization also occur. Signs of acute renal failure or severe colic can occur with bilateral renal artery embolization or embolization of the cranial mesenteric artery, respectively. An embolus to the cerebral arteries can produce central nervous system dysfunction, and embolization of the pulmonary vasculature may cause signs of respiratory distress.

A tentative diagnosis of hypertrophic cardiomyopathy can be made based on the history, physical examination, electrocardiographic findings, and thoracic radiography. Electrocardiographic abnormalities, predominately arrhythmia and conduction disturbances, have been reported to occur in 60% to 70% of cats with hypertrophic cardiomyopathy[4,46–47] (Figure 4). The most commonly reported arrhythmia is premature ventricular contraction; however, atrial fibrillation, atrial tachycardia, atrial premature contraction, ventricular tachycardia, and ventricular bigeminy have all been reported. Reported conduction disturbances include right and left bundle branch blocks, Wolff-Parkinson-White syn-

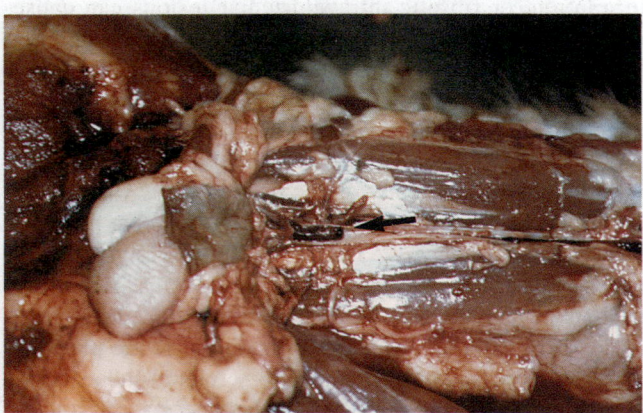

Figure 3—Necropsy examination of a five-year-old male cat presented with acute bilateral hindlimb paresis reveals a thrombus (*arrow*) lodged in the caudal aorta.

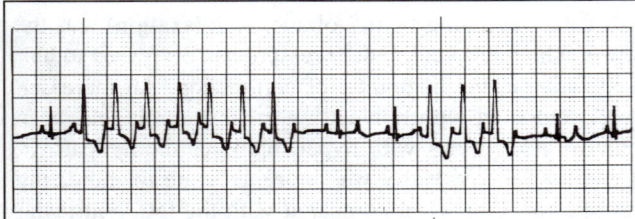

Figure 4—Electrocardiogram (lead II, 25 mm/sec, 1 mV = 1 cm) of a six-year-old neutered cat with hypertrophic cardiomyopathy presented for episodes of ventricular tachycardia.

drome, and varying degrees of atrioventricular block. Although the electrocardiogram is not a sensitive method to assess left atrial or ventricular enlargement,[46] prolongation of the P waves greater than 0.04 second indicating left atrial enlargement and prolongation of the QRS complex greater than 0.04 second with increased R wave amplitude greater than 0.9 mV in lead II indicating left ventricular enlargement may be present.

THORACIC radiographs often show evidence of interstitial and/or alveolar pulmonary edema accompanied by varying degrees of cardiomegaly. If left-sided heart failure is present, the pulmonary vessels also may be enlarged. Pulmonary edema in cats usually is patchy and focal with distribution primarily along the pulmonary vessels rather than located in the perihilar region as seen in dogs. Depending on the severity, the pulmonary edema may make visualization of the cardiac shadow difficult. Cardiac enlargement may be predominately left sided or generalized with pleural and/or pericardial effusion often present with biventricular failure. The classic radiographic description of the heart in feline hypertrophic cardiomyopathy patients is a valentine-heart shape resulting from biatrial enlargement, evident on the ventrodorsal view[48] (Figure 5).

Definitive diagnosis of feline hypertrophic cardiomyopathy requires demonstration of a thickened left ventricular wall and diminished size of the left ventricular chamber. One method is the use of nonselective angiocardiography. Contrast medium is injected intravenously, preferably by use of a centrally placed catheter, and a series of thoracic radiographs are performed at two-second intervals for eight seconds.[49] Angiocardiography effectively demonstrates such typical findings of hypertrophic cardiomyopathy as dilation of the left atrial chamber, hypertrophy of the ventricular wall, diminished capacity of the left ventricular chamber, and enlargement of the papillary muscles.[46,48] In addition, the presence of a thrombus in the left atrium may be visible in some cases.

SEVERAL important disadvantages associated with angiocardiography in hypertrophic cardiomyopathy patients must nonetheless be considered. In order to obtain an angiocardiographic study of suitable quality, heavy sedation or general anesthesia is required. Because most of these patients already are in a state of decompensated heart failure, anesthesia poses significant risk. An additional risk for these patients is the potential for adverse reactions to the contrast agent.[47] Finally, in order to perform the procedure properly, special radiographic equipment is needed to allow frequent and rapid exposure of films. In contrast, echocardiography provides a safe, highly sensitive, noninvasive technique for rapid diagnosis of feline hypertrophic cardiomyopathy.[46,50] In addition to evaluating cardiac structure (wall thickness, chamber volume, papillary muscle size, and valvular competence), parameters of cardiac function can be evaluated. By determining end-diastolic diameter, end-systolic diameter, fractional shortening, stroke volume, and ejection fraction, overall cardiac function can be evaluated. Such parameters also can be periodically reevaluated to assess disease progression with minimal risk to the patient. Consequently, the risks and additional expense of angiocardiography as well the logistical problems involved make echocardiography the preferred means for diagnosing feline hypertrophic cardiomyopathy (Figure 6).

During the diagnostic process, consideration should be given to other potential causes of left ventricular hypertrophy. These include such abnormalities as congenital aortic stenosis, chronic systemic hypertension, hyperthyroidism, and chronic anemia.[51-52] Another advantage of echocardiography is the ability to differentiate hyperthyroid-induced ventricular hypertrophy from hypertrophic cardiomyopathy.[46] Appropriate diagnostic tests should be done when necessary to rule out diagnostic differentials and to screen for coexistent disease, which may affect drug selection.

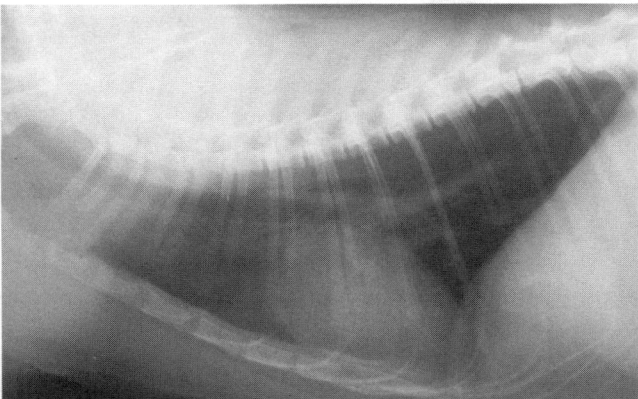
Figure 5A

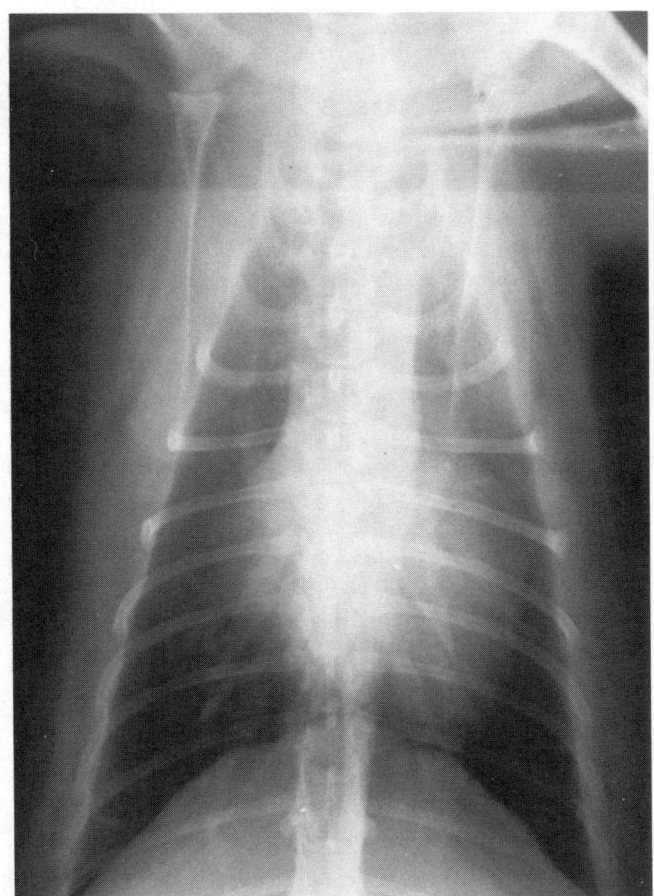
Figure 5B

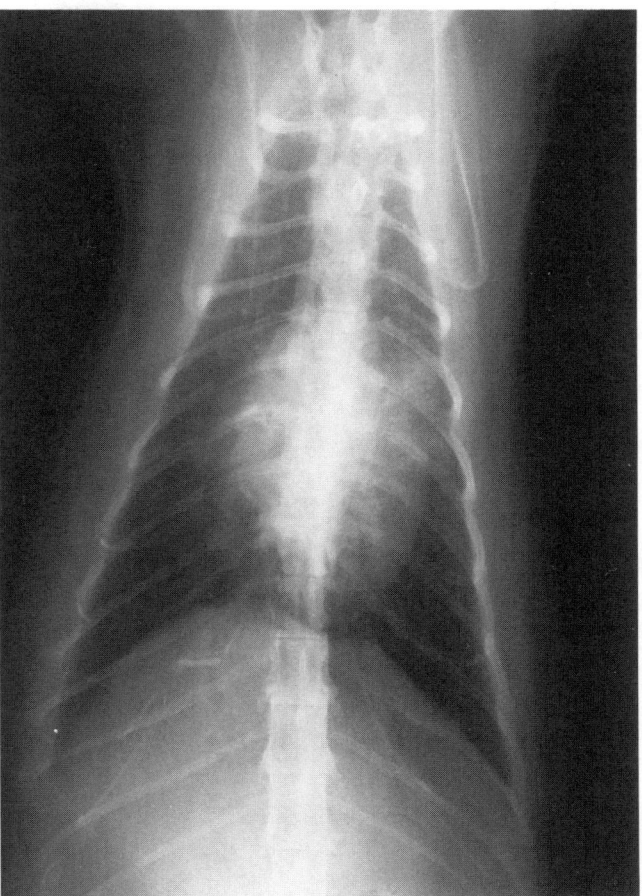
Figure 5C

Figure 5—(**A**) Lateral thoracic radiograph of a three-year-old neutered cat diagnosed with hypertrophic cardiomyopathy displays generalized cardiomegaly. (**B**) Ventrodorsal thoracic radiograph of the same patient as in Figure 5A displays the characteristic valentine-heart shape of the cardiac shadow. (**C**) Ventrodorsal thoracic radiograph of a four-year-old neutered cat diagnosed with hypertrophic cardiomyopathy shows evidence of patchy pulmonary edema in the caudal part of the left cranial lung lobe.

MEDICAL THERAPY

Controlled clinical studies for the treatment of feline hypertrophic cardiomyopathy are lacking. As a result, most drug therapy recommendations have been modified from human protocols. The goals of veterinary therapy, however, are similar: to eliminate pulmonary edema and/or pleural effusion, control arrhythmia, and improve diastolic function. The clinical response to various therapeutic modalities is often variable; and consequently, therapy must be individualized.

DIURETICS are used for relieving signs of pulmonary edema and represent the initial therapeutic step. For mild to moderately severe pulmonary edema, furosemide (1.1 mg/kg intravenously or intramuscularly every 8 to 12 hours) should be administered. After 24 to 36 hours, oral administration is usually initiated and eventually the lowest effective dose is determined. With time, left-sided heart function may deteriorate and right-sided heart failure may develop, necessitating upward dose titration of furosemide (2.2 to 4.4 mg/kg every 8 hours). Refractory right-sided

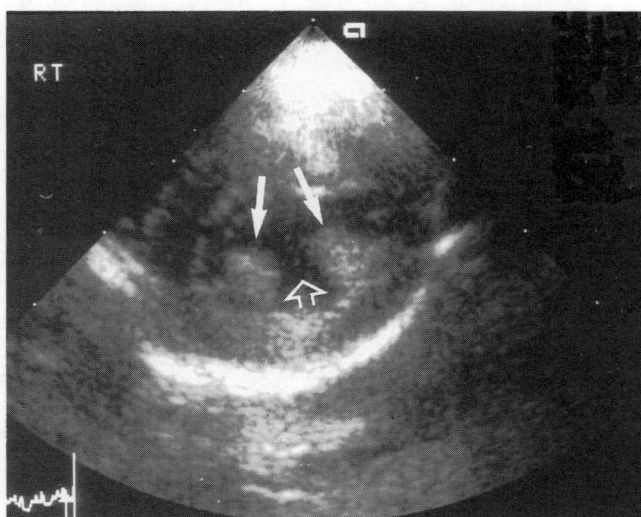

Figure 6A

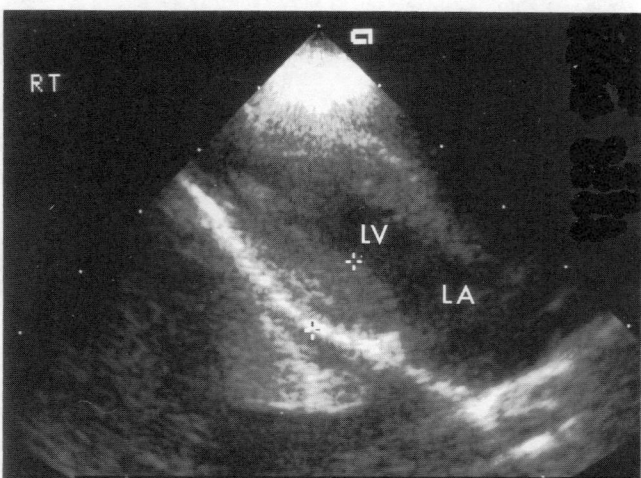

Figure 6B

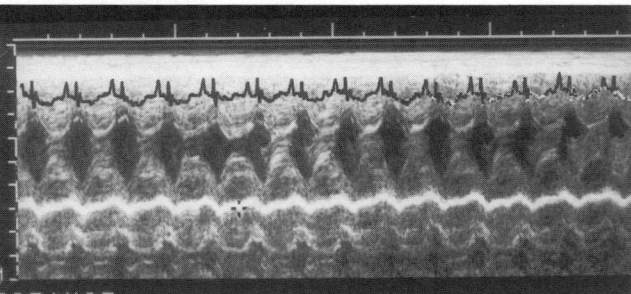

Figure 6C

Figure 6—(**A**) Sagittal two-dimensional echocardiogram of a six-year-old neutered cat demonstrates enlargement of the papillary muscles (*solid arrows*). The left ventricle is indicated by the *open arrow*, and the borders are outlined by *cursors*. (**B**) Sagittal two-dimensional echocardiogram of the same patient as in Figure 6A shows the left ventricle (*LV*), a dilated left atrium (*LA*), and a thickened left ventricular free wall; the borders are outlined by *cursors*. (**C**) M-mode echocardiogram of the same patient as in Figure 6A and 6B demonstrates thickening of the left ventricular free wall, hypercontractility, and decreased size of the left ventricle during systole.

heart failure may respond to the addition of a second diuretic agent acting at a different site in the nephron. Hydrochlorothiazide (1 to 2 mg/kg orally every 12 hours) has been used for this purpose. With combination diuretic therapy, serum electrolytes (particularly sodium and potassium) as well as the parameters of renal function must be monitored closely. Captopril, an angiotensin-converting enzyme (ACE) inhibitor (0.5 to 1 mg/kg every 8 to 12 hours orally), is useful in conjunction with diuretics for treating congestive heart failure.

Since the mid 1960s, β-adrenergic-blocking drugs (BABD) have been the mainstay of medical treatment for human hypertrophic cardiomyopathy. Propranolol, the prototypic β-adrenergic-blocking drug, nonselectively antagonizes $β_1$- and $β_2$-adrenergic receptors. As a result of inhibiting the effects of the sympathetic nervous system on the myocardium, the heart rate, myocardial oxygen demands, left ventricular contractility, and systolic myocardial wall stress diminish, all of which improve cardiac function.[53] Propranolol may also indirectly improve left ventricular diastolic compliance by reducing myocardial ischemia.[53] Controlled clinical studies evaluating the efficacy of propranolol for the treatment of feline myocardial diseases have not been published; therefore, the beneficial effects (if any) remain to be proven. Based on human studies, however, propranolol is recommended for treatment of feline hypertrophic cardiomyopathy. The recommended oral dose regimen is 2.5 mg every 8 to 12 hours for cats weighing less than 6 kg and 5 mg every 8 to 12 hours for cats weighing more than 6 kg. Propranolol can also be used for treating supraventricular and ventricular arrhythmia associated with hypertrophic cardiomyopathy.

CALCIUM channel blockers have provided an effective alternative to propranolol therapy in management of human hypertrophic cardiomyopathy patients.[30,54] It is believed, based on laboratory studies, that abnormal myocardial handling of calcium is a component of hypertrophic cardiomyopathy.[30] An increase in intracellular calcium concentration apparently inhibits complete myocardial relaxation. Calcium channel blockers reduce calcium influx into the myocyte, thereby improving diastolic function. Calcium channel blockers have similar effects to β-adrenergic-blocking drugs in that they decrease heart rate, contractility, systolic pressure gradients, and myocardial oxygen demand.[30] In addition, they also improve myocardial relaxation, induce vasodilation of coronary vasculature, and decrease coronary vasospasm. Clinical trials in veterinary medicine are limited; however, available results are encouraging.[55] In one study, diltiazem hydrochloride was used at a dose of 1.75 to 2.50 mg/kg orally every 8 hours.[55] Further studies are needed to evaluate efficacy of calcium channel blockers completely in management of feline hypertrophic cardiomyopathy.

Long-term management of hypertrophic cardiomyopathy currently entails incorporating diuretics, aspirin, a low-sodium diet, and either propranolol or diltiazem. Periodic reexamination is done with particular attention to the heart rate and frequency of arrhythmia. Ideally, the heart rate should remain below 180 beats/min in the examination room.

THERAPY OF THROMBOEMBOLISM

Medical Management. Initially, medical therapy is directed toward stabilizing the patient. When that goal has been achieved, specific medical therapy for thromboembolism (which is largely empirical) can be initiated. Heparin therapy is advocated to prevent additional clot formation by potentiating the effects of antithrombin III (ATI-II), a serine protease inhibitor. Heparin activates antithrombin III, thereby increasing the neutralization of activated clotting factors, especially factor X and thrombin.[53,56] The dose of heparin required to maintain an effective level of anticoagulation varies greatly. Prolongation of clotting times is considered adequate at 1.5 to 2 times normal.[53,56] A recommended starting dose of heparin is 220 U/kg intravenously, followed 3 hours later by a maintenance dose of 66 U/kg subcutaneously every 6 hours.[56]

Arteriolar dilation with acetylpromazine maleate and hydralazine has been proposed to improve collateral circulation after thromboembolism; however, hydralazine-induced vasodilation is not uniform. Splanchnic, coronary, cerebral, and renal blood flow are increased; while flow to muscle beds is minimally affected.[57-59] Moreover, it has not been shown that hydralazine or acetylpromazine alter platelet-induced vasoconstriction after release of such substances as serotonin and thromboxane A_2.

Use of such thrombolytic agents as streptokinase, urokinase, and tissue plasminogen activator (t-PA) for the purpose of clot dissolution has been investigated. Streptokinase and urokinase are nonspecific activators of plasminogen that cause activation of both circulating and fibrin-bound plasminogen. A fibrinolytic state predisposing to uncontrolled bleeding is a potential complication. Tissue plasminogen activator preferentially binds to fibrin within thrombi, thereby activating plasminogen in the immediate area of the thrombus. In one study, 43% of the cats treated with tissue plasminogen activator survived therapy and were ambulatory within 48 hours.[56] Thrombolytic therapy, however, is not risk free. Fifty percent of the cats in this study died, with 70% of the deaths directly attributable to the reperfusion syndrome (sudden restoration of circulation to an ischemic area). This occurrence raises obvious questions about the safety of tissue plasminogen factor in cats.

At present, cost is another concern with tissue plasminogen factor.

Antiplatelet medication, aspirin being the most common, is often administered prophylactically for the theoretical purpose of preventing thrombus formation. Aspirin induces a functional platelet defect through irreversible acetylation of platelet cyclooxygenase, a key enzyme in the synthesis of thromboxane A_2 from arachidonic acid. Thromboxane A_2, a prostaglandin, is an important stimulus for platelet aggregation and thrombus formation. An apparent paradox exists because aspirin also acetylates endothelial cyclooxygenase and thus prevents formation of prostacyclin, a prostaglandin that inhibits spontaneous platelet aggregation.[60] The inhibitory effect of aspirin on platelet cyclooxygenase is irreversible, presumably because platelets are devoid of a nucleus and are therefore incapable of enzyme synthesis.[61] Consequently, all circulating platelets at the time of aspirin administration are rendered incapable of thromboxane A_2 production for the remainder of their existence.

IN CONTRAST, the effect of aspirin on endothelial cyclooxygenase is reversible.[62] The length of time necessary for feline endothelial cells to synthesize new enzyme is unknown; however, in laboratory studies with rabbits, such synthesis evidently takes less than 2.5 hours.[61] It is thus presumed that aspirin administered to cats at a dose of 25 mg/kg every 3 days provides sufficient time for endothelial cyclooxygenase to regenerate between aspirin doses. Although continuing aspirin therapy indefinitely for feline hypertrophic cardiomyopathy patients is generally recommended, follow-up studies of cats receiving long-term aspirin therapy for prevention of thrombus formation are not encouraging. One study reported additional thromboembolic episodes in 75% of the cats successfully treated with tissue plasminogen activator despite prophylactically administered aspirin.[56] This raises concern that aspirin therapy may have little effect on preventing thrombus formation in feline hypertrophic cardiomyopathy patients. There is experimental evidence, however, demonstrating that cats pretreated with aspirin experienced significantly greater preservation of collateral circulation after induction of a caudal aortic thrombus.[63] This suggests that if a thromboembolic event should occur, preexisting aspirin therapy may shorten the recovery period. Another concern deserving of further study is that the antiplatelet effects of aspirin may be attenuated when used concurrently with propranolol.[64]

Surgical Management. Unless life-threatening vital organ damage is occurring, surgical embolectomy is contraindicated because of the associated mortality. Although actual mortality associated with this procedure in cats is unknown, it exceeds 50% in humans.[34] Most deaths in human patients are related to inherent anesthetic risks superimposed on a severely compromised cardiovascular system. Other potential complications are related to a series of events initiated by the sudden restoration of circulation to an ischemic area (i.e., the previously mentioned reperfusion syndrome).[56] Various substances accumulate in an area of ischemia that, after sudden release into the circulation of a seriously ill patient, can prove fatal. Lactic acid and potassium are two of these substances that, when present in high concentration, can have profound cardiodepressant effects.[34,56,65-66] Activated clotting factors often accumulate distal to the clot, potentially affecting normal coagulation if suddenly released into systemic circulation. Clotted blood from the veins of an ischemic limb can (1) embolize pulmonary vasculature, producing acute respiratory embarrassment, and (2) result in precipitation of myoglobin (released from ischemic myocytes) in renal tubules, causing renal damage.[65-67]

PROGNOSIS

Most cats initially presenting in an acute crisis after a thromboembolic episode die because of the stress placed on an already compromised cardiovascular system. For survivors of the acute crisis, anecdotal reports describe survival times from two to six years, with the most important consideration affecting long-term prognosis being the severity of underlying cardiovascular disease. The presence of severe mitral regurgitation, atrial fibrillation, or biventricular heart failure with pleural effusion merited a poor prognosis. If thromboembolism had occurred, the extent of organ damage was assessed on an individual basis. A clinical study recently confirmed these anecdotal reports by concluding that severity of presenting signs was the only factor affecting prognosis.[68] The median survival time for all hypertrophic cardiomyopathy patients in this study was 732 days; cats experiencing embolic disease or exhibiting signs of heart failure had a poor prognosis (median survival of 61 and 92 days, respectively). The survival time for asymptomatic cats ranged from one day to nearly six years. A correlation also was found between presenting heart rate and prognosis; those cats with resting heart rates slower than 200 beats/min lived significantly longer than those cats with heart rates 200 beats/min or faster.

SUMMARY

Although much information is available on feline hypertrophic cardiomyopathy, most aspects of the disorder still remain a mystery. The cause of the disease has not been conclusively defined, much of the pathophysiology is based on extrapolation, and the appropriate medical therapy is a source of ongoing debate. Only through continuing study, particularly in the areas of the causes and pathophysiology of the disease, will the uncertainties surrounding this disorder be abolished. It is hoped that this form of cardiomyopathy will one day become a relic or at least a disease that can be treated with appropriate conviction.

About the Authors
Dr. Terry Medinger is affiliated with the Pet Practice & Animal Medical Referral Center in Franklin Park, Illinois. Dr. Bruyette practices in Overland Park, Kansas. Both Dr. Medinger and Dr. Bruyette are Diplomates of the American College of Veterinary Internal Medicine.

REFERENCES

1. Maron BJ, Epstein SE: Hypertrophic cardiomyopathy: A discussion of nomenclature. *Am J Cardiol* 43:1242–1244, 1979.
2. Bercu BA, Diettert GA, Danforth WH, et al: Pseudoaortic stenosis produced by ventricular hypertrophy. *Am S Med* 25:814–818, 1958.
3. Van Vleet JF, Ferrans VJ, Weirich WE: Pathologic alterations in hypertrophic and congestive cardiomyopathy in cats. *Am J Vet Res* 41:2037–2048, 1980.
4. Tilley LP, Liu SK, Gilbertson SR, et al: Primary myocardial disease in the cat. A model for human cardiomyopathy. *Am J Pathol* 87:493–513, 1977.
5. Lord PF, Wood A, Tilley LP, et al: Radiographic and hemodynamic evaluation of cardiomyopathy and thromboembolism in the cat. *JAVMA* 164:154, 1974.
6. Rozengurt N, Hayward AHS: Primary myocardial disease of cats in Britain: Pathologic findings in twelve cases. *J Small Anim Pract* 25:617, 1984.
7. Liu SK: Acquired cardiac lesions leading to congestive heart failure in the cat. *Am J Vet Res* 31:2071, 1970.
8. Pion PD, Hird D, Kittleson MD: Epidemiologic evaluation of taurine deficiency and dilated cardiomyopathy in cats. *Proc 8th Annu Vet Med Forum*:1119, 1990.
9. Ciro E, Nichols III PF, Maron BJ: Heterogenous morphologic expression of genetically transmitted hypertrophic cardiomyopathy: Two-dimensional echocardiographic analysis. *Circulation* 67:1227, 1983.
10. Wenger NK, Goodwin JF, Roberts WC: Cardiomyopathy and myocardial involvement in systemic disease, in Hurst JW (ed): *The Heart*, ed 6. New York, McGraw-Hill, 1986, pp 1181–1215.
11. Wynne J, Braunwald E: The cardiomyopathies and myocarditidies, in *Harrison's Principles of Internal Medicine*, ed 12. New York, McGraw-Hill, 1991, pp 975–981.
12. Goodwin JF: An appreciation of hypertrophic cardiomyopathy. *Am J Med* 68:797–800, 1980.
13. Blaufuss AH, Laks MM, Garner K: Production of ventricular hypertrophy simulating idiopathic hypertrophic subaortic stenosis (IHSS) by subhypertensive infusion of norepinephrine (NE) in the conscious dog. *Clin Res* 23:77A, 1975.
14. Witzke DJ, Daye MP: Hypertrophic cardiomyopathy induced by administration of nerve growth factor. *Circulation* 53/54 Suppl 2:11–88, 1976.
15. Goodwin JF, Kirkler DM: Hypothesis: Arrythmia as a cause of sudden death in hypertrophic cardiomyopathy. *Lancet* 2:937–940, 1976.
16. Rouleau JL, Chuck LHS, Hollosi G, et al: Verapamil preserves myocardial contractility in the hereditary cardiomyopathy of the Syrian hamster. *Circ Res* 50:405–412, 1982.
17. Perloff JK: Pathogenesis of hypertrophic cardiomyopathy: Hypothesis and speculation. *Am Heart J* 101:219, 1981.
18. Goodwin JF: Prospects and predictions for the cardiomyopathies. *Circulation* 50:210, 1974.
19. James TN, Marshall TK: Desubitaneis mortibus. XII. Asymmetrical hypertrophy of the heart. *Circulation* 51:1149, 1975.
20. Peterson ME, Taylor S, Greco DS, et al: Acromegaly in 14 cats. *J Vet Intern Med* 4:192–201, 1990.
21. Eigenmann JE, Wortman JA, Haskins ME: Elevated growth hormone levels and diabetes mellitus in a cat with acromegalic features. *JAAHA* 20:747–752, 1984.
22. Morrison SA, Randolph J, Lothrop CD: Hypersomatotropism and insulin-resistant diabetes mellitus in a cat. *JAVMA* 194:91–94, 1989.
23. Ihle SL, Nelson RW: Insulin resistance and diabetes mellitus. *Comp Cont Educ Pract Vet* 13(2):197–205, 1991.
24. Kittleson MD, Pion PD, Lothrop CD: Hypersomatotropism in a cat

presented with hypertrophic cardiomyopathy (hypertrophic cardiomyopathy) and insulin resistance but without diabetes mellitus (DM). *Proc 7th Annu Vet Med Forum*:1038, 1989.
25. Maron BJ, Gottdiener JS, Epstein SE: Patterns and significance of distribution of left ventricular hypertrophy in hypertrophic cardiomyopathy: A wide angle two dimensional echocardiographic study of 125 patients. *Am J Cardiol* 48:418–428, 1981.
26. Peterson EN, Moise NS, Brown CA: Heterogeneity of hypertrophy in feline hypertrophic cardiomyopathy. *J Vet Intern Med* 5:122, 1991.
27. Maron BJ, Bonow RO, Cannon RO: Hypertrophic cardiomyopathy: Interrelations of clinical manifestations, pathophysiology, and therapy. *N Engl J Med* 316:780, 1987.
28. Bonagura JD, Stepien RL, Lehmkuhl LB: Acute effects of esmolol on left ventricular outflow obstruction in cats with hypertrophic cardiomyopathy: A doppler echocardiographic study. *J Vet Intern Med* 5:123, 1991.
29. Wigle ED, Sasson Z, Henderson MA: Hypertrophic cardiomyopathy: The importance of the site and the extent of hypertrophy: A review. *Prog Cardiovasc Dis* 28:1–83, 1985.
30. Bright JM, Golden AL: Evidence for or against the efficacy of calcium channel blockers for management of hypertrophic cardiomyopathy in cats. *Vet Clin North Am [Small Anim Pract]* 21:1023, 1991.
31. Gaasch WH, Levine HJ, Quinones MA, et al: Left ventricular compliance: Mechanisms and clinical implications. *Am J Cardiol* 38:645–653, 1976.
32. Nayler WC, Williams A: Relaxation in heart muscle: Some morphologic and biochemical considerations. *Eur J Cardiol* 7:35, 1978.
33. Golden AI, Bright JM: Use of relaxation half-time as an index of ventricular relaxation in clinically normal cats and cats with hypertrophic cardiomyopathy. *Am J Vet Res* 51:1352, 1990.
34. Maron BJ, Wolfson JK, Epstein SE, et al: Intramural coronary artery disease in hypertrophic cardiomyopathy. *J Am Coll Cardiol* 8:545–547, 1986.
35. Liu SK, Tilley LP, Lord PF: Feline Cardiomyopathy, in Roy PE, Rona G (eds): *Recent Advances in Studies on Cardiac Structure and Metabolism*, ed 10. Baltimore, University Park Press, 1975, pp 627–640.
36. Helenski CA, Ross JN: Platelet aggregation in feline cardiomyopathy. *J Vet Intern Med* 1:24–28, 1987.
37. Rosenthal DS, Braunwald E: Hematologic-oncologic disorders and heart disease, in Braunwald E (ed): *Heart Disease*. Philadelphia, WB Saunders Co, 1980, pp 1792–1800.
38. Lowe GDO, Forbes GD: Blood rheology and thrombosis. *Clin Haemotol* 10(2):343–367, 1981.
39. Riddle JM, Stein PD, Magilligan DJ, et al: Evaluation of platelet reactivity in patients with valvular heart disease. *J Am Coll Cardiol* 1(6):1381–1384, 1983.
40. Mustard JF, Packham MA: Thromboembolism, a manifestation of the response of blood to injury. *Circulation* 62(1):1–21, 1970.
41. Smith RL, Blick EF, Coalson J, et al: Thrombus production of turbulence. *J Appl Physiol* 32(2):261–264, 1972.
42. Weiser MG, Koeiba GJ: Platelet concentration and platelet volume distribution in healthy cats. *Am J Vet Res* 45:518, 1984.
43. Dodds WJ: Species specificities, in de Gaetano G, Garrattini S (eds): *Platelets: A Multidisciplinary Approach*. New York, Raven Press, 1978, pp 45–59.
44. Thompson CB, Jakubowski JA, Quinn PG: Platelet size can determine platelet function independently. *Blood* 63(6):1372–1375, 1984.
45. Tschopp PB: Aggregation of cat platelets in vitro. *Diath Haemor* 23:601–620, 1970.
46. Moise NS, Dietze AE, Mezza LE, et al: Echocardiography, electrocardiography, and radiography of cats with dilatation cardiomyopathy, hypertrophic cardiomyopathy, and hyperthyroidism. *Am J Vet Res* 47:1476–1486, 1986.
47. Harpster NK: Feline myocardial diseases, in Kirk RW (ed): *Current Veterinary Therapy. IX*. Philadelphia, WB Saunders Co, 1986, pp 380–398.
48. Lord PF, Wood A, Tilley LP, et al: Radiographic and hemodynamic evaluation of cardiomyopathy and thromboembolism in the cat. *JAVMA* 164:154–165, 1974.
49. Owens JM, Twedt DC: Nonselective angiocardiography in the cat. *Vet Clin North Am [Small Anim Pract]* 7:309–321, 1977.
50. Soderberg SF, Boon JA, Wingfield WE, et al: M-mode echocardiography as a diagnostic aid for feline cardiomyopathy. *Vet Radiol* 24:66–73, 1983.
51. Morgan RV: Systemic hypertension in four cats: Ocular and medical findings. *JAAHA* 22:615–622, 1986.
52. Kobayashi DL, Peterson ME, Graves TK, et al: Hypertension in cats with chronic renal failure or hyperthyroidism. *J Vet Intern Med* 4:58–62, 1990.
53. Fox PR: Evidence for or against efficacy of beta-blockers and aspirin for the management of feline cardiomyopathies. *Vet Clin North Am [Small Anim Pract]* 21:1011, 1991.
54. Stone PH, Antman EM: *Calcium Channel Blocking Agents in the Treatment of Cardiovascular Disorders*. Mount Kisco, NY, Futura Publishing Co, 1983.
55. Bright JM, Golden AL: A comparison of calcium channel blockers and beta-adrenergic blockers for treatment of feline hypertrophic cardiomyopathy. *Proc 7th Annu Vet Med Forum*:847, 1989.
56. Pion PD, Kittleson MD: Therapy for feline aortic thromboembolism, in Kirk RW (ed): *Current Veterinary Therapy. X*. Philadelphia, WB Saunders Co, 1989, pp 295.
57. Schneeweis A, in *Drug Therapy in Cardiovascular Diseases*. Philadelphia, Lea & Febiger, 1986, p 52.
58. Freis ED: Changing attitudes to hypertension. *Ann Intern Med* 78:141, 1973.
59. Oblad B: A study of the mechanism of the hemodynamic effects of hydralazine in man. *Acta Pharmacol Toxicol* 20:1, 1963.
60. Boothe DM: Prostaglandins: Physiology and clinical implications. *Comp Cont Educ Pract Vet* 6(11):1010–1021, 1984.
61. Kelton JG, Hirsch J, Carter CJ, et al: Thrombogenic effect of high-dose aspirin in rabbits. *J Clin Invest* 62:892–895, 1978.
62. Preston FE, Whipps S, Jackson CJ, et al: Inhibition of prostacyclin platelet thromboxane A_2 after low dose aspirin. *N Engl J Med* 304:76, 1981.
63. Schaub RG, Gates KA, Roberts RE: Effect of aspirin on collateral blood after experimental thrombosis of the feline aorta. *Am J Vet Res* 43:1647, 1982.
64. Allen DG, Johnstone IB, Crane S: Effects of aspirin and propranolol alone and in combination on hemostatic determinations in the healthy cat. *Am J Vet Res* 46:660, 1985.
65. Blaisdell FW, Steel M, Allen RE: Management of acute lower extremity arterial ischemia due to embolism and thrombosis. *Surgery* 84(6):822–834, 1978.
66. Fogarty TJ: Acute arterial occlusion, in Sabiston DC (ed): *Textbook of Surgery*. Philadelphia, WB Saunders Co, 1982, pp 1975–1982.
67. Haimovici H: Myopathic nephrotic-metabolic syndrome associated with massive acute arterial occlusions. *J Cardiovasc Surg* 14:589–600, 1973.
68. Atkins CE, Gallo AM, Kurman ID: A retrospective study of risk factor, presenting signs, and survival in 74 cases of feline idiopathic hypertrophic cardiomyopathy. *J Vet Intern Med* 5:122, 1991.

Heart Failure

Walter E. Weirich, DVM, PhD
Department of Small Animal Clinics
School of Veterinary Medicine
Purdue University

Heart failure is a situation in which the heart cannot deliver enough blood to the tissues to meet their metabolic needs even though venous return is adequate. Before any discussion of heart failure can be appreciated, some of the control mechanisms of normal heart function need to be understood. The heart can be thought of as two pumps in series. The right side of the heart is a low pressure pump which handles volume well. The left ventricle is a high pressure pump that fails quickly if volume is overloaded. Obviously both chambers must pump the same amount of blood or fluid will be trapped somewhere in the circulation.

The mechanisms controlling cardiac function have been described thoroughly and considerable agreement exists between cardiovascular physiologists. Two of these mechanisms will be discussed because they are the most important when considering the clinical signs generated in heart failure states. The first is the Frank-Starling mechanism which describes what occurs as the muscle of the heart is stretched with the filling of the ventricles during diastole. As the fiber length is increased by stretching, an increase in the force of the subsequent contraction occurs. This is beneficial only up to a point. When the fiber has been stretched beyond its optimal length, the force of contraction begins to decrease. Within physiologic limits this contributes greatly to cardiac reserve. As the size of the chamber increases beyond the critical fiber length, the efficiency of cardiac function decreases markedly.

The oxygen demands, which are an indication of energy utilization (efficiency), are most closely related to wall tension generated to produce a given pressure. The law of Laplace describes this pressure/tension relationship:

$$\text{wall tension} = \frac{\text{pressure} \times \text{radius}}{2}$$

From this formula it can be seen that an increase in the radius of the chamber must result in an increase in the wall tension if the same pressure is to be achieved. Therefore when the heart is enlarged (especially by dilatation) the energy consumed as indicated by oxygen utilization increases markedly with the end result being the same amount of pressure generated. The net cost to the heart is lowered efficiency. The Frank-Starling mechanism and increased rate are the most common means of producing an increased cardiac output.

When an individual undertakes an exercise program and increases the degree of physical fitness, the heart responds first by increasing the heart rate, but any sustained effect will be due to an increase in the stroke volume. As the level of fitness increases, the heart rate will rise only after an increase in the severity of exercise. The reason for this is due to the sustained increase in the stroke volume. To enhance the training effect, more severe exercise for longer periods of time must be engaged in to achieve higher levels of physical fitness. This results in an increased depth of cardiac reserve.

A similar series of events takes place when the heart is faced with a need for increased cardiac output because of disease. The most common example is the acquired heart disease, mitral valvular insufficiency. This results in increased rate and stroke volume. Because a portion of each cardiac stroke is lost to the systemic circulation in regurgitant flow into the left atrium, the chief mechanisms for compensation are the increase in the heart rate and stroke volume. This results in what can be referred to as a *high preload state* as the end diastolic volume is increased to provide for the increased stroke volume.

Another method of cardiac compensation is brought into play when a *high afterload state* must be overcome. An example would be pulmonic stenosis. In this situation resting demands for cardiac output are difficult for the heart to meet because the heart must force the stroke volume through an opening that is markedly reduced in size. To accomplish this, the heart will hypertrophy to increase the pressure generated by the affected ventricle, and will sustain systole longer in order to pump the same amount of blood as the opposite ventricle which is faced with a normal afterload. This leads to the significantly increased muscle mass commonly seen in high afterload states.

These two examples of situations where the heart must utilize compensatory mechanisms do not explain all cardiac changes but help describe those most commonly seen in clinical practice. Other mechanisms exist but the reader is referred to the reference list at the end of this article for that information. Heart failure can be further broken down into noncongestive and congestive types.

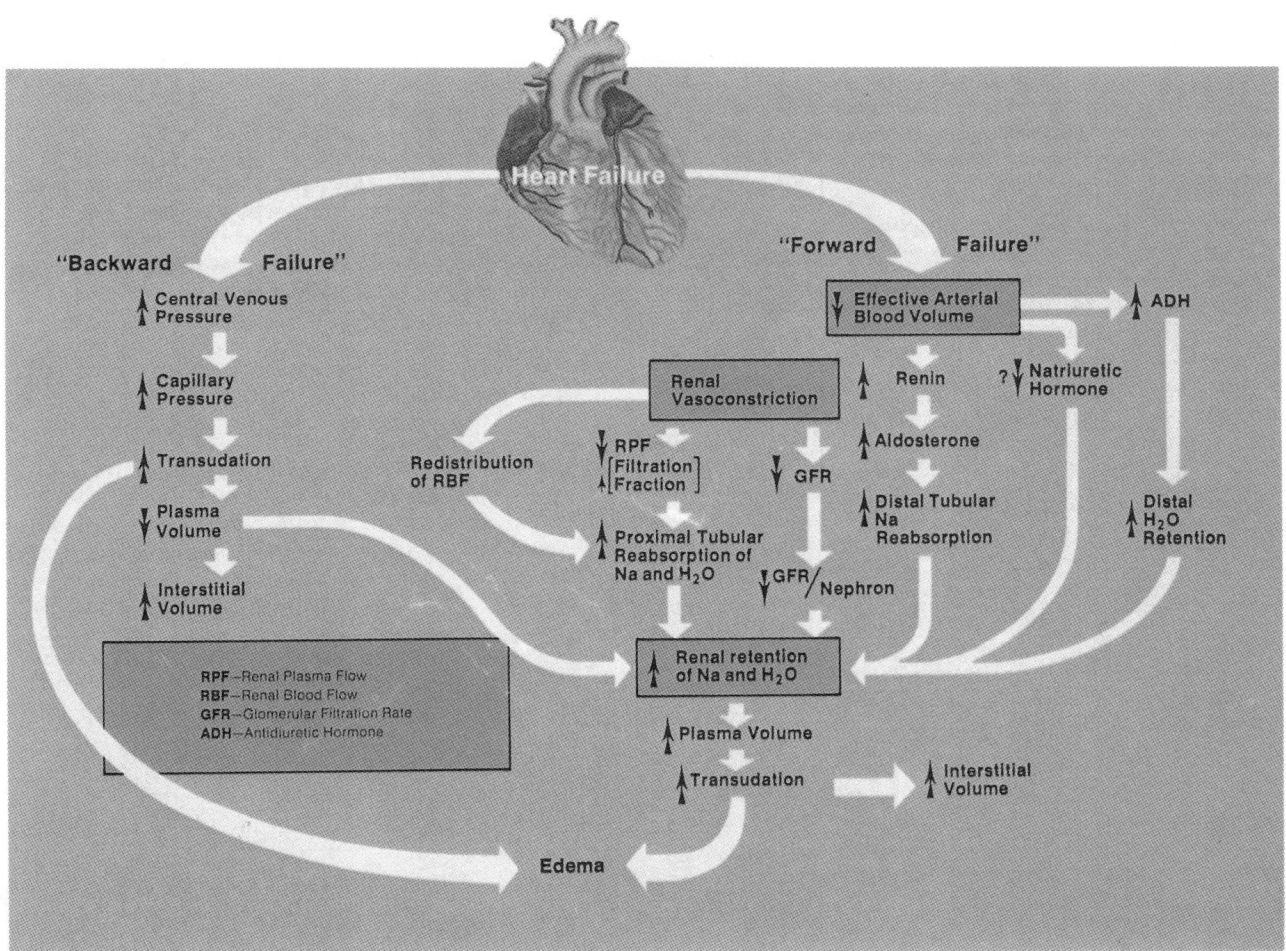

Fig 1—Theories to explain edema formation in heart failure: backward and forward failure. (reprinted with permission of Drs. N. K. Hallenberg, P. J. Cannon and National Laboratories, Animal Health Division, American Hoechst Corporation).

Noncongestive Heart Failure—Noncongestive heart failure occurs in a situation where the heart cannot deliver enough blood to the brain to sustain consciousness, but no vascular bed is congested. An example of noncongestive heart failure would be the syncope that occurs in dogs with aortic stenosis. The stenosis prevents the increase in cardiac output that is necessary to sustain the increased activity. The brain is deprived of sufficient blood flow because of demands elsewhere in the systemic circulation, primarily in the muscles, and very shallow cardiac reserve. A similar situation may occur in severe arrhythmia, but in most instances some degree of congestion is usually present.

Congestive Heart Failure—When congestive heart failure occurs one or more vascular beds are distended with blood to varying degrees. This may lead to edema in the form of fluid in a body cavity or loss of fluid into tissues. The classical description of congestive heart failure refers to it as backward (right heart failure) when the central venous pressure is markedly elevated, or forward (left heart failure) when the cardiac output and pressure generated by the left ventricle are reduced. The clinical signs generated by either of these forms of congestive heart failure will be compatible with the vascular bed involved. Figure 1 depicts schematically the theories developed to explain the congestive state that exists when backward and forward heart failure occur.

The net effect is an increase in the blood and fluid volume in the body. This is an advantage up to a point where the fiber length is longer as a result of increased end diastolic pressure. But a vicious cycle can develop when the optimal fiber length is exceeded, leading to overloading of the circulation. No attempt will be made to describe systematically all the cardiac and vascular difficulties that can lead to congestive heart failure. The thrust of this article is to discuss congestive heart failure as a disease entity in itself.

Clinical Recognition of Heart Failure—Clinical recognition of heart failure and assessment of the degree of involvement of an individual require careful workup and sound clinical judgment. It has been well recognized that a murmur of mitral valvular insufficiency may not cause immediate problems for the animal. In fact, animals may have a murmur in the mitral valve area that is the result of the normal functioning heart and have no organic cardiac disease whatever. Therefore, careful evaluation is indicated to determine if and when therapeutic intervention should be undertaken. The evaluation should include a complete history, physical examination, radiographs of the chest to include the upper abdomen, an electrocardiogram taken at rest, and in certain situations, after exercise. Laboratory studies should include a CBC, BUN, SGPT, sodium, potassium and glucose determinations and a urinalysis.

When noncongestive failure occurs, the animal may be dead on presentation, because sudden death is not uncommon in dogs with increased left ventricular mass. However, if the animal survives this collapsed state, it may be acting nearly normal by the time it is presented. If the syncopal attack is associated with aortic stenosis, the murmur of aortic stenosis will be heard. However, if the collapse is due to an arrhythmia of sudden onset, there may be no physical evidence of what brought on the heart failure. A complete workup is indicated to determine if recognizable cardiac abnormalities exist. If nothing significant is found except in the history, an electrocardiogram after exercise should be done in an attempt to bring out these abnormal clinical signs. It must be realized that some danger exists when performing exercise electrocardiography on these susceptible individuals, as sudden death can occur during exercise.

Congestive heart failure must be evaluated carefully. Staging the disease in a given individual is of considerable importance in determining the following:
1. *What the prognosis may be for that individual.*
2. *If therapy should be instituted.*
3. *If treatment is indicated, what drugs should be used.*

The New York Heart Association has developed a staging method for humans based on how much physical activity they can tolerate without clinical cardiac signs appearing. Dr. S. G. Ettinger uses a similar approach for dogs, however he applies this only to mitral valvular disease. The functional classification listed in Table I is a modification of both of these approaches to staging heart failure regardless of cause.

TABLE I

Functional Classification of Cardiac Patients

Functional Class I: Detectable cardiac abnormality only; no signs of pulmonary or systemic disease related to the cardiac abnormality; normal exercise tolerance.

Functional Class II: Clinical signs occur only after strenuous exercise.

Functional Class III: Clinical signs present after ordinary exercise and may occur after a period of rest.

Functional Class IV: Clinical signs present at rest.

The only way to develop this information is through taking a history. It is very important to question the owner carefully, and it may be helpful to ask the same questions differently in an attempt to obtain information as accurately as possible. Exercise stress testing is possible but it may be difficult to administer a standard dose of exercise. Other historical information is needed to determine if the cardiac lesion is acquired or congenital. The duration and the severity of clinical signs are important in the overall understanding of the individual patient's disease process.

Physical examination is the single most important element in the determination of the animal's clinical status. The points that should be emphasized are auscultation of the heart and lungs, color of the mucous membranes, capillary refill time, evaluation for venous distension, quality of the arterial pulses, and the presence or absence of edema fluid.

Auscultation of the heart may suggest abnormal flow patterns producing a murmur. Congestive heart failure itself may produce alterations of the heart sounds. When a third heart sound is present (rapid ventricular filling sound) in the dog or cat, congestive heart failure is usually present. The third heart sound is heard in these animals when there is high end systolic volume. An accentuated or split second heart sound in the dog indicates elevated pulmonary blood pressure and may precede right heart failure. Abnormal heart rhythms may be heard and may be contributing to the failure state. The extensive hemodynamic deficits that occur in atrial fibrillation, multiple ventricular premature beats and ventricular tachycardia will contribute markedly to the failure state.

The electrocardiogram (ECG) is useful in determining arrhythmias and monitoring digitalis therapy. The electrocardiogram should be recorded on any animal with suspected cardiac disease. Unsuspected arrhythmias and other ECG detectable conduction defects will be brought to light with the use of this diagnostic modality. The most significant use is when serial tracings are recorded over a period of time. The changes seen can identify trends which help in prognosis and monitoring therapy.

Radiography is essential in establishing the size of the cardiac silhouette as well as degree of congestion of the pulmonary vasculature. It is also very helpful because dogs in functional class II may or may not need treatment depending on the radiographic appearance of the heart and lungs. Dogs with mital valve disease will have enlarged left atria (Fig 2 A and B) and an enlarged left ventricle. Right heart changes may also occur and are detailed in Fig 3 A and B. These radiographic findings suggest the heart has compensated, and even though failure is not present, drug therapy may postpone impending failure for a considerable period of time. Animals in late functional class II or beyond should be on some form of cardiovascular support therapy and the drug of choice is one of the digitalis glycosides.

Therapy of Heart Failure—The treatment of early cases is best made with digitalis alone. The animal may have only minimal exercise intolerance and this may not be recognized by the owner. The theory behind the use of this drug support is to prevent rapid cardiac decompensation. It has been shown in research animals as well as in the clinical setting that the rate of hypertrophic changes will be reduced with digitalis therapy. Owners often comment on a marked increase in the animal's physical activity once full digitalization is achieved.

The use of digitalis glycosides is not without some danger, but with careful monitoring there should be little problem with digitalis toxicity. The

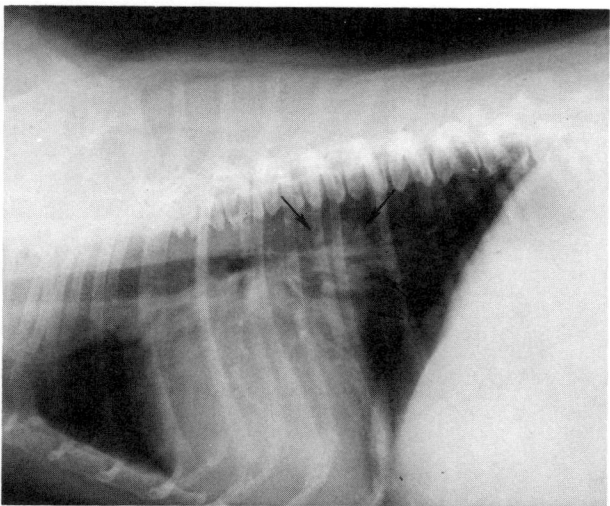

Fig 2A—This lateral radiograph of the thorax of a dog with mitral valvular insufficiency has arrows placed to outline the margins of the enlarged left atrium and tortuous pulmonary veins.

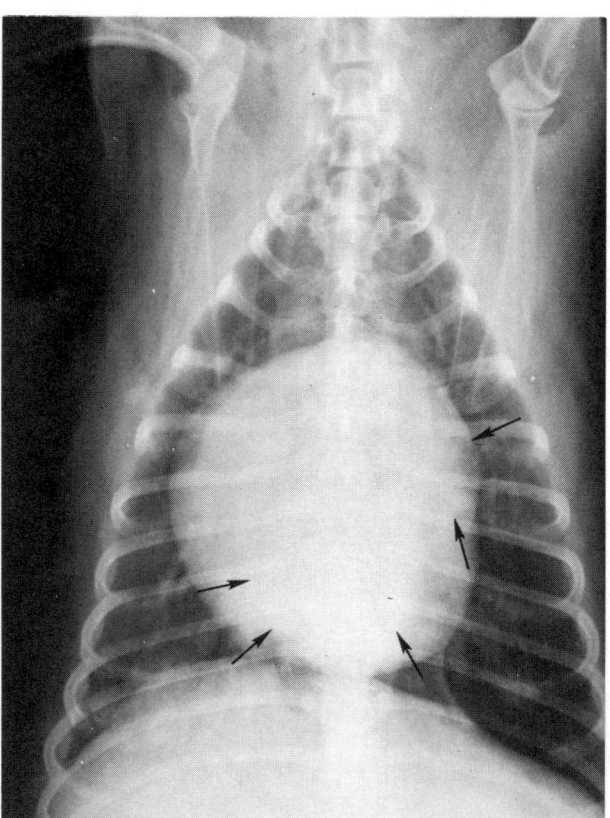

Fig 2B—This ventral dorsal radiograph of the same dog as in Fig 2A has arrows placed to outline the tremendous left atrial enlargement.

client needs to participate fully in the therapeutic regimen and if possible the digitalization should be done at home. The owner needs to be carefully instructed in what is being done, how the animal should respond, and how side effects may appear. Digoxin will give the most consistent results in dogs and cats because little of the drug is protein-

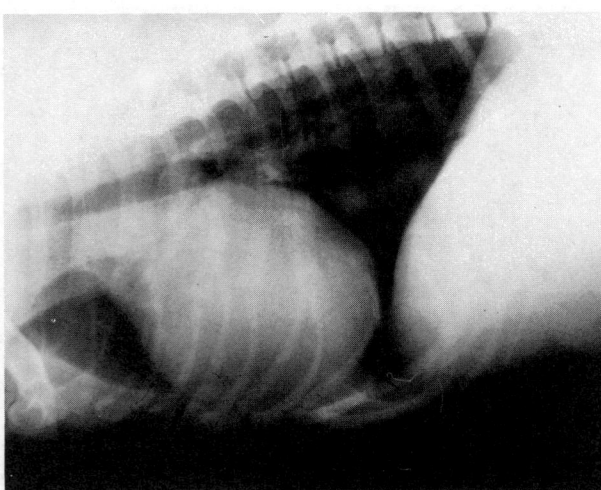

Fig 3A—This dog with pulmonary stenosis has a marked increase in the right ventricular mass. The right heart enlargement has caused the left ventricle to be elevated. The arrows indicate the margins of the right ventricle and the extent of sternal contact.

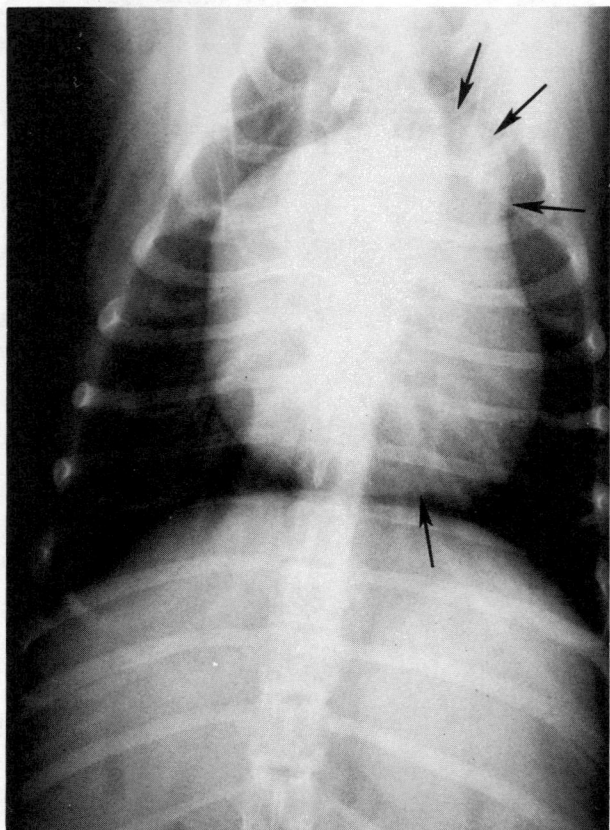

Fig 3B—The backwards *D* pattern is apparent on the ventral dorsal radiograph of the same dog as in Fig 3A. Note the enlarged pulmonary artery and the *bifid apex* seen in dogs with marked right ventricular enlargement.

bound. The dosage from one dog to another will be predictable within reason. Prescribing brand names is important because generic forms of digoxin are not as reliable as brand names such as Lanoxin[a] and Cardoxin.[b] The drug should be given as a maintenance dose only, because there is no need to elevate the intake of the animal to levels of toxicity. The daily dose in dogs is .02mg/kg/day and in cats is .01 mg/kg/day. In both dogs and cats, two doses per day are given.[c] The owner should be instructed to count and record the resting heart beats before each dose is given. An ECG should be run at least at weekly intervals if everything goes well, but more often if problems are noted. These would include anorexia, vomiting, marked cardiac arrhythmia, or bradycardia.

Digitoxin can be used but it is unpredictable because of the extent of protein binding. The dose may have to be increased dramatically to have a digitalizing effect in some dogs. The half-life of digitoxin is shorter than digoxin in the dog and the dose should be given three times a day. The dose in the dog is .02 mg/kg/t.i.d. The monitoring methods are the same as for digoxin. Intravenous digitalis glycosides can be used in emergency situations if an animal is in functional class IV. Ouabain will produce the most rapid effects of all the digitalis glycosides when given intravenously. The dose of ouabain is .01 mg/kg of body weight and may be repeated at 30 minute intervals until the animal has achieved a digitalized state. Careful electrocardiographic monitoring is essential during this process.

As animals become more involved with the congestive failure state (functional classes III and IV) additional modalities of therapy may be indicated. These will include the use of physical management (cage rest and diet), and medical techniques to reduce the animal's blood volume. Reducing the blood volume will aid in reduction of the excessive preload that may be placed upon the myocardial fiber. This can be done in three ways: the use of reduced salt diets, cage rest and diuretics.

Figure 4 describes the presence of various populations of glomeruli within the kidney based on blood flow patterns. The volume of blood flow in the normal dog is greatest in the outer cortex. The blood flow in the inner cortex is less due to the fewer number of glomeruli located in this area. As the blood flow becomes sluggish in heart failure states, the intrarenal blood flow patterns change so that the outer cortical glomeruli are bypassed by much of the blood flow and kidney function is depressed. Prerenal uremia is common.

---

[a] Burroughs Wellcome Co., 3030 Cornwallis Rd., Research Triangle Park, NC 27709

[b] Evsco Pharmaceutical Co., 115 Fourth Av., Needham, MA 02194

[c] Editor's note: Some clinicians recommend the use of a loading dose of digitalis glycoside for 1 day, then using a maintenance dose. In this manner the animal can be *digitalized* in 2 days, as compared to 4-6 days, without giving the loading dose. In the dog, a loading dose of digoxin is .022 mg/kg t.i.d. for 1 day. In the cat, a loading dose is .015 mg/kg t.i.d. (These doses are used in the Section of Cardiology, School of Veterinary Medicine, University of Pennsylvania.)

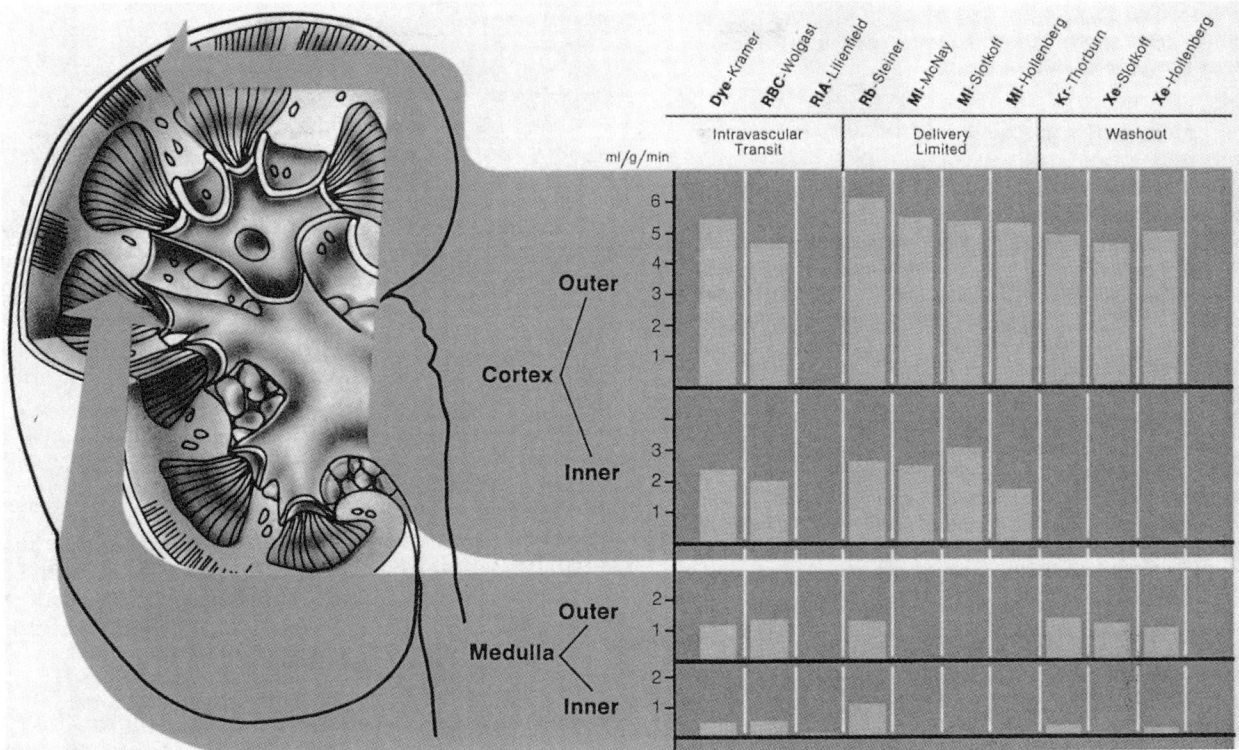

Fig 4—Blood flow measurements in the normal canine kidney are reported by several investigators using techniques indicated on the bar graph. Note that the predominance of blood flow is taking place in the outer cortex where the largest number of glomeruli are located. In forward failure blood flow is shifted to the inner cortical area thereby reducing the kidneys' ability to clear waste products. Furosamide returns more of the blood flow to the cortical glomeruli. (Reprinted with permission of Drs. N. K. Hallenberg, P. J. Cannon and National Laboatories, Animal Health Division, American Hoechst Corporation).

Diuretics such as furosamide have the distinct advantage of altering the blood flow patterns within the kidney to a more normal state, i.e., increasing blood flow to the cortical glomeruli, thereby rendering the kidney much more efficient in clearing waste materials. Therefore, the use of diuretics such as furosamide can be most advantageous if used every day to provide improved kidney function.

The dosage of diuretics will vary depending on the severity of the presenting signs. Furosamide should be utilized at vigorous levels in animals that are severely congested, but this treatment should continue for only short periods of time, such as 24-36 hours. A dog that is presented in functional class IV should be treated with 4.4 mg/kg of body weight and re-evaluated at six hour intervals, repeating this dose if indicated. Once the animal has been stabilized on a full regimen of congestive heart failure therapy to include rest, sodium restricted diet, digitalis glycosides, diuretics, and other drugs, the diuretic dosage may be reduced to 2.2 mg/kg once each day.

Other drugs may be beneficial in the congestive state to aid in relieving the animal's clinical signs. Drugs such as aminophylline or theophylline will produce bronchodilatation, a mild diuretic effect and some mild increase in ventricular inotropy. These are all relatively mild effects but do serve to benefit the patient considerably in many instances. Aminophylline may be given either intramuscularly or orally with considerable benefit to the patient. The dose of 11 mg/kg of body weight is adequate for both aminophylline and theophylline. There is a wide dosage range with reasonable safety, but doses should not exceed 132 mg/kg of body weight or damage to the myocardium can occur.

The ventricle has difficulty in emptying in forward failure, and reduction of the peripheral vascular resistance has been shown to be very beneficial in over 50 dogs at Purdue University, without adverse effects. Nitroglycerin will produce this reduction in vascular resistance.[d] The 2% nitroglycerin ointment appears to be the best dosage form to provide sustained effects. The ointment is massaged into the abdomen or flank areas

---

[d]Editor's note: The use of vasodilators is controversial among veterinary clinicians and some consider it is premature to present vasodilators as a standard means of treatment. These drugs are still considered to be in an experimental stage by some clinicians, until more data is accumulated and analyzed. Adverse effects of nitroglycerin, such as tachycardia and hypotension, are possible.

for absorption by the skin. Dosages will vary and are calculated by the inch of ointment that is squeezed from the tube on the parchment papers provided with the product. Dosage for a small dog will be ¼ inch of ointment b.i.d. to q.i.d. and for larger dogs an inch or more b.i.d. to q.i.d.

Other beneficial drugs are multiple vitamins for dogs that are on diuretics. These would provide additional water soluble vitamins that may be washed away with the increased urine flow. Potassium supplements are given to replace potassium that is lost through heavy use of diuretics and digitalis preparations.

In summary, in congestive heart failure three basic approaches by the clinician can produce benefits for the patient from medical therapy and management. These are:

1. Reduction of the animal's activity which reduces the workload on the heart.
2. An increase in the force of contraction can be accomplished with the use of digitalis glycosides. The efficiency of the force of contractions can be enhanced by the use of nitroglycerin.
3. Reduction of the animal's blood and fluid volume within the body through the use of sodium restricted diets and diuretics.

With these interventions, the congestive state will improve for a period of time. But a rule of thumb is that if the dog is in functional class III or beyond, the average response is 12 months of good quality life. Careful management and the owner's cooperation will allow many of these animals to survive beyond this average period.

REFERENCES

1. Ross, J. N., Jr.: Heart Failure in Shock. *The Textbook of Veterinary Internal Medicine*, S. J. Ettinger, ed. W. B. Saunders Co. Philadelphia, Pa. (1965) 825-864.
2. Ettinger, S. J. and Suder, P. F.: Recognition of Cardiac Disease and Congestive Heart Failure. *Canine Cardiology*, W. B. Saunders Co., Philadelphia, Pa. (1970) 214-221.
3. Hamlin, R. L. and Smith, C. R.: The Heart as a Pump. Hemodynamics and Regulation of Cardiac Output. *Duke's Physiology of Domestic Animals*, M. J. Swenson, ed. Cornell University Press, Ithaca, NY (1977) 81-94.
4. Cohen, M. V., Sonnenblick, E. H. and Kirk, E. S.: Comparative Effects of Nitroglycerin and Isosorbide Dinitrate on Coronary Collateral Vessels and Ischemic Myocardium in Dogs. Am J Card, 37(1976): 243-249.
5. Wyatt, H. L., Mitchell, J. H.: Influences of Physical Training on the Heart of Dogs. Circ Res, 35(1974):883-889.
6. Maron, B. J., Ferrans, V. J. and Roberts, W. C. Ultrastructural Features of Degenerated Cardiac Muscle Cells in Patients with Cardiac Hypertrophy. Am J Path, 79(3) (1975): 387-414.
7. Seiness, E., Christensen, J. and Johansen, H.: Bioavailability of Digoxin Tablets. Clin Pharm and Therap, 14(6)(1973): 949-954.

UPDATE

Many changes have occurred in the diagnosis and treatment of heart failure since original publication of this article in 1979. There now exists a better basic understanding of the nature of heart failure as it occurs in our animal patients. Some of these basic changes in understanding have led to the virtual eradication of dilated cardiomyopathy in cats by the addition of proper amounts of taurine to commercial cat foods. Hypertrophic cardiomyopathy remains a common acquired problem in domestic felines, but we have new treatments for that as well. Mitral valve regurgitation, an acquired heart disease, is still the number one heart disease seen in dogs. In 1979, *patent ductus arteriosus* was the most common congenital heart disease seen in young dogs: Subaortic stenosis has become the most common congenital heart disease in puppies seen at many teaching hospitals. Purebred dog breeders have become activists in understanding the heritable heart diseases that plague their breeds. As a result, a canine heart registry has been established to help eliminate disease and carrier animals from the gene pool for that breed. Over time, this type of approach should reduce the number of affected animals.

The diagnosis of heart disease has become much more sophisticated since 1979. Electrocardiographs (ECG) have become the standard in small animal practice, with many clinicians offering computerized ECG systems. The average veterinary practice can now independently diagnose cardiac arrhythmias in animal patients. A variety of clinical problems are now diagnosed and treated, which, before the widespread use of ECG, went almost totally unrecognized. Ultrasound has nearly replaced cardiac catheterization to diagnose and characterize heart disease in dogs and cats. The use of ultrasound to measure the shortening fraction, chamber size, wall thicknesses and to visualize valvular changes indicates the level of progression in the course of disease.

The most startling changes have occurred in the treatment of heart failure. While afterload reducing drugs were available in 1979, their value in treating heart failure has blossomed in the 1990s. The availability of angiotensin converting enzyme (ACE) inhibitors for afterload reduction has greatly increased the lifespan of dogs that are treated for heart failure. Digoxin and furosemide still have their place in the treatment of heart failure, but the widespread use of reliable ACE inhibitors, in my opinion, has brought about the greatest improvement. With the advent of widespread use of ECG, veterinarians are accurately diagnosing and effectively treating cardiac arrhythmias. The drugs used to treat cardiac arrhythmias remain the same, but their use has increased as the condition becomes more frequently diagnosed.

Calcium channel blockers in the treatment of hypertrophic cardiomyopathy have led to an improved quality and quantity of life in cats with this disease.

The veterinary profession can be proud of the progress that has been made in the understanding, diagnosis and treatment of heart disease in pet animals. We can only hope that the next seventeen years will be as productive as the last.

Feline Aortic Thromboembolism

James A. Flanders, DVM
Department of Clinical Sciences
New York State College of Veterinary Medicine
Cornell University
Ithaca, New York

Thromboembolism is an ischemic condition caused by the acute obstruction of a blood vessel by a platelet aggregate. The platelet aggregate, or embolus, originates from a distant site in the circulatory system and travels in the bloodstream to the point of occlusion. The origin of the embolus is a thrombus, a large aggregate of fibrin and platelets attached to a vascular wall. In feline aortic thromboembolism, the thrombus is attached to the endocardial surface. An embolus breaks loose from the cardiac thrombus and occludes one or more branches of the aorta.

The clinical signs associated with aortic thromboembolism vary with the location of the embolus. Bilateral renal artery embolization produces signs of acute renal failure. Embolization of the cranial mesenteric artery can cause fatal bowel ischemia. Embolization of the cerebral arteries can produce central nervous system dysfunction. Embolization of the pulmonary vasculature can cause signs of respiratory insufficiency. Brachial artery embolization causes forelimb paresis and pain (Figure 1).

In cats, the most common site of embolization is the aortic trifurcation (Figure 2). Embolic occlusion at this site obstructs the internal and external iliac arteries and the median sacral artery. The clinical signs of an embolus at the aortic trifurcation are the five *p*s: pain, paresis, pulselessness, poikilothermy, and pallor. Neuromuscular ischemia secondary to vascular occlusion causes severe pain and paresis. Because of ischemic muscular contracture, the limbs often are held in rigid extension. The femoral pulse, normally palpated on the medial aspect of the proximal thigh, is weak or absent. Poikilothermy (hypothermia of the distal limb) and pale foot pads relate to the degree of circulatory attenuation (Figure 3).

The severity of pelvic limb dysfunction is associated with the extent of vascular obstruction. Some cats present with unilateral paresis or with slight neurologic deficits in both pelvic limbs (Figure 4). If the aortic trifurcation is occluded completely, cats are paralyzed acutely and are in severe pain.

Aortic thromboembolism is one of the most common causes of hindlimb paresis in cats. Hindlimb paresis in cats also can be caused by spinal neoplasia, intervertebral disk protrusion, inflammatory disease, and trauma.[1] Paresis caused by aortic thromboembolism is distinguished by the absence of femoral pulses; cool, pale foot pads; and severe pain.

Most cats with aortic thromboembolism have cardiomyopathy.[2] Large thrombi can develop in the heart chambers of patients with cardiomyopathy (Figure 5). If these thrombi break apart, emboli that can obstruct any branch of the aorta are mobilized.

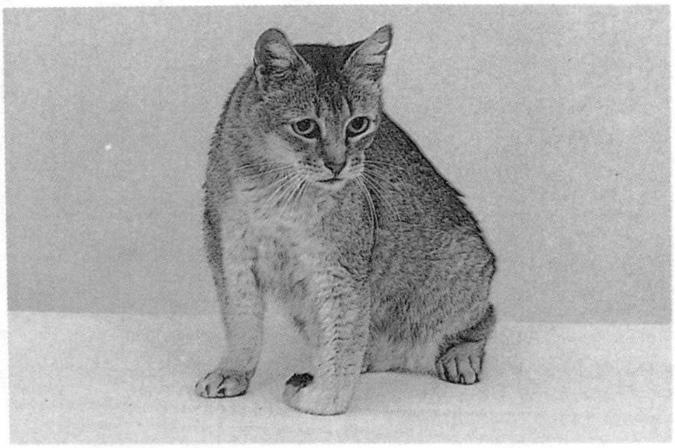

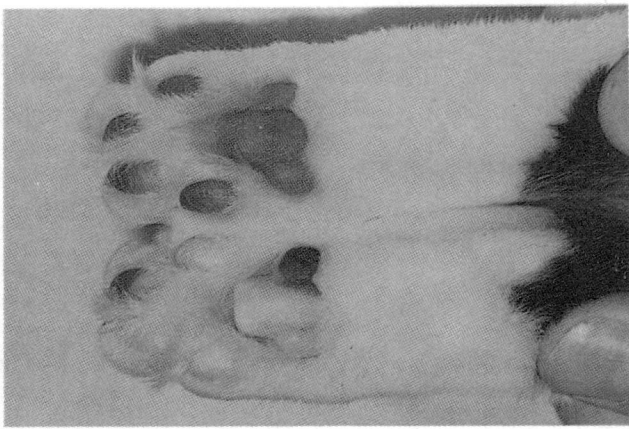

Figure 1—A cat with left forelimb paralysis secondary to brachial artery embolization.

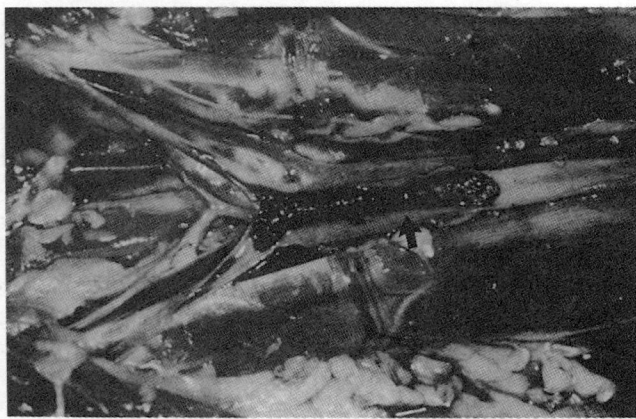

Figure 2—An embolus (*arrow*) occluding the aortic trifurcation. (Courtesy of John King, DVM, New York State College of Veterinary Medicine)

Figure 3—Foot-pad color in a cat with unilateral embolization of the external iliac artery.

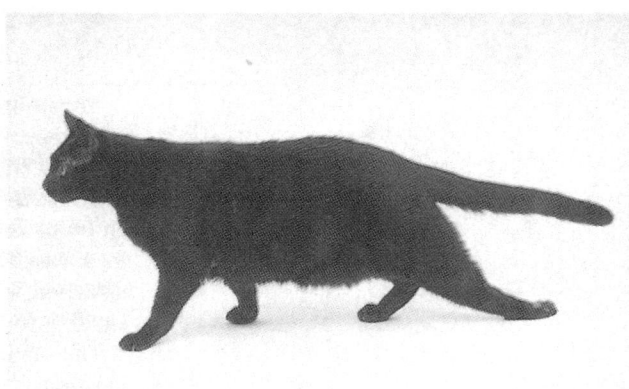

Figure 4—A cat with unilateral hindlimb paralysis secondary to embolization of the left external iliac artery.

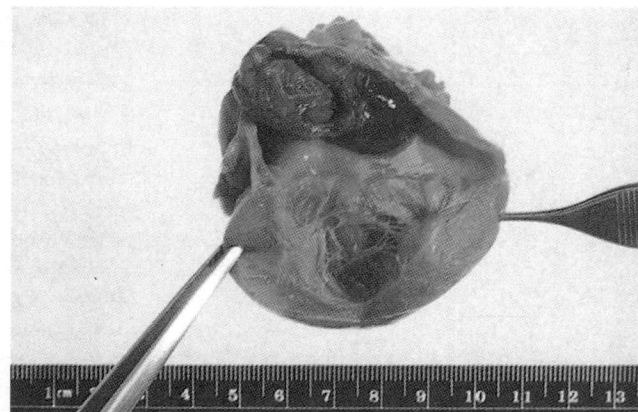

Figure 5—A thrombus in the left atrium of a cat with hypertrophic cardiomyopathy. (Courtesy of N. Sydney Moise, DVM, New York State College of Veterinary Medicine)

Cats paralyzed because of a thromboembolism require specialized treatment. Many patients that survive the acute phase of thromboembolism can, with the appropriate treatment, regain the ability to walk. In order to provide the most effective therapy, the veterinarian must understand the pathogenesis of thromboembolism. The discussion in this article is limited to the cause and treatment of the most common form of thromboembolism in cats, occlusion of the caudal abdominal aorta.

Cardiomyopathy and Thrombus Formation
Feline Cardiomyopathy

Cardiomyopathy is an alteration of the cardiac musculature that results in severe circulatory disturbances. Cardiomyopathy can be secondary to systemic disease (i.e., endocrine, metabolic, or infectious), or it can be primary.[2] The most common form of cardiomyopathy in cats and the type most often associated with thromboembolism is primary cardiomyopathy. Four different types of primary cardiomyopathy have been described in cats.[2] Dilated cardiomyopathy is characterized by extreme dilatation of the ventricles and moderate enlargement of the atrial chambers. Contractility of the heart is poor. Hypertrophic cardiomyopathy consists of greatly thickened ventricular walls and interventricular septum. The left atrium often is hypertrophied and dilated. Because of the extreme mural thickening, cardiac chamber volume and cardiac compliance are decreased. Restrictive cardiomyopathy consists of severe endocardial thickening and fibrosis, which interfere with diastolic filling. The fourth type of feline cardiomyopathy is caused by excessive moderator bands bridging the left ventricular chamber between the septum and the free wall. Restrictive cardiomyopathy and cardiomyopathy associated with excessive moderator bands are much less common than hypertrophic and dilated cardiomyopathy.

Thrombus Pathogenesis

Thrombus formation occurs in all types of feline cardiomyopathy. The physiologic abnormality that predisposes to thrombus formation with cardiomyopathy is not known precisely. In general, thrombus formation results from one or more of the following conditions: exposed vascular subendothelial tissue, abnormal circulatory patterns, and increased blood coagulability.[3] Each of these three conditions occurs in feline cardiomyopathy.

Endocardial Damage

Thrombus formation can occur in the heart chambers if endocardial damage exposes subendocardial collagen. Exposed collagen induces platelet adhesion and aggregation and activates the intrinsic clotting cascade (Figure 6). Activated platelets release adenosine diphosphate, serotonin, and the prostaglandin thromboxane A_2, all of which promote further platelet aggregation and vasoconstriction. Fibrin, the end product of the coagulation cascade, polymerizes within the platelet aggregate to produce an organized thrombus that adheres to the vascular wall.[3]

Endocardial damage, with subsequent subendocardial collagen exposure, is a component of several types of heart disease. Bacterial endocarditis and rheumatic heart disease in humans are well-documented examples of thrombus production on exposed subendocardial collagen.[4] Endocardial damage probably plays a minor role in thrombus formation associated with feline cardiomyopathy. Restrictive cardiomyopathy is the only form of cardiomyopathy that is consistently characterized by inflammatory endocarditis.[5,6] The endocardial inflammation associated with dilated and hypertrophic cardiomyopathy is mild.[5,7,8]

Abnormal Circulatory Patterns

Platelet hyperreactivity secondary to normal circulatory patterns can be a predisposing factor to thrombus formation in feline cardiomyopathy. Platelets stimulated by intravascular turbulence have an increased tendency to aggregate.[9-11] Shear stress exposes the phospholipoprotein on the platelet membrane surface, which provides a site for accumulation and potentiation of clotting factors.[10] Platelets in suspension release adenosine diphosphate and aggregate if gently stirred.[10] In experimental arteriovenous shunts that differed only in the amount of turbulence, significantly more thrombi accumulated distal to the more turbulent site.[11]

Thrombosis can be induced by circulatory stasis as well as by turbulence. An excellent example of static thrombosis is venous thrombosis in humans. As circulation slows,

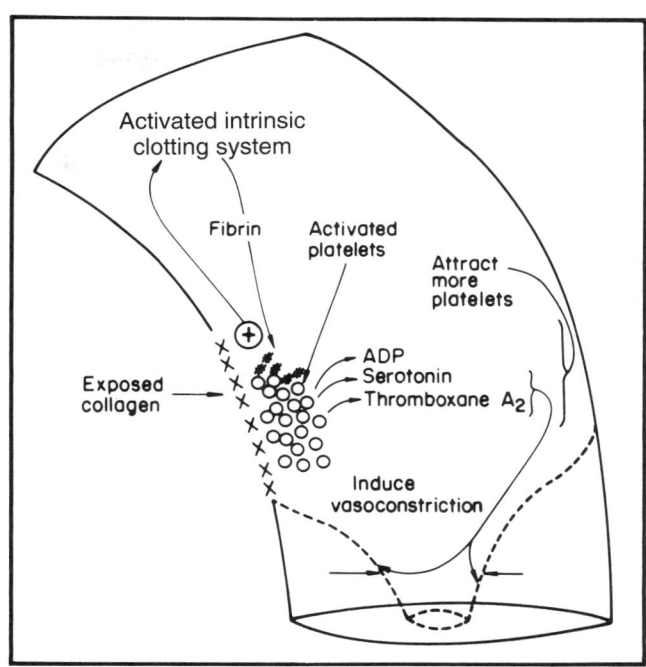

Figure 6—Exposed subendothelial collagen stimulates platelet aggregation and the release of vasoactive substances. Fibrin is produced by activation of the intrinsic clotting system.

red blood cells aggregate and blood viscosity increases.[12,13] Intermittent movement of viscous blood produces a stress on the blood elements, which may induce platelet activation and thrombosis.[12,13] Vascular stasis allows activated coagulation factors to accumulate rather than dilute in the bloodstream.[12] Intracardiac mural thrombi frequently are associated with hypocontractile ventricular wall segments in conjunction with myocardial infarction and congestive cardiomyopathy in humans.[14]

Cardiomyopathy severely affects the circulatory dynamics of the heart. Dilated cardiomyopathy is characterized by a large end-systolic ventricular blood volume. There is stasis of blood in the apical portions of the ventricular chambers, resulting in the formation of intracavitary thrombi.[5,6,15] Thrombi also are present in the atrial appendages.[16] Atrial dilatation is secondary to myocardial degeneration and mitral regurgitation. Aortic thromboembolism occurs in approximately 25% of cats that have dilated cardiomyopathy.[7]

In hypertrophic cardiomyopathy, atrial enlargement is secondary to chronically elevated ventricular end-diastolic pressure resulting from poor ventricular compliance. Also, papillary muscle hypertrophy causes a secondary mitral valve insufficiency because of valve leaflet malalignment.[6,7,17] Valvular turbulence and greatly enlarged, abnormally contracting atria can be predisposing factors to thrombus formation in the atrial appendages.[15-17] Arterial thromboembolism occurs in approximately 50% of cats that have hypertrophic cardiomyopathy.[7]

In restrictive cardiomyopathy, decreased compliance caused by endocardial fibrosis promotes areas of stasis within the ventricular chamber. Turbulence is present at the narrowed inflow and outflow tracts. Twenty-five percent of cats with restrictive cardiomyopathy have thromboembolism.[5]

The circulatory disturbances caused by cardiomyopathy associated with excessive moderator bands have not been well-defined. Characteristics common to congestive and hypertrophic cardiomyopathy have been noted. The meshwork of moderator bands that span the left ventricle causes turbulence. Aortic thromboembolism is evident in approximately 15% of cats with cardiomyopathy caused by excessive moderator bands.[18]

Increased Blood Coagulability

Thrombus formation occurs during periods of increased blood coagulability.[3] Because of an inherently high platelet reactivity, the cat may be in a constant state of increased coagulability. Feline platelets undergo spontaneous aggregation in vitro.[19,20] Feline platelets are relatively large and the platelet volume of cats is greater than that of most species, including humans and dogs.[19,21] Platelet activity is increased as platelet size and volume increase.[19,20] Serotonin, a vasoactive platelet-aggregating substance, is stored in high concentrations in feline platelets.[22] In addition, feline platelets are more responsive to serotonin-induced aggregation than are the platelets of other species.[20]

With such highly reactive platelets, cats may be more prone to produce thrombi, especially if the platelets are stimulated by exposed endocardial surfaces or by abnormal circulatory patterns. An increased susceptibility of platelets to aggregating agents correlates with an increased tendency for thrombosis in humans.[23]

Human Cardiomyopathy and Thromboembolism

Human platelets, compared with those of most animal species, are responsive to aggregating agents.[22] The propensity of human platelets to aggregate might contribute to the relatively high incidence of thromboembolic disease in humans. Cardiac thrombi occur in over 50% of humans with dilated cardiomyopathy.[24] Thromboembolism is associated with restrictive and hypertrophic cardiomyopathy, especially if atrial fibrillation is present[24,25]; however, only 4% of human thromboembolism is related to cardiomyopathy. More common causes of thrombosis in humans are myocardial infarction, rheumatic heart disease, and noncardiac atherosclerotic vascular disease.[26]

Canine Cardiomyopathy and Thromboembolism

Compared with platelets of other species, canine platelets respond moderately to aggregating agents.[22] The incidence of thrombosis in dogs is low.[27] The most common causes of canine thromboembolism are dirofilariasis and bacterial endocarditis.[27] A hypercoagulable state associated with the nephrotic syndrome and with renal amyloidosis has been reported.[28,29] This state is caused by decreased inhibition of the intrinsic coagulation system,[30] not by primary platelet stimulation. Thromboembolism associated with cardiomyopathy in dogs has not been reported.[31,32] The lack of thrombus formation in canine cardiomyopathy might result from decreased platelet reactivity. Another possible explanation is that the hemodynamic disturbances caused by cardiomyopathy in dogs are not as severe as those associated with feline or human cardiomyopathy.

Thromboemboli and Collateral Circulation
Aortic Ligation

In an experiment to help explain the pathogenesis of feline thromboembolism, Imhoff ligated the abdominal aortas of several cats at the level of the iliac trifurcation.[33] Although blood flow through the aorta was interrupted completely, the cats were not in pain and were able to walk after the surgery. The addition of a second ligature 1.5 cm cranial to the first did not change the condition.[33-35] Although the femoral pulses were absent, the hindlimbs remained warm and functional. Slight weakness and hyporeflexia were present, which resolved within 72 hours of aortic ligation.[35]

The maintenance of ambulation in cats with ligated aortas results from the bypass of blood through a preexisting collateral circulation system. Aortograms demonstrate that blood diverts from the caudal aorta through the lumbar vertebral arteries and the cranial and caudal superficial epigastric arteries.[35] Within 72 hours after aortic ligation, vascular perfusion of hindlimb muscles is 90% of the normal value.[35]

Vasoactive Agents

Although aortic ligation does not reproduce the clinical signs of aortic thromboembolism, an experimentally produced aortic thrombus does mimic the clinical syndrome.[33-35] In the procedure, an aortic thrombus is produced by temporary ligation of a segment of the caudal abdominal aorta. Bovine thromboplastin is injected into the occluded aortic segment. The blood in the segment is allowed to clot, and the ligatures are released. Cats with experimentally produced aortic thrombi, unlike those with aortic ligation, have severe paresis, discomfort, and cold limbs, similar to clinical cases.[33,35] Aortograms of cats with experimentally produced thromboembolism are similar to those of natural cases. Both demonstrate poorly developed collateral circulation systems.[33,35,36] It is hypothesized that the difference between ligation and embolus production results from the inhibition of collateral circulation development by a circulating factor from the aortic embolus.[33,35] The vasoactive substance serotonin reproduces the clinical syndrome when injected into an isolated caudal aortic segment.[34,37] Serotonin, a substance contained in platelet cytoplasmic vesicles, causes smooth muscle contraction in vessel walls and produces platelet aggregation. Antiserotonin substances are effective in preventing decreased collateral blood flow in experimentally embolized cats.[37,38]

Serotonin is not the only platelet product that inhibits collateral blood flow. Thromboxane A_2 evidently plays an important role. This agent, a prostaglandin, is produced and released by the platelets in response to many stimuli, including collagen, trauma, adenosine diphosphate, and serotonin.[39] Once it is in the circulatory system, thromboxane A_2 causes intense platelet aggregation and vasoconstriction.[40] The inhibition of collateral circulation caused by giving serotonin is augmented by the release of thromboxane A_2 by stimulated platelets.[41] The collateral circulation of experimentally thrombosed cats is preserved if the activity of thromboxane A_2 is inhibited by giving antiprostaglandin drugs.[42,43]

Neuromuscular Ischemia Induced by Thromboembolism

The circulatory supply to the nerves and muscles of the hindlimbs is greatly reduced when an embolus occludes the aortic trifurcation. In an experimental model, the perfusion of the muscles of the hindlimbs was reduced to 23% of normal 72 hours after embolization.[35]

In clinical cases of aortic thromboembolism, ischemic neuropathy is demonstrated initially by a reduction of nerve conduction velocity and evoked potentials. Ischemic damage to the nerve fibers can vary from minimal change to demyelination and/or axonal degeneration. Remyelination occurs during a period of two to four weeks after the acute ischemic episode. An increase in nerve conduction velocity and evoked potentials over a three-week period correlates well with the degree of recovery of limb movement.[44]

Simultaneous ligation of the caudal aorta and double ligation of the proximal femoral artery produces nerve degeneration similar to that evident in cats severely affected with thromboembolism.[45] Five days after ligation, necrosis of the proximal portions of the peroneal and tibial nerves is almost complete. In many nerve fibers, the myelin sheath is disrupted and the axoplasm is shrunken. The Schwann's cells degenerate, but the basement membrane of the nerve fibers is preserved. Within 21 days after ligation, there is evidence of nerve regeneration. Schwann's cells migrate from less affected areas, phagocytes remove necrotic nerve fibers, and axon regeneration occurs.[45] In cats, axonal regeneration in the tibial and peroneal nerves is present two months after an episode of thromboembolism.[44]

Aortic thromboembolism causes ischemic damage to the muscles of the hindlimbs. Clinically and histologically, the most severely affected muscles are the cranial tibial and gastrocnemius muscles. In some cases, the cranial tibial muscles have no spontaneous electromyogram activity soon after aortic embolization.[44] Histologic changes are characterized by various degrees of localized necrosis. The less severely affected muscle fibers are capable of regeneration, and the necrotic fibers are replaced by scar tissue.[44,46]

Treatment of Aortic Thromboembolism

The definitive treatment for feline aortic thromboembolism is a matter of debate. Early surgical removal of the aortic embolus is recommended by some authors[47-49]; most recent publications recommend cage rest and supportive therapy.[6,32]

Surgical Treatment

Embolectomy is the surgical treatment used for feline aortic thromboembolism. Removal of emboli from the caudal abdominal aorta is the most commonly reported procedure.[47,48,50-52] The caudal abdominal aorta is approached through a ventral midline incision. The area of the iliac trifurcation is packed off; and the proximal aorta, the internal and external iliac arteries, and the sacral artery are temporarily occluded. A transverse or longitudinal arteriotomy is made over the site of the embolus. The embolus is removed with fine forceps, and the ligatures are temporarily loosened to flush out any residual clot through the arteriotomy. Emboli in the renal or mesenteric arteries are milked out through the arteriotomy. The aortic incision is closed with No. 5-0 nonabsorbable suture material. Abdominal closure is routine.

Aortic embolectomy through an abdominal approach is an effective method of embolus removal in cats and humans; however, the technique has been abandoned in humans because it is associated with a mortality rate greater than 50%.[53-55] The major cause of the high mortality rate is believed to be the stress of major surgery on a patient with a severely compromised cardiovascular system.[53,56,57]

The mortality rate associated with abdominal embolectomy in cats has not been determined. Because most cats with thromboembolism have unstabilized cardiomyopathy, the risk of general anesthesia and abdominal surgery is great.[6,32]

Currently, the majority of caudal aortic emboli in humans are removed by the use of Fogarty® catheters (Fogarty® Arterial Embolectomy Catheter—American Hospital Supply) introduced through bilateral femoral arteriotomies (Figure 7).[57] The deflated balloon at the end of the catheter is passed proximal to the aortic obstruction. The balloon is inflated, and the catheter is pulled distally into the femoral artery. The embolus is dislodged by the balloon and pulled out through the arteriotomy site. Analgesia is achieved by tranquilization and local anesthesia.[57]

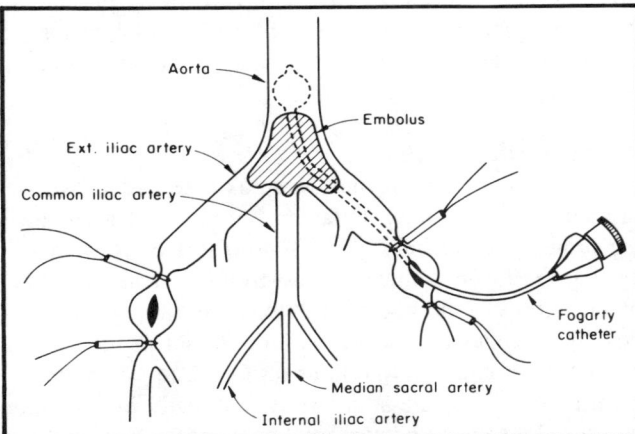

Figure 7—Removal of an embolus in the aortic trifurcation, using a balloon catheter. The catheter is introduced through a femoral arteriotomy and advanced beyond the embolus. The balloon is inflated, and the embolus is dislodged as the catheter is withdrawn.

Several complications unrelated to anesthetic risk have been reported in human patients undergoing embolectomy for lower extremity ischemia. Revascularization of an ischemic limb can mobilize sequestered metabolites, such as lactic acid and potassium. If the release of static blood occurs suddenly, profound cardiac depression can result.[58,59] Prompt revascularization also mobilizes activated clotting factors and liberates clotted blood that has formed in the veins of an ischemic limb. A rapidly mobilized venous clot can embolize the pulmonary vasculature and produce pulmonary insufficiency.[58,59] Myoglobinemia and myoglobinuria occur after blood flow is restored in an ischemic limb. Kidney damage can result from toxic effects of myoglobin on the renal tubules.[60] The human mortality rate associated with Fogarty® catheter embolectomy is 10% to 25%[58,59,61,62]; however, like most feline cases, human patients with rigor and cyanosis in the limbs are considered high risk for lethal complications. In one report, 81% of severely affected patients died after catheter embolectomy.[63]

The use of the Fogarty® catheter for embolectomy in cats requires further investigation. Catheterization of an embolized feline femoral artery is difficult because of the small arterial lumen size. Immobilization of a cat for catheter embolectomy requires heavy sedation or light anesthesia. This poses an increased risk in cats with cardiomyopathy, thereby limiting the use of catheter embolectomy.

Medical Treatment

Many cats with aortic thromboembolism die soon after the onset of clinical signs despite treatment; however, paralyzed cats that survive the initial cardiovascular stress often spontaneously recover the ability to walk.[44,56,64-66] Usually the severity of heart disease, rather than the extent of ischemia, dictates the overall prognosis. In most cats that survive the initial cardiovascular crisis, there is little neurologic improvement for the first week. Slow, steady improvement occurs during the second through fourth weeks as the collateral blood supply develops and nerve and muscle damage is repaired. Although some cats affected with extensive necrosis of the distal limbs do not recover, many cats with bilaterally absent femoral pulses, rigid paretic hindlimbs, and cyanotic foot pads do regain limb function. Some cats retain dropped hocks as the result of ischemic damage of the Achilles tendon[64] (Figure 8).

With medical treatment, the number of cats that survive the initial cardiovascular crisis increases. The return of ambulation might be more rapid. The goals of medical treatment of thromboembolism are supportive care during the acute ischemic crisis, restoration of blood flow to the limbs, and prevention of future embolic episodes. During the acute stage, the main concerns are cardiovascular support and alleviation of pain.

Initial Supportive Care

The stress of embolization can cause cardiovascular decompensation in cats with cardiomyopathy. Severely affected cats might have pulmonary edema or might be hy-

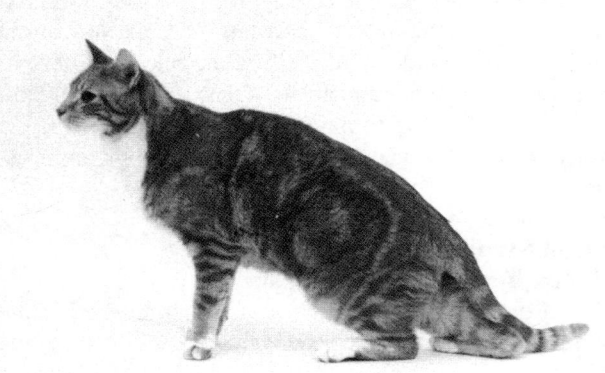

Figure 8—A cat with a residual plantigrade stance 15 months after an episode of thromboembolism.

pothermic and in cardiogenic shock. Carefully monitored oxygen therapy, combined with giving fluids, glucocorticoids, diuretics, and external heat, might be necessary for support. In the initial stages of thromboembolism, generalized supportive therapy is more important than specific antiembolic therapy. If the cat is stable, identification of the type of cardiomyopathy can be attempted. Electrocardiography, thoracic radiography, and echocardiography are useful for differentiating the type of cardiomyopathy and for establishing prognosis. When an accurate diagnosis is made, specific therapy for the various forms of cardiomyopathy can be started.[2]

As a result of ischemic neuromyopathy, cats with thromboembolism are in pain during the first 12 to 24 hours. Attempted movement and muscle palpation tend to exacerbate the pain. Morphine sulfate, given subcutaneously at a dose of 0.1 mg/kg, provides analgesia without excitement for four hours in cats.[67]

Shortening the Recovery Period

The recovery period for cats with aortic saddle embolization can be shortened by rapid clot lysis or by promoting the development of collateral circulation. In humans, a commonly used technique for treating thromboembolisms is thrombolytic enzyme therapy.[68,69]

Thrombolytic Agents

The thrombolytic enzymes streptokinase and urokinase promote clot dissolution by activating plasmin, a circulating proteolytic enzyme.[68,70] Plasmin dissolves clots by digesting the fibrin within the clot. Systemic administration of the thrombolytic agents in humans is through a high-dose intravenous or a low-dose intraarterial method. Both require a constant enzyme infusion for 12 to 120 hours.

Intraarterial enzyme administration directly into the clot permits clot lysis with lower total doses of the thrombolytic agent. The lower dose is believed to decrease hemorrhage at peripheral sites, such as recent surgical scars or vascular cutdown sites.[71,72] Selective arterial catheterization requires heavy sedation or anesthesia in cats. In addition, the necessity of specialized technique and fluoroscopic guidance makes selective arterial delivery of thrombolytic enzymes impractical in cats.

Systemic, high-dose administration of thrombolytic agents might be feasible in cats because placement of intravenous catheters does not require specialized equipment or anesthesia. Close observation of the patient is required during infusion. Clinical status should be assessed frequently, bleeding complications should be watched for, and activation of the fibrinolytic system should be assessed with specific blood tests (activated partial thromboplastin time or prothrombin time).[68] There is a potential for dislodgment of the primary cardiac thrombus by plasmin activity. Portions of the thrombus also can embolize the cerebral, mesenteric, or renal arteries. In addition, the use of monitoring facilities, clotting tests, and enzymes makes treatment of aortic saddle embolization with thrombolytic agents expensive.

In a recent preliminary study involving cats, systemic streptokinase therapy was proven to reduce aortic clot weight after a three-hour infusion. No hemolytic problems were noted during the infusion. Further studies are planned to attempt complete clot lysis with longer thrombolytic infusions.[73]

Heparin Therapy

Heparin therapy is not effective in the lysis of arterial emboli.[68] Heparin provides anticoagulation by potentiating antithrombin III, a plasma globulin that inhibits the formation of thrombin.[74] Thrombin is an enzyme that splits fibrinogen to fibrin. Antithrombin III inhibits fibrin formation so that clot production is inhibited. Heparin, therefore, is effective in preventing clot formation but not in dissolving established arterial thrombi.

Giving heparin might prevent embolus enlargement by inhibiting further clot formation. By minimizing the clot mass, collateral circulation can be established more rapidly. Heparin is commonly used to treat thromboembolism in humans.[58,61,62] Giving the agent to humans before and after surgery improves the results of catheter embolectomy.[56,61,62] Intravenous heparin therapy, followed by long-term oral anticoagulant (warfarin) therapy, is used in lieu of embolectomy in patients with mild clinical signs (i.e., cool, pale, painful limbs without paresis).[58,75] By avoiding embolectomy, the mortality rate of thromboembolism treatment is decreased.[58]

Based on the efficacy of anticoagulation for human thromboembolism, heparin and warfarin therapy might be useful for cats. An effective level of anticoagulation (prolonging the partial thromboplastin time 2.5 times normal) can be achieved by a dosage of 250 to 375 mg of subcutaneous heparin every eight hours.[76] The prophylactic use of low-dose warfarin in cats has not been investigated. Clinical trials are necessary before an effective dosage can be determined.

Vasodilating Drugs

Vasodilating drugs can improve the collateral blood flow in cats with aortic saddle embolization. An effective vasodilator must antagonize the platelet-induced reduction of collateral blood flow associated with embolization. The hypotension associated with many peripheral vasodilators limits their use because the drugs might compromise the cardiovascular status of a cat with aortic saddle embolization. Furthermore, if a vasodilator does not specifically antagonize the platelet-induced inhibition of collateral flow, systemic hypotension actually might decrease the blood flow in an ischemic limb.[77,78]

One category of vasodilators, the calcium channel blockers, has potential in treating feline aortic thromboembolism. Calcium channel blockers produce vasodilation by inhibiting the calcium-dependent contraction of the smooth muscle cells of the vessel wall.[79] Verapamil, one of the calcium channel blockers, has shown some efficacy in treating human patients with hypertrophic cardiomyopathy.[80] Perhaps the most beneficial characteristic of calcium channel blockers in treating cats is their ability to inhibit platelet aggregation.[81] Inhibition of calcium uptake prevents activated platelets from releasing vasoactive and platelet-aggregating substances.

The use of calcium channel blockers for treating feline aortic thromboembolism has not been reported in the literature. A drug that might vasodilate, inhibit platelet aggregation, and improve the cardiac status of a patient with cardiomyopathy certainly merits further investigation.

Prevention of Future Episodes—Antiplatelet Drugs

Drugs that inhibit platelet function or platelet aggregation have been used to treat thrombosis in humans.[3] The most commonly used antiplatelet drug is aspirin.

Aspirin reduces the ischemic effects of aortic thromboembolism by inhibiting platelet thromboxane A_2 production (Figure 9). Aspirin inhibits the activity of the platelet enzyme cyclooxygenase, the enzyme necessary for the conversion of fatty acid precursors into endoperoxides. Endoperoxides are converted into thromboxane A_2 by the action of thromboxane synthetase.[40] By decreasing the vasoconstrictive effects of thromboxane A_2, aspirin allows blood to circumvent aortic obstruction through collateral vessels.[42]

The antiischemic effects of aspirin can be potentiated by giving it less often than every day.[82,83] The inhibitory effect of aspirin on platelet cyclooxygenase is irreversible. All platelets present in the circulatory system when therapeutic levels of aspirin are given are rendered incapable of thromboxane A_2 production for the remainder of their circulation time. Unlike the effect on platelet cyclooxygenase, aspirin has a reversible effect on cyclooxygenase located in the vascular subendothelium. Endothelial cyclooxygenase is used in producing prostacyclin, a prostaglandin that is a potent inhibitor of platelet aggregation.[40] Prostacyclin is the natural check against spontaneous platelet aggregation on blood vessels. Because inhibition of endothelial cyclooxygenase persists for less than 24 hours,[84] giving aspirin every other day allows regeneration of prostacyclin while providing continuous inhibition of thromboxane A_2.

Cats have a low tolerance to aspirin because of their slow

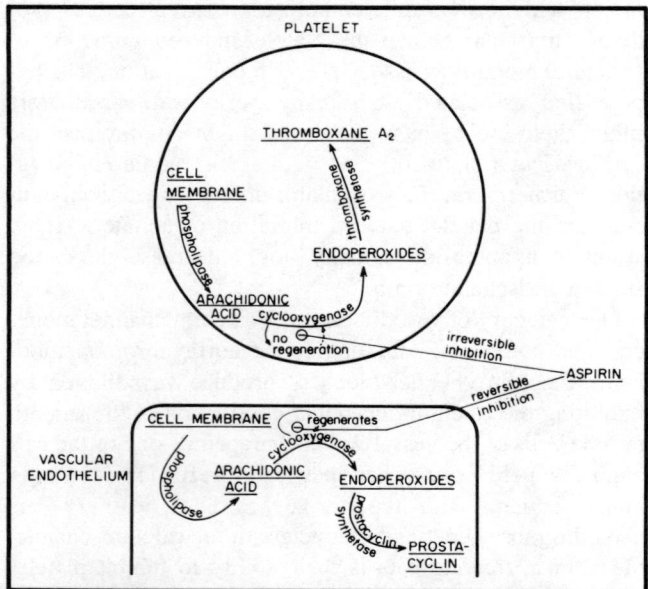

Figure 9—Aspirin irreversibly inhibits the conversion of precursors to thromboxane A_2 in platelets. The effect of aspirin on endothelial prostaglandin production is irreversible.

hepatic metabolism of the drug.[85] Toxic reactions—such as anorexia, emesis, lethargy, and death—can occur at dosages as low as 25 mg/kg orally three times a day.[86] The aspirin dosage required to inhibit platelet aggregation is far below the toxic level: 25 mg/kg every third day.[87] This dosage regimen also allows regeneration of prostacyclin by the vascular endothelium between aspirin doses. The amount of aspirin in a children's aspirin tablet, 1.25 grains, is approximately equal to 25 mg/kg for the average adult cat. For treating thromboembolism, aspirin is administered at a dosage of 25 mg/kg every third day for the remainder of the cat's life.

Giving aspirin is the best prophylactic therapy currently used for feline thromboembolism. Safe dosage for aspirin is known, it can be given orally, it inhibits platelet aggregation, and it preserves collateral circulation. Five cats treated with aspirin at the New York State College of Veterinary Medicine have survived for more than 18 months with no recurrence of thromboembolism.

In the future, new antiprostaglandin drugs, thrombolytic agents, or calcium channel blockers might be added to the treatment regimen for feline thromboembolism. At present, the following protocol is recommended:

1. Supportive care for initial cardiac decompensation—oxygen, diuretics, fluid therapy, glucocorticoids, and external heat
2. Analgesics—subcutaneous morphine sulfate, 0.1 mg/kg, every four to six hours during the first 24 to 48 hours
3. Aspirin—25 mg/kg orally every third day for the remainder of the patient's life.

Prognosis

There are two factors that must be considered before treating thromboembolism. The first is the extent of the ischemia. A poor prognosis must be given if the circulatory occlusion is severe enough to cause gangrenous changes in the limb. The second, and more important, factor is the patient's underlying cardiovascular disease. Many cats with thromboembolism die during the acute crisis because of the stress put on a compromised heart. Those cats that survive the initial phase have a limited life span because of cardiomyopathy. The short- and long-term prognoses must be presented to the owner before thromboembolism treatment begins. Successful treatment might prevent future episodes of thromboembolism, but it might not change the underlying heart disease.

REFERENCES

1. Gilmore DR: Feline pelvic limb paresis/paralysis. *Compend Contin Educ Pract Vet* 5(5):408-412, 1983.
2. Tilley LP, Liu S-K, Fox PR: Myocardial disease, in Ettinger SJ (ed): *Textbook of Veterinary Internal Medicine*, ed 2. Philadelphia, WB Saunders Co, 1983, pp 1029-1051.
3. Rosenthal DS, Braunwald E: Hematologic-oncologic disorders and heart disease, in Braunwald E (ed): *Heart Disease*. Philadelphia, WB Saunders Co, 1980, pp 1792-1800.
4. Deterling RA: Acute arterial occlusion. *Surg Clin North Am* 46(3):587-604, 1966.
5. Liu S-K, Tilley LP: Animal models of primary myocardial diseases. *Yale J Biol Med* 53:191-211, 1980.
6. Fox PR: Feline myocardial diseases, in Kirk RW (ed): *Current Veterinary Therapy VII*. Philadelphia, WB Saunders Co, 1980, pp 337-348.
7. Liu S-K, Tilley LP, Lord PF: Feline cardiomyopathy, in Roy PE, Rona G (eds): *Recent Advances in Studies on Cardiac Structure and Metabolism*, vol 10. Baltimore, University Park Press, 1975, pp 627-640.
8. Van Vleet JF, Ferrans VJ, Weirich WE: Pathologic alterations in hypertrophic and congestive cardiomyopathy of cats. *Am J Vet Res* 41(12):2037-2048, 1980.
9. Riddle JM, Stein PD, Magilligan DJ, McElroy HH: Evaluation of platelet reactivity in patients with valvular heart disease. *J Am Coll Cardiol* 1(6):1381-1384, 1983.
10. Mustard JF, Packham MA: Thromboembolism, a manifestation of the response of blood to injury. *Circulation* 62(1):1-21, 1970.
11. Smith RL, Blick EF, Coalson J, Stein PD: Thrombus production by turbulence. *J Appl Physiol* 32(2):261-264, 1972.
12. Lowe GDO, Forbes CD: Blood rheology and thrombosis. *Clin Haematol* 10(2):343-367, 1981.
13. Dormandy JA: Haemorheological aspects of thrombosis. *Br J Haematol* 45:519-522, 1980.
14. Gould L, Gopalaswamy C, Chardy F, Kim BS: Congestive cardiomyopathy and left ventricular thrombus. *Arch Intern Med* 143:1472-1473, 1983.
15. Goodwin JF, Roberts WC, Wenger NK: Cardiomyopathy, in Hurst JW (ed): *The Heart*, ed 5. New York, McGraw-Hill Co, 1982, pp 1299-1362.
16. Liu S-K: Acquired cardiac lesions leading to congestive heart failure in the cat. *Am J Vet Res* 31(11):2071-2088, 1970.
17. Lord PF, Wood A, Tilley LP, Liu S-K: Radiographic and hemodynamic evaluation of cardiomyopathy and thromboembolism in the cat. *JAVMA* 164(2):154-165, 1974.

18. Liu S-K, Fox PR, Tilley LP: Excessive moderator bands in the left ventricle of 21 cats. *JAVMA* 180(10):1215-1219, 1982.
19. Weiser MG, Kociba GJ: Platelet concentration and platelet volume distribution in healthy cats. *Am J Vet Res* 45(3):518-522, 1984.
20. Tschopp TB: Aggregation of cat platelets in vitro. *Thromb et Diath Haemor* 23:601-620, 1970.
21. Thompson CB, Jakubowski JA, Quinn PG, et al: Platelet size and age determine platelet function independently. *Blood* 63(6):1372-1375, 1984.
22. Dodds WJ: Platelet function in animals: Species specificities, in deGaetano G, Garattini S (eds): *Platelets: A Multidisciplinary Approach*. New York, Raven Press, 1978, pp 45-59.
23. Packham MA, Mustard JF: Platelet aggregation: Relevance to thrombotic tendencies. *Adv Exp Med Biol* 102:51-70, 1978.
24. Roberts WC, Ferrans VJ: Pathologic anatomy of the cardiomyopathies. *Hum Pathol* 6(3):287-342, 1975.
25. Siegel RJ, Prediman KS, Fishbein MC: Idiopathic restrictive cardiomyopathy. *Circulation* 70(2):165-169, 1984.
26. Elliot JP, Hageman JH, Szilagyi DE, et al: Arterial embolization: Problems of source, multiplicity, recurrence, and delayed treatment. *Surgery* 88(6):833-845, 1980.
27. Suter PF: Diseases of the peripheral vessels, in Ettinger SJ (ed): *Textbook of Veterinary Internal Medicine*, ed 2. Philadelphia, WB Saunders Co, 1983, pp 1062-1079.
28. DeBartola SP, Meuter DJ: Renal amyloidosis in two dogs presented for thromboembolic phenomena. *JAAHA* 16:129-135, 1980.
29. Green RA, Russo EA, Greene RT, Kabel AL: Hypoalbuminemia-related platelet hypersensitivity in two dogs with nephrotic syndrome. *JAVMA* 186(5):485-488, 1985.
30. Green RA, Kabel AL: Hypercoaguable state in three dogs with nephrotic syndrome: Role of acquired antithrombin III deficiency. *JAVMA* 181(9):914-917, 1982.
31. Liu S-K, Maron BJ, Tilley LP: Hypertrophic cardiomyopathy in the dog. *Am J Pathol* 94(3):497-507, 1979.
32. Bond B, Tilley LP: Cardiomyopathy in the dog and cat, in Kirk RW (ed): *Current Veterinary Therapy VII*. Philadelphia, WB Saunders Co, 1980, pp 307-315.
33. Imhoff RK: Production of aortic occlusion resembling acute aortic embolism syndrome in cats. *Nature* 192:979-980, 1961.
34. Butler HC: An investigation into the relationship of an aortic embolus to posterior paralysis in the cat. *J Small Anim Pract* 12:141-158, 1971.
35. Schaub RG, Meyers KM, Sande RD, Hamilton G: Inhibition of feline collateral vessel development following experimental thrombolic occlusion. *Circ Res* 39(5):736-743, 1976.
36. Imhoff RK, Tashjian RJ: Diagnosis of aortic embolism by aortography. *JAVMA* 139(2):203-208, 1961.
37. Schaub RG, Meyers KM, Sande RD: Serotonin as a factor in depression of collateral blood flow following experimental arterial thrombosis. *J Lab Clin Med* 90(4):645-653, 1977.
38. Olmstead ML, Butler HC: Five-hydroxytryptamine antagonists and feline aortic embolism. *J Small Anim Pract* 18:247-259, 1977.
39. Davenport DJ, Carakostas MC: Platelet disorders in the dog and cat. *Compend Contin Educ Pract Vet* 4(9):762-772, 1982.
40. Boothe DM: Prostaglandins: Physiology and clinical implications. *Compend Contin Educ Pract Vet* 6(11):1010-1021, 1984.
41. Meyers KM, Seachord CL, Holmser H, et al: A dominant role of thromboxane formation in secondary aggregation of platelets. *Nature* 282:331-333, 1979.
42. Schaub RG, Gates KA, Roberts RE: Effect of aspirin on collateral blood flow after experimental thrombosis of the feline aorta. *Am J Vet Res* 43(9):1647-1650, 1982.
43. Helenski C, Schaub RG, Roberts R: Improvements of collateral circulation after arterial thrombosis with indomethacin therapy. *Thromb Haemost* 44:69-71, 1980.
44. Griffiths IR, Duncan ID: Ischaemic neuromyopathy in cats. *Vet Rec* 104:518-522, 1979.
45. Korthals JK, Wisniewski HM: Peripheral nerve ischemia. Part 1. Experimental model. *J Neurol Sci* 24:65-76, 1975.
46. Karpati G, Carpenter S, Melmed C, Eisen AA: Experimental ischemic myopathy. *J Neurol Sci* 23:129-161, 1974.
47. Palumbo NE, Hubbard RE: Surgical treatment of aortic embolism in the cat. *JAVMA* 148(1):26-28, 1966.
48. Buchanan JW, Baker GJ, Hill JD: Aortic embolism in cats: Prevalence, surgical treatment, and electrocardiography. *Vet Rec* 79 (18):496-506, 1966.
49. DeHoff WD, Greene RW, Greiner TP: Surgical management of abdominal emergencies. *Vet Clin North Am* 2:328-330, 1972.
50. Lucke VM, Sumner-Smith G: Aortic embolism in the cat. *Vet Rec* 79(8):236-239, 1966.
51. Evans MG: Aortic thromboembolism in a cat. *VM SAC* 75(7):1150-1151, 1980.
52. Bryant AR, Lesch M: Posterior aortic thrombosis in a cat. *VM SAC* 72(1):48-49, 1977.
53. Blum L, Rosenthal I: Embolectomy in arteries to extremities. *JAMA* 172(8):794-798, 1960.
54. Schein CJ, Hoffert PW, Hurwitt ES: Aortic embolectomy: A critical evaluation of eleven consecutive cases. *Surgery* 39(6):950-958, 1956.
55. Taylor FW: Saddle embolus of the aorta. *Arch Surg* 62:38-49, 1951.
56. Willman VL, Hanlon CR: Safer operation in aortic saddle embolism. *Ann Surg* 150:568-572, 1959.
57. Fogarty TJ, Cranley JJ, Krause RJ, et al: A method for extraction of arterial emboli and thrombi. *Surg Gynecol Obstet* 116:241-244, 1963.
58. Blaisdell FW, Steele M, Allen RE: Management of acute lower extremity arterial ischemia due to embolism and thrombosis. *Surgery* 84(6):822-834, 1978.
59. Fogarty TJ: Acute arterial occlusion, in Sabiston DC (ed): *Textbook of Surgery*, ed 12. Philadelphia, WB Saunders Co, 1983, pp 1975-1982.
60. Haimovici H: Myopathic nephrotic-metabolic syndrome associated with massive myute arterial occlusions. *J Cardiovasc Surg* 14:589-600, 1973.
61. McPhail NV, Fratesi SJ, Barber GG, Scobie TK: Management of acute thromboembolic limb ischemia. *Surgery* 93(3):381-385, 1983.
62. Busuttil RW, Keehn G, Milliker J, et al: Aortic saddle embolus. *Ann Surg* 197(6):698-705, 1983.
63. Stallone RJ, Blaisdell FW, Cafferata HT, Levin SM: Analysis of morbidity and mortality from arterial embolectomy. *Surgery* 65 (1):207-217, 1969.
64. Holzworth J, Simpson R, Wind A: Aortic thrombosis with posterior paralysis in the cat. *Cornell Vet* 44:468-487, 1955.
65. Freak MJ: Aortic thrombosis with posterior paralysis in the cat. *Vet Rec* 68:816-818, 1956.
66. Joshua JO: A further case of aortic thrombosis in the cat. *Vet Rec* 69:146-147, 1957.
67. Davis LE, Donnelly EJ: Analgesic drugs in the cat. *JAVMA* 153(9):1161-1167, 1968.
68. Sherry S, Bell W, Duckert FH, et al: Thrombolytic therapy in thrombosis: A National Institutes of Health consensus development conference. *Ann Intern Med* 93:141-144, 1980.
69. Bell WR, Meck AG: Guidelines for use of thrombolytic agents. *New Engl J Med* 30(23):1266-1270, 1979.
70. Dotter CT, Rosch J, Seaman AJ: Streptokinase treatment of thromboembolic disease. *Radiology* 102:283-290, 1972.
71. Rush DS, Gewertz BL, Lu C-T, et al: Selective infusion of streptokinase for arterial thrombosis. *Surgery* 93(6):828-833, 1983.
72. Dardik M, Sussman BC, Kahn M, et al: Lysis of arterial clot by intravenous or intra-arterial administration of streptokinase. *Surg Gynecol Obstet* 158:137-140, 1984.
73. Killingsworth CR, Eyster GE, Adams T, et al: Streptokinase treatment of cats with experimentally-induced aortic thrombosis. *Am J Vet Res* 47(6):1351-1359, 1986.
74. O'Reilly RA: Anticoagulant, antithrombotic, and thrombolytic drugs, in Gilman AG, Goodman LS, Gilman A (eds): *The Pharmacologic Basis of Therapeutics*, ed 6. New York, MacMillan Publishing Co, 1980, pp 1347-1366.
75. Abbot WM, McCabe C, Maloney RD, Wirthlin LS: Embolism of the popliteal artery. *Surg Gynecol Obstet* 159:533-536, 1984.
76. Greene CE, Meriwether BA: Activated partial thromboplastin time and activated coagulation time in monitoring heparinized cats. *Am J Vet Res* 43(8):1473-1477, 1982.
77. Thulesius O: Haemodynamic studies on experimental obstruction of the femoral artery in the cat. *Acta Physiol Scand [Suppl 57]* 199:1-95, 1962.
78. Lowe GDO: Vasodilators: Minoxidil and drugs used in peripheral vascular and cerebral disorders. *Br Med J* 286:1262-1264, 1983.
79. Fleckenstein A: Specific pharmacology of calcium in myocardium, cardiac pacemakers, and vascular smooth muscle. *Annu Rev Pharmacol Toxicol* 17:149-166, 1977.
80. Rosing DR, Kent KM, Borer JS, et al: Verapamil therapy: A new approach to the pharmacologic treatment of hypertrophic cardiomyopathy. *Circulation* 60(6):1201-1207, 1979.

81. Schmunk GA, Lefer AM: Anti-aggregatory actions of calcium channel blockers in cat platelets. *Res Commun Chem Pathol Pharmacol* 35(2):179-187, 1982.
82. Wenger TL, Hull JM: Aspirin dosage for cardiovascular effects (letter to the editor). *N Engl J Med* 303(19):1121, 1980.
83. Bradlow BA, Chetty N: Dosage frequency for suppression of platelet function by low dose aspirin therapy. *Thromb Res* 27:99-110, 1982.
84. Kelton JG, Hirsch J, Carter CJ, Buchanan MR: Thrombogenic effect of high-dose aspirin in rabbits. *J Clin Invest* 62:892-895, 1978.
85. Yeary RA, Swanson W: Aspirin dosages for the cat. *JAVMA* 163(10):1177-1178, 1973.
86. Larson JE: Toxicity of low doses of aspirin in the cat. *JAVMA* 143(8):837-840, 1963.
87. Greene CE: Effect of aspirin and propranolol on feline platelet aggregation. *Am J Vet Res* 46(9):1820-1823, 1985.

UPDATE

NEW CLINICAL INFORMATION

In a recent retrospective study of 100 cats with aortic thromboembolism, the investigators found that 63% of the affected cats were neutered males and the average age was 7.7 years.[1] The most common underlying disease was hypertrophic cardiomyopathy (58%), and 88% of the cats had radiographic evidence of cardiomyopathy. Twenty-eight percent of the cats died during initial hospitalization and 35% were euthanatized. The average lifespan of the survivors was 11.5 months, and 50% of the cats reembolized despite warfarin or aspirin therapy. In a retrospective study of cats with hypertrophic cardiomyopathy, 11 cats that developed aortic thromboembolism had an average survival of 61 days.[2]

SURGICAL THERAPY

As mentioned in the paper, aortic thromboembolism is usually a consequence of severe cardiac disease. Surgical therapy, whether it involves surgical or catheter embolectomy, is not recommended for cats with aortic thromboembolism because they are already severely compromised. Medical management is the preferred treatment.

THROMBOLYTIC AGENTS

A relatively new thrombolytic agent, tissue plasminogen activator (TPA), which has been evaluated for treatment of cats with aortic thromboembolism,[3] may lead to hyperkalemia and, therefore, cannot be recommended as therapy for this condition. TPA is theoretically superior to other thrombolytic agents, such as streptokinase or urokinase, because it has a low affinity for circulating plasminogen and a high affinity for fibrin within thrombi. In one clinical study, 43% of cats with aortic thromboembolism treated with TPA were ambulatory within 48 hours. Yet, 50% of the cats in the study died during or soon after therapy, primarily due to severe hyperkalemia caused by a rapid release after clot lysis of ischemic blood trapped distal to the clot.

WARFARIN THERAPY

In a published report of warfarin to treat cats with aortic thromboembolism[4] the average survival was 15.7 months. Yet 43% of those cats reembolized in spite of continuous warfarin therapy. There are many potential complications associated with warfarin dosage. The recommended starting dose of warfarin is 0.5 mg PO every 24 hours. Warfarin therapy should be monitored closely by frequent prothrombin time monitoring to maintain a therapeutic prothrombin time two to three times normal.

The tendency of warfarin to cause an initial hypercoaguable state requires administration of heparin (220 units/kg SC initially followed by 60 to 200 units/kg SC, two to four times daily) for the first three to five days. Cats with liver disease may have prolonged warfarin effects as warfarin is metabolized by the liver. Another consideration should be warfarin pharmacokinetics, which are altered by numerous commonly prescribed drugs such as corticosteroids, barbiturates, cimetidine, metronidazole, and trimethoprim-sulfamethoxazole. Even when closely monitored, 20% of cats receiving warfarin therapy had severe bleeding episodes.[4]

VASODILATORS

The calcium channel blocker diltiazem is effective for treatment of hypertrophic cardiomyopathy in cats.[5] Additionally, diltiazem is a potent vasodilator that improves peripheral perfusion, increases venous oxygen tension, and decreases blood lactate concentration in cats with hypertrophic cardiomyopathy.[5] It is possible that diltiazem may help maintain collateral circulation in cats with aortic thromboembolism. Recommended dose of diltiazem for treatment of cats with hypertrophic cardiomyopathy is 2.5 mg orally twice a day initially, followed by a slow increase to 3.0 mg/kg/day if no clinical complications arise.[5] Alternatively, diltiazem can be administered orally once a day in an extended-release formulation (Dilacor®), one 60 mg pellet (removed from 240 mg capsule).[6]

The use of acepromazine for treatment of cats with aortic thromboembolism is not recommended because it decreases systemic blood pressure and does not antagonize platelet-induced vasoconstriction.

RECOMMENDED THERAPY

Aspirin's simplicity and low incidence of complications give it my personal recommendation as the therapy of choice (25 mg/kg PO every third day) for aortic thromboembolism. While reembolization may still occur with aspirin therapy and the average survival rate is likely to be less than 1 year, we have had reasonable success. Caution is necessary when using aspirin concurrently with propranolol: It has been shown that propranolol negates the antiprostaglandin effects of aspirin.[7] Warfarin may be the preferred anticoagulant when propranolol is a necessary part of the treatment of the underlying heart disease in a cat with thromboembolism. In general, however, diltiazem is more effective than propranolol for therapy of hypertrophic cardiomyopathy in cats.[5]

REFERENCES

1. Laste NC, Harpster NK: A retrospective study of 100 cases of feline distal aortic thromboembolism: 1977–1993. *JAAHA* 31:492–500, 1995.

2. Atkins CE, Gallo AM, Kurzman ID, Cowen P: Risk factors, clinical signs and survival in cats with a clinical diagnosis of idiopathic hypertrophic cardiomyopathy: 74 cases (1985–1989). *JAVMA* 201:613–618, 1992.
3. Pion PD: Feline aortic thromboemboli and the potential utility of thrombolytic therapy with tissue plasminogen activator. *Vet Clin North Am (Small Anim Pract)* 18:79–86, 1988.
4. Harpster NK, Baty CJ: Warfarin therapy of the cat at risk of thromboembolism, in Bonagura J (ed): *Kirk's Current Veterinary Therapy XII*. Philadelphia, WB Saunders Co, 1995, pp 868–873.
5. Bright JM, Golden L, Gompf RE, Walker MA, Toal RL: Evaluation of the calcium channel-blocking agents diltiazem and verapamil for treatment of feline hypertrophic cardiomyopathy. *J Vet Intern Med* 5:272–282, 1992.
6. Moise NS: personal communication, 1996.
7. Allen DG, Johnstone IB, Crane S: Effects of aspirin and propranolol alone and in combination on hemostatic determinants in the healthy cat. *Am J Vet Res* 46:660–663, 1985.

Pharmaceutical Treatment of Acute Spinal Cord Trauma

Louisiana State University
Elmarie Meintjes, BVSc, MS, MRCVS
Giselle Hosgood, BVSc, MS, FACVS
Joanna Daniloff, PhD

FOCAL POINT

★ It is critical to initiate aggressive and appropriate treatment within hours after insult to prevent the continued neuronal destruction that follows acute spinal cord trauma.

KEY FACTS

- The use of high doses of methylprednisolone seems to be essential, but initiation of treatment more than 8 hours after injury is not only ineffective but detrimental to the spinal cord, p. 628.

- Overdosage of glucocorticoids as well as combined use with nonsteroidal antiinflammatory agents can result in severe adverse effects, p. 628.

- Calcium channel blockers may be beneficial in limiting secondary injury and should be used in conjunction with vasopressors, p. 628.

- The nonglucocorticoid tirilazad mesylate seems to be safer and more effective than methylprednisolone and may be available commercially in the near future, p. 630.

Spinal cord concussion or laceration as a result of vertebral fracture, luxation, or disk extrusion is one of the most frequent neurologic disorders seen in small animal practice.[1] The complex set of primary and secondary pathologic changes that follow mammalian spinal cord injury have been extensively described but are not yet completely understood,[2-6] and much controversy exists. Injury to the spinal cord, however, often results in relatively predictable pathology and pathophysiology.[1,7,8]

Ischemic, biochemical, and cellular changes following mechanical trauma are believed to contribute to damage known as *secondary injury*.[9-11] A possible mechanism for the continued cellular destruction that is seen after injury may involve vasogenic edema[12] and a dramatic decrease in spinal cord blood flow in segments cranial and caudal to the lesion.[11,13] This progressive decline in spinal cord blood flow is probably caused by an injury-initiated molecular cascade involving a massive increase in intracellular calcium,[1,14] liberation of vasoactive prostanoids and thromboxane A_2, and microvascular lipid peroxidative reactions with release of excessive amounts of cytotoxic free radicals.[1,5,15] The ultimate consequence is continued neuronal cell death and loss of sensorimotor function.

Control of the chemical and vascular changes that result in secondary injury should limit the loss of function. Therefore, acute spinal cord injury is an emergency, and early treatment is critical to limit the degeneration after injury.[9,16,17] Treatment should be directed at prevention of the spread of biochemical neuronal destruction[10] and at decompression of the spinal cord and/or stabilization of the vertebral column.[18] In addition, adequate nursing and supportive care for paraplegic or tetraplegic animals is vital for recovery and should never be neglected.[18-20]

Numerous pharmacologic agents for the treatment of acute spinal cord injury have been described, but there are many opposing views regarding the efficacy of

> **Problems Associated with the Use of Dexamethasone**
>
> ■ Uncertain efficacy
> ■ Severe side effects
>   Gastrointestinal hemorrhage
>   Ulceration
>   Pancreatitis
>   Immunosuppression
>   Colonic perforation

these agents (Table I). This article assesses recent developments in the use of drugs that specifically target the treatment of secondary injury.

TREATMENT METHODOLOGIES
Glucocorticoids

Since the 1960s, glucocorticoids have been used extensively in the clinical treatment of spinal cord trauma, mainly because of the theory that they would reduce edema.[21] The dose, timing, optimum duration of treatment, overall effectiveness, and mechanisms of action, however, remain controversial.[17,22,23] Possible mechanisms of action include suppression of edema, enhancement of spinal cord blood flow, inhibition of the inflammatory response that is associated with long-lasting vasospasm, and protection from cytotoxic free radicals.[7,15]

Dexamethasone

Dexamethasone sodium phosphate at 2.2 mg/kg is the drug most commonly used in the clinical treatment of dogs with acute intervertebral disk herniation.[24] The use of repeated high doses of dexamethasone (4 mg/kg) has also been reported, but such side effects as gastrointestinal hemorrhage, ulceration, pancreatitis, and immunosuppression are common complications.[19,25,26] One of the most catastrophic complications, colonic perforation and death, occurred in dogs within 5 to 10 days after neurosurgery and the administration of dexamethasone sodium phosphate at 2.2 mg/kg.[21,27]

In addition, it is uncertain whether any beneficial effects are achieved from the use of dexamethasone. Cats with a ventral compression injury at the second lumbar vertebra (L2) were treated intravenously with 2.2 mg/kg of dexamethasone sodium phosphate twice daily the first day, with a decreasing dose to 0.5 mg/kg twice daily for 3 days after injury. In these animals, neurologic recovery scores (horizontal ladder walking) and electrophysiologic responses (somatosensory-evoked potentials) were the same as those for cats that received no treatment.[28] In summary, because of the frequency of severe side effects in addition to the uncertain efficacy, the use of dexamethasone for treating acute spinal cord injuries is not recommended.

Methylprednisolone

Administration of a high-dose methylprednisolone sodium succinate regimen within 8 hours after trauma has been reported to inhibit spinal tissue lipid peroxidation. This mechanism of action is believed to be the major reason for its therapeutic benefit.[29,30] Methylprednisolone also supports energy metabolism, reverses the intracellular calcium accumulation, prevents progressive ischemia, and increases electrophysiologic responses in the spinal cord after injury.[21,31,32] These beneficial effects are achieved only with doses of methylprednisolone sodium succinate that are higher (30 mg/kg) than antiinflammatory doses (0.25 mg/kg).[30,32,33] Significant gastrointestinal complications have not been reported when the high dose is given over a short period (48 hours).[34]

In rats, a 30 mg/kg intravenous bolus of methylprednisolone sodium succinate was given 1 hour after a compression injury at the level of the first thoracic vertebra (T1). This was followed by an intravenous dose of 5.4 mg/kg/hour for 3 hours. The study reported that somatosensory evoked potentials were preserved with the use of this regimen.[35]

In cats with compression trauma at L2, treatment was begun 30 minutes after injury with a 30 mg/kg intravenous bolus of methylprednisolone sodium succinate; 6 hours later, an additional 15 mg/kg intravenous bolus was given, followed by a continuous intravenous infusion of 2.5 mg/kg/hour for 48 hours.[36] Based on evaluation of general mobility, running, and stair-climbing, the treated cats scored significantly higher than the placebo-treated cats at 4 weeks after injury.[36] A single intravenous dose of methylprednisolone sodium succinate (30 mg/kg) given as soon as possible after injury, with a maintenance dose of 15 to 20 mg/kg intravenously every 2 to 3 hours, has also been reported as the optimum dosage to inhibit spinal lipid peroxidation and enhance motoneuron function in cats.[30]

In a report of 86 dogs with rear limb paresis or paralysis (onset of 3 to 36 hours) due to intervertebral disk herniation, 92% of the dogs recovered completely after treatment with high-dose methylprednisolone sodium succinate and decompressive surgery.[37] Fifty-two dogs had deep pain perception before surgery and 34 had no deep pain perception. A 30 mg/kg intravenous bolus of methylprednisolone sodium succinate was given before surgery, with a continuous intravenous infusion of 5.4 mg/kg/hour for the next 23 hours.[37] Methylprednisolone seemed to significantly increase the success rate of decompressive surgery for intervertebral disk herniation in dogs.[37]

Prednisolone

An initial intravenous dose of 20 mg/kg prednisolone sodium phosphate followed 3 hours later by 10 mg/kg intravenously and another 10 mg/kg intravenously 3

TABLE I
Compounds that May Ameliorate Secondary Injury after Experimental Mechanical Damage (Contusion, Compression, Transection) to the Spinal Cord

Compound	Species	Dosage	Mechanism of Action	Reference
Available drugs				
Methylprednisolone sodium succinate	Cats	30 mg/kg IV within 8 hours after injury; 15 mg/kg IV 2 and 6 hours later; infusion of 2.5 mg/kg/hr IV up to 48 hours after injury	Inhibits lipid peroxidation	36
	Dogs	30 mg/kg IV bolus followed by 5.4 mg/kg/hr IV infusion for 23 hours		37
Prednisolone sodium phosphate	Dogs	20 mg/kg IV; 10 mg/kg 3 and 6 hours later; 9 hours later, infusion of 2 mg/kg/hr IV for 24 hours	May reduce edema and inflammatory response	18
Diltiazem	Cats	100 μg/kg IV bolus with 5 μg/kg/min IV infusion for 4 hours (dissolve in 0.9% saline)	Prevents decrease in spinal cord blood flow because of reduction in intracellular Ca^- influx	11
Nifedipine	Cats	10 μg/kg IV bolus followed by 1 μg/kg/min IV infusion	Same as diltiazem	11
Nimodipine	Baboons	0.04 mg/kg/hr IV infusion for 7 days	Same as diltiazem	41
Ibuprofen	Cats	10 mg/kg IV bolus at time of injury with 5 mg/kg IV 90 minutes later	Cyclooxygenase inhibitor that maintains spinal cord blood flow within normal limits	11
Experimental drug				
Tirilazad mesylate	Cats	0.3 to 30 mg/kg IV bolus 30 minutes after injury with 0.15 to 15 mg/kg IV bolus at 2½ and 6 hours after injury followed by infusion of 1.6 to 160 mg/kg to reach total dose within 48 hours	Nonglucocorticoid that inhibits lipid peroxidation	48

hours later has been suggested for dogs.[18] Nine hours after initiation of treatment, a continuous intravenous infusion should be given at the rate of 2 mg/kg/hour for 24 hours. The total dose should be approximately 90 mg/kg during a 30-hour treatment period.[18] If the animal's neurologic status deteriorates after discontinuation of glucocorticoid therapy, a continuous intravenous infusion should be reinstated, but not for more than an additional 24 hours.[18] Although side effects were not seen with this regimen, no controlled studies have been performed to establish its benefits.[18]

Additional Considerations on the Use of Glucocorticoids

There is unequivocal evidence that methylprednisolone beneficially modifies the course of events after severe spinal cord injury[21]; however, several drawbacks have been described. The effective dose range of methylprednisolone is very narrow, with 60 mg/kg causing loss of beneficial effect and 90 mg/kg promoting lipid peroxidation.[30] The potential for immunosuppression and gastrointestinal disturbances also exists when the drug is administered over a longer period.[17,23] Finally, the finding that initiating treatment after 8 hours may actually exacerbate neuronal necrosis and inhibit axonal sprouting has caused more controversy.[17,38]

In spinal cord injury models, several drugs (e.g., the calcium-channel antagonist flunarizine[31]) tested in combination with methylprednisolone have produced superior results.[17] Combining some drugs with methylprednisolone, however, can be deleterious.[17] For example, the combination of the narcotic antagonist naloxone and methylprednisolone does not reduce edema as much as either drug alone and seems to be toxic by enhancing lipid peroxidation.[39,40] In addition, the combination of glucocorticoids, particularly dexamethasone,[24] with nonsteroidal antiinflammatory drugs (e.g, phenylbutazone, ibuprofen, or flunixin meglumine) may have serious and sometimes lethal side effects related to gastrointestinal bleeding and perforation. One must be aware of the sensitivity of dogs as well as cats to nonsteroidal antiinflammatory drugs and to the combination of nonsteroidal antiinflammatory drugs and glucocorticoids—both impair normal defense mechanisms of the bowel wall. No experimental data exist to suggest that using such a combination is beneficial.

Calcium-Channel Antagonists

Calcium-channel antagonists (e.g., nimodipine, diltiazem hydrochloride, nifedipine, and flunarizine hydrochloride) have recently been used with significant success in experimental spinal cord injuries, possibly because of the inhibitory effect of these drugs on cellular calcium entry. Nimodipine (0.04 mg/kg/hour, intravenous infusion for 7 days after insult) significantly increased local spinal cord blood flow and improved axonal function (as measured with somatosensory evoked potentials) following a compression injury at L1 in baboons.[41] Pretreating cats with diltiazem (100 µg/kg intravenous bolus, followed by a 5 µg/kg/minute intravenous infusion) or nifedipine (10 µg/kg intravenous bolus, followed by a 1 µg/kg/minute intravenous infusion) for 30 minutes before a contusion injury (blunt impact) at L3 largely prevented the spinal cord blood flow decrease after injury.[11] Similar results were not obtained, however, with verapamil.[11]

Flunarizine (0.1 mg/kg intravenously) was administered 5 and 120 minutes after a contusion injury to the exposed spinal cord of cats, and somatosensory evoked potentials were recorded 4 hours later. This treatment resulted in a 52% recovery of the preinjury amplitude versus a 17% recovery in cats without treatment.[31] Furthermore, when flunarizine and methylprednisolone sodium succinate (30 mg/kg 5 minutes after injury) were administered together, a significantly higher (62%) recovery of preinjury amplitude was reported.[31]

Therefore, it is likely that treatment for acute spinal injuries will be enhanced by the inclusion of calcium-channel antagonists in conjunction with vasopressors (such as high-dose dopamine at 10 µg/kg/min in dogs) to maintain systemic blood pressure.[42] Experience in the clinical use of these agents in both dogs and cats, however, is limited, and specific adverse effects are not well described.

Narcotic Antagonists

The potential use of the narcotic antagonist naloxone has been tested because of its established ability to counteract endorphin-mediated hypotension that follows acute spinal injury.[40,43] Although these studies resulted in amelioration of neurologic deficits, another study could not substantiate these effects.[44] Furthermore, because naloxone is expensive and inferior to methylprednisolone, clinical use of the drug is precluded.[38]

Osmotic Diuretics

Although osmotic diuretics (e.g., mannitol, dextran, and glycerol) are useful in reducing brain edema, there is no evidence that these agents are effective in the treatment of spinal cord injury. In fact, treatment with osmotic diuretics can contribute to hemorrhage in the gray matter[18] and impede neurologic recovery.[28] Such treatment can also produce serious side effects that include hypokalemia, tissue dehydration, and rebound increases in cerebrospinal fluid pressure.[20] Despite the fact that carbonic anhydrase inhibitors (e.g., furosemide) reduce cerebrospinal fluid pressure, they can also induce hypokalemia.[22]

Dimethyl Sulfoxide

Electron microscopy indicated that dimethyl sulfoxide given 1 hour after contusion injury in dogs protected myelin sheaths and axons, reduced edema, and accelerated return of motor function.[45] Dimethyl sulfoxide may exert its effect by reducing thrombin-stimulated serotonin release and acting as a hydroxyl radical (released during lipid peroxidation) scavenger.[5,20] Several side effects, however, have been reported and include production of a destructive methyl radical, fever, hemolysis, and renal toxicity.[5,20]

In cats, at 42 days after a compression injury at L2 and administration of decreasing doses (1.5, 1.5, 1.0,

0.7, and 0.5 g/kg, intravenously) of dimethyl sulfoxide for 4 days, no therapeutic effect could be demonstrated by somatosensory evoked potentials and horizontal ladder walking.[28] Many other studies on the effects of dimethyl sulfoxide have been performed. Although positive results have been reported, the majority are negative; therefore, the use of dimethyl sulfoxide remains controversial.

Miscellaneous Drugs

Numerous agents, such as superoxide dismutase,[18] iron chelators (e.g., deferoxamine[18]), antioxidants (e.g., vitamin E and selenium[11]), nonsteroidal antiinflammatory drugs (e.g., ibuprofen and flunixin[11,15]), and aspartate-receptor antagonists (e.g., ketamine) have potential value in the clinical treatment of spinal cord trauma.[11,18] Deferoxamine inhibits the iron-catalyzed formation of hydroxyl radicals by chelating iron, is well tolerated, and has minimal toxicity.[5] Allopurinol inhibits formation of superoxide radicals formed by the xanthine oxidase pathway by inhibiting the xanthine oxidase.[5] Combined administration of deferoxamine (50 mg/kg/day) and allopurinol (50 mg/kg/day) for 3 days before aortic crossclamping in pigs significantly reduced the incidence of paraplegia.[46] Although used as a pretreatment in this study, these two drugs may be clinically useful after trauma to prevent the spread of secondary injury.

Nonsteroidal antiinflammatory drugs, such as ibuprofen and flunixin, help prevent vasoconstriction and platelet aggregation.[15] Cats were treated with ibuprofen, a cyclooxygenase inhibitor at 10 mg/kg intravenously 30 minutes before a contusion injury at L2. A 5-mg/kg intravenous bolus was also administered 1.5 hours after injury. The treated cats (in contrast to the untreated controls) were reported to maintain spinal cord blood flow within normal limits during the 4-hour observation period after trauma.[11] The effect of anesthetics (e.g., nitrous oxide, isoflurane, fentanyl, and ketamine) on neurologic outcome following spinal cord injury in rats has been tested; no significant improvement was demonstrated.[47]

Tirilazad Mesylate: The Future Drug of Choice?

The nonglucocorticoid tirilazad mesylate is currently under investigation for its potential ability to limit secondary injury. This agent is a potent inhibitor of iron-dependent lipid peroxidation.[48,49] It is a 21-aminosteroid that lacks glucocorticoid or mineralocorticoid activity; therefore it is especially useful for treatment of central nervous system trauma.[49,50]

More than a 100-fold range of doses (1.6 to 160.0 mg/kg/48 hours, intravenously) promoted functional recovery by 4 weeks in cats with a spinal cord compression injury at L2.[48] Nearly 75% of normal neurologic function was restored and no adverse effects were reported. Furthermore, tirilazad mesylate (3 mg/kg intravenous bolus 4 hours after the insult) partially reversed ischemia within 30 minutes in cats with a contusion injury at L3, a result not seen with the 30 mg/kg intravenous methylprednisolone regimen.[50,51]

The preceding advantages should make the clinical use of tirilazad mesylate more appealing than the glucocorticoid drugs currently available. Tirilazad mesylate is already commercially available in Sweden and Denmark and is in phase 3 trials for FDA approval in the United States. It is currently being administered within 8 hours following spinal cord injury in a human clinical trial (NASCIS 3).[38]

DISCUSSION

The numerous studies that have used currently available drugs for the treatment of acute spinal cord injury have provided controversial results. A successful treatment protocol remains elusive as a result, in part, of the lack of understanding of the complex set of events that inhibit recovery and of the factors that support regeneration. Because effective treatment protocols for spinal cord injury have not been established, the topic continues to be intensely investigated. Areas of study include clarifying the pathophysiology of the acutely traumatized spinal cord,[1,8,16] developing experimental spinal cord injury models for evaluating neurologic changes that follow treatment,[52–57] and describing therapeutic interventions that limit secondary injury and stimulate regeneration of axonal fibers.[58–62]

Supportive care of animals with spinal cord injuries is essential. To limit the spread of secondary cellular destruction, however, treatment must be initiated within hours after trauma. The faster and highly effective action of methylprednisolone provides a distinct advantage over the slower, more potent action of dexamethasone. Methylprednisolone is therefore the drug of choice in treating acute spinal cord injury.

Even methylprednisolone sodium succinate, however, can be detrimental if treatment is initiated more than 8 hours after injury or if the dose is too high (more than 30 mg/kg initial intravenous dose). In animals in which surgery (that may result in further spinal cord trauma) is performed more than 8 hours after injury, it is unclear whether or not methylprednisolone should be administered; no standard protocol can be defined.

A decision to administer methylprednisolone should be made on an individual basis. It is probably necessary to distinguish between the magnitude of damage caused by the initial trauma and that of the surgical procedure that will be performed. If neurologic signs indicate that major trauma has already been inflicted, treatment with methylprednisolone should be initiated as soon as possible and continued only for the recommended period, regardless of surgical intervention. Because of the strong indications that initiating treatment more than 8 hours after acute trauma may actually exacerbate neuronal necrosis and inhibit axonal sprouting, it may be ill-advised to administer high-dose methylprednisolone if a much longer period has elapsed (despite the timing of surgical intervention). In most cases, it is unlikely that the surgical trauma is of significant magnitude in relation to the initial trauma.

The use of calcium-channel antagonists seems to be beneficial and may potentiate the beneficial effects of methylprednisolone. Clinical experience with the use of these drugs, however, is limited. Calcium-channel antagonists should be used in conjunction with vasopressors (such as dopamine) to maintain systemic blood pressure. Although clinical studies are lacking, this treatment regimen could be introduced into current veterinary protocols with minimal risk and possibly considerable benefit.

Nonsteroidal antiinflammatory drugs may prevent spinal cord ischemia after injury. When used in conjunction with glucocorticoids, however, nonsteroidal antiinflammatory drugs may have serious and even lethal gastrointestinal complications.

All drugs currently available have limited beneficial effects and several side effects. A promising drug that should be available commercially in the near future is tirilazad mesylate. This compound does not have glucocorticoid activity, has a broad range of effective doses, and lacks adverse side effects.

About the Authors

When this article was submitted, Drs. Meintjes and Daniloff were affiliated with the Department of Veterinary Anatomy and Fine Structure and Dr. Hosgood was affiliated with the Department of Veterinary Clinical Sciences, School of Veterinary Medicine, Louisiana State University, Baton Rouge, Louisiana. Dr. Meintjes is currently in practice at Parkway Animal Hospital in Cary, North Carolina. Dr. Hosgood is a Diplomate of the American College of Veterinary Surgeons.

REFERENCES

1. Braund KG, Shores A, Brawner WR: The etiology, pathology and pathophysiology of acute spinal cord trauma. *Vet Med* 85:684–691, 1990.
2. Blight AR: Remyelination, revascularization, and recovery of function in experimental spinal cord injury. *Adv Neurol* 59:91–103, 1993.
3. Rymer WZ: Spinal cord injury, physiology and transplantation. *Adv Neurol* 59:157–162, 1993.
4. Povlishock JT: Traumatically induced axonal injury: Pathogenesis and pathobiological implications. *Brain Pathol* 2:1–12, 1992.
5. Rochat MC: An introduction to reperfusion injury. *Compend Contin Educ Pract Vet* 13(6):923–930, 1991.
6. Collins GH, West NR: Prospects for axonal regrowth in spinal cord injury. *Brain Res Bull* 22:89–92, 1989.
7. Janssen L, Hansebout RR: Pathogenesis of spinal cord injury and newer treatments: A review. *Spine* 14:23–32, 1989.
8. Osterholm JL: The pathophysiological response to spinal cord injury—the current status of related research. *J Neurosurg* 40:5–33, 1974.
9. Young W: Secondary injury mechanisms in acute spinal cord injury. *J Emerg Med* 11(Suppl 1):13–22, 1993.
10. Kliot M, Lustgarten JH: Strategies to promote regeneration and recovery in the injured spinal cord. *Neurosurg Clin N Am* 1:751–759, 1990.
11. Hall ED, Wolf DL: A pharmacological analysis of posttraumatic spinal cord ischemia. *J Neurosurg* 64:951–961, 1986.
12. Griffiths IR: Vasogenic edema following acute and chronic spinal cord compression in the dog. *J Neurosurg* 42:155–165, 1975.
13. Koyanagi I, Tator CH, Lea PJ: Three-dimensional analysis of the vascular system in the rat spinal cord with scanning electron microscopy of vascular corrosion casts. Part 2: Acute spinal cord injury. *Neurosurgery* 33:285–292, 1993.
14. Happel RD, Smith KP, Banik NL, et al: Calcium accumulation in experimental spinal cord trauma. *Brain Res* 211:476–479, 1981.
15. Sorjonen DC, Vaughn DM: Membrane interactions in central nervous system injury. *Compend Contin Educ Pract Vet* 11(3):248–254, 1989.
16. Janssens LAA: Mechanical and pathophysiological aspects of acute spinal cord trauma. *J Small Anim Pract* 32:572–578, 1991.
17. Young W: Strategies for the development of new and better pharmacologic treatments for acute spinal cord injury. *Adv Neurol* 59:249–256, 1993.
18. Shores A, Braund KG, Brawner WR: Management of acute spinal cord trauma. *Vet Med* 85:724–739, 1990.
19. Braund KG, Shores A, Brawner WR: Recovering from spinal cord trauma: The rehabilitative steps, complications, and prognosis. *Vet Med* 85:740–743, 1990.
20. Berg J, Rucker NC: Pathophysiology and medical management of acute spinal cord injury. *Compend Contin Educ Pract Vet* 7(8):646–654, 1985.
21. Hall ED: The neuroprotective pharmacology of methylprednisolone. *J Neurosurg* 76:13–22, 1992.
22. De La Torre JC: Spinal cord injury. Review of basic and applied research. *Spine* 6:315–335, 1981.
23. Galandiuk S, Raque G, Appel S, Polk HJ: The two-edged sword of large-dose steroids for spinal cord trauma. *Ann Surg* 218:419–425, 1993.
24. Bellah JR: Colonic perforation after corticosteroid and surgical treatment of intervertebral disk disease in a dog. *JAVMA* 183:1002–1003, 1983.
25. Kiwerski JF: Application of dexamethasone in the treatment

of acute spinal cord injury. *Injury* 24:457–460, 1993.
26. Nacimiento AC, Bartels M, Herrmann HD: Dexamethasone prevents loss of axonal conduction and reflex activity and reduces spread of structural damage in acute spinal cord trauma (abstract). *Soc Neurosci* 5:727, 1979.
27. Hoerlein BF, Spano JS: Non-neurological complications following decompressive spinal cord surgery. *Arch Am Coll Vet Surg* 4:11–16, 1982.
28. Hoerlein BF, Redding RW, Hoff EJ, McGuire JA: Evaluation of dexamethasone, DMSO, mannitol, and solcoseryl in acute spinal cord trauma. *JAAHA* 19:216–226, 1983.
29. Hall ED: The effects of glucocorticoid and nonglucocorticoid steroids on acute neuronal degeneration. *Adv Neurol* 59:241–248, 1993.
30. Braughler JM, Hall ED: Correlation of methylprednisolone levels in cat spinal cord with effects on $(NA^+ + K^+)$-ATPase, lipid peroxidation, and alpha motor neuron function. *J Neurosurg* 56:838–844, 1982.
31. De Lay G, Laybaert L: Effect of flunarizine and methylprednisolone on functional recovery after experimental spinal injury. *J Neurotrauma* 10:25–35, 1993.
32. Xu J, Qu ZX, Hogan FL, Perot PJ: Protective effect of methylprednisolone on vascular injury in rat spinal cord injury. *J Neurotrauma* 9:245–253, 1992.
33. Ross IB, Tator CH, Theriault E: Effect of nimodipine or methylprednisolone on recovery from acute experimental spinal cord injury in rats. *Surg Neurol* 40:461–470, 1993.
34. Bracken MB, Shepard MJ, Collins WF, et al: Methylprednisolone or naloxone treatment after acute spinal cord injury: 1-year follow-up data. Results of the Second National Acute Spinal Cord Injury Study. *J Neurosurg* 76:23–31, 1992.
35. Akdemir H, Pasaoglu H, Arman F, et al: Effects of TRH and high-dose corticosteroid therapy on evoked potentials, and tissue Na^+ and K^+ and water content in experimental spinal injury. *Res Exp Med* 194:297–304, 1993.
36. Braughler JM, Hall ED, Means ED, et al: Evaluation of an intensive methylprednisolone sodium succinate dosing regimen in experimental spinal cord injury. *J Neurosurg* 67:102–105, 1987.
37. Siemering GB, Vroman ML: High dose methylprednisolone sodium succinate: An adjunct to surgery in canine intervertebral disk herniation. Scientific meeting abstract. *Vet Surg* 21:406, 1992.
38. Bracken MB, Holford TR: Effects of timing of methylprednisolone or naloxone administration on recovery of segmental and long-tract neurological function in NASCIS 2. *J Neurosurg* 79:500–507, 1993.
39. Young W, DeCrescito V, Flamm ES, et al: Pharmacological therapy of acute spinal cord injury: Studies of high dose methylprednisolone and naloxone. *Clin Neurosurg* 34:675–697, 1988.
40. Baskin DS, Simpson RJ, Browning JL, et al: The effect of long-term high-dose naloxone infusion in experimental blunt spinal cord injury. *J Spinal Disord* 6:38–43, 1993.
41. Pointillard V, Gense D, Gross C, et al: Effects of nimodipine on posttraumatic spinal cord ischemia in baboons. *J Neurotrauma* 10:201–213, 1993.
42. Guha A, Tator CH, Piper I: Effect of a calcium channel blocker on post-traumatic spinal cord blood flow. *J Neurosurg* 66:423–429, 1987.
43. Flamm ES, Young W, Demopoulos HB, et al: Experimental spinal cord injury: Treatment with naloxone. *Neurosurgery* 10:227–231, 1982.
44. Hoerlein BF, Redding RW, Hoff EJ, McGuire JA: Evaluation of naloxone, crocetin, thyrotropin releasing hormone, methylprednisolone, partial myelotomy, and hemilaminectomy in the treatment of acute spinal cord trauma. *JAAHA* 21:67–77, 1985.
45. Kajihara K, Kawanaga HM, De La Torre JC, Mullan S: Dimethyl sulfoxide in the treatment of experimental acute spinal cord injury. *Surg Neurol* 1:16–22, 1973.
46. Quayumi AK, Janusz MT, Dorovini-Zis K, et al: Additive effect of allopurinol and deferoxamine in the prevention of spinal cord injury caused by aortic clamping. *J Thorac Cardiovasc Surg* 107:1203–1209, 1994.
47. Grissom TE, Mitzel HC, Bunegin L, Albin MS: The effect of anesthetics on neurological outcome during the recovery period of spinal cord injury in rats. *Anesth Analg* 79:66–74, 1994.
48. Anderson DK, Braughler JM, Hall ED, et al: Effects of treatment with U74006F on neurological outcome following experimental spinal cord injury. *J Neurosurg* 69:562–567, 1988.
49. Hall ED, Yonkers PA, Mccall JM, Braughler JM: Effects of the 21-aminosteroid U74006F on experimental head injury in mice. *J Neurosurg* 68:456–461, 1988.
50. Hall ED: Effects of the 21-aminosteroid U74006F on posttraumatic spinal cord ischemia in cats. *J Neurosurg* 68:462–465, 1988.
51. Francel PC, Long RA, Malik JM, et al: Limiting ischemic spinal cord injury a free radical scavenger 21-aminosteroid and/or cerebral fluid drainage. *J Neurosurg* 79:742–751, 1993.
52. Helgren ME, Goldberger ME: The recovery of postural reflexes and locomotion following low thoracic hemisection in adult cats involves compensation by undamaged primary efferent pathways. *Exp Neurol* 123:17–34, 1993.
53. Gorska T, Bem T, Majczynski H, Zmylslowski W: Unrestrained walking in cats with partial spinal lesion. *Brain Res Bull* 32:241–249, 1993.
54. Behrmann DL, Bresnahan JC, Beattie MS, Shah B: Spinal cord injury produced by consistent mechanical displacement of the cord in rats: Behavioral and histological analysis. *J Neurotrauma* 9:197–217, 1992.
55. Wietholter H, Eckert S, Stevens A: Measurements of atactic and paretic gait in neuropathies of rats based on analysis of walking tracts. *J Neurosci Methods* 32:199–205, 1990.
56. Parker AJ, Clarke KA: Gait topography in rat locomotion. *Physiol Behav* 48:41–47, 1990.
57. Goldberger ME, Bregman BS, Vierck CJJ, Brown M: Criteria for assessing recovery of function after spinal cord injury: Behavioral methods. *Exp Neurol* 107:113–117, 1990.
58. Schnell L, Schneider R, Kolbeck R, et al: Neurotropin-3 enhances sprouting of corticospinal tract during development and after spinal cord lesion. *Nature* 367:170–173, 1994.
59. Caubit X, Arsanto J-P, Figarella-Branger D, Thouveny Y: Expression of polysialyted neural cell adhesion molecule (PSA-N-CAM) in developing, adult, and regenerating spinal cord of the urodele amphibians. *Int J Dev Biol* 37:327–336, 1993.
60. Dong YQ: The therapeutic effect of pulsed electric field on

experimental spinal cord injury. *Chung Hua Wai Ko Tsa Chih* 149:437–441, 1992.

61. Kuhlengel KR, Bunge MB, Bunge P, Burton H: Implantation of cultured sensory neurons and Schwann cells into lesioned neonatal rat spinal cord. II. Implant characteristics and examination of corticospinal tract growth. *J Comp Neurol* 293:74–91, 1990.

62. Caroni P, Schwab ME: Antibody against myelin-associated inhibitor of neurite growth neutralizes nonpermissive substrate properties of CNS white matter. *Neuron* 1:85–96, 1988.

Emergency Management of Traumatic Pulmonary Contusions

Veterinary Referral Associates, Gaithersburg, Maryland
Susan G. Hackner, BVSc, MRCVS

KEY FACTS

☐ Pulmonary contusion results in structural and functional changes in the lung, which can lead to hypoxemia and respiratory failure.

☐ Lesions tend to be progressive, and the extent of lung injury frequently is not apparent at presentation.

☐ Radiographic signs of contusion may not be evident until several hours after injury.

☐ Early detection of contusion often relies on a high index of suspicion and careful patient monitoring.

☐ Successful treatment depends on adherence to the basic principles of trauma management and on early recognition of the contusion and associated injuries.

A pulmonary contusion is an anatomic and physiologic lesion of the lung that occurs after a compression–decompression injury to the chest wall.[1–3] Pulmonary contusion is observed most commonly after blunt thoracic trauma; the most frequent cause of such trauma is motor vehicle accidents.[2,4] Other causes include animal interactions, human abuse, falls, and crush injuries.[2] Although pulmonary contusion may be subtle and overlooked when more dramatic injuries are present, it has the potential to progress and develop into respiratory insufficiency. For this reason, pulmonary contusion deserves careful consideration in the management of patients with blunt thoracic trauma.

Thoracic injury is common following trauma in dogs and cats and tends to be underestimated. The incidence of thoracic injury in dogs with fractures resulting from motor vehicle trauma has been evaluated in several studies and is reported to range from 38.9% to 59.5%.[5–7] Pulmonary contusion is the most common lesion, accounting for approximately 50% of all thoracic injuries. It frequently occurs in association with other chest injuries, such as pneumothorax, hemothorax, rib fractures, flail chest, diaphragmatic hernia, myocardial contusion, and cardiac tamponade.[2,5–7] The final outcome of patients with pulmonary contusion frequently depends on early recognition of the associated injuries.

Pulmonary contusion can be mild and associated with few clinical or radiographic abnormalities or it can be extensive and result in significant respiratory compromise and hypoxemia. Lesions tend to worsen within 24 to 36 hours after injury.[8–12] Because of the insidious nature of pulmonary contusion, attention is frequently diverted to other injuries; thus, therapy for the pulmonary contusion is delayed and high mortality results. The mortality of human patients with pulmonary contusions has been reported to range from 20% to 50%.[11,12] Mortality probably is similar in dogs and cats. It is therefore important for clinicians to maintain a high index of suspicion for pulmonary contusion in trauma patients and to be familiar with the early recognition and management of such injuries.

PATHOPHYSIOLOGY

Pulmonary contusion results in structural and physiologic changes in the lung. If extensive, these changes result in hypoxemia and, possibly, acute respiratory failure. Hypoxemia, or decreased partial pressure of oxygen in the blood, may be caused by four mechanisms: hypoventilation, gas diffusion abnormalities, intrapulmonary shunt, and ventilation–perfusion mismatching.[13] Each of these mechanisms contributes to the development of hypoxemia following pulmonary contusion.

The extent of direct pulmonary contusion resulting from blunt trauma is related to the magnitude, duration, and velocity of the applied force and the area to which it is applied.[2] Indirectly, the forces of acceleration, deceleration, compression, torsion, and shear contribute to the injury.[2] The extent of lung injury varies from mild bruising in one lobe to extensive involvement of both lungs.

The forces acting on the lung cause structural disruption with rupture of the alveoli and adjacent blood vessels.[8–10,14] Intraalveolar and interstitial hemorrhage occurs. The surrounding parenchyma is also damaged at a cellular level, which causes progressive leakage of plasma constituents into the interstitium and air spaces.[8–10,14,15] As injury occurs, arachidonic acid is liberated from cell membranes. Arachidonic acid is a precursor of prostaglandins, hydroxy fatty acids, and leukotrienes, which may influence pulmonary function by increasing capillary permeability, causing airway constriction, and effecting pulmonary vasoconstriction.[14,15] Lipoxygenase attracts granulocytes, which contain lysosomal enzymes and produce oxygen radicals, thereby mediating parenchymal injury.[14,15]

The lesion of pulmonary contusion is therefore initially caused by hemorrhage, which is followed by an increasing infiltration of edema fluid, nucleated cells, and inflammatory mediators. The effects are decreased compliance and an increased diffusion distance for oxygen and carbon dioxide.[10,11,15] The progressive involvement of larger areas of the lung by edematous changes accounts, at least partially, for the progressive deterioration seen clinically.[10,11]

The early response of the traumatized vascular bed is vasoconstriction of varying intensity.[8,16,17] This vasoconstriction occurs largely in response to local hypoxia, either via a direct effect on vascular smooth muscle or via the release of mediator substances (e.g., leukotrienes).[16] The decrease in local perfusion may also be caused by mechanical disruption, such as congestion, platelet aggregation, or fibrin microthrombi.[16] The overall effect is to minimize the perfusion of unventilated lung, thus limiting ventilation–perfusion mismatching and preventing a rise in shunt fraction in the early stages of injury.[16,17]

Air spaces adjacent to the traumatized region have normal perfusion per unit volume but are less compliant (because of edema and disruption of the surfactant layer) and are thus poorly ventilated.[8,17–19] As a result, ventilation–perfusion mismatching increases in this part of the lung, and venous admixture is increased. The resultant hypoxemia responds to an increased inspired oxygen concentration.[8,18,20] As the edema worsens (because of the effects of inflammatory mediators) and involves progressively larger portions of lung, however, mismatching is further increased and shunting may become a significant problem.[11,19] The hypoxemia becomes progressively refractory to high concentrations of inspired oxygen and to mechanical ventilation, even when high positive end expiratory pressures are used.[10,12,19]

Hypoventilation may exacerbate hypoxemia. Respiratory effort may be decreased because of pain. Bronchial constriction and airway obstruction by hemorrhage can reduce effective ventilation, and concurrent thoracic injuries (such as hemothorax, pneumothorax, or flail chest) can contribute to the decreased compliance.[9,11]

Severe hypoxemia has systemic effects. If partial pressure of oxygen in arterial blood (PaO_2) falls below 60 mm Hg, tissue hypoxia and acidosis, cardiac arrhythmia, mental depression, and eventual loss of consciousness may result.[20]

Most patients with pulmonary contusion have an increased respiratory rate and a resultant decreased partial pressure of carbon dioxide ($PaCO_2$). With severe pulmonary contusion, however, carbon dioxide retention can occur.[10,11] Mechanisms of hypercapnia include hypoventilation and profound ventilation–perfusion mismatching.[11,21] Severe hypercapnia with a $PaCO_2$ greater than 60 mm Hg can lead to cerebral edema.[22]

Decreased cardiac output has been demonstrated following pulmonary contusion in experimental dogs.[9] This is a significant hemodynamic effect because it occurs when tissue demands for oxygen are greatest.[9,23] Furthermore, in the presence of a large intrapulmonary shunt, decreased cardiac output will exaggerate arterial tissue hypoxia because of admixture of venous blood with especially low oxygen tension. This impairment in cardiac function is presumably the result of myocardial contusion and hypovolemia and can be corrected with appropriate fluid therapy.[9]

Severe contusions can result in increased pulmonary vascular resistance and pulmonary artery hypertension.[10,24,25] These conditions impose a higher workload on the right ventricle, which may lead to right-sided heart failure. The changes in pulmonary vascular resistance have proved to be among the earli-

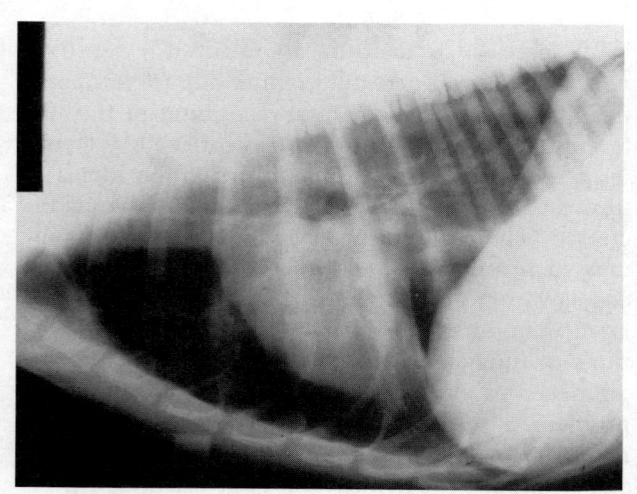

Figure 1—Lateral (**A**) and ventrodorsal (**B**) thoracic radiographs taken six hours after a dog was hit by a car. Areas of pulmonary contusion are seen as patchy alveolar and interstitial patterns, especially in the left lung lobes. Note the displacement of the mediastinum (mediastinal shift) toward the left. The displacement is caused by hypoinflation of the more severely injured lobes. In the lateral radiograph, this displacement is seen as an elevation of the cardiac silhouette and is easily mistaken for a pneumothorax.

est and most sensitive hemodynamic responses following injury as well as being an important early predictor of survival in human patients.[24,25]

Resolution of pulmonary contusion generally occurs within three to seven days.[1] Studies in human patients, however, have shown that pulmonary functional disturbances may persist for several weeks, which explains the discrepancy between normal radiographs and a delayed clinical recovery in some cases.[4] Some degree of pulmonary fibrosis may be a sequela of contusion.[19] Bacterial pneumonia is a relatively common complication in humans, although the incidence in canine and feline patients is unknown.[24] Experimentally, contusion alone does not impair lung antibacterial defenses.[26] The administration of large volumes of crystalloids or large doses of corticosteroids or the addition of mechanical ventilation can, however, significantly reduce bacterial clearance.[26]

DIAGNOSIS

The diagnosis of pulmonary contusion is based on a history of trauma, physical examination findings, and thoracic radiography. Arterial blood gas analysis is an extremely useful and sensitive tool for monitoring the severity of respiratory compromise and thus guiding therapy. When severe injury occurs, patients are in shock and in deteriorating condition at the time of presentation. Resuscitation must therefore be initiated before a definitive diagnosis can be made. It is important to remember that signs of contusion may not be evident on initial assessment; periodic reassessment is therefore mandatory to assure that respiratory impairment is not overlooked.

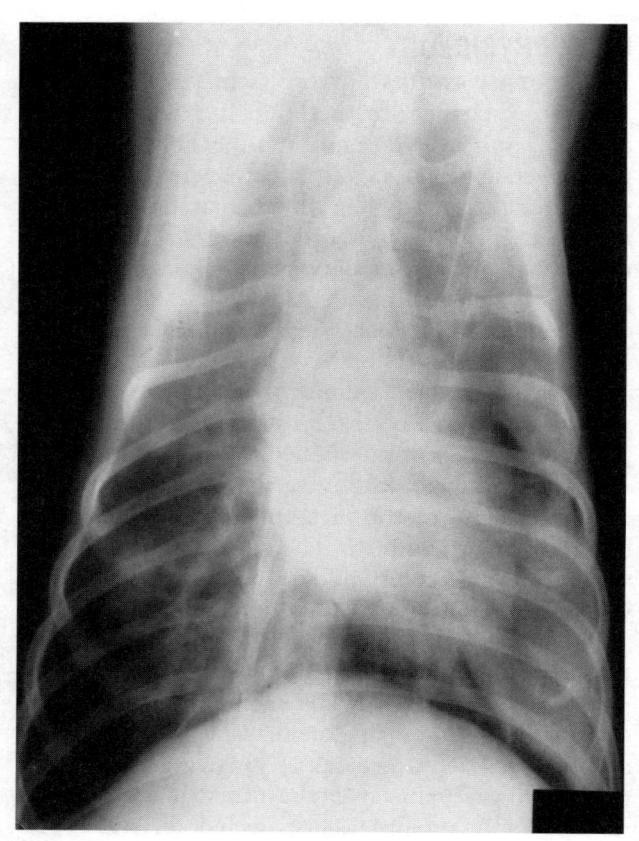

Pulmonary contusion should be suspected in any patient with a history of thoracic trauma. Clinical signs vary with the extent of injury. Animals may show signs of only mild respiratory compromise, such as an increased respiratory rate. With significant injury, dyspnea, tachypnea, orthopnea, and open-mouth breathing are common. Hemoptysis or the presence of blood or blood-tinged fluid in the oropharynx and trachea indicates severe contusion. Thoracic auscultation may reveal moist rales, bronchovesicular sounds, and/or bronchial sounds.[19]

Radiographs are one of the most important and practical means of diagnosing lung contusions and associated thoracic injury. Contusions appear radiographically as diffuse or patchy areas of alveolar and interstitial patterns that do not follow an anatomic pattern[19] (Figure 1). Experimental studies in dogs have shown, however, that radiographs do not reliably predict the presence of contusion when taken within one hour of injury; contusion may not be evident for four to six hours.[27] Radiographs taken within six hours of injury may only confirm other thoracic disorders (e.g., hemothorax or pneumothorax, rib fracture, and ruptured diaphragm) and serve as a baseline for later evaluation of contusion or pleural space disease. Although pulmonary contusion frequently occurs without accompanying damage to the chest wall, the presence of rib fractures is an indication of likely underlying contusion even though the pulmonary involvement may not yet be evident. It is important to take additional radiographs when respiratory compromise continues.

The most sensitive means for detecting respiratory compromise is monitoring arterial blood gases.[19,22,27,28] Because many veterinary practices do not have the necessary equipment, local hospitals can be contacted for assistance. Proper handling of arterial blood samples is essential to ensure accurate results.[29]

The severity of hypoxemia is determined by measuring PaO_2. Normal values range from 80 to 100 mm Hg.[20,28] Cyanosis is usually not seen until values are below 50 mm Hg.[20] Patients with PaO_2 levels below 60 mm Hg require oxygen supplementation.[28] If PaO_2 levels are below 60 mm Hg, even with an inhaled oxygen content that exceeds 50%, mechanical ventilation is required.[12]

$PaCO_2$ monitors effective ventilation.[13,20] Normal values range from 35 to 45 in dogs and 30 to 40 in cats.[28] $PaCO_2$ is usually low in patients with pulmonary contusion because of hyperventilation. Pain or a flail segment may reduce this response. In the absence of significant head trauma, hypoventilation (and an increased $PaCO_2$) indicates severe contusion. Patients with $PaCO_2$ exceeding 50 mm Hg require mechanical ventilation.[12,28]

Arterial blood gases also are necessary for the detection of ventilation–perfusion mismatching, which is indicated by an increased alveolar-arterial oxygen gradient (A-a gradient). The A-a gradient can be calculated according to the following formula (if the patient is breathing room air): A-a gradient = $(150 - PaCO_2/0.8) - PaO_2$.[13] An A-a gradient greater than 15 indicates a ventilation–perfusion mismatch.[20]

MANAGEMENT

Pulmonary contusion seldom occurs as an isolated injury. Patients are often in shock and may have other significant injuries. The management of contusion therefore cannot be addressed as a single entity. Rather, successful treatment depends on adherence to the basic principles of trauma management as well as on early and appropriate management of the injured lung.

The basis for successful management of trauma is early detection and correction of life-threatening emergencies. It is important to realize that significant thoracic injury can occur without damage to the chest wall. Detection should therefore depend on prediction and exclusion rather than on direct manifestation of injury. The immediate priorities of therapy apply equally to all trauma patients. These priorities are to establish a patent airway and to ensure adequate ventilation and circulation. Rapid and simple measures of initial resuscitation must be used.

Immediate Establishment of Adequate Ventilation

In patients with ventilatory compromise that becomes evident shortly after trauma, seven conditions should be considered initially: airway obstruction, open pneumothorax, flail chest, tension pneumothorax, massive hemothorax, severe pulmonary contusion, and diaphragmatic hernia. These conditions can be quickly assessed by listening to the animal's breathing; examination of the oropharynx; observation of the rate, pattern, and degree of chest movements; and inspection, auscultation, and percussion of the thorax.

The oropharynx should be cleared of blood and secretions. Severe contusion may result in large amounts of blood-tinged foamy saliva, thereby requiring immediate endotracheal intubation and suction of the airways. In one report, the most significant cause of acute death was obstruction of the airways by blood clots.[12] Airway suction can be achieved by passing a suction catheter down into one mainstem bronchus and then the other, and aspirating intermittently. Instilling small amounts of sterile saline will aid in breaking up clots and mucus. Unconscious animals should be immediately intubated and ventilated mechanically. Emergency tracheostomy is reserved for conditions of mechanical obstruction, such as severe facial or laryngeal edema, in which endotracheal intubation is not possible.

With an open pneumothorax, the wound should be covered with a dressing or gloved hand (thus converting it to a closed pneumothorax) until definitive closure is possible. Patients with flail chest should be placed in lateral recumbency, with the injured side down. Such positioning will reduce paradoxical chest motion, alleviate pain, and prevent further injury to the lung. The most significant pathologic effects of flail chest are caused by the underlying contusion; definitive stabilization of the segment is not required in the emergency setting.[21,30] Rapid needle thoracentesis will eliminate the lethal potential of a tension pneumothorax and identify the presence of a hemothorax.

If chest excursions are adequate, oxygen should be administered to the patient at 3 to 10 L/minute via face mask.[30] A nasopharyngeal or intratracheal catheter can be used to deliver oxygen at 1 to 2 L/minute.[30] The placement of these catheters is described elsewhere.[31]

Intubation and mechanical ventilation are required when the preceding procedures do not ensure adequate ventilation. Indications for mechanical ventilation will be discussed subsequently.

Immediate Establishment of Adequate Perfusion

A gross assessment of the circulatory status of the patient can be made by evaluating pulse rate and quality, mucous membrane color, capillary refill time and looking for evidence of external hemorrhage. The management of circulatory compromise depends on the cause(s), with particular attention to cardiogenic and hypovolemic factors.

Immediately at presentation, an indwelling intravenous catheter should be placed, blood drawn for baseline hematocrit and total protein determinations, and fluid therapy initiated. Electrocardiography is essential in patients with thoracic trauma to aid in the diagnosis of cardiac tamponade (due to hemopericardium) and myocardial contusion. Cardiac tamponade requires immediate pericardiocentesis to restore adequate hemodynamics. Severe external hemorrhage should be controlled.

Much controversy exists in the literature regarding the optimal fluid therapy for patients with pulmonary contusion. Early studies claim that the use of isotonic crystalloid solutions in large volumes for resuscitation, with resultant hemodilution and lowering of plasma oncotic pressure, predisposes patients with contusion to a more severe and progressive lesion.[10,32] These studies demonstrate the hazard of fluid overload on the lungs and perhaps emphasize that the injured lung is more sensitive to overload than the normal lung. They fail, however, to demonstrate conclusively that isotonic crystalloid fluids per se have a negative effect or that colloid solutions have a positive, protective effect. Subsequent studies have shown that reduced pulmonary function and hypoxemia were unrelated to plasma oncotic pressure and hemodilution.[33,44]

It is generally agreed that fluid therapy should be administered to restore optimum cardiac output and tissue perfusion. Fluid restriction and forced dehydration should be avoided. Careful monitoring is essential, however, to avoid overload. The fluid volume required depends on the individual patient needs. Volumes administered, regardless of the fluid type, should be based on physiologic end points, such as physical indicators of perfusion, urine output (0.5 to 1.0 ml/kg/hr), arterial blood pressure, central venous pressure, pulmonary artery wedge pressure, and/or cardiac output. As a guide, animals in shock can receive replacement crystalloid solutions at rates of up to 90 to 100 ml/kg/hr in dogs and 45 to 50 ml/kg/hr in cats; continuous assessment of the response to fluid loading is mandatory.

The use of hypertonic saline solutions in the treatment of shock has been extensively reviewed.[35-37] These solutions offer many beneficial effects for the resuscitation of patients in shock, including a rapid increase in cardiac output, blood pressure, splanchnic blood flow, and blood volume, with less net fluid administration. Hypertonic saline solutions do not increase extravascular lung water or compromise pulmonary function or respiratory system mechanics.[38-41] They are therefore a useful adjunctive therapy directed at rapidly restoring circulatory function without deleterious pulmonary effects. A combination of 7.5% NaCl with 6% dextran-70 has been shown to be superior to saline alone.[36,40] This combination is administered at 3 to 5 ml/kg intravenously over five minutes[37] and is used in conjunction with standard resuscitative measures to achieve recovery from shock.

Inotropic or vasopressor agents may be required for cardiovascular support in some patients, especially those with severe myocardial contusions. These agents, however, should not be used as substitutes for appropriate fluid therapy. Patients that have significant hemodilution or ongoing hemorrhage require blood transfusion to restore adequate oxygen-carrying capacity.

Ongoing Monitoring

During and after resuscitation, the patient's vital signs and response to treatment should be closely monitored. Electrocardiography, hemodynamic monitoring, pulse oximetry, and blood gas determinations are extremely useful in the continued objective assessment of critical patients. Periodic reassessment and, if necessary, adjustments in therapy are mandatory. Thoracic radiography should be considered only when the condition of the patient has stabilized. The information provided rarely warrants the potential risk to the patient.[33,42]

Management of Pulmonary Injury

After stabilization of immediate life-threatening emergencies, therapy of the pulmonary contusion can be addressed. Most therapies are supportive and are aimed at maintaining adequate oxygenation. The aggressiveness of treatment depends on the severity of the lesion. When the injury is mild and not accompanied by respiratory compromise, patients can recover with cage rest alone.[20] Animals with dyspnea and hypoxemia require oxygen therapy, either in an oxygen cage or via a nasopharyngeal catheter. Frequent changes in position are recommended for patients that are in lateral recumbency.

The use of corticosteroids is controversial. Much

research points to their beneficial effects.[43–47] When large doses of methylprednisolone were given shortly after injury, pulmonary vascular resistance and the size of the lesions were reduced.[43,47] Trials in humans showed lower mortality and decreased incidence of complications in patients treated with steroids.[44,45] The incidence of bronchial infection was not increased. Other studies, however, have demonstrated that large doses of corticosteroids may aggravate pulmonary failure after hypovolemic shock and decrease lung bacterial clearance.[26,48] The studies alluded to used large doses of methylprednisolone (30 mg/kg). One study evaluating dexamethasone (total dose of 15 mg intravenously) in dogs with experimentally induced contusions failed to show any beneficial effects of the drug.[1] If corticosteroids are used, it is recommended that they be administered shortly after injury. There is no evidence that continued steroid therapy is beneficial, and such use is likely to increase the risk of infection and gastrointestinal ulceration.

Aminophylline has been recommended by some authors for treating patients with pulmonary contusion.[2,19,49] Although bronchodilator therapy may have beneficial effects, such therapy is unlikely to produce dramatic improvement, because bronchoconstriction is not a major factor in the pathogenesis of respiratory compromise in these patients.[16,17]

The benefits of analgesia are clear for patients with pulmonary contusion. Pain associated with thoracic trauma inhibits ventilatory effort and can lead to progressive respiratory distress. In addition, pain reduces coughing, promotes atelectasis, and predisposes to pulmonary infection.[50–52] Effective analgesia has been shown to improve ventilatory function, decrease morbidity and mortality, and allow patients to be effectively managed without mechanical ventilation.[50–52]

Serious caution must be exercised with the use of narcotics for analgesia because of their potential to depress central respiratory drive. Clinicians must titrate the dose to find a balance that assures sufficient analgesia to allow the patient to cough and breathe deeply but not so much as to depress the patient's respiratory drive. In practice, this balance is difficult to achieve. For this reason, epidural analgesia, using morphine or fentanyl, is preferred and is routinely used in human patients with pulmonary contusion.[51–53] This technique results in less significant respiratory depression; in addition, any depression that results from systemic absorption (early depression) or direct effects on the brain (late depression) are easily reversed. Techniques and dosages for epidural analgesia in small animal patients have been described.[54]

If intravenous or intramuscular narcotics are used, I recommend agonist-antagonist or partial agonist opioids, such as butorphanol (0.2 to 1.0 mg/kg in dogs and 0.1 to 0.4 mg/kg in cats, given intravenously, intramuscularly, or subcutaneously every 2 to 4 hours) or buprenorphine (0.005 to 0.02 mg/kg in dogs and 0.005 to 0.01 mg/kg in cats, given intravenously or intramuscularly every 4 to 12 hours). The use of a pure opioid agonist, such as oxymorphone, is contraindicated in animals with concurrent head trauma that may have resulted in increased intracranial pressure.

Diuretics are not recommended for treating pulmonary contusion unless fluid overload and pulmonary edema occur.[2,15] One must be aware, however, that because the use of diuretics can cause dehydration and exacerbate tissue hypoxia, strict attention must be paid to fluid balance and urine output. If pulmonary edema occurs, furosemide can be administered as an intravenous bolus (1 to 2 mg/kg) or by continuous-rate infusion (0.1 to 0.2 mg/kg/hour).

Antibiotic therapy is not indicated unless bronchopneumonia develops. In this situation, bacterial culture of tracheal fluid is indicated. Other therapies, such as naloxone and flunixin meglumine, have been suggested for use in patients with pulmonary contusion but remain experimental and can therefore not be recommended at this time.[15]

It is important to realize the potential of impending respiratory decompensation in the patient with pulmonary contusion. Initially, the animal may appear stable, but signs of hypoxemia may develop with time. Changes in respiratory pattern should be closely observed. Arterial blood gas measurements, if available, should be monitored until stabilization is assured.

Mechanical Ventilation

Patients with severe contusions may require intubation and mechanical ventilation. Mechanical ventilation should be instituted in patients that

- are unconscious
- are unable to maintain a patent airway or that have evidence of large amounts of blood in the airways
- are hypoventilating and that have a $PaCO_2$ exceeding 50 mm Hg. When blood gas analysis is not possible, a subjective assessment can be made. Hypoventilation can also be determined by attaching a respirometer to a well-fitting face mask in conscious animals. The volume of gas breathed in one minute is then measured.[22] Normal minute volume is 150 to 250 ml/kg[28]
- have a PaO_2 less than 60 mm Hg with an inhaled oxygen content exceeding 50%
- have clinical signs of respiratory deterioration and fatigue
- have evidence of increased intracranial pressure.

In emergency situations, mechanical ventilation can be provided manually for a limited period with an Ambu bag or an anesthetic machine. Prolonged ventilation, however, requires a mechanical ventilator and equipment and personnel for intensive monitoring. Ventilator therapy is therefore generally limited to referral institutions. Because of the practical limitations of ventilator therapy in veterinary medicine, mechanical ventilation is restricted to those patients in which adequate ventilatory function cannot be achieved despite rigorous oxygen therapy and analgesia.

Mechanical ventilation is generally initiated with intermittent positive pressure ventilation, which approximates manual ventilation. This method can overcome inadequate respiratory efforts by the patient and can counter decreased compliance. Success of ventilator therapy is judged by arterial blood gas analysis.[22,28] Pulse oximetry and capnography are extremely useful tools for the continuous monitoring of respirator patients. If response is inadequate, positive end expiratory pressure (PEEP) is required. The patient must exhale against a mild positive pressure (usually 5 to 15 cm H_2O), thus countering early airway closure. Reviews of ventilatory techniques are available elsewhere.[55]

PROGNOSIS

The prognosis for patients with pulmonary contusion depends on the severity of lung injury, the number and severity of other injuries, and the hemodynamic status of the patient at presentation. The mortality of canine and feline patients with pulmonary contusions has not been reported. In human patients, factors associated with high morbidity and mortality are the presence of shock, severe blood loss, severe head trauma, flail chest, and other severe thoracic injuries.[34,50,56,57] In addition, combined thoracoabdominal injury is associated with high mortality, particularly when the diaphragm is ruptured.[56]

Recovery, with radiographic resolution of the contusion, is reported to occur within three to seven days.[1] The incidence of bacterial pneumonia following pulmonary contusion has not been reported in dogs and cats. Pneumonia seems to be more common in patients with severe lesions, especially if the patient is mechanically ventilated or is anesthetized for corrective surgery of other injuries. Some degree of pulmonary fibrosis may be a sequela of severe contusion.[19]

About the Author
Dr. Hackner is Director of the Critical Care Unit, Veterinary Referral Associates, Gaithersburg, Maryland. Dr. Hackner is a Diplomate of both the American College of Veterinary Internal Medicine and the American College of Veterinary Emergency and Critical Care.

REFERENCES

1. Trinkle JK, Furman RW, Hinshaw MA, et al: Pulmonary contusion—Pathogenesis and effect of various resuscitative measures. *Ann Thorac Surg* 16(6):568–573, 1973.
2. Jones KW: Thoracic trauma. *Surg Clin North Am* 60(4):957–981, 1980.
3. Trinkle JK: Pulmonary contusion. *Ann Thorac Surg* 16:568–573, 1973.
4. Spackman CJA, Caywood DD: Management of thoracic trauma and chest wall reconstruction. *Vet Clin North Am Small Anim Pract* 17(2):431–447, 1987.
5. Selcer BA, Buttrick M, Barstad R, et al: The incidence of thoracic trauma in dogs with skeletal injury. *J Small Anim Pract* 28:21–27, 1987.
6. Tamas PM, Paddleford RR, Krahwinkel DJ: Thoracic trauma in dogs and cats presented for limb fractures. *JAAHA* 21:161–166, 1985.
7. Spackman CJA, Caywood DD, Feeney DA, et al: Thoracic wall and pulmonary trauma in dogs sustaining fractures as a result of motor vehicle accidents. *JAVMA* 185(9):975–977, 1984.
8. Oppenheimer L, Craven KD, Forkert L, et al: Pathophysiology of pulmonary contusions in the dog. *J Appl Physiol* 47(4):718–728, 1979.
9. Moseley RV, Vernick JJ, Doty DB: Response to blunt chest injury: A new experimental model. *J Trauma* 10(8):673–683, 1970.
10. Fulton RL, Peter ET: The progressive nature of pulmonary contusion. *Surgery* 67(3):499–506, 1970.
11. Nichols RJ, Pierce HJ, Greenfield LJ: Effects of experimental pulmonary contusion on respiratory exchange and lung mechanics. *Arch Surg* 96:723–729, 1968.
12. Shin B, McAslan C, Hankins JR, et al: Management of lung contusion. *Am Surg* 45:168–175, 1979.
13. West JB (ed): *Respiratory Physiology: The Essentials*, ed 4. Baltimore, Williams & Wilkins, 1990, pp 51–68.
14. Brigham KL: Mechanisms of lung injury. *Clin Chest Med* 3:97–103, 1982.
15. Berkwitt L, Berzon JL: Thoracic trauma—Newer concepts. *Vet Clin North Am Small Anim Pract* 15(5):1031–1039, 1985.
16. Wagner RB, Slivko B, Jamieson PM, et al: Effect of lung contusion on pulmonary hemodynamics. *Ann Thorac Surg* 52:51–58, 1991.
17. Craven KD, Oppenheimer L, Wood LDH: Effects of contusion and flail chest on pulmonary perfusion and oxygen exchange. *J Appl Physiol* 47(4):729–737, 1979.
18. Rutherford RB, Valenta J: An experimental study of "traumatic wet lung." *J Trauma* 11(2):146–163, 1971.
19. Crowe DT: Traumatic pulmonary contusions, hematomas, pseudocysts, and acute respiratory distress syndrome: An update—Part I. *Compend Contin Educ Pract Vet* 5(5):396–402, 1983.
20. Hawkins EC, Ettinger SJ, Suter PF: Diseases of the lower respiratory tract (lung) and pulmonary edema, in Ettinger SJ (ed): *Textbook of Veterinary Internal Medicine*, ed 3. Philadelphia, WB Saunders Co, 1989, pp 816–866.
21. Calhoon JH, Grover FL, Trinkle JK: Chest trauma—approach and management. *Clin Chest Med* 13(1):55–67, 1992.

22. Court MH: Respiratory support of the critically ill small animal patient, in Murtaugh RJ, Kaplan PM (eds): *Veterinary Emergency and Critical Care Medicine.* St Louis, Mosby Year Book, 1992, pp 575–592.
23. Edwards JD, Redmond AD, Nightingale P, et al: Oxygen consumption following trauma: A reappraisal in severely injured patients requiring mechanical ventilation. *Br J Surg* 75:690–692, 1988.
24. Bugge-Asperheim B, Svennevig JL, Birkeland S: Hemodynamic and metabolic consequences of lung contusion following blunt chest trauma. *Scand J Thorac Cardiovasc Surg* 14:295–299, 1980.
25. Zapol WM, Snider MT: Pulmonary hypertension in severe acute respiratory failure. *N Engl J Med* 296:476–480, 1977.
26. Richardson JD, Woods D, Johanson WG, et al: Lung bacterial clearance following pulmonary contusion. *Surgery* 86(5):730–735, 1979.
27. Erickson DR, Shinozaki T, Beekman E, et al: Relationship of arterial blood gases and pulmonary radiographs to the degree of pulmonary damage in experimental pulmonary contusion. *J Trauma* 11(8):689–694, 1971.
28. Haskins SC: Management of pulmonary disease in the critical patient, in Zaslow IM (ed): *Veterinary Trauma and Critical Care.* Philadelphia, Lea & Febiger, 1984, pp 339–384.
29. Haskins SC: Sampling and storage of blood for pH and blood gas analysis. *JAVMA* 170:429–433, 1979.
30. Hunt CA: Chest trauma—The approach to the patient with chest injuries. *Compend Contin Educ Pract Vet* 1(7):537–541, 1979.
31. Fitzpatrick RK, Crowe DT: Nasal oxygen administration in dogs and cats: Experimental and clinical investigations. *JAAHA* 22:293–300, 1986.
32. Fulton RL, Peter ET: Physiologic effects of fluid therapy after pulmonary contusion. *Am J Surg* 126:773–778, 1973.
33. Bongard FS, Lewis FR: Crystalloid resuscitation of patients with pulmonary contusions. *Am J Surg* 148:145–149, 1984.
34. Johnson JA, Cogbill TH, Winga ER: Determinants of outcome after pulmonary contusion. *J Trauma* 26(8):695–698, 1986.
35. Velasco IT, Pontieri V, Rocha-e-Silva M, et al: Hyperosmotic saline and severe hemorrhagic shock. *Am J Physiol* 239:H664–H673, 1980.
36. Velasco IT, Oliveisa MA: A comparison of hyperosmotic and hyperoncotic resuscitation from severe hemorrhagic shock in dogs. *Circ Shock* 21:338–341, 1987.
37. Miller MW, Schertel ER, DiBartola SP: Conventional and hypertonic fluid therapy: Concepts and application, in Murtaugh RJ, Kaplan PM (eds): *Veterinary Emergency and Critical Care Medicine.* St Louis, Mosby Year Book, 1992, pp 618–628.
38. Martias MA, Youres RN, Lin CA, et al: Hypovolemic shock resuscitation with hyperosmotic 7.5% NaCl. *Circ Shock* 26:147–155, 1988.
39. Johnston WE, Alford PT, Prough DS, et al: Cardiopulmonary effects of hypertonic saline in canine oleic acid-induced pulmonary edema. *Crit Care Med* 13:814–817, 1985.
40. Kreimeir U, Brückner UB, Niemczyk S, et al: Hyperosmotic saline dextran for resuscitation from traumatic-hemorrhagic hypotension: Effect on regional blood flow. *Circ Shock* 32:83–99, 1990.
41. Auler JOC, Zin WA, Martins MA, et al: Respiratory system mechanics in patients treated with isotonic or hypertonic saline solutions. *Circ Shock* 36:243–248, 1992.
42. Thomson SR, Huizinga WKJ, Hirshberg A: Prospective study of the yield of physical examination compared with chest radiography in penetrating thoracic trauma. *Thorax* 45:616–619, 1990.
43. Franz JL, Richardson JD, Grover FL, et al: Effect of methylprednisolone sodium succinate on experimental pulmonary contusion. *J Thorac Cardiovasc Surg* 68(5):842–844, 1974.
44. Svennevig JL, Bugge-Asperheim B, Bjorgo S, et al: Methylprednisolone in the treatment of lung contusion following blunt chest trauma. *Scand J Thorac Cardiovasc Surg* 14:301–305, 1980.
45. Svennevig JL, Bugge-Asperheim B, Geiran O, et al: High-dose corticosteroids in thoracic trauma. *Acta Chir Scand* 526(Suppl):110–118, 1985.
46. Lennquist S, Jansson I, Bäckstrand B, et al: Posttraumatic respiratory distress syndrome and high-dose corticosteroids. *Acta Chir Scand* 526(Suppl):104–108, 1985.
47. Vaage J: Effects of high-dose corticosteroids on the pulmonary circulation. *Acta Chir Scand* 526(Suppl):73–82, 1985.
48. Lucas CE, Ledgerwood AM: Pulmonary response to massive steroids in seriously injured patients. *Ann Surg* 194:256–261, 1981.
49. Short CE, Ivin K: Management of thoracic trauma in the cat. *Feline Pract* 12(6):11–20, 1982.
50. Freedland M, Wilson RF, Bender JS, et al: The management of flail chest injury: Factors affecting outcome. *J Trauma* 30(12):1460–1468, 1990.
51. Wisner DH: A stepwise logistic regression analysis of factors affecting morbidity and mortality after thoracic trauma: Effect of epidural analgesia. *J Trauma* 30(7):799–804, 1990.
52. Cicala RS, Voeller GR, Fox T, et al: Epidural analgesia in thoracic trauma: Effects of lumbar morphine and thoracic bupivacaine in pulmonary function. *J Trauma* 18(2):229–231, 1990.
53. Mackersie RC, Shackford SR, Hoyt DB, et al: Continuous epidural fentanyl analgesia: Ventilatory function improvement with routine use in treatment of blunt chest injury. *J Trauma* 27(11):1207–1210, 1987.
54. Clark GN: Epidural analgesia, in Kirk RW (ed): *Current Veterinary Therapy. XI.* Philadelphia, WB Saunders Co, 1992, pp 95–98.
55. Pascoe PJ: Short-term ventilatory support, in Kirk RW (ed): *Current Veterinary Therapy. IX.* Philadelphia, WB Saunders Co, 1986, pp 269–271.
56. Svennevig JL, Bugge-Asperheim B, Geiran OR, et al: Prognostic factors in blunt chest trauma—Analysis of 652 cases. *Ann Chir Gynaecol* 75:8–14, 1986.
57. Clark GC, Schecter WP, Trunkey DD: Variables affecting outcome in blunt chest trauma: Flail chest versus pulmonary contusion. *J Trauma* 28(3):298–303, 1988.

Feline High-Rise Syndrome

KEY FACTS

- The term *high-rise syndrome* describes the traumatic injuries sustained by cats falling at least two stories.
- Injuries associated with the feline high-rise syndrome most commonly include thoracic trauma, facial and oral trauma, and limb injuries.
- The two most important factors affecting the extent of injury include the length of the fall and the landing surface.
- In treated cats, the survival rate is 90%.

The University of Pennsylvania,
Philadelphia, Pennsylvania
Amy S. Kapatkin, DVM

Tinton Falls Veterinary Specialists,
Tinton Falls, New Jersey
David T. Matthiesen, DVM

IN CATS, the term *high-rise syndrome* was first used in 1976 to describe traumatic injuries resulting after falls of two or more stories (24 or more feet).[1] In 1987, Whitney and Mehlhaff reviewed 132 cases for survival rates and types of injuries sustained in relationship to the height of the fall; the same authors also proposed a theory to explain the correlations.[2] High-rise syndrome (also known as jumper's syndrome and high-flyer syndrome) has been described in humans[3-14]; an unpublished study of 81 dogs has also recently been done.[15]

The New York City Department of Buildings defines a story as a length of 12 to 15 feet. A high-rise syndrome cat is one that has fallen two or more stories[2]; a high-rise syndrome dog is one that has fallen one or more stories.[15]

Injuries involved in a high-rise syndrome fall sustained by cats include thoracic trauma, facial and oral trauma, limb and spinal fractures and luxations, abdominal trauma, and shock. In treated cats, the survival rate is 90%.[2]

THORACIC TRAUMA

Thoracic trauma is the most common injury and the most common cause of death associated with high-rise syndrome in cats[1,2]; however, this is not true in humans or dogs.[3-15] Head injury is the leading cause of death of high-rise syndrome humans[2,14]; most high-rise syndrome dogs are euthanatized.[15]

Radiography of the chest should always be included in the diagnostic workup for high-rise syndrome cats, even if the patient is eupneic. Some cats are so distressed on presentation that the clinician may need to perform thoracentesis during treatment for shock. After shock and oxygen therapy, most cats can withstand radiography if minimally stressed.

Of the cats studied by Whitney and Mehlhaff, thoracic injuries were present in 90%, pulmonary contusions in 68%, and pneumothorax in 63%[2] (Figure 1). Hemothorax was not as significant in this group of cats.[2] Twenty-five percent of the cats with air aspirated from the thorax required multiple thoracenteses, but only one cat required tube thoracostomy.[2] Thoracentesis is not a totally benign procedure and should not be done on eupneic cats before radiography unless pneumothorax is strongly suspected based on clinical findings. If pneumothorax is suspected, the cat should undergo thoracentesis immediately. In general, most cats with pulmonary contusions or pneumothorax can be treated conservatively.

High-rise syndrome dogs have fewer chest injuries than do their feline counterparts.[15] In one study, pneumothorax occurred in less than one third of the dogs and pulmonary contusions were noted in less than 50% of the dogs.[15] Incidence of thoracic injuries in high-rise syndrome humans ranges from 10% to 40%.[6,9,10,13,14]

FACIAL AND ORAL TRAUMA

In the study by Whitney and Mehlhaff, 56% of high-rise syndrome cats sustained soft tissue facial abrasions; hard

Figure 1—Lateral radiograph of a cat that fell six stories. Severe pneumothorax was present. The cat was treated for shock, and thoracentesis was performed.

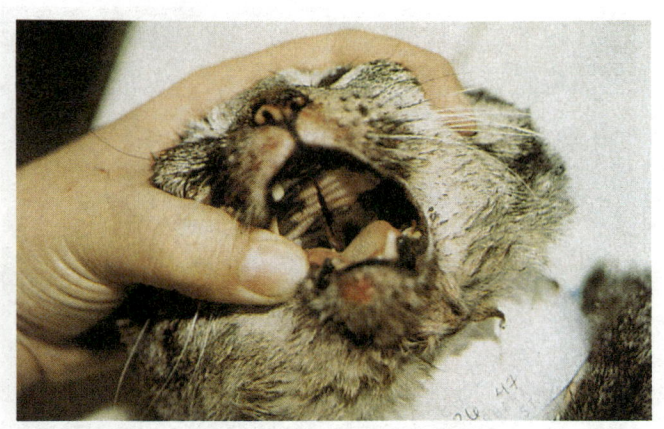

Figure 2—A three-year-old Domestic Shorthair that sustained a hard palate fracture after falling four stories.

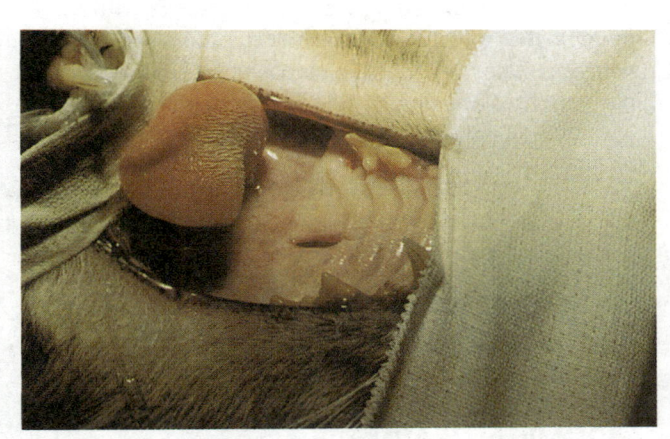

Figure 3—Oronasal fistula occurring secondary to a split hard palate that failed to heal completely. This type of complication associated with a hard palate injury is unusual; most cats with hard palate injuries can be successfully treated with a conservative approach, as was done for the patient in Figure 2.

palate (Figure 2), dental, and mandibular fractures also occurred in 17% of the cats.[2] Temporomandibular luxations are also relatively common.

Because cats usually fall in a splayed-leg position, they often land on all four limbs, which causes either direct injury to the head or secondary injury as a result of bouncing. Cats therefore sustain more facial injuries (from the face absorbing the shock) than do dogs.[1,2,15] Another study found dental fractures to be the most common type of oral trauma in dogs (occurring in 14% of the dogs), whereas hard palate fractures did not occur and mandibular fractures occurred in only 3% of the dogs.[15]

Hard palate fractures in cats should be managed conservatively with a soft diet for at least one month after injury. Antibiotics are optional and may lessen the possibility of secondary infection. All cats in the study by Whitney and Mehlhaff healed without surgery.[2] If a hard palate fracture persists and results in oronasal fistula (Figure 3), then one of the described procedures for flap surgery should be used for repair.[16] The split-palatal U flap technique is a new procedure useful for treating chronic or recurrent oronasal fistulas secondary to hard palate injury.[17]

Depending on the type and location of the fracture, mandibular fractures can be handled in various ways. Symphyseal fractures are usually repaired with 18- to 20-gauge orthopedic wire placed in a cerclage wire fashion. The wire is placed caudal to the canine teeth. Unilateral or bilateral mandibular ramus fractures can be treated with tape muzzles, dental composite of the canine teeth, or an external fixation device. Pinning the mandible is contraindicated because of the shape and position of the teeth. Plating can be used for midbody or caudal ramus fractures. Care must be taken in placing screws to avoid endangering the roots of the teeth.

Dental fractures should be evaluated with a dental probe. Any tooth with a fracture occurring above the gum line with pulpal exposure should be extracted or endodontically treated. Teeth fractured below the gum line usually are not salvageable and should be removed.

LIMB AND SPINAL FRACTURES AND LUXATIONS

High-rise syndrome cats sustain various musculoskeletal injuries. According to Whitney and Mehlhaff, fractures occurred in 39% of the cats and luxations occurred in 18%.[2] Approximately 17% of the cats sustained multiple injuries of the extremities.[2]

Forelimb and hindlimb injuries had similar incidence, with each occurring in 17% of the cats.[2] Fractures of the

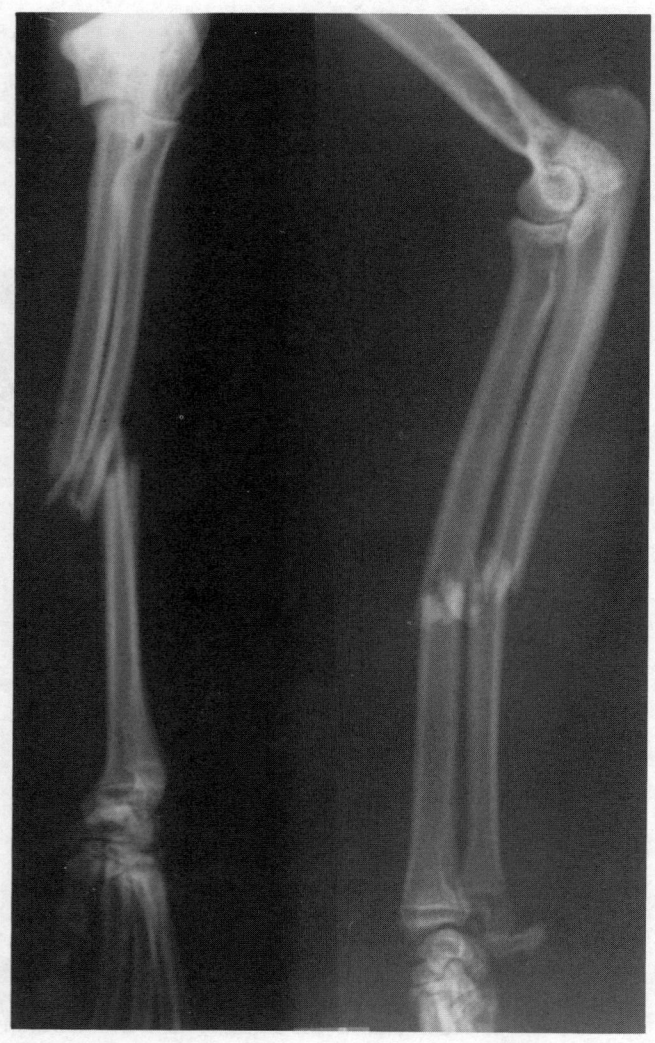

Figure 4—Radiograph of a comminuted radius and ulna fracture in a cat that fell eight stories. Most forelimb fractures involve the radius and ulna; humeral, carpal, and metacarpal fractures occur less frequently.

forelimb were distal to the elbow in 92% of the cats, with most fractures involving the radius and ulna[2] (Figure 4). Most hindlimb fractures involve the femur and tibia (Figures 5 and 6). Ninety-three percent of femoral fractures occurred in cats younger than one year of age, with a high number of fractures involving the growth plate.[2]

Many fractures secondary to fall injuries are open (Figure 7) and require immediate clipping, debridement, flushing, and splinting.[2] After initial management, many open fractures can be managed with an external fixation device because of multiple fracture comminutions and contamination. Depending on the type and location of the fracture as well as the owner's financial commitment, other methods of fixation include plating, intramedullary pinning and cerclage wiring, or closed fracture management in a splint. In the Whitney and Mehlhaff study, the most common reason for euthanasia (in 17 of 132 cats) was cost-prohibitive treatment involved in treating multiple fractures of extremities.[2]

The incidence of luxation injuries was similar for forelimbs and hindlimbs.[2] Traumatic carpal luxations were the most common (Figure 8), followed by tarsal, coxofemoral, and temporomandibular joint luxations.[2] Carpal luxations can be splinted for six weeks with some success. In most cats, however, arthrodesis using a plate or a transarticular external fixation device is the preferred method of treatment.

SPINAL INJURY in high-rise syndrome cats is unusual; only two cats in one study had fractures of the thoracic and lumbar spine (Figure 9). Both had concurrent spinal cord trauma and paresis.[2] One cat had a caudal vertebral fracture with no neurologic clinical signs.[2] Stabilization of vertebral fractures in cats include fixation with pins and methylmethacrylate, dorsal spinous or vertebral body plating, vertebral body cross pinning, or stapling. The advantages and disadvantages of these methods have been well documented.[18]

Another study found that high-rise syndrome dogs sustain similar injuries to the extremities but have increased incidence of long-bone fractures (occurring in 45% of the dogs) and spinal injuries (occurring in 16% of the dogs).[15] Such injuries are more common because dogs land unevenly on one or more extremities and absorb the impact of the fall in a different way than do cats.[2,15]

ABDOMINAL TRAUMA

In the study by Whitney and Mehlhaff, abdominal trauma was reported in 7% of the cats.[2] More common abdominal injuries include hemoperitoneum, diaphragmatic herniation, and urinary tract trauma. Cats with radiographic evidence of hydroperitoneum or hemoperitoneum should undergo abdominocentesis and, if necessary, diagnostic peritoneal lavage. Assessment of the urinary bladder in all high-rise syndrome cats is important. Abdominocentesis and a negative or positive cystogram are usually necessary to diagnose urinary tract injury definitively. If the bladder is ruptured and the cat is unstable for surgery, temporary abdominal drains can be placed while the cat's cardiovascular system is stabilized. A urinary catheter should also be placed with a urinary collection system because a significant amount of urine may still pass by means of the urethra. Drainage can be achieved by means of multiple Penrose drains, sump drains, or a peritoneal dialysis catheter. Definitive repair of the bladder or urethra is necessary as soon as possible.

The clinician should assess whether hemoperitoneum is present, and packed cell volume should be carefully moni-

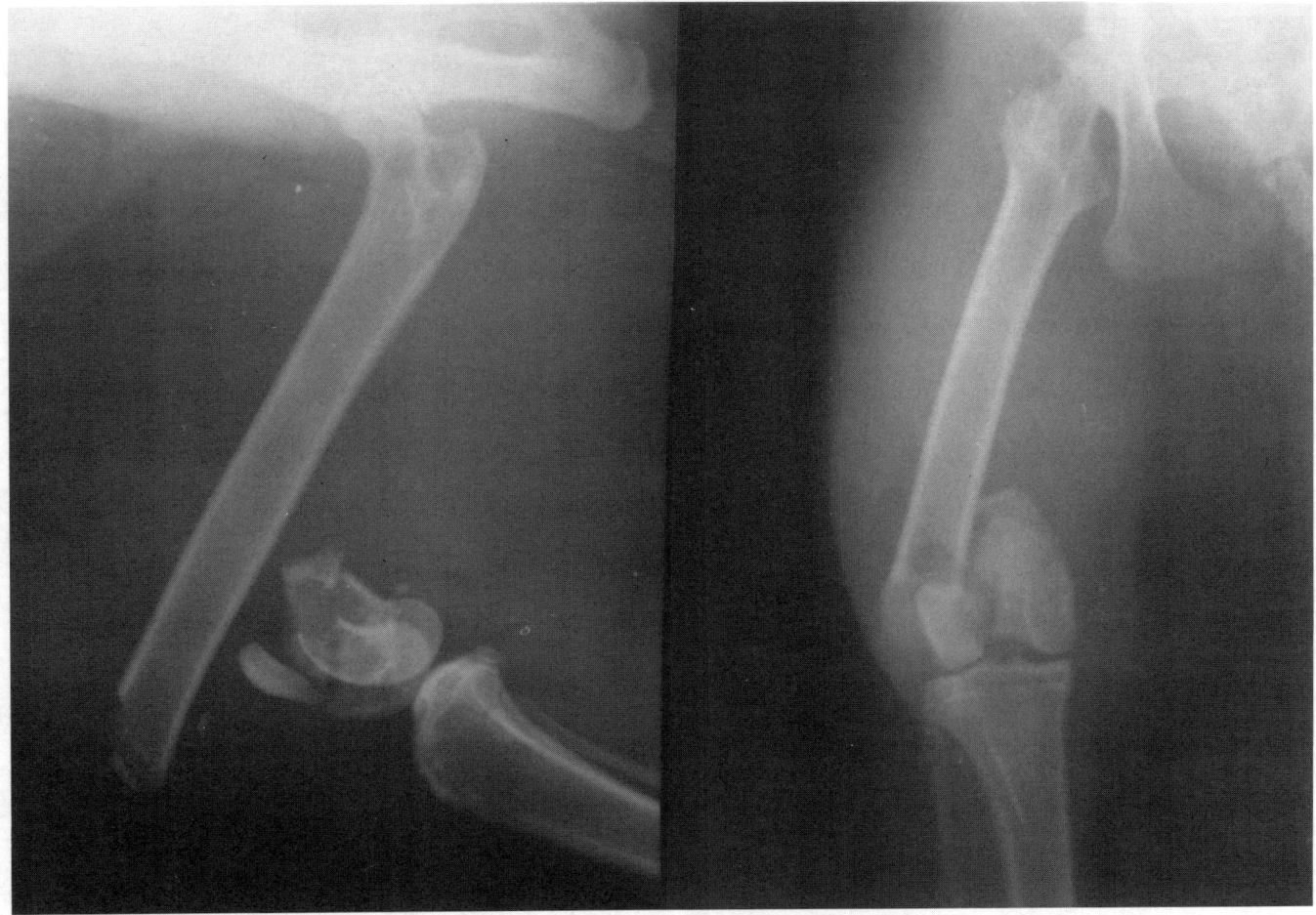

Figure 5A

Figure 5B

Figure 5—(**A**) and (**B**) Radiograph of a comminuted, intercondylar femoral fracture sustained by a cat after an eight-story fall. High-impact injuries often result in marked fracture comminution and displacement.

tored until it is considered stable. No cat in the Whitney and Mehlhaff study required transfusion or surgery for abdominal hemorrhage.[2] Another study reports that dogs have a higher incidence of abdominal injuries than do cats (occurring in 15% of the dogs).[15] Similar to cats, dogs rarely require surgical intervention.[15] Visceral injury is more common in high-rise syndrome humans and often results in fatality.[3,6,10–14]

SHOCK

In the Whitney and Mehlhaff study, life-sustaining treatment was required in 37% of the cats and nonemergency treatment was required in 30% of the cats; the need for treatment resulted largely from shock and thoracic trauma.[2]

While placing a catheter during treatment for shock, a packed cell volume and blood gas analysis should be done. Standard treatment for shock also includes administration of fluids, steroids, and antibiotics.

After initial assessment of the patient, a cardiac monitor should be placed and the temperature of the patient should be monitored. At this time, the clinician should also evaluate the need for thoracentesis.

In one study, 44% of the dogs required emergency treatment; however, the need for thoracentesis was less common than for cats.[15] It should be noted that none of the dogs fell more than six stories in the study.[15] It is likely that dogs that fell more than six stories died before reaching the hospital.[15]

CONCLUSIONS

Many factors contribute to the type of injuries sustained by cats with high-rise syndrome. The length of the fall and the surface on which the cat lands are the two main factors influencing the type and severity of injuries. Other factors include landing position, air drag, and obstacles breaking the fall.[2,5–8,11,13–15]

Biophysical principles explain the reason that the rate of injury of cats falling as many as seven stories is linear but levels off after that distance—a point just past terminal ve-

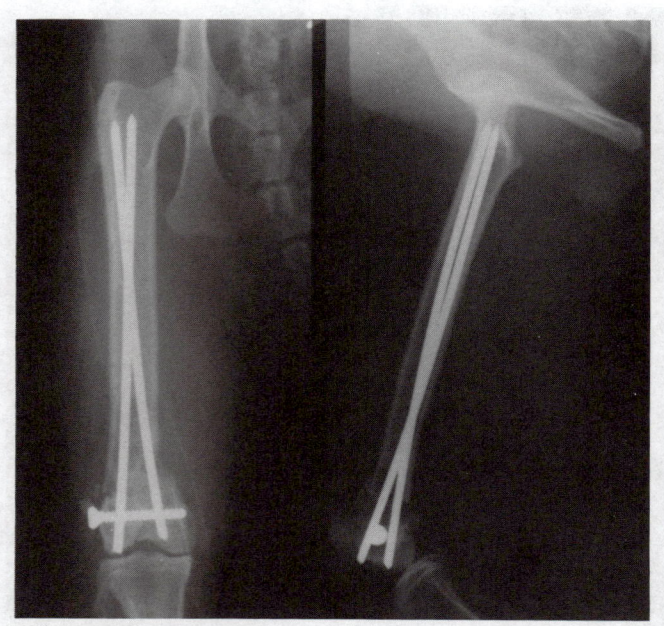

Figure 6A   **Figure 6B**

Figure 6—(**A**) and (**B**) Radiograph of the femoral fracture in the cat in Figure 5 repaired with a lag screw and two dynamic cross pins. Because of the degree of comminution, the fracture was controlled, collapsed, and reduced to a stable position.

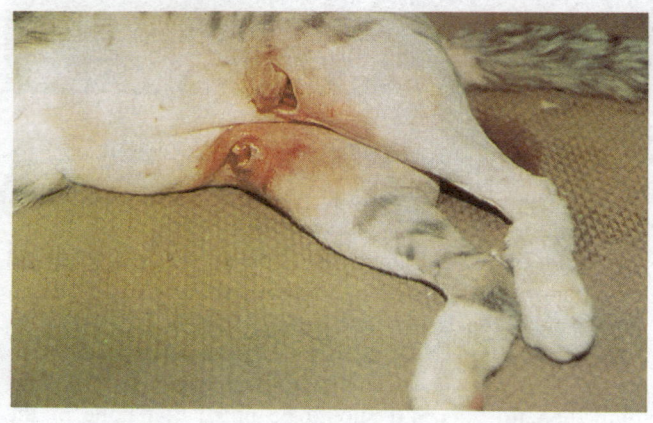

Figure 7—Bilateral, open, supracondylar femoral fractures occurred in this cat after a nine-story fall. Because of the high impact caused by acceleration forces, falling often results in open fractures.

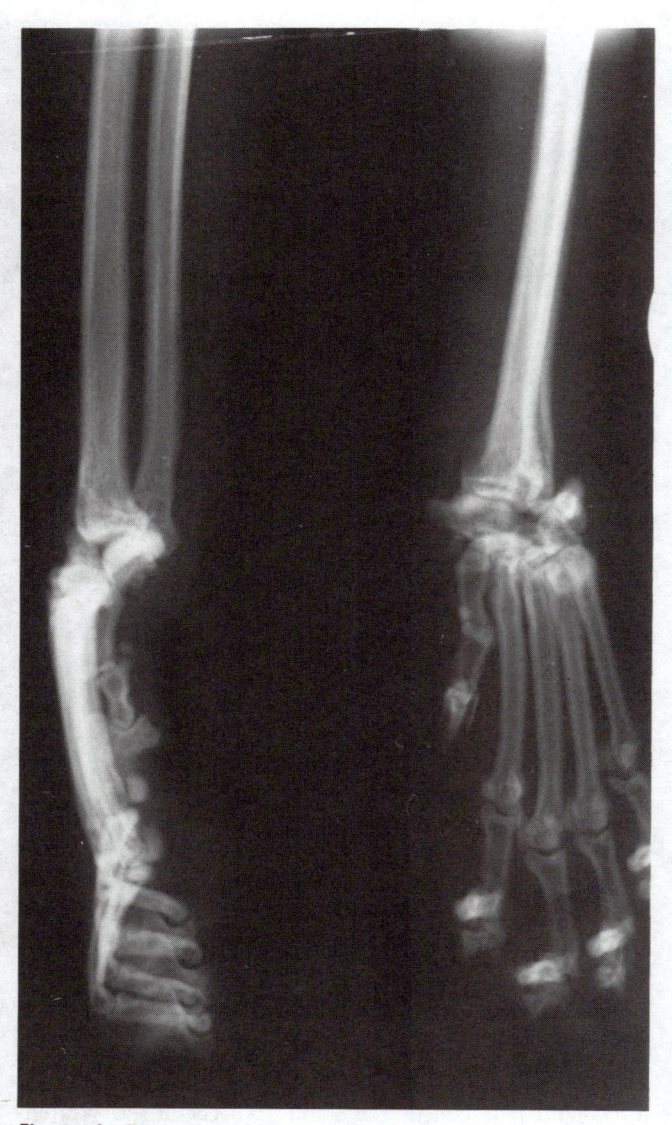

Figure 8—Radiograph of a traumatic carpal luxation–hyperextension injury in a cat after a fall. The radiocarpal bone is luxated caudally. The injury was treated by pancarpal arthrodesis.

locity.[2,13-15] A human falling in a vacuum reaches terminal velocity at 120 miles per hour after falling 32 stories.[2,13-15] Cats have the unique ability to achieve terminal velocity at approximately 60 miles per hour after falling approximately five stories. Until it achieves terminal velocity, a cat experiences acceleration and reflexively extends its limbs, thereby making them potentially more susceptible to injury.[2] As soon as terminal velocity is reached and the cat's vestibular system is less stimulated, the cat may relax and orient its limbs more horizontally. As cats position themselves in a splayed-leg position, increased air drag occurs, simultaneously eliminating the effect of postural torque rotation and tumbling on terminal velocity.[2] During landing, a cat distributes the force of impact evenly throughout its body in much the same manner as a parachutist does and thereby minimizes injury.[2] A fall to a pliant surface, such as mud or snow, diminishes the severity of injuries in all species studied[2,5-8,11,13-15]; however, most cats in an urban setting fall to concrete or asphalt.

SURVIVAL RATE of treated cats is 90%.[2] In the Whitney and Melhaff study, the mean height of falls was

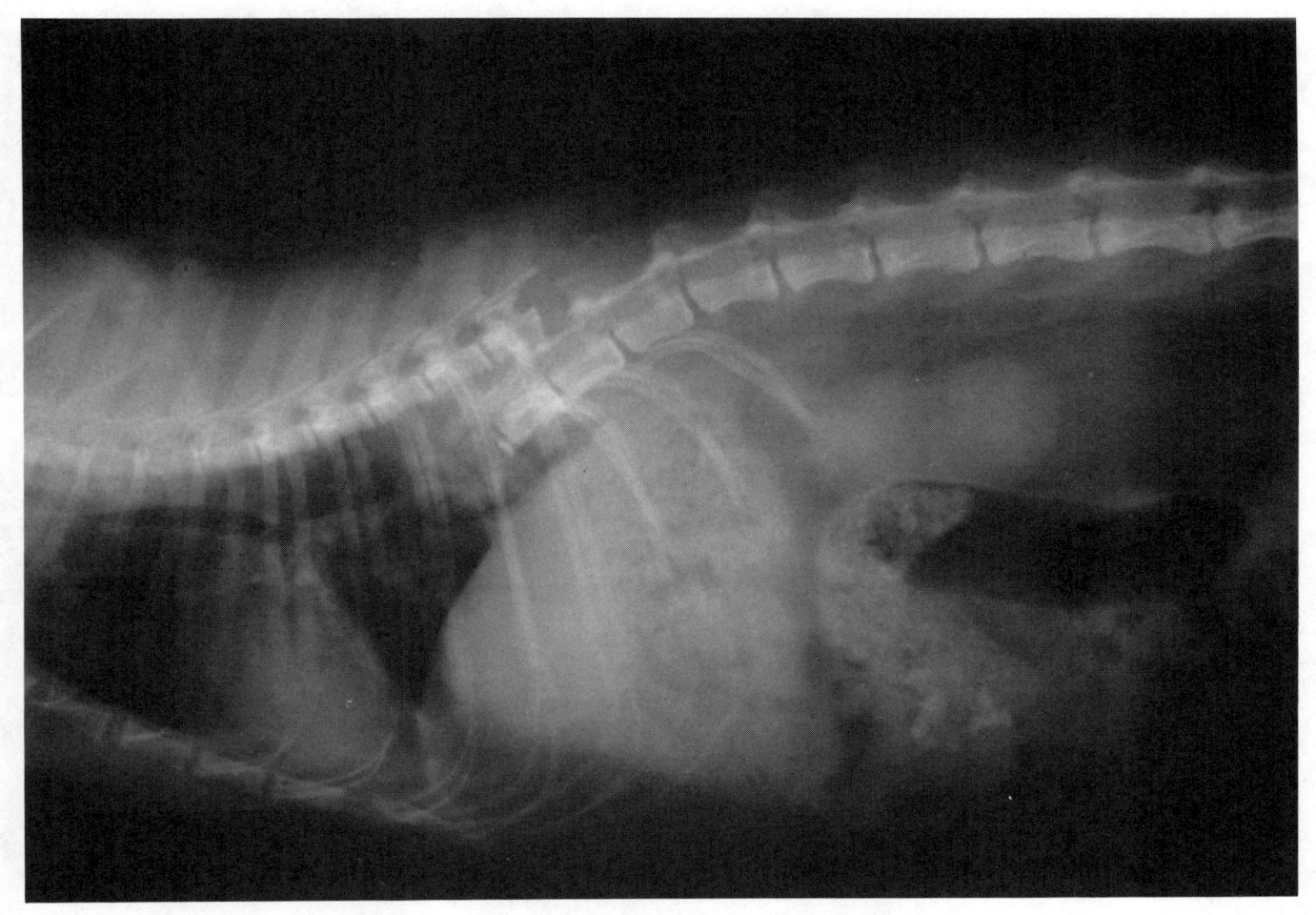

Figure 9—Radiograph of a fracture-luxation of the tenth thoracic vertebrae with severe displacement after a four-story fall. Because of severe spinal cord injuries, the cat was euthanatized. Ordinarily, because of biophysical properties, spinal injuries are rare in high-rise syndrome cats.

5½ stories; surviving cats fell a range of 2 to 32 stories.[2] Treated high-rise syndrome dogs had a 99% survival rate[15]; however, as mentioned previously, no dog in the study fell more than six stories. Predictably, injuries in dogs falling one to three stories were moderate; injuries in dogs falling four to six stories were more severe.[15] Because deceleration forces are directly related to the mass of the falling object, most dogs sustain a greater deceleration force than do cats falling the same distance.[14] Fatality in humans falling more than six stories reached nearly 100%. Head trauma followed by abdominal hemorrhage are the main causes of death in humans.[2,14]

High-rise syndrome is common in urban areas.[1-15] Survival rate is excellent for cats with early diagnosis and treatment.

About the Authors

Dr. Kapatkin is affiliated with the School of Veterinary Medicine at the University of Pennsylvania in Philadelphia. Dr. Matthiesen, a Diplomate of the American College of Veterinary Surgeons, is affiliated with Tinton Falls Veterinary Specialists, Tinton Falls, New Jersey.

REFERENCES

1. Robinson GW: The high-rise trauma syndrome in cats. *Feline Pract* 6(5):40-43, 1976.
2. Whitney WO, Mehlhaff CJ: High-rise syndrome in cats. *JAVMA* 191(11):1399-1403, 1987.
3. Barlow B, Niemirska M, Gandhi RP, Leblanc W: Ten years of experience with falls from a height in children. *J Pediatr Surg* 18(4):509-511, 1983.
4. Bergner L, Mayer S, Harris D: Falls from heights: A childhood epidemic in an urban area. *Am J Pediatr Health* 61(1):90-96, 1971.
5. Ciccone R, Richman R: The mechanism of injury and the distribution of three thousand fractures and dislocations caused by parachute jumping. *J Bone Joint Surg* 30A(1):77-97, 1948.
6. Goonetilleke A: Injuries caused by falls from heights. *Med Sci Law* 20(4):262-275, 1980.
7. Kravitz H, Driessen G, Gomberg R, Korach A: Accidental falls from elevated surfaces in infants from birth to one year of age. *Pediatrics [Suppl]* 44:869-876, 1969.
8. Layton TR, Villella ER, Kelly EG: High free-fall with survival. *J Trauma* 21(11):983-985, 1981.
9. Lewis WS, Lee AB, Grantham SA: Jumper's syndrome: The trauma of high free-fall as seen at Harlem Hospital. *J Trauma* 5(5):812-818, 1965.

of high free-fall as seen at Harlem Hospital. *J Trauma* 5(5):812–818, 1965.
10. Reynolds BM, Balsano HA, Reynolds FX: Falls from heights: A surgical experience of 200 consecutive cases. *Ann Surg* 174(2):304–308, 1971.
11. Sieben RL, Leavitt JD, French JH: Falls as childhood accidents: An increasing urban risk. *Pediatrics* 47(5):886–892, 1971.
12. Smith MD, Burrington JD, Woolf AD: Injuries in children sustained in free falls: An analysis of 66 cases. *J Trauma* 15(11):987–991, 1975.
13. Snyder RG: Human tolerances to extreme impacts in free-fall. *Aerospace Med* 34(8):695–709, 1963.
14. Warner KG, Demling RH: The pathophysiology of free-fall injury. *Ann Emerg Med* 15:1088–1093, 1986.
15. Gordon LE, Thacher CT, Kapatkin AS: Unpublished data, High-rise syndrome in dogs: A retrospective study of 81 cases. New York, Animal Medical Center, 1986–1991.
16. Nelson AW, Wykes PM: Upper respiratory system, in Slatter DH (ed): *Textbook of Small Animal Surgery*. Philadelphia, WB Saunders Co, 1985.
17. Manfra Marretta S, Grove TX, Grillo JF: Split palatal U-flap: A new technique for repair of caudal hard palate defects. *J Vet Dent* 8(1):5–8, 1991.
18. Walker TL, Tomlinson J, Sarjonen DC, Kornegay JN: Diseases of the spinal column, in Slatter DH (ed): *Textbook of Small Animal Surgery*. Philadelphia, WB Saunders Co, 1985.

Principles of Head Trauma Management in Dogs and Cats—Part I

KEY FACTS

- Head trauma patients often have other concurrent injuries that must be evaluated and treated.
- Hemorrhage and edema occur immediately after serious head trauma and lead to various secondary autolytic processes.
- Oxygen-free radical-induced brain injury probably plays an important role in secondary brain tissue damage.
- Understanding the development of increased intracranial pressure after head trauma is crucial to the selection of appropriate therapeutic measures.
- Level of consciousness and brain stem reflexes are important in initial assessment and monitoring of head trauma patients.

Texas A&M University
Curtis W. Dewey, DVM, MS

University of Georgia
Steven C. Budsberg, DVM, MS

John E. Oliver, Jr., DVM, MS, PhD

INJURY to the brain in dogs and cats is a common occurrence that is usually associated with automobile trauma; missile injuries (e.g., gunshot wounds), animal bites, falls, and malicious human behavior can also result in such injury.[1-11] Management of the brain-injured pet is an extreme challenge to the emergency veterinarian who must assess, treat, and attempt to predict the outcome of damage to an organ system more complex than any other system in the body. Head injury in animals and humans often connotes a poor to grave prognosis; of paramount importance in treatment of the head-injured dog or cat is preservation of vital brain stem structures.[2,3,11] Proper application of the principles to be discussed may increase the number of successful outcomes in animals with head injuries. Also, application of standardized guidelines for monitoring the progress of neurologic recovery may improve the veterinarian's accuracy and precision in making prognostic decisions.

FUNCTIONAL NEUROANATOMY

A complete description of the anatomy of the brain is beyond the scope of this article. To understand the principles that will be discussed, however, the divisions of cerebrum, cerebellum, and brain stem (diencephalon, midbrain [mesencephalon], pons, and medulla oblongata) are sufficient (Figure 1). From external to internal, the dura mater, arachnoid, and pia mater constitute the soft tissue coverings of the brain (meninges); cerebrospinal fluid occupies the space between the pia mater and arachnoid.[12,13] Focal damage to individual brain subdivisions results in characteristic, localizing neurologic deficits. Head trauma, however, often involves damage to more than one anatomic subdivision of the brain, which results in various possible clinical signs.[14,15]

Focal, cerebral hemispheric damage is often characterized by depression, behavioral changes, contralateral visual deficits (decreased or absent menace response), contralateral facial hypalgesia, and contralateral conscious proprioceptive deficits.[14-16] Although many patients are too depressed and/or in too much pain to move a great deal immediately following cerebral trauma, if the animal is willing and able (no spinal or significant orthopedic injuries) to ambulate, gait is usually normal. A subtle hemiparesis may be observed. The patient may pace compulsively and may headpress when confronted with a wall.

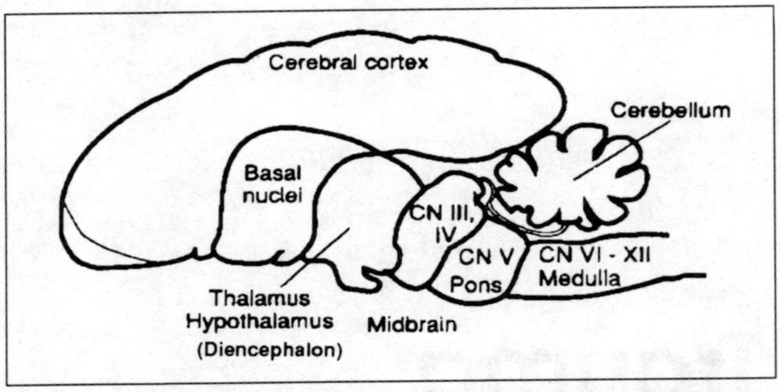

Figure 1—Schematic representation of major brain subdivisions. (CN = cranial nerve) (From Shell LG: The cranial nerves of the brain stem. Prog Vet Neurol 1(3):233-244, 1990. Reprinted with permission.)

Circling, when observed, is usually toward the side of the lesion and is typically in a wide arc.[14-16] More generalized cerebral dysfunction (e.g., cerebral edema) can result in more extensive disturbances of consciousness (e.g., stupor or coma), although such severe clinical signs are more often associated with brain stem dysfunction.[17-19] Brain stem reflexes and cranial nerve function, with the exception of menace deficits, are normal with cerebral trauma.[14-16]

Although anatomically a part of the brain stem, focal diencephalic (thalamus and hypothalamus) damage often produces neurologic signs similar to those seen with focal cerebral damage. Because the diencephalon constitutes part of the ascending reticular activating system (ARAS) of the brain stem, large lesions in this area can produce stupor and coma. The ascending reticular activating system is a meshwork of neurons and associated axonal fibers located from the caudal diencephalon to the medulla. Because this system is of vital importance in maintaining the animal in a wakeful state, lesions affecting the system produce alterations in consciousness ranging from depression to coma.[14-19]

DAMAGE to the mesencephalon, pons, and medulla are often associated with severe disturbances of consciousness (stupor or coma), depressed or absent brain stem reflexes, and depressed or absent cranial nerve functions ipsilateral to the lesion. Upper motor neuron signs to front- and hindlimbs on one side (spastic hemiparesis) or, with larger lesions, to all four limbs (spastic tetraparesis) are common. If the animal is ambulatory, the gait will be grossly abnormal, which is in contrast to the normal gait associated with cerebral lesions.[14-19]

Peripheral or central lesions of the vestibular system, which controls an animal's balance, typically produce signs such as head tilt ipsilateral to the side of the lesion, asymmetric ataxia, positional strabismus (eye ipsilateral to the side of the lesion deviates ventrally when the head is elevated), and nystagmus with the fast phase usually away from the side of the lesion. Peripheral vestibular lesions (middle or inner ear damage) may cause deficits in cranial nerve VII in addition to cranial nerve VIII and an ipsilateral Horner's syndrome, which is characterized by ptosis, miosis, and enophthalmos; other cranial nerves should be unaffected. Mental status and postural reactions (proprioception) should be normal. Nystagmus is typically rotatory or horizontal and does not change direction with different positions of the head. Central (medullary) vestibular disease is present if, in addition to the signs discussed previously, there are signs indicative of brain stem dysfunction. These signs include proprioceptive deficits; hemiparesis or tetraparesis; involvement of cranial nerves V, VI, IX, X, or XII; and abnormal mental status. Also, vertical nystagmus, nystagmus with the fast phase toward the side of the lesion, and nystagmus that changes direction are indicative of central vestibular disease.[13-15,20,21]

Because the cerebellum is well protected in the cranial vault, it is unusual to see isolated cerebellar trauma.[15] Cerebellar trauma is characterized by ataxia with preservation of strength; dysmetria (movements that are too long or too short) of the head and limbs; menace deficits with normal vision and normal palpebral reflexes when diffuse lesions are present; and intention tremors, which are tremors, including cerebellar nystagmus, that worsen when the animal initiates a movement.[15,22] Acute cerebellar trauma can result in decerebellate rigidity.[7-9,15,22] Lesions of the cerebellar medulla and caudal cerebellar peduncle can result in a head tilt and vestibular ataxia away from the side of the lesion (paradoxic vestibular disease).[15,22]

PATHOPHYSIOLOGY OF HEAD TRAUMA
Initial Trauma

Brain trauma can be classified as concussion, contusion, or laceration injuries.[1,4,8-11] Concussion injury, the least serious of the three, is typified by a brief loss of consciousness, often followed by a short period of confusion. In concussion injury, there is no significant brain parenchymal damage.[1,4,8-11]

Contusion and laceration injuries are associated with physical damage to brain parenchyma, with accompanying brain hemorrhage and edema. Laceration injuries are commonly associated with skull fractures.[1,4,8-11]

Hemorrhage and Edema

Immediately after the traumatic event, hemorrhage and edema occur in and around the brain.[1,4,7,11] If these processes are of sufficient magnitude and left untreated, they set in motion a vicious cycle of events that lead to increasing intracranial pressure.[4,6] Subarachnoid and intraparenchymal hemorrhages are purportedly the main forms of hemorrhage associated with head injury in dogs and cats; clinically significant epidural and subdural hemorrhage is believed to be very uncommon.[1,4,6,9,11] Brain edema caused

Pupil Size	Reactivity	Prognosis
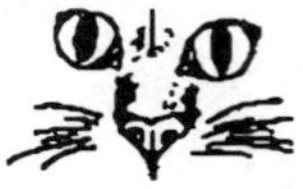 Normal (midrange)	Normal	Good
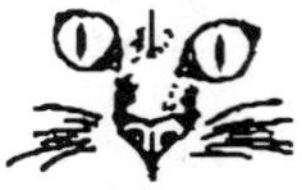 Bilateral Miosis	Poor to Non-responsive	Guarded (variable, depending on other signs)
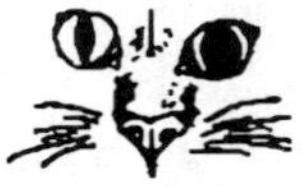 Unilateral Mydriasis	Poor to Non-responsive (mydriatic side)	Guarded to Poor
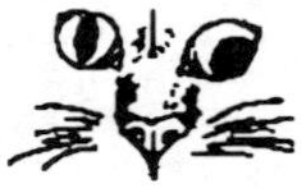 Unilateral Mydriasis with Ventrolateral Strabismus	Poor to Non-responsive (mydriatic side)	Guarded to Poor
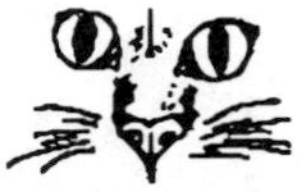 Normal (midrange)	Non-responsive	Poor to Grave
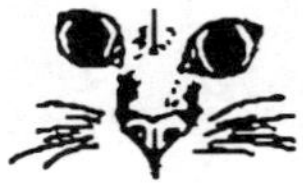 Bilateral Mydriasis	Poor to Non-responsive	Poor to Grave

Figure 5—Pupillary size and reactivity in relation to prognosis in head trauma victims (ranked from top to bottom in order of increasing severity).

one in which the animal has an altered perception of the environment and thus inappropriate responses to external stimuli; such a patient may frantically struggle and vocalize as if hallucinating. Stupor describes an animal that remains in a sleep state unless aroused by a strong stimulus. Coma is a state of deep unconsciousness from which the patient cannot be aroused.[13–15,31,32] Stupor and coma are associated with generalized cerebral disturbances or, more commonly, dysfunction of the ascending reticular activating system of the brain stem.[13–15,18,19,31,32]

Pupillary size and response should be evaluated initially to assess the integrity of the mesencephalon and periodically thereafter to monitor for improvement or deterioration of neurologic status (Figure 5). Unilateral, slowly progressing pupillary abnormalities (hours to days), in the absence of direct ocular injury, are characteristic of brain stem compression and/or herniation caused by progressive brain swelling. Acute onset of bilateral pupillary abnormalities are indicative of brain stem hemorrhage (Figure 5).[5,6] It is important for the clinician to distinguish between these two conditions because compression or herniation may respond to therapy whereas brain stem hemorrhage probably will not.[5,6] Unresponsive mid-range or mydriatic pupils usually reflect an irreversible brain stem lesion and a grave prognosis.[4,5,6,8] Severe, bilateral miosis indicates extensive brain dysfunction but is not, by itself, of localizing value.[1,4,5,6,9] Return of pupils to normal size and reactivity is a favorable prognostic sign, but progression from bilaterally miotic to bilaterally mydriatic or mid-range fixed pupils indicates worsening of the brain disturbance.[4,7,8] An early sign of unilateral tentorial herniation is an ipsilateral dilated pupil with ventrolateral strabismus secondary to compression of the oculomotor nerve and/or nucleus[1,5,6,9] (Figure 5).

Oculocephalic reflexes are evaluated to assess the integrity of the medial longitudinal fasciculus of the brain stem (the area of the brain stem that coordinates eye movements with movement of the head) and the nuclei and nerves of cranial nerves III, IV, and VI.[1–11,13–15,31,32] Normally, moving an animal's head from side to side initiates normal physiologic nystagmus with the fast phase toward the direction of head movement (doll's eye reflex). Similar to pupillary size and response, loss of normal oculocephalic reflex activity is an early sign with brain stem hemorrhage and a late sign with brain stem compression and herniation.[5,6,33,34]

Further evaluation should include assessment of remaining cranial nerves, motor ability, and tendon reflex activity

TABLE II
The Small Animal Coma Scale for Evaluating Head Trauma Victims[a]

Category/Description	Score
Motor activity	
Normal gait; normal spinal reflexes	6
Hemiparesis, tetraparesis, or decerebrate activity	5
Recumbent; intermittent extensor rigidity	4
Recumbent; constant extensor rigidity	3
Recumbent; constant extensor rigidity with opisthotonos	2
Recumbent; hypotonia of muscles; depressed or absent spinal reflexes	1
Brain stem reflexes	
Normal pupillary light responses and oculocephalic reflexes	6
Slow pupillary light reflexes; normal to reduced oculocephalic reflexes	5
Bilateral unresponsive miosis; normal to reduced oculocephalic reflexes	4
Pinpoint pupils; reduced to absent oculocephalic reflexes	3
Unilateral, unresponsive mydriasis; reduced to absent oculocephalic reflexes	2
Bilateral, unresponsive mydriasis; reduced to absent oculocephalic reflexes	1
Level of consciousness	
Occasional periods of alertness and response to environment	6
Depression or delirium; capable of responding to environment	5
Semicomatose; responsive to visual stimuli	4
Semicomatose; responsive to auditory stimuli	3
Semicomatose; responsive to noxious stimuli	2
Comatose; unresponsive to repeated noxious stimuli	1

Total Score	Likely Prognosis
3–8	Grave
9–14	Poor to guarded
15–18	Good

[a]From Shores A: Treatment and prognosis of head trauma. *Proc 13th Kal Kan Symp*:29–36, 1990. Modified with permission.

(e.g., patellar reflexes). Information concerning motor activity, brain stem reflexes, and level of consciousness should be graded according to the Small Animal Coma Scale (SACS) (Table II) and recorded. The Small Animal Coma Scale is a modification of the Glasgow Coma Scale used in human head trauma management. The Small Animal Coma Scale can be used for initial assessment and continued monitoring of the patient's neurologic status.[1,11,35]

The animal's posture (e.g., decerebrate rigidity or decerebellate rigidity) should be noted for both lesion localization and prognostic reasons. For example, decerebrate rigidity (opisthotonos with hyperextension of all four limbs) signifies interruption of communicating pathways between brain stem structures and higher control centers. In the comatose patient, decerebrate rigidity is usually associated with a poor prognosis. Decerebellate rigidity (opisthotonos with forelimb extension and hindlimb flexion), however, is usually associated with a fair to good prognosis.[1,7,8,9]

The respiratory pattern of the head-injured patient can be of localizing and prognostic value.[1,4,8,9,11] Also, if an abnormal respiratory pattern appears or worsens, more aggressive therapy is indicated. Cheyne-Stokes respiration is characterized by periods of hyperventilation, which taper off gradually to periods of apnea of variable duration. Respirations then resume and gradually accelerate to the point of hyperventilation. Cheyne-Stokes respiration is seen with damage to deep cerebral hemispheric structures, basal ganglia, internal capsules, and the diencephalon.[1,4,8,9,11]

Central neurogenic hyperventilation, typical of lower mesencephalon and pontine damage, is characterized by rapid and regular respirations at a rate of approximately 25/minute.[1,4,8,9,11]

More irregular respiratory patterns are seen with severe damage to the caudal pons and medulla and are associated with poor to hopeless prognoses. Apneustic breathing describes a cyclic respiratory pattern of a prolonged inspiratory phase followed by expiration and an apneic phase; this cycle typically repeats itself one to one and a half times per minute. Cluster breathing refers to closely grouped respirations followed by periods of apnea. Very ataxic, chaotic, or gasping respirations usually represent agonal breathing subsequent to extensive damage to medullary respiratory centers.[1,4,8,9,11]

The veterinarian must be cautious not to attribute signs of pulmonary trauma or hypoxemia to neurologic dysfunction. On the other hand, pulmonary edema, congestion, and hyperemia (in the absence of direct pulmonary damage) may develop after head trauma, presumably as a result of alterations in autonomic outflow from the brain stem to the lungs.[36]

Radiographs of the skull are indicated in most cases of head trauma.[11,17] Although skull radiographs do not allow evaluation of soft tissue structures within the cranial vault, they may indicate the presence and severity of skull fractures.[37] Computed tomography (CT) is considered the best method for evaluation of skull fractures and magnetic resonance imaging (MRI) is regarded as the best method for achieving superior detail of brain parenchymal injury.[5,11]

SUMMARY

The head trauma patient poses a medical and sometimes surgical emergency. The emergency clinician must evaluate and administer therapy for concurrent, life-threatening injuries. A good understanding of functional neuroanatomy and the events leading to elevated intracranial pressure is essential for proper assessment and management of the patient with head injury. Accurate neurologic assessment of the head-injured dog or cat is important both for prognostic reasons and for guiding the clinician in making therapeutic decisions.

ACKNOWLEDGMENTS

The authors thank Lynn Reece, AHT, Small Animal Medicine Laboratory Technician, Department of Small Animal Medicine, University of Georgia College of Veterinary Medicine, for all of her work in the preparation of the tables and figures; the authors also thank Mamie Watson for her special contribution to the manuscript.

About the Authors

Dr. Dewey is a Clinical Associate Professor in the Department of Small Animal Medicine and Surgery at Texas A&M University. Drs. Budsberg and Oliver are affiliated with the Department of Small Animal Medicine, College of Veterinary Medicine, University of Georgia, Athens, Georgia. Dr. Budsberg, who is a Diplomate of the American College of Veterinary Surgeons, is Associate Professor in the Department of Small Animal Medicine. Dr. Oliver, who is a Diplomate of the American College of Veterinary Internal Medicine (Neurology), is Full Professor in the Department of Small Animal Medicine.

REFERENCES

1. Shores A: Craniocerebral trauma, in Kirk RW (ed): *Current Veterinary Therapy X*. Philadelphia, WB Saunders Co, 1989, pp 847–853.
2. Pitts LH, Martin N: Head injuries. *Surg Clin North Am* 62(1):47–60, 1982.
3. Levati A, Farina ML, Vecchi G, et al: Prognosis of severe head injuries. *J Neurosurg* 57:779–783, 1982.
4. LeCouteur R: Central nervous system trauma, in Kornegay JN (ed): *Contemporary Issues in Small Animal Practice: Neurologic Disorders*. New York, Churchill Livingstone, 1986, pp 147–167.
5. Oliver JE: Neurologic emergencies in small animals. *Vet Clin North Am [Small Anim Pract]* 2(2):341–357, 1972.
6. Oliver JE: Intracranial injury, in Kirk RW (ed): *Current Veterinary Therapy VII*. Philadelphia, WB Saunders Co, 1980, pp 815–820.
7. Colter S, Rucker NC: Acute injury to the central nervous system. *Vet Clin North Am [Small Anim Pract]* 18(3):545–561, 1988.
8. LeCouteur R: Neurologic Emergencies (in Small Animals). Lecture Notes V.M. 260, University of Georgia, Small Animal Teaching Hospital, 1981.
9. Selcer RR: Trauma to the central nervous system. *Vet Clin North Am [Small Anim Pract]* 10(3):619–639, 1980.
10. Griffiths IR: Central nervous system trauma, in Oliver JE, Hoerlein BF, Mayhew IG (eds): *Veterinary Neurology*. Philadelphia, WB Saunders Co, 1987, pp 303–310.
11. Shores A: Treatment and prognosis of head trauma. *Proc 13th Kal Kan Symp*:29–36, 1990.
12. Evans HE, Christensen GC: *Miller's Anatomy of the Dog*. Philadelphia, WB Saunders Co, 1979, pp 842–902.
13. DeLaHunta A: *Veterinary Neuroanatomy and Clinical Neurology*. Philadelphia, WB Saunders Co, 1987, pp 6–52.
14. Oliver JE, Mayhew IG: Neurologic examination and the diagnostic plan, in Oliver JE, Hoerlein BF, Mayhew IG (eds): *Veterinary Neurology*. Philadelphia, WB Saunders Co, 1987, pp 7–56.
15. Oliver JE: Localization of lesions: The anatomic diagnosis. *Prog Vet Neurol* 1(1):28–39, 1990.
16. Chrisman CL: The functional neuroanatomy of the cerebrum and rostral brain stem. *Prog Vet Neurol* 1(2):117–122, 1990.
17. Selcer RR: Functional neuroanatomy of the caudal brain stem and cerebellum. *Prog Vet Neurol* 1(3):226–231, 1990.
18. Shores A, Roudebush P: Altered states of consciousness: Coma and stupor, in Ettinger SJ (ed): *Textbook of Veterinary Internal Medicine*. Philadelphia, WB Saunders Co, 1989, pp 578–623.
19. Colter SB: Stupor and coma. *Prog Vet Neurol* 1(2):137–145, 1990.
20. Schunk KL: Disorders of the vestibular system. *Vet Clin North Am [Small Anim Pract]* 18(3):641–664, 1988.
21. Schunk KL: Diseases of the vestibular system. *Prog Vet Neurol* 1(3):247–254, 1990.
22. Kornegay JN: Ataxia of the head and limbs: Cerebellar diseases in dogs and cats. *Prog Vet Neurol* 1(3):255–274, 1990.
23. Crowe DT: Triage and trauma management, in Murtaugh RJ, Kaplan PM (eds): *Veterinary Emergency and Critical Care Medicine*. St. Louis, CV Mosby, 1992, pp 77–121.
24. Siesjo BK: Cell damage in the brain: A speculative synthesis. *J Cereb Blood Flow Metab* 24(1):155–185, 1981.
25. Sorjonen DC, Vaughn DM: Membrane interactions in central nervous system injury. *Compend Contin Educ Pract Vet* 11(3):248–254, 1989.
26. McCord JM: Oxygen-derived free radicals in postischemic tissue injury. *N Engl J Med* 312(3):159–163, 1985.
27. Freeman BA, Crapo JD: Biology of disease: Free radicals and tissue injury. *Lab Invest* 47(5):412–426, 1982.
28. Ikeda Y, Long DM: The molecular basis of brain injury and brain edema: The role of oxygen free radicals. *J Neurosurg* 27(1):1–8, 1990.
29. Opie LH: Reperfusion injury and its pharmacologic modification. *Circulation* 80(4):1049–1062, 1989.
30. White BC, Krause GS, Aust SD, et al: Postischemic tissue injury by iron-mediated free radical lipid peroxidation. *Ann Emerg Med* 14(8):804–809, 1985.
31. Fenner WR: The neurologic evaluation of patients, in Ettinger SJ (ed): *Textbook of Veterinary Internal Medicine*. Philadelphia, WB Saunders Co, 1989, pp 549–577.
32. Fenner WR: Neurologic disorders, in Sherding RG (ed): *The Cat: Diseases and Clinical Management*. New York, Churchill Livingstone, 1989, pp 1163–1215.
33. Mueller-Jensen A, Neunzig HP, Emskotter TH: Outcome prediction in comatose patients: Significance of reflex eye movement analysis. *J Neurol Neurosurg Psychiatry* 50:389–392, 1987.
34. Shell LG: The cranial nerves of the brain stem. *Prog Vet Neurol* 1(3):233–244, 1990.
35. Shores A: Development of a coma scale for dogs: Prognostic value in craniocerebral trauma. *Proc 6th Annu Vet Med Forum*:251–253, 1988.
36. Crittendon DJ, Beckman DL: Traumatic head injury and pulmonary damage. *J Trauma* 22(9):766–769, 1982.
37. Greene CE, Braund KG: Diseases of the brain, in Ettinger SJ (ed): *Textbook of Veterinary Internal Medicine*. Philadelphia, WB Saunders Co, 1989, pp 578–623.

Principles of Head Trauma Management in Dogs and Cats— Part II

Texas A&M University
Curtis W. Dewey, DVM, MS
University of Georgia
Steven C. Budsberg, DVM, MS
John E. Oliver, Jr., DVM, MS, PhD

KEY FACTS

❏ Recent evidence suggests that much of the injury to the brain incurred after head trauma is theoretically reversible if secondary autolytic processes can be attenuated.

❏ Hypertonic solutions (given alone or in combination with crystalloid or colloid solutions) seem to be more effective than crystalloid or colloid administration alone for shock therapy in head trauma victims.

❏ Considerable controversy exists regarding current therapies for head trauma patients.

❏ A number of new therapies aimed at reduction of oxygen free radical–induced brain tissue damage have shown promise.

❏ Surgical intervention is sometimes required in the management of brain-injured pets.

After serious head trauma occurs, there is a narrow window of time during which therapy is effective in preventing further damage to nervous tissue. Recent evidence supports the assertion that much of the brain tissue damage that occurs immediately after trauma is reversible axonal injury. If the surrounding biochemical environment is favorable, some compromised axons can recover with time[1–4]; however, secondary inflammatory mediators (e.g., arachidonic acid metabolites and oxygen free radicals) produced after trauma can convert reversible nervous tissue injury to irreversible injury within hours.[2,3] Therapy that counteracts such effects reduces the likelihood of irreversible brain damage and associated permanent dysfunction or death.[5–7] When confronted with a brain-injured animal, the emergency veterinarian should immediately begin therapy that is appropriate for the patient's suspected degree of brain insult. The first veterinarian the brain-injured patient encounters after the traumatic incident is very likely to dictate the eventual outcome for that patient.

A major dilemma of head trauma management is that there are few pharmacologic agents or protocols that have been clearly demonstrated to be clinically effective in improving eventual outcome.[5,8,9] A paradox exists because although the need for immediate therapy after brain injury is recognized, there is uncertainty regarding the therapy that should be used. Various complex pathophysiologic events contribute to brain tissue damage after trauma; effective therapy must therefore target a number of these processes.[8–11] Few veterinarians would argue that head trauma victims seem to respond, at least temporarily, to multimodality drug therapy. In the past 10 years, an explosion of knowledge in the area of head trauma pathophysiology and potential therapies has occurred.[2,4,10] Many of these new therapies for

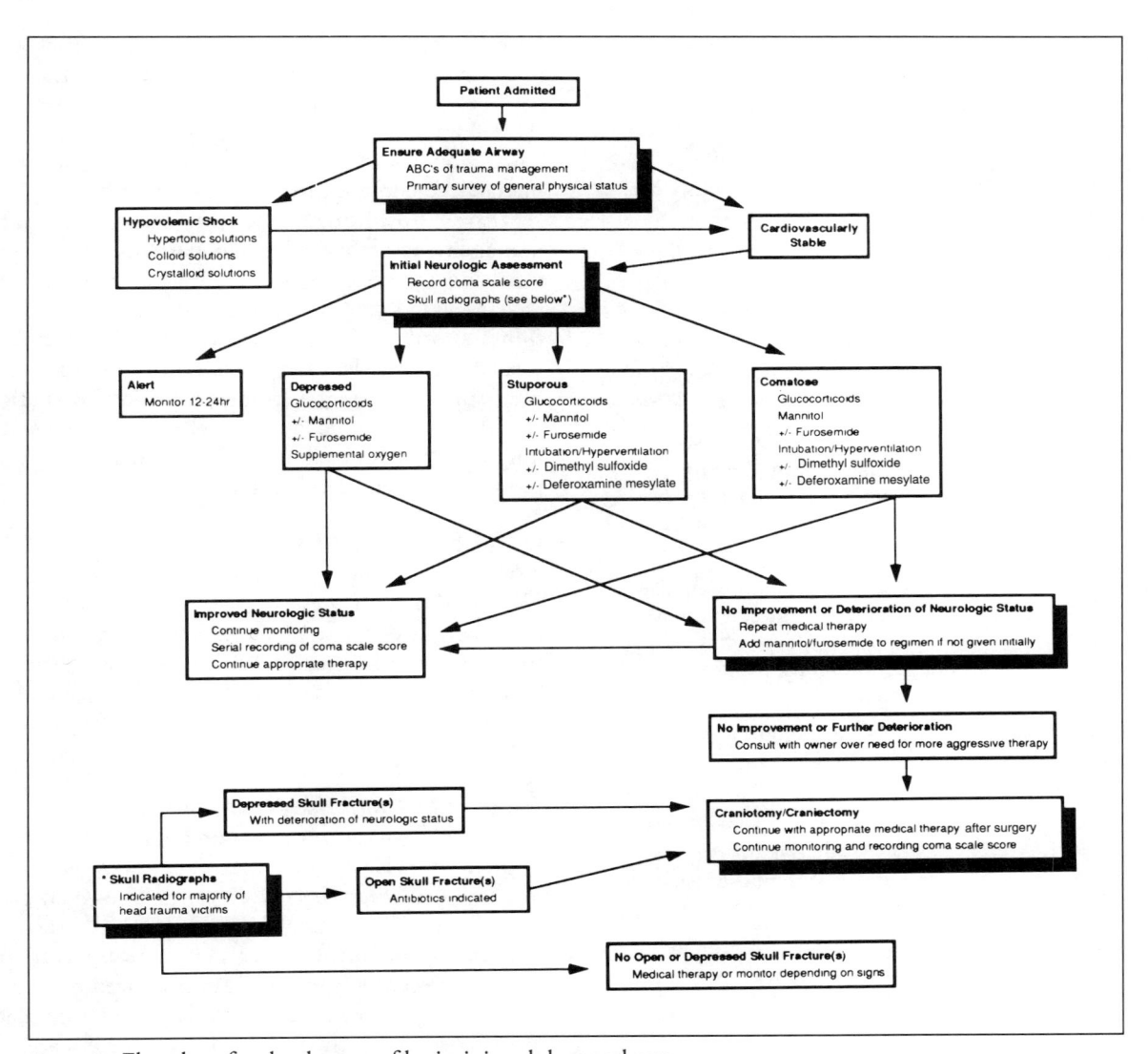

Figure 1—Flowchart for the therapy of brain-injured dogs and cats.

the head trauma victim are available to the practicing veterinarian.

When considering implementation of a medical or surgical therapeutic option, there is a tendency to overemphasize potential side effects of a drug or procedure if it has not been proven effective. In most cases of head trauma, however, the consequences of unattenuated secondary autolytic brain tissue destruction are far more disastrous than are the side effects of a potentially beneficial but unproven therapy. This article discusses new therapeutic developments as well as conventional head trauma management.

MEDICAL TREATMENT

The main objective of medical treatment for brain-injured dogs and cats is to protect the brain from further insult by secondary autolytic processes.[2,4,7] The various procedures and therapeutic agents discussed in this article are directed at combating the development and reducing the effects of brain ischemia, brain edema, and progressive elevations in intracranial pressure.[6–12] These interrelated pathologic processes result in further destruction of brain tissue. Figure 1 is a flowchart for therapy of brain-injured dogs and cats, and Table I provides a listing of the drugs and dose regimens commonly used in brain-injured dogs and cats.

The exact therapeutic plan chosen for an individual patient depends on the severity of the general physical and neurologic injuries, the location of the lesion or lesions, the cause of brain trauma (e.g., automobile trauma or gunshot injury), the rate of progression of signs, the response to initial therapy, and the economic constraints of the owners.[13,14] Preference with regard to specific drugs also plays a role in the therapeutic plan. For example, some clinicians avoid the

TABLE I
Names and Dose Regimens of Drugs Commonly Used in Brain-Injured Pets

Drug Name	Dose Regimen
Hypertonic saline (7%)	4–5 ml/kg intravenously over 3–5 minutes
Prednisone-prednisolone	10–30 mg/kg initially, followed by gradually tapering doses every 6–8 hours
Dexamethasone (sodium phosphate)	1–4 mg/kg intravenously initially, followed by gradually tapering doses every 6–8 hours
High-dose methylprednisolone	30 mg/kg intravenously initially, 15 mg/kg intravenously at 2 and 6 hours, then 2.5 mg/kg/hr for 42 hours
Mannitol (25%)	0.25–2.0 g/kg intravenously over 20 minutes; repeat every 3–8 hours, depending on patient response, osmolality, and electrolyte status
Dimethyl sulfoxide (10%–40%)	0.5–1.0 g/kg intravenously over 30–45 minutes every 8–12 hours
Furosemide	2–5 mg/kg intravenously; repeat every 6 hours depending on patient response, osmolality, and electrolyte status
Deferoxamine mesylate	One time dose of 25–50 mg/kg intramuscularly

use of mannitol because of the potential side effects, whereas others regard it as a first-line drug for brain injury because of its ability to lower intracranial pressure rapidly. In short, each brain-injured patient is unique and requires individualized therapy.

During treatment of the brain-injured pet, continued monitoring of the patient's general physical and neurologic status is essential; the monitoring interval is dictated by the severity of injuries and neurologic dysfunction as well as the rate at which the patient is improving or deteriorating. A dog or cat that has sustained a concussion injury and is in stable condition can be monitored every four to six hours in the absence of neurologic deterioration; however, an animal with significant disturbance of consciousness (i.e., severe depression or coma) with or without other significant injuries should initially be monitored every 15 to 60 minutes.[13–14] Neurologic progression or deterioration should be recorded periodically in the form of a coma scale score.[13–16] Broad-spectrum antibiotics with effective central nervous system penetration (e.g., trimethoprim-sulfadiazine and chloramphenicol) are indicated with suspected or confirmed open skull fractures, with open and potentially contaminated wounds on other areas of the body, and as prophylactic agents for intracranial surgery.[13,14]

During hospitalization, nursing care is vital to management of brain-injured patients.[9,13] Adequate nutrition is necessary because brain-injured patients have elevated caloric requirements. Recumbent patients should be placed in well-padded areas and turned often (at least every six hours) to avoid decubital sores. Frequent turning of recumbent patients also decreases the chance of atelectasis in dependent lung lobes. Bedding should be cleaned as necessary to prevent urine and fecal scalding.[13–17]

Initial Emergency Therapy

Many head trauma victims are in a state of hypovolemic shock on presentation to the emergency veterinarian. Because hypoxia and hypotension are extremely detrimental to an already compromised brain, establishing adequate oxygen delivery and cardiovascular support are immediate therapeutic requirements.[2,5–14,16]

Oxygenation and Hyperventilation

Hyperoxygenation is recommended for most brain-injured animals.[11–14,16,18,19] Methods of oxygen supplementation include oxygen cages, nasal oxygen catheters (Figure 2), transtracheal oxygen catheters, and tracheal intubation.[13,14,16] Oxygen cages are least effective for oxygen delivery to a brain-injured patient because they provide an environment of approximately 40% oxygen, which quickly drops to 20% after the cage door is opened. Because most brain-injured animals require constant monitoring, oxygen cages do not allow for concomitant close patient observation and maintenance of a high-oxygen environment.[16,20]

Although administration of oxygen to the patient by means of a nasal or transtracheal catheter is of questionable efficacy in reducing brain swelling, it should be done if the patient is not going to be intubated and hyperventilated.[13,16] Because one potential hazard of nasal oxygen catheter placement is invasion of the cranial cavity by the catheter through a rostral skull fracture, placement of a transtracheal catheter may be preferable.[16,20] Inadvertent compression of the jugular veins must be kept at a minimum during placement of a transtracheal catheter. With nasal and transtracheal oxygen catheters, an inspired oxygen concentration of 40% is provided with flow rates of 100 ml/kg/min and 50 ml/kg/min, respectively. It has been reported that oxygen concentrations as high as 95% can be delivered to the patient with propor-

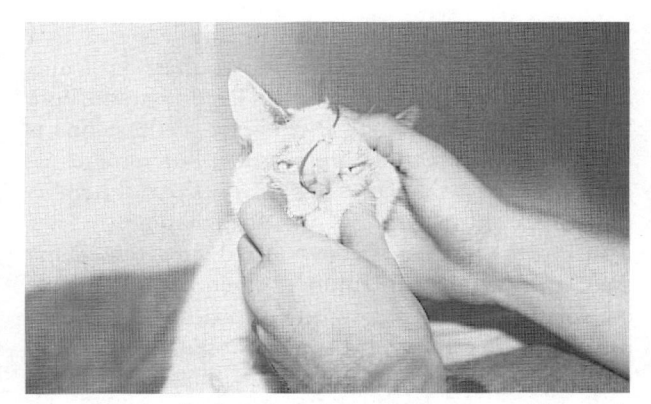

Figure 2—Nasal administration of oxygen to a cat with cerebral trauma.

tionally higher flow rates.[16,20] The most effective means of reducing or preventing the brain swelling secondary to hypercapnia is controlled hyperventilation and hyperoxygenation with 100% oxygen (a 95% oxygen with 5% carbon dioxide mixture has also been recommended) through an endotracheal or tracheostomy tube.[8,11,13]

Hyperventilation reduces cerebral blood volume as much as 36%, whereas hypoventilation has been associated with increases in cerebral blood volume as high as 170%.[10] A tracheostomy tube may be useful in patients with oscillating states of consciousness, in which an endotracheal tube cannot be predictably maintained.[13] If the patient's level of consciousness permits, an endotracheal or tracheostomy tube should be passed and the animal is placed on a mechanical ventilator.

If blood gas measurement or capnography is available, arterial blood PCO_2 levels or end tidal carbon dioxide concentration ($ETCO_2$) should be maintained between 25 and 35 mm Hg; PCO_2 levels in this range can usually be achieved with a ventilatory rate of 10 to 20 breaths/min.[8,13,14,16,21] It is generally recommended that human patients with a coma score of 8 or less be intubated and ventilated with 100% oxygen.[10] The head of the patient should be kept elevated at approximately a 30° angle to ensure adequate venous return of blood from the head.[16,21] Oxygen humidification is recommended with nasal, transtracheal, and endotracheal oxygen administration.[20]

Emergency Fluid Therapy

The goal of fluid support in brain-injured pets is to administer the minimum amount of fluid necessary to maintain hydration and normal blood pressure. It is standard emergency protocol to administer shock doses (40 to 90 ml/kg/hr) of isotonic crystalloid fluids (e.g., lactated Ringer's solution or 0.9% sodium chloride) to hypotensive brain-injured animals. Administration of such large volumes of isotonic fluids to brain-injured patients has, however, been associated with worsening of brain edema and further increases in intracranial pressure.[11,14,16,19,21]

Hypertonic (hypertonic saline) and colloid (e.g., dextran and hetastarch) solutions have recently been investigated as potential alternative resuscitative fluids for head trauma victims.[16,22–37] Hypertonic saline (7%) has received considerable attention and is considered by many veterinarians to be the resuscitative fluid of choice for brain-injured dogs and cats.[16,22] The administration of small volumes (4 to 5 ml/kg) of hypertonic saline to hypotensive animals has been shown to increase myocardial contractility and cardiac output, improve peripheral perfusion, increase urine output, and improve mesenteric and coronary blood flow.[22,23,25,26] Hypertonic saline administration has also been shown to protect against increases in cerebral edema and intracranial pressure, even with subsequent administration of isotonic crystalloid solutions.[22–25,27–30] The cardiovascular stabilizing effects of hypertonic saline are believed to be the result of osmotic expansion of the vasculature as well as vagally mediated reflexes initiated by stimulation of osmoreceptors in the lungs, although the latter mechanism of action has recently been questioned.[23–25] The stabilizing effects of hypertonic saline are transient (15 to 60 minutes); however, there is some evidence that the effects can be prolonged by concurrent administration of 6% dextran 70 or hetastarch.[22–25]

Hypertonic saline should not be used in the presence of dehydration, if uncontrolled hemorrhage is strongly suspected or confirmed, if the patient is already hypernatremic or otherwise in a hyperosmolar state (e.g., ketoacidotic), or if the patient is hypothermic. Hypertonic saline should also be avoided in patients with congestive heart failure or anuric renal failure.[22–24,31] There is some controversy concerning the use of hypertonic saline in patients with acute brain injury because it is usually impossible to tell whether ongoing hemorrhage is occurring within the cranial vault. Hypertonic saline should be given slowly intravenously for a period of three to five minutes.[22–24] In dogs, dosing of hypertonic saline may be repeated, if necessary, to a total dose of 10 ml/kg (4 to 5 ml/kg is the maximum dose in cats).[24] Osmolality and the serum sodium level must be within normal limits if the maximum dose is exceeded because hypernatremia and hyperosmolality have been associated with high mortality.[22,24,38] A recent experimental study showed that a maintenance infusion of a slightly hypertonic solution (1.8% saline) supported systemic pressure and reduced rises in intracranial pressure after a focal brain injury.[33] Combinations of hypertonic and isotonic fluids should be administered to maintain mean arterial pressure at approximately 100 mm Hg.[21]

High-molecular-weight dextran (dextran 70) has not demonstrated the same protective effects against brain swelling that hypertonic saline has shown. Dextran has been reported to be associated with anaphylactic reactions (as well as coagulopathy and renal failure), but the incidence of such complications is apparently low.[22,23,30,34]

Because dextrans decrease platelet function, their use should be avoided in thrombocytopenic patients.[23,24] Six percent hetastarch at an intravenous dose of 20 ml/kg has been shown to have cardiovascular stabilizing and brain protective effects similar to those of hypertonic saline.[24,34–37] Although hypertonic saline and hetastarch succeed in reducing or preventing brain edema and elevations in intracranial pressure, they fail to increase oxygen delivery and overall perfusion to damaged brain tissue.[28,36]

The neurologic examination of the hypotensive brain-injured patient often inaccurately reflects the true neurologic status of the patient; therefore, once normal blood pressure is regained, the patient may appear dramatically improved neurologically. Because of this fact, the neurologic status of the hypotensive patient should not be the sole basis for deciding whether to pursue therapy.[8]

Glucocorticoids

Administration of glucocorticoids (e.g., dexamethasone, prednisone, and prednisolone) remains a standard yet controversial aspect of medical therapy for veterinary patients with head trauma.[5–7,11–14,19,21,39] Proposed benefits of glucocorticoid administration include stabilization of plasma membranes (including lysosomal membranes) in the central nervous system, increased energy supply to central nervous system tissue, reduced production of cerebrospinal fluid, reduced central nervous system edema, promotion of diuresis, and reduced oxygen free radical formation.[5,6,11,13,14,39,40,41]

The primary rationale for glucocorticoid administration is to reduce brain swelling through the aforementioned mechanisms. The type and dose of glucocorticoid used vary considerably among clinicians. Dexamethasone, which is the least expensive and most widely used glucocorticoid, is given initially at an intravenous dose of 1 to 4 mg/kg; the same dose (or a gradually tapering dose) is given six to eight hours later, and tapering doses are administered every six to eight hours for the next 48 to 72 hours, depending on the clinical response of the patient.[5,7,13,39] Some authors recommend even lower doses of dexamethasone (in the range of 0.2 to 0.4 mg/kg) if the patient is not in shock; if the patient is in shock, initial doses of 1 to 4 mg/kg are recommended.[11,12,21]

Prednisone-prednisolone can be administered in a similar schedule at equipotent doses that, on a milligram basis, are five to eight times larger than the dose level of dexamethasone.[42] Prednisone-prednisolone is more expensive than dexamethasone, but some clinicians believe that it causes less gastrointestinal hemorrhage than equivalent doses of dexamethasone.

Although they are effective in reducing the edema associated with brain tumors, glucocorticoids have consistently failed to show any statistically significant beneficial effects (experimentally or clinically) on the outcome of acute brain trauma or spinal cord trauma at the doses commonly given to patients with brain disorders.[5,10–14,41,43–46] Research in human head trauma management has shown no beneficial effect of standard glucocorticoid therapy on reduction of intracranial pressure, reduction of cerebral edema, or improvement of overall clinical response.[10,44–46]

High-Dose Methylprednisolone Protocol

A recent and promising development in the area of glucocorticoid therapy for central nervous system trauma is the high-dose methylprednisolone protocol. Large intravenous doses of methylprednisolone sodium succinate have been shown experimentally and clinically to reduce nervous tissue destruction and ischemia and to improve neurologic outcome in spinal cord or brain trauma.[41,47–57] Currently, the recommended high-dose protocol is an initial dose of 30 mg/kg followed by 15 mg/kg two and six hours after the initial dose. These bolus doses should be injected slowly intravenously over a period of several minutes. After the second follow-up dose has been given six hours after the initial dose, the patient is placed on a continuous intravenous infusion at a dosage of 2.5 mg/kg/hr for the next 42 hours; at the end of this time, steroid administration is discontinued.[41,47]

Because some concentrations of methylprednisolone are incompatible with diluent (e.g., lactated Ringer's solution, 0.9% sodium chloride, or 5% dextrose in water), compatibility information should be gathered before the continuous intravenous infusion is prepared.[58] A total methylprednisolone dose of 165 mg/kg is thus administered within a 48-hour period.[41,47] Because this dose level of methylprednisolone far exceeds those necessary to activate steroid receptors, it is believed that the mechanisms of action may be unrelated to direct glucocorticoid (hormonal) effects. The main therapeutic effect of the high-dose methylprednisolone protocol may be attenuation of oxygen free radical–mediated damage (peroxidation) of central nervous system membrane lipids.[41,47]

High-dose methylprednisolone has been shown to decrease injury-induced spinal lipid peroxidation in vitro and in vivo.[41,47–51] Other postulated beneficial effects of the high-dose methylprednisolone protocol (some of which may be directly related to antioxidant activity) include support of cellular energy metabolism, prevention or reversal of intracellular calcium accumulation, inhibition of formation of arachidonic acid metabolites, and attenuation of postinjury central nervous system ischemia and acidosis.[41,47-53] Studies on human and feline spinal cord trauma suggest that high-dose methylprednisolone therapy is most effective if given within the first few hours after trauma; virtually no effect was noted if therapy was begun more than eight hours after trauma.

Deleterious side effects of glucocorticoid administration (e.g., hemorrhagic gastroenteritis, gastric and colonic perforation, and pancreatitis) were rare when high-dose methylprednisolone was given to cats and humans.[48,55,56] Administering prednisolone sodium succinate instead of methylprednisolone sodium succinate at the same high-dose schedule mentioned previously has been suggested as an acceptable alternative.[7] In vivo and in vitro experiments with mice have shown, however, that high-dose prednisolone sodium succinate is only half as potent as high-dose methylprednisolone sodium succinate as a neuroprotective agent and antioxidant when given at equivalent doses.[57]

More recently, synthetic 21-aminosteroid nonglucocorticoid analogs of methylprednisolone have been developed. It is hoped that these analogs will have central nervous system protective effects similar to high-dose methylprednisolone without the potential deleterious side effects of the glucocorticoids.[59-62]

Mannitol

Mannitol (25%) is an osmotic diuretic that has been shown to be effective in reducing brain edema and intracranial pressure.[5,7,10,11,21,40,63] Mannitol draws extravascular fluid into the intravascular space, thereby relieving brain edema by a local dehydrating action and a general osmotic diuretic action. Other proposed beneficial effects of mannitol include reduction of cerebrospinal fluid production, oxygen free radical scavenging action, and cerebral arteriolar vasoconstriction.[10,11,21,40,41,64] Mannitol is recommended at a dose of 0.25 to 2.0 g/kg given slowly intravenously during a period of 20 to 30 minutes.[5-7,10,11,19,21,40,63] Because mannitol tends to form crystals at room temperature (22°C [72°F]), warming the drug to 37°C (99°F) before administration is recommended.[11,40] An in-line filter should also be used when administering mannitol.[11,40]

Mannitol exerts an antiedema effect within 30 to 60 minutes, and the effect lasts for two to four hours. The efficacy of doses at the lower end of the range is reported to be similar to that of higher doses, but the effect lasts for a shorter period.[5,11,21,40] On administration, mannitol causes a mild, transient rise in intracranial pressure; this effect is minimized if the drug is given slowly during a period of 20 minutes. A rebound phenomenon has also been described with mannitol use in brain-injured animals. This phenomenon refers to a rise in intracranial pressure above baseline as the level of mannitol in the blood subsides. The rebound phenomenon is less pronounced with mannitol than with other osmotic diuretics that penetrate the extravascular compartment. Mannitol administration can be repeated every three to eight hours, depending on clinical response, for a maximum of three doses in 24 hours.[6,7,11,13,21,40]

Several precautions must be taken if mannitol is to be used. Mannitol administration is strictly contraindicated in patients that are dehydrated or in hypovolemic shock. Serum electrolytes and serum osmolality should be monitored, especially if multiple mannitol doses are to be administered. Serum osmolality should be maintained below 320 mosm/L, and serum electrolytes should be maintained in the normal range. Urine output should be monitored during mannitol therapy, which, in recumbent stuporous or comatose patients, may necessitate indwelling urethral catheterization with a closed urinary collection system. If no urine is produced within one hour of mannitol administration, furosemide should be given at 2 to 5 mg/kg to induce diuresis. Mannitol is contraindicated in patients with congestive heart failure, anuric renal failure, and pulmonary edema.[5,6,8,10-14,21,38,40,41,64]

The use of mannitol in brain-injured dogs and cats is highly controversial and poses inherent risks.[6,7,11-14] The controversy centers around the safety of administration of mannitol in a situation in which ongoing, undetectable intracranial hemorrhage may be occurring. In such cases, there are several theoretical pitfalls associated with administration of the drug. Because osmotic particles may equilibrate between extravascular and intravascular blood in areas of active hemorrhage, one concern is that the extravascular hemorrhage may increase in these areas as a result of the osmotic action of mannitol. Because the agent draws fluid intravascularly and therefore increases blood volume within brain vasculature, another concern is that increased blood flow may exacerbate ongoing hemorrhage. Finally, by decreasing brain size, mannitol may provide more room for further extravasation of epidural or subdural hemorrhage.[6,7,11-14]

These theoretical contraindications to the use of mannitol in brain-injured pets have not been confirmed through experimentation as actual phenomena.[13] Some authors recommend routine use of mannitol in head trauma patients, whereas others recommend use of the drug only in extreme or deteriorating situations. Because subdural and clinically significant epidural hematomas are reportedly rare and edema is common, we advocate the use of mannitol for reducing intracranial pressure (despite other medical therapies), especially if the patient is severely depressed or comatose or if the patient's condition is deteriorating rapidly. If the patient's neurologic status deteriorates rapidly after administration of mannitol, the veterinarian should be prepared for an emergency craniotomy-craniectomy to alleviate uncontrolled intracranial hemorrhage and edema or accept a potentially hopeless turn of events.

Furosemide

Furosemide, a loop diuretic, has been shown to reduce intracranial pressure in head trauma victims. The agent presumably exerts its effects by causing diuresis, decreasing cerebrospinal fluid production, and reducing astroglial swelling.[8,9,11–13,19,21,64–66] Some evidence suggests that administration of furosemide in conjunction with mannitol provides a synergistic effect in reducing intracranial pressure.[8,19,21,64] It has also been suggested that administering furosemide at a dose of 2 to 5 mg/kg intravenously a few minutes before intravenous infusion of mannitol may prevent the initial rise in intracranial pressure associated with mannitol administration as well as the rebound of intracranial pressure associated with decreasing serum levels of mannitol.[21,67]

Furosemide administration can be repeated every six hours, depending on the clinical response. To minimize dangers of hypotension and electrolyte abnormalities, furosemide therapy should not be extended beyond 24 hours. Serum electrolytes and osmolality and urine output must be monitored with prolonged furosemide therapy (repeated doses), especially if mannitol is administered concurrently. As with mannitol, the use of furosemide is strictly contraindicated in hypotensive or dehydrated patients.[8,11,13,21] A combination of albumin and furosemide has been shown experimentally to have effects similar to those of mannitol and furosemide in reducing intracranial pressure without the undesirable side effect of systemic dehydration.[66]

Dimethyl Sulfoxide

Despite conflicting opinions concerning its efficacy in central nervous system trauma, dimethyl sulfoxide has persisted for years as a potentially useful neuroprotective agent in veterinary medicine.[5–7,9,11,12,41,68] Dimethyl sulfoxide has been effective in reducing intracranial pressure and improving the outcome of brain injury, both experimentally and clinically.[9,68–72] Dimethyl sulfoxide reportedly exerts beneficial neuroprotective effects by reducing oxygen and glucose requirements of brain tissue (i.e., reduced cerebral metabolic rate), scavenging oxygen free radical species, stabilizing lysosomal membranes, directly decreasing brain edema by stabilizing capillary endothelial cells, and indirectly reducing brain edema through antiinflammatory and diuretic properties.[41,68,69,71,72] Dimethyl sulfoxide is recommended at a dose of 0.5 to 1.0 g/kg intravenously during a period of 30 to 45 minutes every 8 to 12 hours.[41,73]

Although a number of potential toxic side effects (e.g., intravascular hemolysis and prolonged bleeding times) have been noted with dimethyl sulfoxide therapy, such signs rarely occur with therapeutic doses and are usually of little clinical significance. The most commonly reported toxic side effects are intravascular hemolysis and associated hemoglobinuria, but these signs rarely appreciably alter the patient's packed cell volume. The degree of hemolysis depends on the concentration and rate of administration of dimethyl sulfoxide; hemolysis occurs most commonly with dimethyl sulfoxide concentrations exceeding 20%. Recommended dimethyl sulfoxide concentrations range from 10% to 40%.[68,71,73] The main disadvantage of using concentrations at the low end of the range is that a large fluid bolus must be given, and this is contraindicated in the presence of elevated intracranial pressure. We believe that dimethyl sulfoxide therapy is warranted for brain-injured pets because of reports of efficacy as well as the low level of toxicity associated with its use.

Barbiturates

Barbiturates have been demonstrated to decrease intracranial pressure after brain injury, but evidence of improvement in neurologic function and overall outcome is lacking.[9,10,18,74–76] High-dose barbiturate therapy, or induction of a barbiturate coma, has been advocated in human head trauma victims with intracranial pressures refractory to conventional medical therapy.[9,10,18] Barbiturates are believed to reduce intracranial pressure by reducing oxygen and glucose demands of neural tissue (decreased metabolic rate) and by reducing cerebral blood flow by decreasing systemic arterial pressure and increasing cerebral vascular resistance.[7,9,10,40,41] Barbiturates have also demonstrated oxygen free radical scavenging ability, but this ability is reportedly of minor significance.[74,76]

Because they can cause profound hypotension, barbiturates must be used with extreme caution, especially if other potentially hypotensive drugs (e.g., mannitol and furosemide) have been administered.[9,10,75] Barbiturate coma can be induced with an initial intravenous loading dose of sodium pentobarbital (3 to 5 mg/kg) given to effect and followed by 1 to 3 mg/kg of the drug to effect, as needed.[64]

The objective of barbiturate therapy is to minimize

brain electrical activity (as measured by an electroencephalogram) while adequate systemic blood pressure is maintained. It has been suggested, however, that this objective can be more reliably obtained through use of a continuous intravenous infusion protocol instead of intermittent boluses.[77] In human head trauma medicine, barbiturate coma is considered a potentially dangerous therapy necessitating very close monitoring of systemic and intracranial pressures; in veterinary medicine, this danger is magnified by the often limited ability to monitor patients intensively.[10] Also, because of this limitation, the proper time for discontinuing high-dose barbiturate therapy is an arbitrary estimation (24 to 48 hours) and is not based on a measurable clinical response (i.e., declining intracranial pressure).

There is evidence that induction of barbiturate coma in the presence of an expanding intracranial mass lesion (e.g., enlarging hematoma) is ineffective in reducing intracranial pressure and may adversely affect brain perfusion.[78] Although we recommend judicious use of sodium pentobarbital for such problems as uncontrolled seizure activity or vocalizing and thrashing brain-injured patients, induction and maintenance of barbiturate coma should be done only when all other measures have failed.

Antioxidant Drugs

In addition to the drugs with suspected or proven antioxidant activity that have already been discussed, there are several experimental drugs with a principal therapeutic action that is aimed at attenuation or prevention of damage to brain tissue induced by oxygen free radicals. There is abundant evidence that oxygen free radical production after brain trauma is a major contributor to brain tissue autolysis and brain edema.[79] Superoxide radical production has been demonstrated to continue for at least one hour after experimental brain injury in cats.[80]

Deferoxamine mesylate is a potent iron chelator that readily crosses the blood–brain barrier and cellular membranes. The agent inhibits iron-dependent, oxygen free radical–producing reactions by forming a chemically inert complex with iron; this complex is then excreted in the urine. Deferoxamine mesylate does not interfere with the oxygen transport function of hemoglobin.

Although clinical studies are lacking, experimental evidence has shown deferoxamine mesylate to be effective in reducing cold-induced brain edema in cats and in improving neurologic outcome in dogs subjected to a brief period of cardiac arrest. The recommended dose of deferoxamine mesylate is 25 to 50 mg/kg intramuscularly or very slowly intravenously. Intravenous injection of the drug has been associated with profound hypotension; therefore, if the intravenous route is chosen, the drug should be given over at least a 20-minute period. Deferoxamine mesylate should not be given concurrently with phenothiazine drugs because the combination has been associated with such neurologic side effects as visual deficits and loss of consciousness. Based on experimental evidence of efficacy and the low incidence of side effects, we advocate the use of deferoxamine mesylate very early in the therapy of brain-injured pets.[74,81–85]

Superoxide dismutase and catalase are two endogenously occurring enzymes that convert the more reactive superoxide radical to successively less reactive molecules. Most experimental evidence shows that administration of exogenous superoxide dismutase and catalase provides no beneficial effect unless given in advance of brain injury. Recent studies with liposome-encapsulated forms of these agents show more promise; liposome encapsulation enhances intracellular entry of these agents.[80–83,86–90]

Allopurinol inhibits the enzyme xanthine oxidase.[7] Xanthine oxidase is important in reperfusion injury, which is a major pathway for oxygen free radical production after brain ischemia. Although clinical studies have not been reported, experimental studies have shown allopurinol and its longer lived metabolite, oxypurinol, to improve neurologic outcome in animal models of brain ischemia.[75,81,82,91] Superoxide dismutase, catalase, and allopurinol appear promising as potential neuroprotective agents, but their use cannot be recommended at this time.

Miscellaneous Drugs

A number of other potential therapeutic agents are under investigation. It has been suggested (and supported experimentally) that release or activation of endogenous opioids after trauma may contribute to secondary damage of tissue of the central nervous system. There are conflicting reports concerning efficacy of opiate antagonists (e.g., naloxone hydrochloride) in preventing posttraumatic destruction of the brain and spinal cord. Extremely high doses (2 to 5 mg/kg) of naloxone hydrochloride were used in the studies that showed beneficial effects of naloxone hydrochloride therapy.[8,11,41,56,92,93]

Thyrotropin-releasing hormone reportedly acts as an opiate antagonist and has been investigated as a potential therapeutic agent; however, evidence concerning the efficacy of this hormone is also conflicting.[11,41] Calcium channel blockers (e.g., verapamil, diltiazem hydrochloride, and nimodipine) have also been studied as potential neuroprotective agents. They reportedly reduce cerebral vasospasm and improve brain perfusion; however, other evidence suggests that calcium channel blockers increase intracranial pressure. Calci-

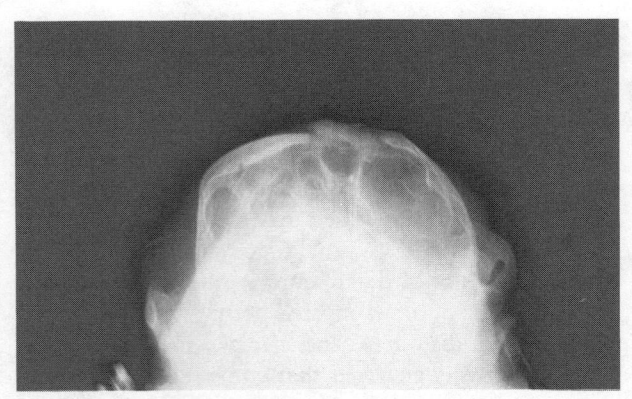

Figure 3—Depressed skull fracture of a dog with deteriorating neurologic status.

um channel blockers are known to have vasodilatory and negative inotropic effects; they therefore must be used with caution. The efficacy or inefficacy of calcium channel blockers remains controversial.[10,11,41,74]

Tromethamine is a buffering agent that penetrates the central nervous system and is theoretically superior to sodium bicarbonate for treatment of central nervous system acidosis after trauma. There is also some evidence that tromethamine has beneficial effects on decreasing intracranial pressure.[8]

SURGICAL TREATMENT
Indications for Surgery

Surgical intervention is warranted for management of open skull fractures and skull fractures depressed more than the width of the calvarium in the fracture area (Figure 3), for retrieval of potentially contaminated bone fragments or foreign material (e.g., bullets) lodged in brain parenchyma, for debridement of associated damaged brain tissue, for persistent leakage of cerebrospinal fluid, and as a decompressive maneuver associated with deteriorating neurologic status despite aggressive medical therapy.[7,9,11,13,14,16,19,94] In the absence of neurologic deterioration, surgery for open or depressed skull fractures, cerebrospinal fluid leakage, or embedded bone or foreign material may be postponed for 24 to 48 hours if time is needed for patient stabilization.[14,19] If the patient is cardiovascularly stable, surgery should be done as soon as possible.

In cases of embedded bone fragments or foreign material in brain parenchyma, the surgeon must take into account the portion of the brain to be explored and debrided. Potential benefits of surgery in reducing the chance of brain infection must be weighed against potential risks of surgery causing severe neurologic dysfunction or death.[94]

Anesthetic Considerations

There is no ideal anesthetic agent or protocol for intracranial surgery. Because intracranial pressure is intimately tied to ventilation and oxygenation (and inhalation anesthetic agents tend to increase intracranial pressure), the sooner the patient is intubated and hyperventilated with 100% oxygen, the better. Preanesthetic agents should be avoided because even slight respiratory depression and the associated hypoventilation produced by a 10- to 15-minute preanesthetic period could be detrimental when combined with the effects of inhalation anesthetics. Barbiturates (e.g., thiopental sodium) alone or in combination with narcotics (e.g., oxymorphone hydrochloride) and/or benzodiazepines (e.g., diazepam and midazolam hydrochloride) should be used for rapid induction. These drugs offer some protection against brain swelling at commonly used doses.[21,95,96]

Propofol, a new phenolic intravenous anesthetic drug, has been shown to be a safe and effective neuroanesthetic agent.[97] Depolarizing and nondepolarizing neuromuscular blocking agents are also acceptable neuroanesthetic drugs. Ketamine hydrochloride is contraindicated as an induction agent because it causes increased intracranial pressure. Phenothiazine tranquilizers (e.g., acepromazine maleate) and xylazine hydrochloride are contraindicated because they may precipitate seizures.

Intubation should proceed quickly and smoothly because patient struggling and coughing caused by ineffective intubation attempts result in significant increases in intracranial pressure. Methoxyflurane, halothane, isoflurane, and nitrous oxide elevate intracranial pressure by increasing cerebral blood flow; however, hyperventilation and hyperoxygenation easily overcome this undesirable effect of all the inhalation anesthetics except halothane.

Halothane has exhibited toxic effects on oxidative pathways of brain cells and, when used in brain-injured patients, has been associated with greater incidence of brain herniation than other inhalation anesthetics. Because of adverse effects on brain autoregulatory mechanisms, halothane anesthesia in brain-injured patients is not recommended. Isoflurane is the inhalation anesthetic of choice for brain-injured patients.[21,95,96]

Hyperventilation and hyperoxygenation should follow the guidelines previously discussed. Patients should be slowly weaned from 100% oxygen in order to avoid oxygen toxicity; oxygen toxicity has been reported to occur in dogs within 24 hours of oxygen administration.[98] Dextrose supplementation of anesthesia fluids should be avoided because hyperglycemia may worsen brain ischemia.[96] A commercial or homemade head stand should be used to position the patient for intracranial surgery. Proper positioning involves elevating the head and avoiding compression of the jugular veins[99] (Figure 4).

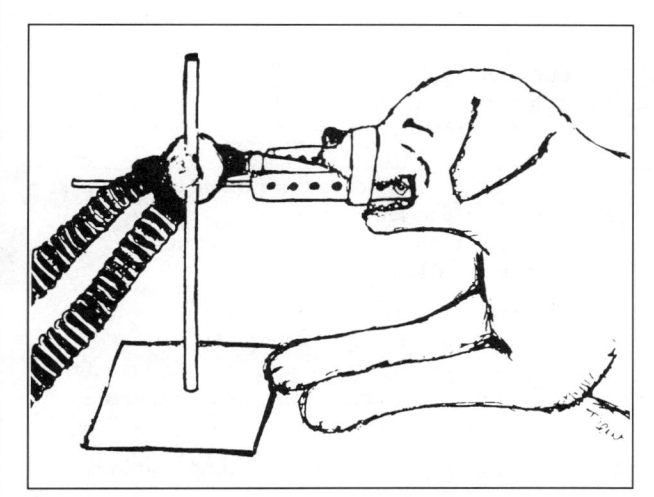

Figure 4—Proper positioning of a patient for intracranial surgery.

Surgical Procedure

The specifics of intracranial surgery are beyond the scope of this article; more detailed information can be obtained from excellent discussions in other literature.[100,101] The most common approach to the brain in the head trauma patient is the rostrotentorial or lateral approach.[13,14,16,19,101] Approaches to the rostral and caudal fossae have also been described but are not commonly used.[101,102] After reflection of the skin and temporalis muscle on one side, the limits of the rostrotentorial craniotomy-craniectomy are defined by four bur holes through the calvarium as shown in Figure 5.[14] The bur holes are connected and the resultant bone flap is removed, thereby exposing the cerebrum. Evacuation of intracranial hematomas and removal of foreign material, bone fragments, and devitalized brain tissue can then be done. Care must be taken not to lacerate the dorsal sagittal and transverse venous sinuses or the middle meningeal artery.[101] If possible, the dura is closed to avoid herniation of brain tissue through a dural opening and to prevent potential development of a cerebrospinal fluid fistula.[95,103] If dural closure is impossible, a temporalis fascial graft can be used as a dural substitute. Inert, synthetic dural substitutes may soon be available.[104] Whether to replace the bone flap is based primarily on the degree of brain swelling seen at surgery. When extensive brain swelling exists, the bone flap is not replaced.[19]

A number of fairly new neurosurgical instruments that are commonly used in human brain surgery are becoming more readily available to veterinary neurosurgeons in university and private referral practices. Among these new instruments are the carbon dioxide laser and the ultrasonic aspirator.[99]

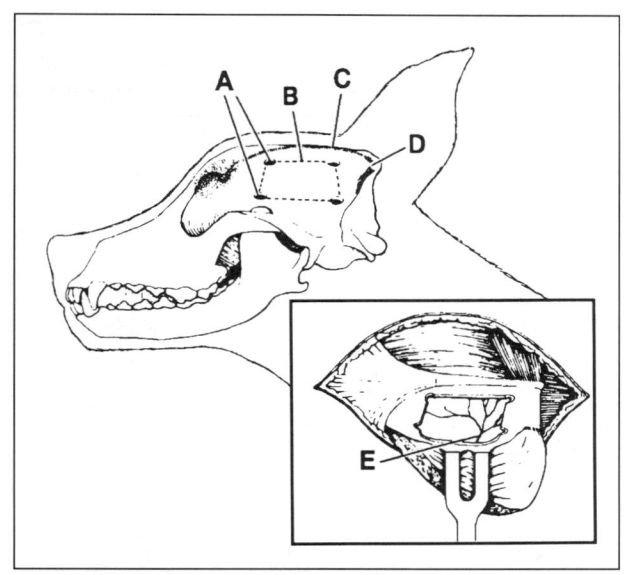

Figure 5—Anatomic guidelines for bur holes and a lateral rostrotentorial craniotomy in the treatment of brain trauma. A = rostral pair of bur holes. B = lines for connecting the bur holes to perform the craniotomy. C = dorsal sagittal venous sinus. D = transverse venous sinus. E = middle meningeal artery. (From Shores A: Craniocerebral trauma, in Kirk RW (ed): *Current Veterinary Therapy. X.* Philadelphia, WB Saunders Co, 1989, pp 847-853. Reprinted with permission.)

MONITORING OF INTRACRANIAL PRESSURE

Intracranial pressure monitoring is commonly done in human head trauma patients. Progressive elevation of intracranial pressure has been associated with poor outcomes in brain-injured humans. Aggressive medical and/or surgical therapy based on increasing intracranial pressure (instead of gross neurologic signs of deterioration) has resulted in lower morbidity and mortality.[105,106] Intracranial pressure can be measured by intraventricular, subarachnoid, subdural, and epidural catheters.[64,107] With the recent advent of a fiber-optic intracranial pressure monitor, pressure readings can now be taken directly from brain parenchyma.[108,109] Each of the monitoring systems has advantages and disadvantages[107] (Table II[10]). Recent research with the fiber-optic monitor in dogs suggests that this device could be a useful adjunct to veterinary head trauma therapy[108]; however, the expense of the monitor may limit its use in veterinary medicine. Use of an easily implantable, inexpensive epidural monitoring system in dogs and cats has recently been suggested.[16] Although it is still in the experimental stage, intracranial pressure monitoring is likely to become an integral part of head trauma management in veterinary patients.

TABLE II
**Advantages and Disadvantages of Common Types of
Intracranial Pressure Monitors Used in Human Victims of Head Trauma[10]**

Monitor	Advantages	Disadvantages
Ventricular catheters	Accurate and reliable	Requires brain penetration and may be difficult to place in some instances Highest infection rate of current monitors External transducer required
Subarachnoid bolts	No brain penetration Very low infection rate	External transducer required Firm fixation into skull required May be unreliable under some clinical conditions Must be placed coplanar to brain surface for optimum function
Epidural monitors	No brain or dural penetration Very low infection rate	Requires bur hole, dural stripping, and intact skull Must be accurately placed for optimum function
Fiber-optic parenchymal monitors	Easily placed Functions well in parenchymal, subarachnoid, or intraventricular spaces Wave forms and responses equivalent to ventricular catheters Very low infection rate Does not require a fluid column	Minimal brain penetration Cannot be re-zeroed once placed Expensive

PROGNOSIS AND COMPLICATIONS

Prediction of morbidity and mortality is extremely difficult in brain-injured animals and humans, especially those with severe neurologic dysfunction. The veterinarian should formulate a prognosis based on several observable or measurable factors for optimum accuracy. Such factors include level of consciousness, brain stem reflexes, motor ability, respiratory pattern, presence and extent of other injuries, responsiveness to therapy, and age and general physical status.[13,14,110–113] In management of head trauma in humans, the Glasgow Coma Scale has been shown to be very accurate in predicting outcome, especially in terms of mortality.[109-112] It is hoped that the Small Animal Coma Scale (SACS) will prove to be a reliable prognostic indicator for brain-injured dogs and cats.[13,14]

Although no single clinical sign or observation is an absolute indicator of a poor to hopeless outcome, some signs highly suggest irreversible damage that will culminate in permanent dysfunction or death. Such signs include coma persisting for more than 48 hours despite therapy, decerebrate rigidity, and ataxic or apneustic respiratory patterns in comatose patients.[5,13,16,17,79]

Potential complications associated with brain injury in dogs and cats include nosocomial pneumonia and sepsis, disorders of coagulation (including disseminated intravascular coagulation), cerebrospinal fluid fistula formation, intracranial infection with open skull fractures or missile injuries to the brain, and development of epileptic seizure activity.[9,10]

SUMMARY

Because the events leading to secondary autolytic brain tissue destruction subsequent to head trauma are diverse and complex, effective therapy is also diverse and complex. When presented with a brain-injured patient, the emergency veterinarian must immediately begin therapy because irreversible brain tissue destruction can occur within hours of the primary traumatic insult. Although most available drugs used for brain injury are controversial in terms of efficacy, the potential benefits of most of these agents warrant judicious administration.

Several new drugs and protocols are available to the practicing veterinarian. The emergency veterinarian should be familiar with the effects of anesthetic agents on the compromised brain and the indications for surgical intervention in brain-injured dogs and cats. Diligent effort should be made to arrive at an accurate prognosis in head-injured patients for appropriate decisions to be made.

About the Authors

Dr. Dewey is a Clinical Associate Professor in the Department of Small Animal Medicine and Surgery at Texas A&M University. Drs. Budsberg and Oliver are affiliated with the Department of Small Animal Medicine, College of Veterinary Medicine, University of Georgia, Athens, Georgia. Dr. Budsberg, who is a Diplomate of the American College of Veterinary Surgeons, is Associate Professor in the Department of Small Animal Medicine. Dr. Oliver, who is a Diplomate of the American College of Veterinary Internal Medicine (Neurology), is Full Professor in the Department of Small Animal Medicine.

REFERENCES

1. Steward O: Reorganization of neuronal connections following CNS trauma: Principles and experimental paradigms. *J Neurotrauma* 6(2):99–152, 1989.
2. Becker DP, Verity MA, Povlishock J, et al: Brain cellular injury and recovery—Horizons for improving medical therapies in stroke and trauma [specialty conference]. *West J Med* 158:670–684, 1988.
3. Erb DE, Povlishock JT: Axonal damage in severe traumatic brain injury: An experimental study in cat. *Acta Neuropathol* 76:347–358, 1988.
4. Rogers MC, Kirsch JR: Current concepts in brain resuscitation. *JAMA* 261(21):3143–3147, 1989.
5. Oliver JE: Intracranial injury, in Kirk RW (ed): *Current Veterinary Therapy. VII.* Philadelphia, WB Saunders Co, 1980, pp 815–820.
6. Selcer RR: Trauma to the central nervous system. *Vet Clin North Am Small Anim Pract* 10(3):619–639, 1980.
7. Colter S, Rucker NC: Acute injury to the central nervous system. *Vet Clin North Am Small Anim Pract* 18(3):545–561, 1988.
8. Narayan RK: Emergency room management of the head-injured patient, in Becker DP, Gudeman SK (eds): *Textbook of Head Injury.* Philadelphia, WB Saunders Co, 1990, pp 23–65.
9. Pitts LH, Martin N: Head injuries. *Surg Clin North Am* 62(1):47–60, 1982.
10. Luerssen TG, Marshall LF: The medical management of head injury, in Vinken PJ, Bruyn GW, Klawans HL (eds): *Handbook of Clinical Neurology: Head Injury.* New York, Elsevier Science Publishers B.V., 1990, pp 207–247.
11. LeCouteur R: Central nervous system trauma, in Kornegay (ed): *Contemporary Issues in Small Animal Practice: Neurologic Disorders.* New York, Churchill Livingstone, 1986, pp 147–167.
12. Fenner WR: Head trauma and nervous system injury, in Kirk RW (ed): *Current Veterinary Therapy. IX.* Philadelphia, WB Saunders Co, 1986, pp 830–836.
13. Shores A: Treatment and prognosis of head trauma. *Proc 13th Kal Kan Symp*:29–36, 1990.
14. Shores A: Craniocerebral trauma, in Kirk RW (ed): *Current Veterinary Therapy. X.* Philadelphia, WB Saunders Co, 1989, pp 847–853.
15. Shores A: Development of a coma scale for dogs: Prognostic value in cranio-cerebral trauma. *Proc 6th Annu Vet Med Forum*: 251–253, 1988.
16. Crowe DT: Triage and trauma management, in Murtaugh RJ, Kaplan PM (eds): *Veterinary Emergency and Critical Care Medicine.* St. Louis, CV Mosby, 1992, pp 77–121.
17. Young B, Ott L, Twyman D, et al: The effect of nutritional support on outcome from severe head injury. *J Neurosurg* 67:668–676, 1987.
18. Taboada J: The diagnostic and therapeutic approach to stupor and coma. *Proc 9th ACVIM Forum*:19–22, 1991.
19. Oliver JE: Neurologic emergencies in small animals. *Vet Clin North Am Small Anim Pract* 2(2):341–357, 1972.
20. Crowe DT: Managing respiration in the critical patient. *Vet Med* 84(1):55–76, 1989.
21. Dayrell-Hart B, Klide AM: Intracranial dysfunctions: Stupor and coma. *Vet Clin North Am Small Anim Pract* 19(6):1209–1222, 1989.
22. Gibbons G: Hypertonic solutions in the treatment of shock. *Proc 8th ACVIM Forum*:69–72, 1990.
23. Miller MW, Schertel ER, DiBartola SP: Conventional and hypertonic fluid therapy: Concepts and applications, in Murtaugh RJ, Kaplan PM (eds): *Veterinary Emergency and Critical Care Medicine.* St. Louis, CV Mosby, 1992, pp 618–628.
24. Schertel ER: Fluid therapy for noncardiogenic shock. *Proc 14th Kal Kan Symp*:27–31, 1991.
25. Maningas PA: Hypertonic sodium chloride solutions for the prehospital management of traumatic hemorrhagic shock: A possible improvement in the standard of care? *Ann Emerg Med* 15(2):1411–1414, 1986.
26. Velaseo IT, Pontiera V, Rocha E, et al: Hyperosmotic NaCl and severe hemorrhagic shock. *Am J Physiol* 239:H664–H673, 1980.
27. Todd MM, Tommasino C, Moore S: Cerebral effects of isovolemic hemodilution with a hypertonic saline solution. *J Neurosurg* 63:944–948, 1985.
28. Prough DS, Johnson JC, Stullken EH, et al: Effects on cerebral hemodynamics of resuscitation from endotoxic shock with hypertonic saline versus lactated Ringer's solution. *Crit Care Med* 13(12):1040–1044, 1985.
29. Prough DS, Johnson JC, Poole GV, et al: Effects on intracranial pressure of resuscitation from hemorrhagic shock with hypertonic saline versus lactated Ringer's solution. *Crit Care Med* 13(5):407–411, 1985.
30. Gunnar W, Jonasson O, Merlatti G, et al: Head injury and hemorrhagic shock: Studies of the blood brain barrier and intracranial pressure after resuscitation with normal saline solution, 3% saline solution, and dextran-40. *Surgery* 103(4):398–407, 1988.
31. Gross D, Landau EH, Assalia A, et al: Is hypertonic saline resuscitation safe in "uncontrolled" hemorrhagic shock? *J Trauma* 28(6):751–756, 1988.
32. Halvorsen L, Gunther RA, Dubick MA, et al: Dose response characteristics of hypertonic saline dextran solutions. *J Trauma* 31(6):785–794, 1991.
33. Shackford SR, Zhuang J, Schmoker J: Intravenous fluid tonicity: Effect on intracranial pressure, cerebral blood flow, and cerebral oxygen delivery in focal brain injury. *J Neurosurg* 76:91–98, 1992.
34. Kirby R: Clinical advantages of 6% hetastarch during fluid resuscitation. *Proc 2nd Int Vet Emerg Crit Care Symp*: 331–332, 1990.
35. Armistead CW, Vincent JL, Preiser JC, et al: Hypertonic saline solution-hetastarch for fluid resuscitation in experimental septic shock. *Anesth Analg* 69:714–720, 1989.
36. Poole GV, Johnson JC, Prough DS, et al: Cerebral hemodynamics after hemorrhagic shock: Effects of the type of resuscitation fluid. *Crit Care Med* 14(7):629–633, 1986.
37. Tommasino C, Moore S, Todd MM: Cerebral effects of isovolemic hemodilution with crystalloid and colloid solutions. *Crit Care Med* 16(9):862–868, 1988.
38. Bingham WF: The limits of cerebral dehydration in the

treatment of head injury. *Surg Neurol* 25(3):340–345, 1986.
39. Metz SR, Taylor SR, Kay WJ: The use of corticosteroids for treatment of neurologic disease. *Vet Clin North Am Small Anim Pract* 12(1):41–60, 1982.
40. Greene CE: Principles of medical therapy, in Oliver JE, Hoerlein BF, Mayhew IG (eds): *Veterinary Neurology*. Philadelphia, WB Saunders Co, 1987, pp 393–408.
41. Rucker NC: Management of spinal cord trauma. *Prog Vet Neurol* 1(4):397–411, 1990.
42. Chastain CB: Use of corticosteroids, in Ettinger SJ (ed): *Textbook of Veterinary Internal Medicine*. Philadelphia, WB Saunders Co, 1989, pp 413–428.
43. Tornheim PA, McLaurin RL: Effect of dexamethasone on cerebral edema from cranial impact in the cat. *J Neurosurg* 48:220–227, 1978.
44. Dearden NM, Gibson JS, Chir B, et al: Effect of high-dose dexamethasone on outcome from severe head injury. *J Neurosurg* 64:81–88, 1986.
45. Braakman R, Schouten HJA, Dishoek MJ, et al: Megadose steroids in severe head injury: Results of a prospective double-blind clinical trial. *J Neurosurg* 58:326–330, 1983.
46. Saul TG, Ducker TB, Salcman M, et al: Steroids in severe head injury. *J Neurosurg* 54:596–600, 1981.
47. Braughler JM, Hall ED, Means ED, et al: Evaluation of an intensive methylprednisolone sodium succinate dosing regimen in experimental spinal cord injury. *J Neurosurg* 67:102–105, 1987.
48. Braughler JM, Hall ED: Effects of multi-dose methylprednisolone sodium succinate administration on injured cat spinal cord neurofilament degradation and energy metabolism. *J Neurosurg* 61:290–295, 1984.
49. Braughler JM, Hall ED: Lactate and pyruvate metabolism in injured cat spinal cord before and after a single large intravenous dose of methylprednisolone. *J Neurosurg* 59:256–261, 1983.
50. Braughler JM, Hall ED: Correlation of methylprednisolone levels in cat spinal cord with its effects on (Na+ + K+)-ATPase, lipid peroxidation, and alpha motor neuron function. *J Neurosurg* 56:838–844, 1982.
51. Hall ED, Wolf DL, Braughler JM: Effects of a single large dose of methylprednisolone sodium succinate on experimental posttraumatic spinal cord ischemia: Dose-response and time-action analysis. *J Neurosurg* 61:124–130, 1984.
52. Hall ED: The neuroprotective pharmacology of methylprednisolone. *J Neurosurg* 76:13–22, 1992.
53. Hsu CY, Dimitrijeviz MR: Methylprednisolone in spinal cord injury: The possible mechanism of action. *J Neurotrauma* 7(3):115–119, 1990.
54. Braughler JM, Hall ED: Current application of "high-dose" steroid therapy for CNS injury: A pharmacological perspective. *J Neurosurg* 62:806–810, 1985.
55. Bracken MB, Shepard MJ, Collins WF, et al: A randomized, controlled trial of methylprednisolone or naloxone in the treatment of acute spinal-cord injury: Results of the second national acute spinal cord study. *N Engl J Med* 322(20):1405–1411, 1990.
56. Bracken MB, Shepard MJ, Collins WF, et al: Methylprednisolone or naloxone treatment after acute spinal cord injury: 1-year follow-up data: Results of the second national acute spinal cord injury study. *J Neurosurg* 76:22–31, 1992.
57. Hall ED: High-dose glucocorticoid treatment improves neurologic recovery in head-injured mice. *J Neurosurg* 62:882–887, 1985.
58. Trissel LA: *Handbook on Injectable Drugs*, ed 6. Houston, American Society of Hospital Pharmacists, pp 498–503, 1990.
59. Dimlich RVW, Tornheim PA, Kindel RM, et al: Effects of a 21-aminosteroid (U-74006F) on cerebral metabolites and edema after severe experimental head trauma: *Adv Neurol* 52:365–375, 1990.
60. Hall ED, Yonkers PA, McCall JM, et al: Effects of the 21-aminosteroid U74006F on experimental head injury in mice. *J Neurosurg* 68:456–461, 1988.
61. Hall ED, McCall JM, Chase RL, et al: A nonglucocorticoid steroid analog of methylprednisolone duplicates its high-dose pharmacology in models of central nervous system trauma and neuronal membrane damage. *J Pharmacol Exp Ther* 242(1):137–142, 1987.
62. Braughler JM, Pregenzer JF, Chase RL, et al: Novel 21-amino steroids as potent inhibitors of iron-dependent lipid peroxidation. *J Biol Chem* 262(22):10438–10440, 1987.
63. Miller JD, Leech P: Effects of mannitol and steroid therapy on intracranial volume-pressure relationships in patients. *J Neurosurg* 42:274–281, 1975.
64. Becker D, Remondino RL: Intracranial pressure monitoring, in Shoemaker WL, Ayres S, Grenvik A, et al (eds): *Textbook of Critical Care*. Philadelphia, WB Saunders Co, 1989, pp 291–295.
65. Cottrell JE, Marlin AE: Furosemide and human head injury. *J Trauma* 21(9):805–806, 1981.
66. Albright AL, Latchaw RE, Robinson AG: Intracranial and systemic effects of osmotic and oncotic therapy in experimental cerebral edema. *J Neurosurg* 60:481–489, 1984.
67. Bouzarth WF, Goldman HW: Emergency management of trauma: Trauma to the head, in Schwartz GR, Safar P, Stone JH, et al (eds): *Principles and Practice of Emergency Medicine*. Philadelphia, WB Saunders Co, 1986, pp 1297–1308.
68. Brayton CF: Dimethyl sulfoxide (DMSO): A review. *Cornell Vet* 76:61–90, 1986.
69. delaTorre JC, Rowed DW, Kawanaga HM, et al: Dimethyl sulfoxide in the treatment of experimental brain compression. *J Neurosurg* 38:345–353, 1973.
70. James HE, Cornell W, delBigio M, et al: Dimethyl sulfoxide in brain edema and intracranial pressure. *Ann NY Acad Sci*:253–360, 1983.
71. Waller FT, Tanabe CT, Paxton HD: Treatment of elevated intracranial pressure with dimethyl sulfoxide. *Ann NY Acad Sci*:286–292, 1983.
72. Brown FD, Johns L, Mullan S: Dimethyl sulfoxide therapy following penetrating brain injury. *Ann NY Acad Sci*:245–251, 1983.
73. Sorjonen DC, Knecht CD: Principles of neurologic treatment. *Prog Vet Neurol* 1(1):73–82, 1990.
74. Muir WW: Brain hypoperfusion post-resuscitation. *Vet Clin North Am Small Anim Pract* 19(6):1151–1166, 1989.
75. Clubb RJ, Maxwell RE, Chou SN: Experimental brain injury in the dog. *J Neurosurg* 52:189–196, 1980.
76. Wauquier A, Edmonds HL, Clincke HC: Cerebral resuscitation: Pathophysiology and therapy. *Neurosci Biobehav Rev* 11:287–306, 1987.
77. Selman WR, Spetzler RF, Anton AH, et al: Management of prolonged therapeutic barbiturate coma. *Surg Neurol* 15:9–10, 1981.
78. Bricolo AP, Glick RP: Barbiturate effects on acute experimental intracranial hypertension. *J Neurosurg* 55:397–406, 1981.
79. Dewey CW, Budsberg SC, Oliver JE: Principles of head trauma management in dogs and cats—Part I. *Compend Contin Educ Pract Vet* 14(2):199–207, 1992.
80. Ikeda Y, Brelsford KL, Ikeda K, et al: Effect of superoxide

dismutase in cats with cold-induced edema. *Adv Neurol* 52:203–210, 1990.
81. Muir WM: Reperfusion injury: Pathophysiology and therapy. *Proc 2nd Int Vet Emerg Crit Care Symp*:47–51, 1990.
82. Rochat MC: An introduction to reperfusion injury. *Compend Contin Educ Pract Vet* 13(6):923–930, 1991.
83. Ikeda Y, Long DM: The molecular basis of brain injury and brain edema: The role of oxygen free radicals. *J Neurosurg* 27(1):1–8, 1990.
84. Ikeda Y, Ikeda K, Long DM: Protective effect of the iron chelator deferoxamine on cold-induced brain edema. *J Neurosurg* 71:233–238, 1989.
85. Ikeda Y, Ikeda K, Long DM: Comparative study of different iron-chelating agents in cold-induced brain edema. *Neurosurgery* 24(6):820–823, 1989.
86. Kontos HA, Wei EP: Superoxide production in experimental brain injury. *J Neurosurg* 64:803–807, 1986.
87. Liu TH, Beckman JS, Freeman BA, et al: Polyethylene glycol conjugated superoxide dismutase and catalase reduce ischemic brain injury. *Am J Physiol* 256:H589–H593, 1989.
88. Levasseur JE, Patterson JL, Ghatak NR: Combined effect of respirator-induced ventilation and superoxide dismutase in experimental brain injury. *J Neurosurg* 71:573–577, 1989.
89. Schettini A, Lippman R, Walsh EK: Attenuation of decompressive hypoperfusion and cerebral edema by superoxide dismutase. *J Neurosurg* 71:578–587, 1989.
90. Ikeda Y, Anderson JH, Long DM: Oxygen free radicals in the genesis of traumatic and peritumoral brain edema. *Neurosurgery* 24(5):679–685, 1989.
91. Itoh T, Kawakami M, Yamauchi Y, et al: Effect of allopurinol on ischemia and reperfusion-induced cerebral injury in spontaneously hypertensive rats. *Stroke* 17(6):1284–1287, 1986.
92. McIntosh TK, Hayes RL, DeWitt DS, et al: Endogenous opioids may mediate secondary damage after experimental brain injury. *Am J Physiol* 253:E565–E574, 1987.
93. McIntosh TK, Head VA, Faden AI: Alterations in regional concentrations of endogenous opioids following traumatic brain injury in the cat. *Brain Res* 425:225–233, 1987.
94. Roy R, Cooper PR: Penetrating injuries of the skull brain, in Vinken PJ, Bruyn GW, Klawans HL (eds): *Handbook of Clinical Neurology: Head Injury*. New York, Elsevier Science Publishers B.V., 1990, pp 299–315.
95. Shores A: Neuroanesthesia: A review of the effects of anesthetic agents on cerebral blood flow and intracranial pressure in the dog. *Vet Surg* 14(3):257–263, 1985.
96. Cornick JL: Anesthetic management of patients with neurologic abnormalities. *Compend Contin Educ Pract Vet* 14(2):163–172, 1992.
97. Freedman M, Levy ER: Propofol intravenous anaesthesia for neurosurgery. *S Afr Med J* 74:10–12, 1988.
98. Moon PF, Concannon KT: Mechanical ventilation, in Kirk RW, Bonagura JD (eds): *Current Veterinary Therapy Therapy. XI*. Philadelphia, WB Saunders Co, 1992, pp 98–104.
99. Shores A: Instrumentation for intracranial surgery. *Prog Vet Neurol* 2(3):175–182, 1991.
100. Oliver JE: Surgical approaches to the canine brain. *Am J Vet Res* 29(2):354–378, 1968.
101. Oliver JE, Raffe MR: The nervous system, in Harvey CE, Newton D, Schwartz A (eds): *Small Animal Surgery*. Philadelphia, JB Lippincott Co, 1990, pp 479–492.
102. Kostolich M, Dulisch ML: A surgical approach to the canine olfactory bulb for meningioma removal. *Vet Surg* 16(4):273–277, 1987.
103. Bullock R, Teasdale G: Surgical management of traumatic intracranial hematomas, in Vinken PJ, Bruyn GW, Klawans HL (eds): *Handbook of Clinical Neurology: Head Injury*. New York, Elsevier Science Publishers B.V., 1990, pp 249–288.
104. Sakas DE, Charnvises K, Borges LF, et al: Biologically inert synthetic dural substitutes. *J Neurosurg* 73:936–941, 1990.
105. Saul TG, Ducker TB: Effect of intracranial pressure monitoring and aggressive treatment on mortality in severe head injury. *J Neurosurg* 56:498–503, 1982.
106. Marmarou A, Anderson RL, Ward JD, et al: Impact of ICP pressure instability and hypotension on outcome in patients with severe head trauma. *J Neurosurg* 75:559–566, 1991.
107. Aucoin PJ, Kotilainen HR, Gantz NM, et al: Intracranial pressure monitors: Epidemiologic study of risk factors and infections. *Am J Med* 80:369–376, 1986.
108. Shores A, Jevens D, DeCamp CE: Intraoperative brain pressure monitoring in the dog. *Proc 9th ACVIM Forum*: 831–833, 1991.
109. Ostrup RC, Luerssen TG, Marshall LF, et al: Continuous monitoring of intracranial pressure with a miniaturized fiberoptic device. *J Neurosurg* 67:206–209, 1987.
110. Narayan RK, Greenberg RP, Miller JD: Improved confidence of outcome prediction in severe head injury. *J Neurosurg* 54:751–762, 1981.
111. Miller JD, Butterworth JF, Gudeman SK: Further experience in the management of severe head injury. *J Neurosurg* 54:289–299, 1981.
112. Young B, Rapp RP, Norton JA: Early prediction of outcome in head-injured patients. *J Neurosurg* 54:300–303, 1981.
113. Davis RA, Cunningham PS: Prognostic factors in severe head injury. *Surg Gynecol Obstet* 159:597–604, 1984.

UPDATE

Recent experimental evidence implicates sodium as the major osmotic agent contributing to brain edema; in light of this evidence, hetastarch may be preferable to hypertonic saline for shock fluid therapy.[1] Humans with head trauma and hyperglycemia have a poorer neurologic outcome than do euglycemic patients.[2] Because large doses of glucocorticoids can exacerbate hyperglycemia, blood glucose levels should be checked before initiating glucocorticoid therapy. Finally, potentially operable post-traumatic intracranial hemorrhage may be more common in dogs and cats than was previously recognized.[3,4] With the increased availability and affordability of computed tomography in veterinary practice,[5] surgical intervention may begin to play a larger role in the management of dogs and cats with head trauma.

REFERENCES

1. Menzies SA, Betz AL, Hoff JT: Contributions of ions and albumin to the formation and resolution of ischemic brain edema. *J Neurosurg* 78:257–266, 1993.
2. Young B, Ott L, Dempsey R, et al: Relationship between admission hyperglycemia and neurologic outcome of severely brain-injured patients. *Ann Surg* 210(4):466–473, 1989.
3. Dewey CW, Downs MO, Aron DN, et al: Acute traumatic intracranial hemorrhage in dogs and cats: A retrospective evaluation of 23 cases. *VCOT* 6:153–159, 1993.
4. Dewey CW, Downs MO, Crowe DT: Management of a dog with an acute traumatic subdural hematoma. *JAAHA* 29:551–554, 1993.
5. Hathcock JT, Stickle RL: Principles and concepts of computed tomography. *Vet Clin North Am Small Anim Pract* 23:399–415, 1993.

Coxofemoral Luxations in Dogs

KEY FACTS

- The principal stability of the coxofemoral joint comes from the joint capsule (which extends from the acetabulum to the neck of the femur) and the ligament of the head of the femur (which runs from the fovea capitis of the femur to the acetabular fossa).
- Dislocation of the hip is the most common luxation in dogs.
- The method of repair is generally determined by the duration and extent of injury, species, size, presence of other diseases or fractures, economics, and preference of the surgeon.
- Surgeons must be familiar with more than one method of repair because a preferred method occasionally cannot be used.

Pfizer Animal Health Group
North America Region,
Dallas, Texas

Steven M. Fox, MS, DVM

HIP LUXATIONS are common traumatic injuries encountered in small animal practice. They account for as many as 90% of luxations in dogs.[1] The primary cause is blunt trauma with resultant disruption of the joint capsule and round ligament of the head of the femur. Although closed reduction is often possible after acute injury, the high percentage of subsequent reluxations necessitates the use of surgical techniques to maintain coxofemoral reduction.

ANATOMY

The hip is a ball-and-socket joint that allows a wide range of motion, principally flexion and extension.[2] Primary stability of the joint comes from (1) the joint capsule, which extends from the acetabulum to the neck of the femur, and (2) the teres (or round) ligament of the head of the femur, which runs from the fovea capitis of the femur to the acetabular fossa. Secondary support for the hip joint comes from a proposed hydrostatic stability factor[3] and from numerous surrounding muscles that function as flexors, extensors, abductors, adductors, and internal rotators of the limb.

The gluteal and thigh muscles are the most developed and numerous of these muscle groups and are the most important for weight bearing and locomotion. The gluteal muscles lie dorsal and cranial to the hip joint. In addition to extending the hip joint, the gluteal muscles rotate the hip internally and abduct the femur. Ventral and cranial to the hip joint, the iliopsoas muscle originates from the ventral lumbar vertebrae and ilium and inserts on the lesser trochanter of the femur. This muscle rotates and flexes the hip joint internally.

The pelvic acetabulum is a deep socket that surrounds the femoral head. Coverage is subjectively assessed via ventrodorsal radiographs and measured with the acetabular angle of Weiberg.[4] The thickened aspect of the subchondral acetabular bone is referred to as the acetabular sourcil.[5] The sourcil is thickest on the craniodorsal aspect of the acetabulum, the area of greatest intraarticular stress.[5] It has been experimentally demonstrated that the joint capsule and the ligament of the femoral head are the key structures in preventing coxofemoral luxation in dogs.[6]

One study demonstrated that luxation does not occur if the joint capsule, round ligament, or cartilaginous acetabular rim is removed separately.[6] If the joint capsule and round ligament are both removed, coxofemoral luxation occurs in a high percentage of animals.

Vascular supply to the canine hip joint is extensive and involves multiple anastomoses.[7] The capsular arterial ring yields arteries that enter the femoral neck and anastomose with terminal branches of the nutrient artery from the femoral shaft.[8] Vessels have been observed in the ligament of the head of the femur; these vessels make a small contribution to the blood supply of the femoral head.[8] The acetabulum receives its blood from the iliolumbar, cranial gluteal, and caudal gluteal arteries.[7] The cranial gluteal artery supplies the craniodorsal aspects of the acetabulum; the caudal gluteal artery supplies the caudodorsal acetabulum.

CAUSE

A common cause of luxation is strong, traumatic impact to the rump.[9] As the dog starts to fall in the direction of the impact force, the affected leg becomes adducted. As the hip moves ventrolaterally toward the ground, the long-lever action of the adducted femoral shaft forces the femoral head out of the acetabulum as far as the round ligament and joint capsule allow. When the greater trochanter strikes the ground, the kinetic energy is transmitted through the femoral neck to the femoral head. The head is driven over the dorsal rim of the acetabulum and thus shears the round ligament and joint capsule.

Occasionally, the ligament avulses the femoral head or acetabulum or fractures part of the dorsal acetabular rim. Because of gluteal muscle contraction, the femoral head comes to rest in a craniodorsal position.

BACKGROUND

Dislocation of the hip is the most common luxation in skeletally mature dogs.[10] Although it may be a sequela of hip dysplasia or a postoperative complication of total hip replacement, dislocation is usually a result of trauma. Young dogs with an open proximal femoral physis usually sustain a Salter-Harris fracture through the physis as a result of the same trauma that produces luxation in older dogs. The femoral head epiphysis fuses to the neck in dogs at 11 to 12 months of age; before this time, the ratio of probability that femoral neck fracture will occur rather than hip dislocation is approximately 2:1.[11]

COXOFEMORAL luxations are generally classified as craniodorsal, dorsal, caudodorsal, and ventral.[10] After trauma, the femoral head is most frequently displaced craniodorsal to the acetabulum. This direction of displacement results from the strong pull of the gluteal muscles.

Although coxofemoral luxations are not regarded as emergencies, they should be treated as soon as possible. At least two radiographic views of the pelvis are essential to confirm or refute the clinical diagnosis and to identify other injuries, such as avulsion fracture of the femoral head, fracture of the dorsal acetabular rim, or concurrent pelvic fracture. Thoracic radiographs may also be necessary to determine whether pneumothorax, traumatic lung pathology, diaphragmatic hernia, or rib fracture is present; such radiographs are especially important if the trauma is from a motor vehicle or of unknown origin.

DIAGNOSIS

Hip luxations can usually be detected by physical examination. The patient may bear weight on the affected limb with the toes rotated laterally. This rotation is caused by craniodorsal displacement and external rotation of the proximal femur. The patient should be palpated for other abnormalities, such as hip fractures and stifle injuries. The greater trochanter, which can be palpated in all but very obese dogs, is displaced from its ventral point of triangulation with the ipsilateral tuber ischium and wing of the ilium.

IN A CRANIODORSALLY luxated hip, the greater trochanter is more in line with the ipsilateral tuber ischium and wing of the ilium. It also rides higher than the normal position of the contralateral greater trochanter. Hip joint congruity can be further assessed by comparative placement of the practitioner's thumbs between the ischium and greater trochanter on each side of the pelvis. In a normal hip, the thumb is displaced by external rotation of the leg. If the thumb is not displaced, fracture or luxation of the hip joint has occurred. In addition, medial rotation of the femur is restricted as a result of the luxated hip.

When the femoral head luxates craniodorsally, the femoral head, neck, and greater trochanter come to rest parallel to the shaft of the ilium and are held in position by the gluteal muscles. Medial rotation of the femur is restricted as the femoral head and neck abut the shaft of the ilium. Craniodorsal hip luxation also results in a shortened hindleg, which is evident when both limbs are extended with the patient in dorsal recumbency.

TREATMENT

Coxofemoral luxations that have been present for less than 72 hours can usually be replaced by closed reduction unless there are indications for open reduction.[12] Such indications include avulsion fractures of the fovea capitis or acetabulum, dorsal rim acetabular fractures, and cases in which closed reduction cannot be achieved. Femoral head fractures must be detected because small osteochondral fragments may lie in the acetabulum and interfere with joint action.

Osteochondral fragments are not always visible on plain radiographs, and their presence is likely if there is failure to achieve reduction of the femoral head into the acetabulum. Hemorrhage in the acetabulum rapidly organizes and hinders attempts at reduction. In addition, infolding of the joint capsule or proliferation of the torn joint capsule and round ligament may fill the acetabulum and thus prevent closed reduction. Once reduced, the round ligament can proliferate and reattach.[12]

The longer the hip joint remains luxated, the more likely is pathologic change to the femoral head and acetabulum.

This change may increase the difficulty of treatment and the possibility of lameness after satisfactory reduction. Stability may be harder to establish as a result of marked muscle atrophy. The gluteal muscles and muscles of the lower limb are affected. When these muscles are weak, the tension exerted to maintain the femoral head in the acetabulum is much less than normal. In most untreated patients, the hip remains painful, its motion is restricted, and the leg is carried or used for balance only.[13]

SEVERAL METHODS are available to treat coxofemoral luxations. The chosen repair is generally determined by the duration and extent of injury related to the luxation, species, size, presence of other diseases or fractures, economics, and preference of the surgeon. Surgeons must be familiar with more than one method because the preferred method occasionally cannot be used. If severe hip dysplasia is present in a dog with hip luxation, reduction may be inappropriate and other surgical techniques may be necessary.

Closed Reduction

Closed reduction should be attempted as soon as possible after the injury. The patient is anesthetized and placed in lateral recumbency with the affected leg uppermost. In small dogs, countertraction is maintained by the surgeon's hand in the inguinal region of the dog. In large dogs, this traction is maintained by an assistant pulling on a strap or towel placed under the tail and affected leg.

The luxated limb is grasped by the stifle, rotated laterally, abducted, and pulled distally to bring the femoral head to the acetabulum. As the femoral head moves distally over the rim of the acetabulum, the femur is rotated medially and adducted to a normal position. With the help of an assistant, the surgeon's second hand grasps the greater trochanter and guides it into the acetabulum. An audible clunk often accompanies the reduction.

After the hip has been reduced, the joint is manipulated through a full range of motion and pressure is placed on the greater trochanter to evacuate clotted blood from the acetabulum. Unsuccessful reduction often results from the presence of debris in the acetabulum or inversion of the joint capsule into the joint space. In ventral and caudal luxations, the clinician should place the femoral head in the craniodorsal position and follow the standard reduction technique. Proper reduction is confirmed by radiographs and manipulation of the joint through a full range of motion. Several methods are available to reduce the likelihood of reluxation.

The most common technique for maintaining reduction of a luxated coxofemoral joint is use of an Ehmer sling or figure-of-eight flexion bandage[14] (Figure 1). When properly applied, the bandage holds the flexed hindlimb in ab-

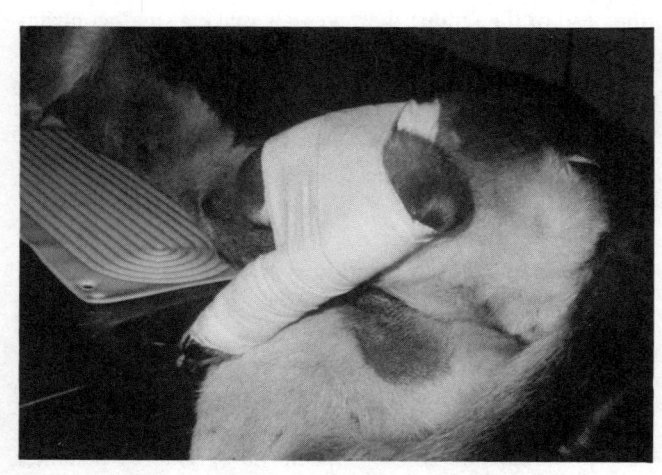

Figure 1—If properly applied, the Ehmer sling provides sufficient padding to the plantar aspect of the metatarsal bones and holds the hock in abduction.

duction and internal rotation and gives the femoral head maximum acetabular coverage.[15] The more effective the restraint, however, the less comfortable the bandage apparently is for the patient. After reduction of the hip joint, the Ehmer sling should remain in place for one to three weeks.

Because of the natural canine resistance to hyperflexion, there is considerable pressure at the edges of the bandage, which may cut into the underlying soft tissue. Resistance to hyperflexion by the encircling tape produces pressure on the plantar aspect of the metatarsus; such pressure may lead to edema and swelling. Sufficient padding thus must be applied around the metatarsal area before application of the figure-of-eight tape. The foot should be examined daily for swelling[16] (Figure 2).

AN ALTERNATIVE to the flexion bandage is the DeVita pin, which can be inserted to provide additional dorsal support to the hip joint and lessen the likelihood of reluxation.[17] The DeVita pin, which can be used in conjunction with closed or open reduction methods, is a Steinmann pin introduced through a stab incision just below the ischiatic tuberosity. The pin is advanced slowly to avoid damage to the sciatic nerve. It is advanced tangential to the femoral neck and embedded in the wing of the ilium[17] (Figure 3).

The most common error in the use of the DeVita pin is inserting it too far medially at the ischium.[13] Embedment in the ilial wing may be difficult if there is minimal concavity to the ilial bone. The pin is removed in two to six weeks. If the pin is left in place for four to six weeks, a channel of scar tissue forms and provides permanent reinforcement of the dorsal acetabular rim after removal of the pin.[13]

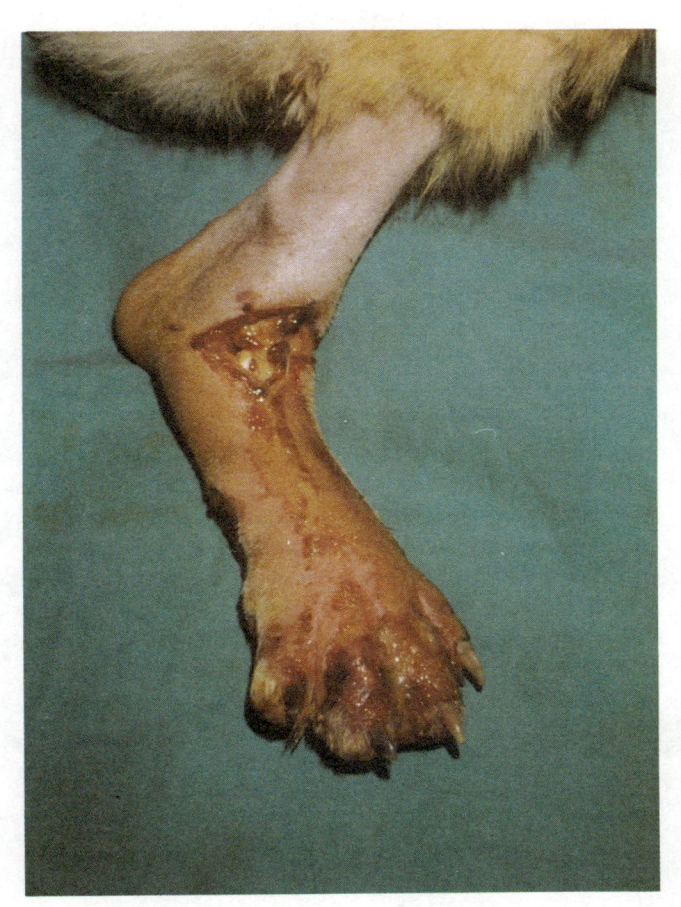

Figure 2—Distal limb trauma caused by an incorrectly applied Ehmer sling and inattentive follow-up.

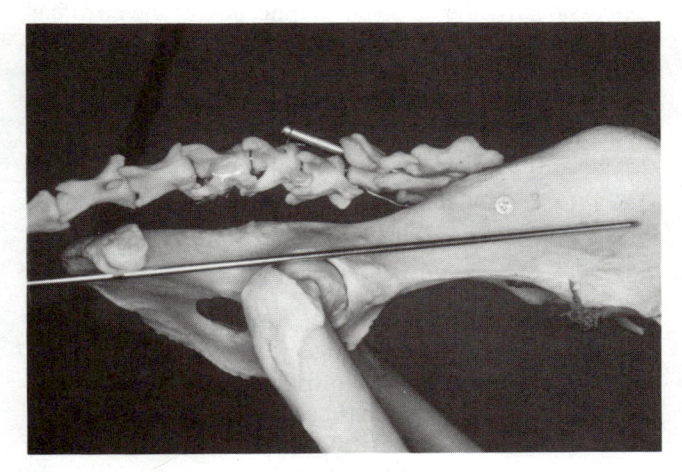

Figure 3—The DeVita pin is placed in a caudal-to-cranial direction; it is inserted under the tuber ischium, tangential to the femoral head and neck, and into the wing of the ilium. A threaded-tip pin is best for this purpose.

Because the DeVita pin can damage the sciatic nerve, slow insertion is essential to allow the nerve to move as the pin advances. Pin migration may be a problem; a threaded pin tip reduces this possibility. Other techniques for reducing migration have been presented.[13] On one occasion, a draining sinus tract beneath the tuber ischium was reported to develop after DeVita pin placement.[18]

Open Reduction

If the femoral head does not reduce adequately or reluxates easily from the acetabulum when slight stress is applied to the hip after closed reduction, open reduction is necessary. Open reduction is best achieved via a cranial or dorsal approach,[19] which allows removal of debris from the acetabulum and suturing of the joint capsule. Acetabular debris, such as blood clots or fibrous tissue, is removed as necessary. Remnants of the round ligament of the head of the femur may require removal, and the inverted joint capsule is everted. The joint is reduced, and tears or incisions in the joint capsule are sutured with a simple interrupted, horizontal, or cross-mattress pattern of a nonabsorbable material.

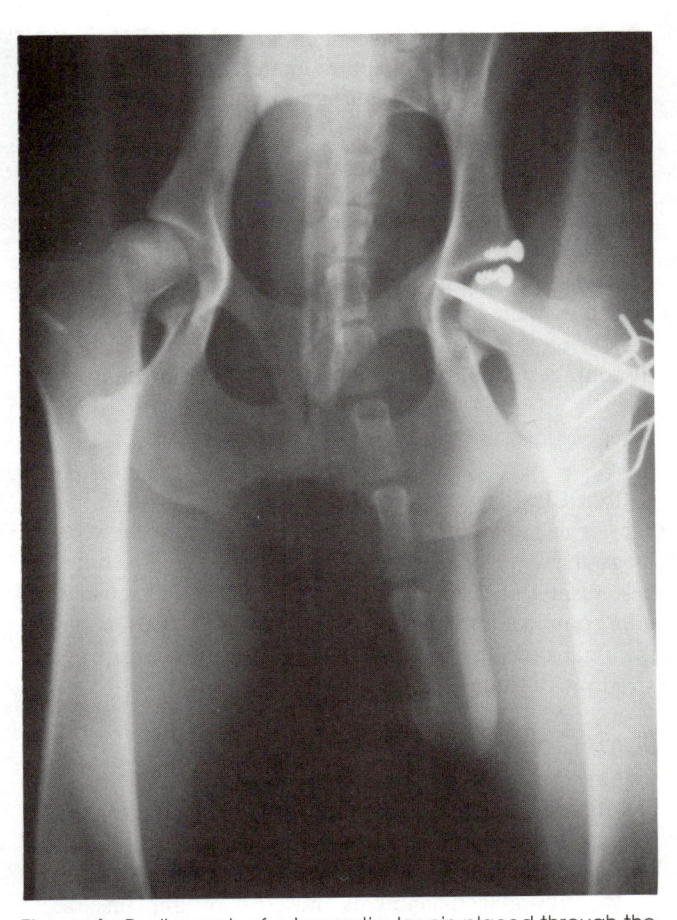

Figure 4—Radiograph of a transarticular pin placed through the coxofemoral joint to maintain reduction. The screws in the acetabulum were placed to anchor the capsulorrhaphy. The greater trochanter has been relocated and attached with Kirschner wires and a tension band.

Occasionally, the anatomic architecture of the coxofemoral joint is damaged such that surgery is necessary to maintain reduction. The various reported techniques can be classified as: (1) replacement of the ligament of the head of the femur, (2) substitution for a damaged or missing joint capsule, (3) alteration of the dorsal acetabular rim, or (4) creation of extramuscular forces around the coxofemoral joint to maintain permanent reduction.

Replacement of the Ligament of the Femoral Head

Replacement of the round ligament by natural body tissue (skin or fascia lata) or a prosthetic device (nonabsorbable sutures and a toggle) has been described.[12,20-22] A tunnel is drilled through the femoral shaft cortex just below the greater trochanter, traversing the femoral head and neck, and emerging at the point of attachment of the round ligament of the femoral head. The tunnel is most accurately drilled by beginning at the origin of the round ligament.[12] The graft or prosthesis is then passed through the tunnel and secured at a predrilled hole in the acetabulum.

The use of a postreduction, temporary transarticular pin ensures femoral head placement in the acetabulum. The implant is removed in approximately two weeks.[23-25] A transarticular Steinmann pin is introduced ventrolateral to the greater trochanter and pushed through the femoral neck and head to emerge through the fovea capitis of the femoral head (Figure 4). The luxation is reduced, and the pin is pushed three to seven millimeters through the acetabular fossa until it can be felt (by an assistant performing rectal examination) emerging through the acetabulum. The pin is placed with the hip held in flexion and abduction.[25] The pin is bent on the lateral aspect of the femur to aid removal, discourage migration, and reduce local tissue trauma.

PROBLEMS with this technique include bending, breakage, or migration of the pin and perforation of the rectum. Dogs that weigh less than 30 kilograms demonstrate the best results after transarticular pinning.[25] The most common complication, pin breakage, reportedly does not affect the final outcome and can be avoided by using properly sized pins (Table I).[25]

Joint Capsule Substitution

Joint capsule integrity ensures hip reduction.[6] In some coxofemoral luxations, secure capsulorrhaphy cannot be accomplished because there is extensive damage to the joint capsule. In such cases, surrounding soft tissue (e.g., rectal femoral and gemellus muscles) or implants (e.g., screws placed in the acetabular rim) can be used to anchor sutures of the capsulorrhaphy.

Several extracapsular suture stabilization techniques have been described to substitute for or augment coxofemoral capsulorrhaphy.[26-28] The web and prosthetic capsule technique involves two screws in the dorsal edge of the acetabulum and one in the craniodorsal aspect of the femur.[26] Nonabsorbable suture material is looped in figure-of-eight fashion between the screw in the femur and the screws in the acetabular rim. Reaction to the suture material is apparently limited to the development of scar tissue that envelopes the sutures. The effect is a thick mass of scar tissue that substitutes for the joint capsule.[26]

A modification of the web technique involves substituting the femoral screw with a tunnel drilled in the femoral neck just lateral and distal to the joint capsule attachment (Figure 5). Spiked washers are placed under the screws to prevent slippage of the suture over the screw head.[27,28] Two nonabsorbable sutures are passed through the tunnel and around the screws. Although the technique is designed to augment hip joint capsulorrhaphy and trochanteric transposition, I have had success using the technique in primary repair of acute and chronic coxofemoral luxations. An Ehmer bandage is not routinely used after surgery.

Acetabular Rim Alteration

Several procedures have been used to maintain coxofemoral reduction by extension of the acetabular rim.[29-31] A plastic Schaffer sleeve was used by Helper and Schiller.[29] Marvich placed a bone screw parallel to the neck of the femur, protruding from the acetabular rim.[30] Durr placed two threaded, three-inch Kirschner wires into the acetabular roof over the trochanter and head of the femur.[31] These procedures are technically demanding; each has been replaced by less time-consuming techniques that provide better results.

Other techniques have been used for primary repair or, more often, to supplement the described procedures. Rather than substituting the ligament of the head of the femur, the joint capsule, or the acetabular rim, these techniques impose forces around the coxofemoral joint to maintain reduction.

Muscular Force Augmentation

Relocation of the greater trochanter increases gluteal

TABLE I
Transarticular Pin Selection According to Body Weight

Weight (kg)	Pin Diameter	
	Inches	Millimeters
4 to 7	1/16	1.6
8 to 11	5/64	2.0
12 to 19	3/32	2.3
20 to 29	7/64	2.7
Greater than 30	1/8	3.1

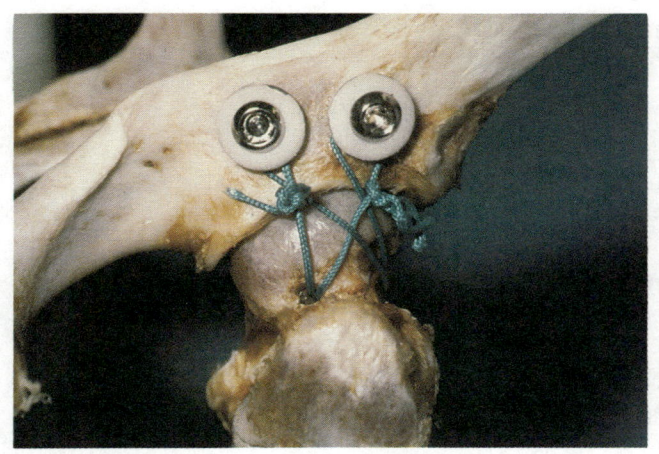

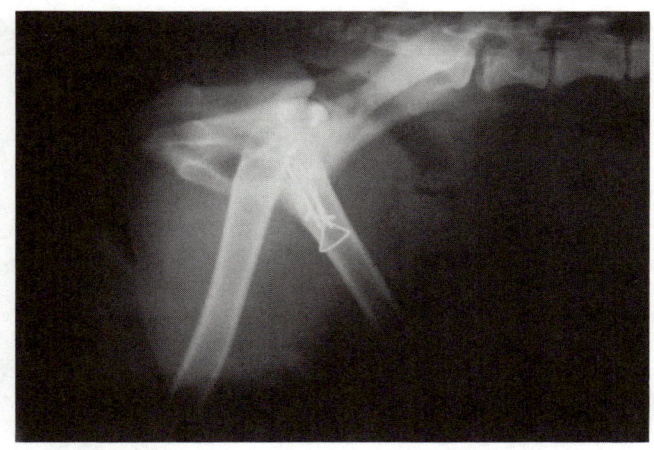

Figure 5A

Figure 5B

Figure 5—(**A**) Skeleton model demonstrating extracapsular suture stabilization with 2.7-mm screws and spiked washers. The suture tunnel is drilled through the femoral neck. Heavy nonabsorbable sutures are used. (**B**) Postoperative lateral radiograph of the technique. The greater trochanter has been repositioned as in Figure 4.

muscle tension, abducts and internally rotates the femur, and firmly seats the femoral head in the acetabulum.[32,33] After reduction of the hip, the greater trochanter is repositioned approximately one or two centimeters distal and slightly cranial to its original site. It is fixed in this position by two small pins and a tension band wire. I believe that a cancellous bone interface enhances healing and thus prefer to make a distal bed for the osteotomized greater trochanter. Occasionally, the small pins cause soft tissue trauma and require removal after bone healing.

FOR LUXATIONS that can be reduced without joint exploration, Hansmeyer has attempted to tighten the muscle forces around the hip by placing a purse-string suture around the greater trochanter.[34] After exposure of the greater trochanter by reflection of subcutaneous tissue, a No. 4 chromic gut purse-string suture is placed into the deep musculature surrounding the greater trochanter and drawn as tight as possible. Suture passage caudal to the greater trochanter must be made carefully in order to avoid the sciatic nerve.

A recently described technique of prearticular stabilization involves the use of heavy double-mattress sutures tied between the tendons of insertion of the smaller psoas and middle gluteus muscles.[35] The principle is to avoid reluxation by limiting the range of rotatory movement of the femoral head. The sutures lie just craniolateral to the joint and prevent extensive outward rotation of the femoral head. The sutures are tied while the joint is rotated inward. Unlike other procedures, this technique provides ventral rather than dorsal support to the coxofemoral joint.

Immobilization of the reduced coxofemoral luxation can be achieved via trochanteric pinning[36] or an external fixator.[37,38] In trochanteric pinning, a Steinmann pin is inserted through the greater trochanter. The pin is directed so that it passes proximal to the head of the femur and enters the acetabular portion of the pelvis on the craniodorsal border of the acetabulum. Complications associated with this technique are similar to those of transarticular pinning.[36]

A five-pin external fixator has also been used to maintain the hip in reduction. Fixation pins are placed laterally into the wing of the ilium, shaft of the ilium, and ischium as well as dorsally into the caudal ischium. With the hip reduced, the fifth fixation pin is drilled into the greater trochanter. All pins are connected with Kirschner clamps to a ¼-inch, contoured, soft aluminum rod. The apparatus is removed in approximately two weeks.

Femoral Head and Neck Excision

Excision arthroplasty can be used as a salvage procedure for chronic, nonreducible coxofemoral luxation. If correctly performed, the procedure should result in a pain-free joint. A false fibrous joint forms as early as two weeks after the operation.[39] This joint has a smaller range of motion and is less stable than the normal ball-and-socket hip joint. The motion of the leg is thus not normal, and some lameness is anticipated.

The most common postoperative findings include shortening of the limb and restricted movement of the hip pseudarthrosis.[39] Long-term problems are mild to moderate discomfort after excessive exercise and stiffness on cold, damp days.[40] Although few patients demonstrate lameness or pain in the operated hip, muscle atrophy is frequent. In small-breed dogs, patellar instability has been a sequela of the procedure.[39,40] In dogs that weigh more than 20 kilograms, excision arthroplasty coupled with a bi-

TABLE II
Repair of Coxofemoral Luxation

Technique	Number of Cases	Successful Results (%)	Complications and Observations	Reference
Closed reduction	34	56	Reluxation	43[a]
Closed reduction with Ehmer bandage	37	70.27	No lameness	44[a]
		16.2	Reluxation	
Closed reduction with Ehmer bandage	1588	14.7	Reluxation	42
Closed reduction	74	47.3	Reluxation	45
Capsulorrhaphy	21	9.5	Reluxation	45
Trochanteric transposition and capsulorrhaphy with Ehmer bandage	16	56.25	Normal range of motion and gait	33
		25	Reluxation	
Trochanteric transposition and capsulorrhaphy with Ehmer bandage	78	83.8	Reported as normal or nearly normal	32[a]
Trochanteric transposition	8	12.5	Reluxation	45
Capsule prosthesis	22	66.6	Reported as normal or nearly normal	27[a]
			Transient, acute postoperative setback; possible suture breakage at 4 to 10 weeks; technique limits range of motion	
Extracapsular suture stabilization	5	100	None	28[a]
Prearticular stabilization and capsulorrhaphy	11	72.7	Excellent (as good as before luxation)	35
		27.2	Good; limp after heavy exercise	
Trochanteric pinning	15	—	Encouraging results	36[a]
Transarticular pinning	7	14.3	Reluxation	45
Transarticular pinning	40	25	Excellent; no lameness	25
		5	Very good; lame with heavy activity	
		2	Good; occasionally favored limb (pin breakage in 11 cases did not affect outcome)	
Transarticular pinning	7	100	Reported sound	24[a]
Skin substitute	9	67	No lameness; one case of sinus tract	20
Toggle pinning	4	25	No lameness; reluxation	45
Acetabular rim prosthesis	10	90	Complete recovery with no lameness (largest dog weighed 22 kg)	29[a]
Bone screw with Ehmer bandage	13	—	Good; one screw loosened	30[a]
Kirschner wires	17	100	Reduction maintained; wire broke in one case and migrated in one case	31[a]
Purse-string sutures	34	100	Good; gratifying results	34[a]
External fixator	18	100	Good; no reluxation	37[a]
External fixator	5	60	Reluxation	45
Excision arthroplasty	94	82.6	Excellent (76% to 100% limb usage); 27 cases of coxofemoral luxation	40[a]
Excision arthroplasty	177	93	Satisfactory (number of coxofemoral luxations not given); muscle atrophy; restricted range of motion; limb shortening	39[a]
Excision arthroplasty	7	37	No gait abnormality	46
		25.7	Favored limb or slight, permanent gait abnormality (Early intervention [from diagnosis] is best: excellent is an average of less than one month, poor is an average of more than six months. Lightweight dogs do better: excellent is an average of less than 8.03 kg, poor is an average of more than 16.7 kg.)	
Excision arthroplasty and biceps muscle sling	150	59	Excellent; total weight bearing	47[a]
		33	Good; slight lameness (number of coxofemoral luxations not given)	

[a]Data were subjective or left to interpretation, or results were not clearly defined.

ceps femoris muscle sling (using the caudal pass technique) has better results than femoral head excision alone.[41]

CONCLUSION

Table II demonstrates that many coxofemoral luxations do not respond to one-time external manipulation and closed reduction. Because there was no significant difference between the recurrence rates of surgical reduction as the initial procedure and those of surgical reduction after failure of closed reduction, it is reasonable to recommend closed reduction as an initial treatment even though the risk of recurrence is higher.[45] The need for surgery may thus be avoided.

Because of the high success rates of the various open reduction techniques, some clinicians may prefer to use such techniques initially. This choice often depends on the skill of the clinician. If the instrumentation is available, I prefer the extracapsular suture stabilization technique for open reduction. Without bone screw instrumentation, transarticular pinning is preferred. If possible, the joint capsule should be reconstructed; an Ehmer type bandage is recommended if a DeVita pin is not used.

About the Author

Dr. Fox is the Technical Services Veterinarian in the Companion Animal Division of Pfizer Inc.'s Animal Health Group, North America Region, in Dallas, Texas.

REFERENCES

1. Fry PD: Observations on the surgical treatment of hip dislocation in the dog and cat. *J Small Anim Pract* 15:661–670, 1974.
2. Miller ME: *Anatomy of the Dog*. Philadelphia, WB Saunders Co, 1964.
3. Smith GK, Darryl NB, Gregor TP: New concepts of coxofemoral joint stability and the development of a clinical stress-radiographic method for quantitating hip joint laxity in the dog. *JAVMA* 196:59–70, 1990.
4. Weiberg G: Shelf operation in congenital dysplasia of the acetabulum and in subluxation and dislocation of the hip. *J Bone Joint Surg* 35A:65–71, 1953.
5. Pauwels F: *Biomechanics of the Normal and Diseased Hip*. New York, Springer Verlag, 1976.
6. Smith WS, Coleman CR, Olix ML, Slager RF: Etiology of congenital dislocation of the hip. *J Bone Joint Surg* 45:491–500, 1963.
7. Kaderly RE, Anderson WD, Anderson BG: Extraosseus vascular supply to the mature dog's coxofemoral joint. *Am J Vet Res* 43:1208–1214, 1982.
8. Rivera LA, Abdelbake YZ, Titkemeyer CW, Hulse DA: Arterial supply to the canine hip joint. *J Vet Orthop* 1:20–24, 1979.
9. Wadsworth PL: Biomechanics of the luxation of joints, in Bojrab MJ (ed): *Pathophysiology in Small Animal Surgery*. Philadelphia, Lea & Febiger, 1981, pp 804–811.
10. Herron MR: Coxofemoral luxations in small animals. *J Vet Orthop* 1:30–37, 1979.
11. Campbell JR, Wyburn RS: Coxofemoral luxation in the dog. *Vet Rec* 77:1173–1177, 1965.
12. Piermattei DL: A technique for surgical management of coxofemoral luxations. *Small Anim Clin*:373–386, 1963.
13. Pettit GD: Coxofemoral luxations. *Vet Clin North Am* 1:503–522, 1971.
14. Ehmer EE: Special casts for the treatment of pelvic and femoral fractures and coxofemoral luxations. *North Am Vet* 15:31–35, 1934.
15. Knecht DD: Principles and application of traction and coaptation splints. *Vet Clin North Am [Small Anim Pract]* 5:177–195, 1975.
16. Fox SM: External coaptation bandages: How and when to use them. *Vet Med* 83:153–163, 1988.
17. DeVita J: A method of pinning for chronic dislocation of the hip joint. *Proc 89th Annu Meet AVMA*:191–192, 1952.
18. Leeds EB, Renegar WR: The use of the DeVita pin in the multi-traumatized canine patient with a concurrent coxofemoral luxation. *J Vet Orthop* 1:35–45, 1979.
19. Piermattei DL, Greeley RG: *An Atlas of Surgical Approaches to the Bones of the Dog and Cat*. Philadelphia, WB Saunders Co, 1979.
20. Zakiewicz M: Recurrent hip luxation in the dog: Skin as a substitute ligament. *Vet Rec* 81:538–539, 1969.
21. Knowles AT, Knowles JO, Knowles RP: An operation to preserve the continuity of the hip joint. *JAVMA* 123:508–515, 1953.
22. Lawson DP: Toggle fixation for recurrent dislocation of the hip in the dog. *J Small Anim Pract* 67:57–59, 1965.
23. Gendreau CL, Rouse GP: Surgical management of the hip. *Sci Proc AAHA*:393–395, 1975.
24. Bennett D, Duff SR: Transarticular pinning as a treatment for hip luxation in the dog and cat. *J Small Anim Pract* 21:373–379, 1980.
25. Hunt CA, Henry WE: Transarticular pinning for repair of hip dislocation in the dog: A retrospective study of 40 cases. *JAVMA* 187:828–834, 1985.
26. Leighton RL: A novel technique to manage coxofemoral luxations in dogs. *Vet Med* 80:53–58, 1985.
27. Branden TD, Johnson ME: Technique and indications of a prosthetic capsule for repair of recurrent and chronic coxofemoral luxations. *Vet Comp Orthop Traumatol* 1:26–29, 1988.
28. Allen SW, Chambers JN: Extracapsular suture stabilization of canine coxofemoral luxation. *Compend Contin Educ Pract Vet* 8(7):457–462, 1986.
29. Helper LC, Schiller AG: Repair of coxofemoral luxations in the dog and cat by extension of the acetabular rim. *JAVMA* 143:709–711, 1963.
30. Marvich JM: Use of a bone screw in repair of traumatic coxofemoral luxations. *VM SAC* 67:302–304, 1972.
31. Durr JL: The use of Kirschner wires in maintaining reduction of dislocations of the hip joint. *JAVMA* 130:78–81, 1957.
32. DeAngelis M, Prata R: Surgical repair of coxofemoral luxation in the dog. *JAAHA* 9:175–182, 1973.
33. Hammer DL: Recurrent coxofemoral luxation in fifteen dogs and one cat. *JAVMA* 177:1018–1020, 1980.
34. Hansmeyer LL: Fixation after reduction of luxation of the coxofemoral joint in dogs. *J S Afr Vet Assoc* 34:459–460, 1963.
35. Mehl NB: A new method of surgical treatment of hip dislocation in dogs and cats. *J Small Anim Pract* 29:789–795, 1988.
36. Horne RD: Trochanteric pinning procedure for reduction of coxofemoral luxations. *VM SAC* 66:331–334, 1971.
37. Stader O: Dislocations of the hip. *North Am Vet* 36:1026–1030, 1955.
38. Ellis A: Unpublished data, Veterinary Orthopedic Society, Copper Mountain, CO, 1985.
39. Duff R, Campbell JR: Long term results of excision arthroplasty of the canine hip. *Vet Rec* 101:181–184, 1977.
40. Berzon JL, Howard PE, Covell SJ, et al: A retrospective study of the efficacy of femoral head and neck excisions in 94 dogs and cats. *Vet Surg* 3:88–92, 1980.
41. Lippincott CL: Excision arthroplasty of the femoral head and neck utilizing a biceps femoris muscle sling. II. The caudal pass. *JAAHA* 20:377–384, 1984.
42. Greene JE, Hoerlein BF, Hayes HW, et al: Orthopedic surgery. *North Am Vet* 34:50–51, 1953.
43. Stead AC: Changes in the hip joint of the dog following traumatic luxation. *J Small Anim Pract* 11:591–600, 1970.
44. Campbell JR, Lawson DD, Wyburn RS: Coxofemoral luxation in the dog. *Vet Rec* 77:1173–1177, 1965.
45. Bone DL, Walker M, Cantwell HD: Traumatic coxofemoral luxation in dogs: Results of repair. *Vet Surg* 13:263–270, 1984.
46. Gendreau C, Cawley AJ: Excision of the femoral head and neck: The long-term results of 35 operations. *JAAHA* 13:605–608, 1977.
47. Lippincott CL: Excision arthroplasty of the femoral head and neck. *Vet Clin North Am [Small Anim Pract]* 4:857–871, 1987.

UPDATE

Since original publication of this article, I have taken the opportunity to necropsy two dogs repaired by the extracapsular technique described by Allen and Chambers.[28] Both of these cases showed scoring of the femoral head from the heavy, figure-eight sutures. Thereafter, I changed preference to the toggle technique, using Ø Novafil and a short toggle made from Steinman pin stock. More than ten cases repaired in this manner, together with capsular reconstruction, have yielded excellent results. I would advise that the toggle pin technique is quicker and less technically demanding for the general surgeon.

Diagnosis of Soft Tissue Injuries Associated with Pelvic Fractures

KEY FACTS

- Pelvic fractures resulting from trauma frequently affect other organ systems.
- Abdominal trauma (including injuries to the urinary tract and abdominal organs), thoracic trauma, and peripheral nerve damage are commonly associated with pelvic fractures.
- An organized, systematic approach should be followed in the evaluation of pelvic fractures.
- Survey radiographs of the thorax and abdomen should be standard procedure in pelvic fracture cases.
- Although simple paracentesis is a valuable diagnostic technique if a large volume of free peritoneal fluid is present, diagnostic peritoneal lavage is the most reliable technique in detecting abdominal injuries.
- Follow-up physical examinations are very important in assessing the stability of the patient and in diagnosing injuries that may have gone unnoticed during initial evaluation.

University of California, Davis
Frank J. M. Verstraete, DrMedVet, MMedVet(Chir), FAVD

University of Pretoria
Nic E. Lambrechts, BVSc

PELVIC fractures and fracture-dislocations in dogs and cats are commonly seen in veterinary practice; 20% to 30% of all fractures in small animals are pelvic fractures.[1,2] A study by Kolata and Johnston revealed that the pelvis was the most frequently injured bone in urban dogs that had been hit by cars[2]; most pelvic fractures in dogs are caused by such accidents.[3–5] Böhmer reported that falls from great heights are the most commonly identified cause of pelvic fractures in cats.[6]

The magnitude of the traumatic insult required to fracture the pelvic bones is such that coincidental multiple injuries can be expected to occur.[6–8] Soft organ injuries were found in 16.5% of dogs with skeletal injury.[2]

A survey by Jackson and Brasmer (cited by Tarvin[9]) indicated that other injuries occur in more than 50% of canine pelvic fracture cases. In a study of numerous cases of pelvic fractures in cats, a 58.6% incidence of additional injuries was found.[6] The musculoskeletal system was involved in 56.4% of these cases, the abdomen and thorax in 23.2% of the cases, and the nervous system in 20.4% of the cases (see Soft Tissue Conditions Associated with Pelvic Fractures).

SOFT TISSUE INJURIES
Thoracic Injuries

The high incidence of thoracic injury associated with pelvic trauma is well documented. Brasmer mentions a study in which radiographic signs of thoracic trauma were found in 48 of 100 dogs with pelvic fractures.[10] Clinical signs, however, were detected in only 18 of these dogs.

Spackman and coworkers reported a 38.9% incidence of thoracic wall and pulmonary trauma in dogs sustaining fractures (including a considerable number of pelvic fractures) as a result of motor vehicle accidents.[11] Another study noted a 33% incidence of thoracic trauma in conjunction with hindlimb fractures in dogs.[12] Most of the thoracic injuries were multiple. The most common injury was pulmonary contusion (51.5%) followed by pneumothorax (15.1%) and pleural effusion (13.1%).

Thoracic injuries were diagnosed in 14.2% of cats with pelvic fractures, thereby accounting for 78.9% of all concomitant nonneurologic soft tissue injuries.[6] The thoracic injuries in the cats consisted mainly of hemothorax and pneumothorax.

Urinary System Injuries

Urinary tract trauma is commonly associated with pelvic fractures, although reported incidence rates vary.[8,13–17] Urinary tract injuries were diagnosed in only 0.5% of cats with pelvic fractures.[6] One study in dogs suggested a 4% incidence[17]; however, a prospective investigation of 100 dogs with pelvic fractures demonstrated urinary tract trauma in

> **Soft Tissue Conditions Associated with Pelvic Fractures**
>
> **Abdominal injuries**
> Abdominal hernia
> Avulsion of the bladder neck from the urethra
> Avulsion of the ureter
> Bladder herniation
> Bladder mucosa damage
> Bladder rupture
> Bowel necrosis
> Bowel perforation
> Mesenteric damage and ischemia
> Rectal tear
> Ruptured gallbladder and common bile duct
> Ruptured parenchymatous organs
> Urethral rupture
>
> **Cardiovascular conditions**
> Iliac arterial hemorrhage
> Myocardial ischemia and contusion
>
> **Peripheral nerve damage**
> Avulsion of lumbosacral roots
> Femoral nerve injury
> Lumbosacral trunk injury
> Sacral roots and pelvic plexus injury
> Sciatic nerve injury
>
> **Thoracic injuries**
> Diaphragmatic hernia
> Pleural effusion and/or hemothorax
> Pneumothorax
> Pulmonary contusion
>
> **Other soft tissue injuries**
> Contusion
> Hemorrhage
> Laceration

39 cases.[16] Sixteen of these cases required surgical repair. This discrepancy in reported incidence rates coincides with the reported incidence of urinary tract trauma in humans, which ranges from 0.7% to 25%.[18] It may be that such injuries sometimes remain undetected.[16]

A range of injuries (resulting from pelvic fractures) to the urinary system have been described. Selcer noted a high incidence of relatively minor damage to bladder mucosa.[16] Rupture of the bladder evidently is the most common type of serious urinary system injury in dogs and cats as well as being the most common soft tissue injury associated with pelvic fracture.[14,16] Burrows and Bovee reported that 46.2% of bladder ruptures were associated with pelvic fractures.[19] It has been suggested that this complication is more common in male dogs,[14,15] but this was refuted by Selcer.[16] Other injuries to the urinary system associated with pelvic fractures are avulsion of the bladder neck from the urethra,[2] rupture of the urethra,[4,15–17] avulsion of the ureters,[16] and renal trauma.[6] Rupture of the urethra occurs almost exclusively in male animals.[13,15,16] Herniation of the bladder (caudally into the pelvic cavity, through the abdominal wall, through a separated pubic symphysis, and through a rectal laceration) has been reported in association with pelvic fractures.[16,20–22]

Three mechanisms of injury are evidently involved in bladder trauma. First, intravesicular pressure increases quickly in a bladder distended as a result of rapid elevation of abdominal pressure after blunt trauma of the caudal abdomen[2,7,14–16]; this is apparently the most common mechanism.[15] Second, penetrating bone fragments from the fractured pelvis cause direct trauma[2,7,14–16,18]; avulsion of the bladder neck from the prostatic urethra may occur with this form of injury.[2] Finally, bruising of the bladder wall may result in localized areas of necrosis. Extravasation of urine becomes evident after a few days and may be precipitated by forceful palpation or manual bladder expression.[16]

With most bladder ruptures, urine leaks into the peritoneal space.[15] The associated pathophysiology has been well documented.[19] Urethral lacerations, ruptures, and traumatic obstructions mainly result from pubic fractures and fragment impingement.[23] Urine leakage associated with these injuries occurs mainly extraperitoneally, resulting in cellulitis and tissue necrosis.[14,15,17] If urine leakage continues, a fistulous tract may develop after several days.[14,15,17]

Peripheral Nerve Damage

Peripheral nerve damage is commonly found in pelvic fracture cases.[9] Böhmer reported an incidence of 13.9% of lumbosacral plexus damage in cats with pelvic fractures.[6] In another survey of 34 dogs and cats, 11% were found to have peripheral nerve injury.[24]

TWO MECHANISMS of injury apparently exist. The first mechanism is acute injury to the spinal roots, lumbosacral trunk, or sciatic nerve that results in an immediate and static neurologic deficit.[24–26] Avulsion of the lumbosacral roots is rare,[26] but sacroiliac luxations with cranial displacement of the ilium may cause damage to the L6 and L7 roots.[24,26] Lumbosacral trunk injury may be associated with ilial fractures with craniomedial displacement of bone fragments.[24] Direct damage to the pelvic part of the sciatic nerve is more rare because of its less intimate bony association; such damage has, however, been associated with acetabular fractures.[24]

The second mechanism, sciatic nerve entrapment, is likely to manifest after a delay period.[25] Sciatic nerve entrapment may occur secondary to ischial or acetabular fractures.[24,26] According to Chambers and Hardie, sciatic nerve entrapment in a healing fracture may occur as a result of intimate contact, callus formation, or both; alternatively, either ischial callus or craniolateral displacement of the ischial fragment can cause narrowing of the tunnel between the sciatic tuberosity and greater trochanter, thereby compressing the nerve.[26]

Injuries to other nerves, such as the femoral nerve, evidently are rare. Damage to the sacral roots and pelvic plexus may result in urinary retention or incontinence.[27]

Gastrointestinal Injuries

Reports of gastrointestinal injury directly attributable to pelvic fractures are rare.[4,28,29] It is conceivable, however, that abdominal organ injuries associated with blunt abdominal trauma may be found in patients with pelvic fractures.[7]

Lacerations of the rectum occur in the caudal four to six centimeters of the organ.[30] Laceration by pubic fracture fragments and entrapment of the organ between pubic fracture fragments have been named as the two most common mechanisms of direct injury.[22,29,30]

Other Injuries

Injury to the reproductive system evidently occurs infrequently.[13] Prostatic laceration was reported in two dogs,[2] and rupture of the pregnant uterus is possible.[13]

Herniation through the abdominal wall is possible in conjunction with pelvic fracture.[4,6,27] Vascular injury is a main concern in humans, where extraperitoneal hemorrhage is largely responsible for the high mortality associated with pelvic fracture.[7] This complication also may occur in small animals.[27]

CARDIAC ARRHYTHMIA has been diagnosed in multiple trauma cases involving dogs. When it arises in conjunction with pelvic fracture in dogs, cardiac arrhythmia is attributed to myocardial contusion and myocardial ischemia resulting from shock as well as neurogenic causes.[31]

Soft tissue trauma associated with pelvic fractures is common. These injuries are not limited to the pelvic region and often are not readily apparent. The following discussion suggests a rational diagnostic approach to soft tissue injuries associated with pelvic fractures.

DIAGNOSTIC MODALITIES

Because pelvic trauma can cause injury in other areas of the body, the veterinarian must completely evaluate the patient and not limit the diagnostic field to the pelvis and immediate areas.[9] Several authors have emphasized the importance of accurately diagnosing an acutely injured animal.[7,9,10,32,33] A number of injuries will not readily be apparent[16] and should be excluded during the diagnostic procedure. The protocol for examining the trauma patient, as outlined by Brasmer,[10] is highly recommended; initial evaluation and emergency care as described in this work are beyond the scope of this article.

The following diagnostic outline concentrates especially on injuries *integral* to pelvic fractures as well as a few of the more important injuries *coincidental* to pelvic fractures. Figure 1 summarizes the diagnosis of soft tissue injuries associated with pelvic fractures.

History and Physical Examination

The history may be taken during physical examination.[32] The following information should be obtained: the nature of the traumatic incident, the amount of time that has lapsed between the traumatic incident and the examination, the ability of the animal to ambulate, whether the animal has passed urine or feces, and whether the animal is hemorrhaging.[32-38]

PELVIC FRACTURE patients experience severe pain and should be examined humanely; analgesia should be provided as soon as possible. Physical examination should start with a visual inspection. The chest wall should be inspected for visible abnormalities as well as the rate and quality of chest wall movement. The body wall, inguinal area, and perineum should be inspected for bruising, tire marks, abdominal distention, asymmetry, and localized swellings. Crowe has found that approximately 10% of patients with marked abdominal bleeding have a circular, red discoloration of the umbilical region.[39] Measuring abdominal girth at admission and afterward has been recommended as a method of detecting abdominal distention.[33]

The thorax should properly be auscultated for cardiac arrhythmia, abnormal lung sounds, displaced cardiac sounds, and borborygmi. The latter two indicate diaphragmatic hernia, as does the presence of dyspnea.

An abdominal or intercostal hernia as well as rib fractures may be diagnosed by superficial palpation of the body wall. Perineal or inguinal bruising may be associated with a ruptured urethra. Diffuse abdominal muscle splinting or areas of localized pain should be noted.

Deep palpation should be done gently, as vigorous palpation may cause dislodgment of blood clots and lead to further hemorrhage.[32] An abdomen that feels empty on palpation is suggestive of diaphragmatic hernia. Palpation should be done systematically, and the presence or absence of normally palpable structures should be noted. Areas of pain as well as abnormal intraabdominal or retroperitoneal masses may indicate abdominal injury. The absence of a palpable bladder may indicate a rupture of that organ. In dogs, however, it may be that the bladder is empty and located within the pelvic canal. A palpable and distended bladder may be found in conjunction with a ruptured urethra.[14] Palpation of the abdomen may indicate the presence of free fluid. If a large volume of fluid is present, ballottement of the abdomen may indicate a fluid wave. Additional tests that are useful for detecting smaller amounts of free peritoneal fluid

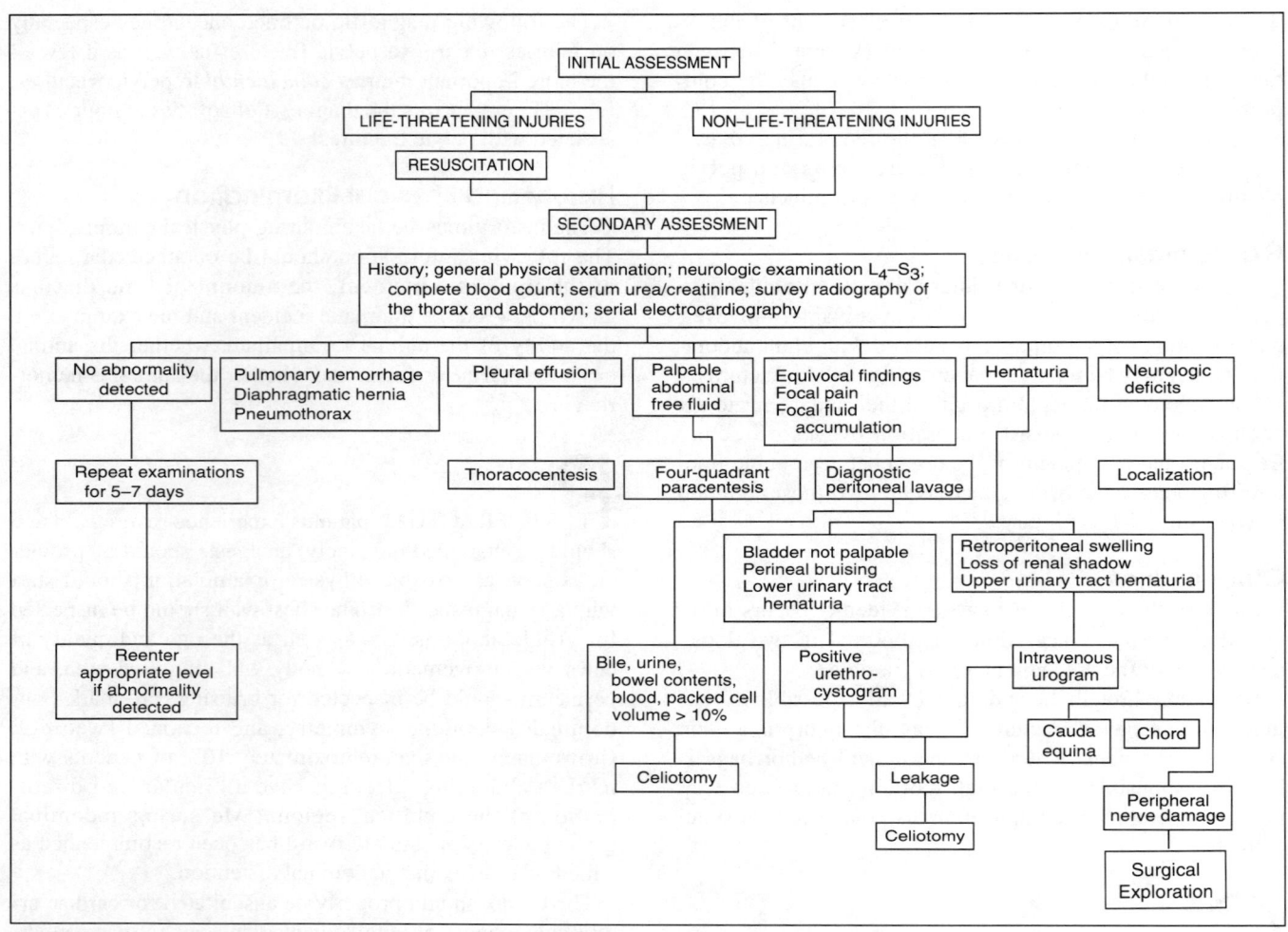

Figure 1—Summary of the diagnosis of soft tissue injuries associated with pelvic fractures.

have been recommended by Crowe and include the puddle test and the shifting dullness test.[34]

Physical examination of a pelvic fracture patient is incomplete without rectal examination, provided that the patient is an adequate size. The nature of the pelvic fracture can be palpated and the degree of displacement and presence of sharp bone fragments can be noted with a gloved and lubricated finger. In dogs, an empty bladder may be palpable in the pelvic canal. The prostate and pelvic urethra should be palpated in male dogs. Blood on the glove after completion of the examination may indicate a rectal tear.

Assessment of peripheral nerve damage is based primarily on knowledge of the sensory and motor distribution of the nerves of the pelvic limb.[25] Cutaneous, sensory, and voluntary motor deficits are the most common peripheral nerve deficits found with peripheral nerve damage associated with pelvic fractures.[24] Reflex abnormalities and severe pain also may be present.[24] Anal tone should be noted during rectal examination. Tail sensation and voluntary tail movement also should be assessed.[6,24] Assessment of peripheral nerve damage should be repeated because of its prognostic significance.[9,10]

Repeat Physical Examination

Secondary evaluation may disclose an obvious problem, such as an abdomen filled with a large volume of free fluid in an anemic patient. A few additional tests are then required to confirm the diagnosis, and immediate therapeutic action is indicated. Frequently, however, physical examination does not yield abnormal findings. In humans and small animals, lack of reliability of initial abdominal examination after blunt trauma has been emphasized.[34,40] Additional tests, continuous monitoring, and repeat physical examinations are thus indicated. Examples of conditions that may only manifest after some time has lapsed are:

- Progressive abdominal distention[33,37]
- Perineal discoloration and swelling as a result of extravasation of urine associated with urethral injury[23]

- Developing peritonitis, which becomes apparent after a few days in cases of intestinal necrosis resulting from bruising or mesenteric avulsion[28,32,38]
- Persistent absence of intestinal sounds, which is a very reliable sign of intraabdominal injury[38]
- Renal bleeding or retroperitoneal extravasation of urine[32] manifested as a progressively enlarging mass around the kidneys
- Cardiac arrhythmia (developing 12 to 48 hours after the insult) associated with multiple trauma.[31]

Clinical Pathology

An intravenous catheter should be placed during the workup and while the animal is being monitored.[34] When the catheter is inserted, blood samples may be collected for various tests. Packed cell volume and total plasma protein are important baseline values, although they are not reliable tests for assessing acute blood loss.[10,35,36,38] Serial measurements, however, may be helpful in monitoring continued hemorrhage.[10,35,36,38]

White blood cell counts may be of diagnostic value. Leukocytosis resulting from neutrophilia with minimum left shift may be evident three hours after hemorrhaging has begun.[41] Although leukocytosis may be a nonspecific finding in trauma cases,[37,38,40] severe leukocytosis with left shift can be associated with peritonitis,[38] extravasation of urine (associated with a ruptured urethra),[14,17] and splenic injury.[37] Peritonitis resulting from bile duct or intestinal rupture is reflected only by neutrophilic leukocytosis with left shift three to five days after occurrence. Endotoxemia resulting from absorption of bacterial endotoxins through intestinal ischemia, however, may induce early (within one hour), transient neutropenia.[41] Blood gas values of arterial blood reveal defective respiratory gas exchange at an early stage and thus aid in management of the defect.[42]

SERUM UREA NITROGEN and creatinine invariably increase in shocked animals because of reduced renal blood flow. Persistent azotemia after restoration of normal blood volume and pressure, however, is clinically significant. Persistent azotemia could indicate postshock renal failure, compromised renal blood supply, postrenal obstruction, or postrenal leakage of urine.

Potassium should be monitored for two reasons: (1) imbalances caused by intravenous fluid administration, crush syndrome, and shock can compromise cardiac function; (2) postrenal obstruction or leakage can cause life-threatening hyperkalemia. Serum bilirubin is elevated during bile leakage.[38] Conjugated bilirubin assay, however, is a more sensitive parameter than measurement of total bilirubin levels.

Catheterization and Urinalysis

An animal's ability to urinate and produce normal-appearing urine does not rule out the possibility of bladder rupture.[14,19,34] In many cases, however, the animal is able only to void small amounts of blood-tinged urine.[14,19] Hematuria is common in patients with urinary tract injury associated with pelvic fractures.[13–16] Hematuria at the beginning of urination may be associated with a lesion of the urethra or prostate, whereas hematuria at the end of urination may suggest a lesion in the bladder or kidneys.[15] In cases of pelvic fracture in humans, however, microscopic hematuria in the absence of other urologic signs has not been found to be a reliable indicator of significant urinary system injury.[18] Unless frank hematuria (as identified on a dipstick) is present, hematuria must be confirmed by urine sediment because myoglobinuria caused by muscle trauma also gives positive results.

URINE may be collected for routine urinalysis by catheterization or cystocentesis.[34] In addition, free-flow sampling may reveal urethral injury. Diagnostic catheterization is not recommended if urethral rupture is suspected because of the risk of further damage and introduction of infection.[13,17] Successful collection of urine through the catheter does not rule out bladder rupture. An amount of urine may remain in the ruptured bladder or the catheter may pass through the tear in the bladder wall into the urine in the abdominal cavity.[13,14,19,34] Injecting sterile saline solution and subsequently attempting to aspirate the fluid has not been found to be a reliable diagnostic technique.[19] Inflating the bladder with air (or preferably carbon dioxide gas) and listening for the sound of gas escaping from the bladder into the peritoneal cavity has been suggested for diagnosis of bladder rupture.[13,19,43]

Radiographic Evaluation

The high incidence of thoracic and urologic injury associated with pelvic fractures in small animals warrants routine thoracic and abdominal survey radiographs.[12,16,34,35] The timing of radiographic evaluation is very important. Early radiographic assessment of thoracic and abdominal trauma is indicated, but such assessment should not interfere with resuscitation or cause unnecessary stress for the patient.[14,15,38,43] Furthermore, thoracic injury may not be radiographically evident immediately after trauma has occurred.[12] Pulmonary hemorrhage cannot be reliably diagnosed on radiographs taken within one hour of injury because signs may take 2 to 12 hours to develop.[33]

Thoracic radiographs should be evaluated systematically.[44] Localized increased pulmonary densities on air bronchograms indicate pulmonary hemorrhage, which is reportedly the most common thoracic injury associated with pelvic fractures. Pneumothorax is usually easily identified, and its severity must be assessed. Other conditions that may be diagnosed include pleural effusion and diaphragmatic herniation.

Abdominal survey radiographs are of diagnostic value and may reveal generalized increased density, which indicates free peritoneal fluid; such fluid may be blood, urine, bile, or exudate. An increased density in a particular region may be associated with localized hemorrhage or localized peritonitis. In cases of localized peritonitis, free peritoneal gas also may be found; the gas originates from a ruptured, hollow viscus. Repeat radiographs may be indicated because radiographic signs may take considerable time to develop.[36,38,44] Organ enlargement may result from subcapsular hemorrhage.[36]

THE RETROPERITONEAL space should carefully be evaluated. Increased density and loss of the renal shadow may be associated with extravasation of urine or hemorrhage. If the renal shadow is not visible or if gross hematuria is clinically evident, intravenous urography is indicated.[7,13-16,18,34,36,38,44] Intravenous urography also demonstrates injury to the ureters.[16,44] If the bladder shadow is not visible, if signs of free fluid in the abdomen are present, or if there is clinical suspicion of bladder rupture or urethral damage, a positive-contrast retrograde cystourethrogram is indicated.[14-17,34,36,42,44] Negative contrast has not been found to be reliable,[19] and use of air may result in fatal air embolism.[13] Care should be taken to pass the catheter aseptically and atraumatically to avoid introducing infection and minimize further trauma.[7,13] If catheterization is difficult, the integrity of the bladder also can be assessed in the end stage of an intravenous urogram.[16,45]

Paracentesis and Diagnostic Peritoneal Lavage

Needle paracentesis is indicated if evidence of a considerable amount of free peritoneal fluid is found during examination.[34,46,47] Needle abdominal paracentesis is done using the four-quadrant technique. After aseptic preparation, a hypodermic needle is inserted and fluid, if present, is allowed to flow freely into the needle hub. A free flow of at least 0.5 ml of liquid (i.e., blood, urine, bile, or exudate) mixed with intestinal contents is considered a positive result.[34-36,38,46-48] If urine is retrieved, it usually is blood tinged and turbid.[19] Gentle manipulation of the abdomen or redirection of the needle may be helpful.[35,38] Fluid samples may be submitted for cytology and analysis.[33,38,47] A negative finding, however, may be insignificant because abdominal injury was only detected by needle paracentesis in 47% of cases in one study.[47]

The accuracy of paracentesis can be increased to 83% by using a multiholed peritoneal dialysis catheter in a midline position caudal to the umbilicus instead of a needle and the four-quadrant localization.[47] Diagnostic peritoneal lavage, however, has been shown to be the most reliable method of detecting visceral injuries, with a reported accuracy of 95% in both small animals and humans.[47,49] This technique does not, however, detect retroperitoneal conditions.[46,48]

After aseptic preparation of the periumbilical skin and infiltration of a local anesthetic, the animal is placed in left lateral recumbency. Care should be taken if the bladder is palpably distended, and catheterization may be indicated. A peritoneal dialysis catheter or a large-bore intravenous catheter with additional holes cut on the side can be used.[34,50] There are three techniques of introducing the diagnostic peritoneal lavage catheter.[40] The closed method consists of inserting the catheter percutaneously and through the linea alba. With the semiopen technique, which is the preferred method, a small skin incision is made immediately caudal to the umbilicus. With a trocar-tipped stylet in place, the catheter is gently pushed through the linea alba and into the peritoneal cavity. The open method involves minilaparotomy on the patient in dorsal recumbency.[50] Both the skin and linea alba are incised with a scalpel blade; the linea alba edges are held apart by two stay sutures, and the catheter is introduced without using a stylet. The catheter is directed caudodorsally. Lukewarm lactated Ringer's solution (20 ml/kg) is infused through the catheter into the peritoneal cavity by means of a drip set. The patient is gently rolled from side to side, and the fluid is subsequently siphoned from the abdomen. After the catheter has been withdrawn, the skin and the linea alba are closed with a single interrupted suture.[34,35,38,46,48,50]

IF THE RETURNED FLUID is clear, serious abdominal injury can be ruled out[34,46]; it has recently been suggested that laboratory analysis is unnecessary in such cases.[51] A grossly bloody lavage fluid indicates abdominal bleeding. Measurement of the packed cell volume or the number of red blood cells, however, is a more objective means of assessing abdominal bleeding. A packed cell volume of 10% or a red blood cell count of 100,000/mm^3 generally is considered to be significant for severe hemorrhage, whereas a packed cell volume of less than 5% indicates mild hemorrhage.[40,47,48,52] With equivocal results, continued monitoring of the patient's vital signs and repeat diagnostic peritoneal lavage is indicated.[48,50]

A white blood cell count and cytologic examination of the sediment is indicated if the fluid appears turbid.[34,48] A white blood cell count of more than 1000/mm^3 indicates peritoneal irritation usually associated with intestinal perforation, although urine or pancreatic secretions can produce a similar response.[52] This finding should be correlated with physical signs and the results of cytologic examination. Intracellular or free bacteria, degenerative neutrophils, and vegetable fibers indicate visceral leakage.[34,48] These findings rule out an elevated white blood cell count reflecting severe systemic leukocytosis in the absence of abdominal injury.[50] A white blood cell count from lavage fluid is of no diagnostic value if done within four hours of injury because it takes time for the white blood cell count to elevate after peritoneal irritation.[51]

Chemical analysis of lavage fluid, however, may be of great diagnostic value. Free bilirubin in the nonicteric patient indicates bile leakage.[34,47,48] Urinary leakage is indicated when creatinine and urea nitrogen values in the lavage fluid are higher than in the correponding serum values.[34,48] Care must be taken when evaluating serum urea nitrogen, creatinine, and bilirubin values in conjunction with diagnostic peritoneal lavage. Dialysis fluid dilutes these substances and thus makes quantitative determinations impossible. Evaluation of the substances is of far more value if done after paracentesis. The value of amylase determination has recently been questioned,[33,49] although high amylase values in lavage fluid usually are associated with pancreatic damage.[47,48] Interpretation of Clinicopathologic Analysis of Peritoneal Fluid summarizes the most important types of analysis and interpretation of peritoneal fluid.

Exploratory Celiotomy

Exploratory celiotomy, although relatively traumatic, is the definitive diagnostic modality.[53] Diagnostic peritoneal lavage is an important gauge in determining the timing of celiotomy in abdominal trauma cases.[46]

Other Diagnostic Modalities

Various other tests that may be indicated in selected cases have been described. Electromyographic examination may be of diagnostic value in determining the level of peripheral nerve lesions,[26] although it takes several days for abnormal findings to become evident.[24,25] Electrocardiography is indicated during monitoring of multiple trauma cases[31] and may also reveal the presence of electrolyte imbalance disorders, such as hyperkalemia.[54] Cystoscopy has recently been named as the procedure of choice for accurate assessment of urinary tract damage, especially in female animals.[55]

DIAGNOSTIC ultrasonography is a noninvasive diagnostic tool that is able to demonstrate the presence of free intraperitoneal fluid, solid organ hematomas, and retroperitoneal fluid accumulation.[40] Laparoscopy has recently been advocated as being more accurate for surgical decision making than diagnostic peritoneal lavage in humans.[56] Computed tomography and nuclear magnetic resonance imaging have been found to be useful in complementing diagnostic peritoneal lavage in humans[40] but are not readily accessible for veterinary use.

SUMMARY

The practitioner must be aware that soft tissue injuries are not the only types of injuries that occur in conjunction with pelvic fractures. Coincidental and possibly serious injuries in distant parts of the body also occur, thereby supporting a comprehensive examination.

After initial assessment and (if indicated) resuscitation of the pelvic fracture patient, a detailed examination is needed to diagnose concomitant soft tissue injuries, which are known to occur. The cornerstones of examination are as follows: the physical examination, during which assessment of vital signs, careful abdominal palpation, and rectal examination are done; survey radiographic studies of the thorax and abdomen, which should be complemented by positive-contrast studies if urinary tract injury is suspected; diagnostic peritoneal lavage, which has been found to be an extremely reliable method of diagnosing abdominal injuries; and finally, repeat physical examinations.

Whether to place emphasis on repeat physical examinations or on diagnostic peritoneal lavage in the management of pelvic fracture patients depends on clinical acumen and practice circumstances. We believe that repeat physical ex-

---

Interpretation of Clinicopathologic Analysis of Peritoneal Fluid

Bile duct rupture (exudate)
- Bilirubin crystals
- Color
- Greenish-gray material phagocytosed by macrophages
- Macrophage, neutrophil, and mesothelial cell reaction

Blood
- Erythrophagocytosis (later development)
- Mild cellular macrophage and mesothelial cell reaction
- Thrombocytes (early, active hemorrhage)

Intestinal rupture (exudate)
- Color and odor
- Macrophage, neutrophil, and mesothelial cell reaction
- Undigested food particles
- Varied bacterial spectrum (many free)

Urinary tract rupture (transudate or modified transudate)
- Ammonia odor on heating
- Creatinine-to-urea ratio in lavage fluid greater than serum creatinine-to-urea ratio
- Mild macrophage, neutrophil, and mesothelial cell reaction

aminations are very important and should be done on a routine basis provided that they do not further compromise the patient's condition.

ACKNOWLEDGMENTS

The authors thank Drs. P. H. Turner and F. Reyers for their assistance in preparing this article.

About the Authors

Dr. Verstraete is affiliated with the Department of Surgical and Radiological Sciences, School of Veterinary Science, University of California at Davis. He is a Diplomate of the American Veterinary Dental College and the European College of Veterinary Surgeons. Dr. Lambrechts is at the Department of Surgery, Faculty of Veterinary Science, University of Pretoria at Onderstepoort, South Africa.

REFERENCES

1. Brinker WO, Piermattei DL, Flo GL: *Handbook of Small Animal Orthopedics and Fracture Treatment.* Philadelphia, WB Saunders Co, 1983, p 51.
2. Kolata RJ, Johnston DE: Motor vehicle accidents in urban dogs: A study of 600 cases. *JAVMA* 167:938–941, 1975.
3. Kolata RJ: Trauma in dogs and cats: An overview. *Vet Clin North Am [Small Anim Pract]* 10:515–522, 1980.
4. Denny HR: Pelvic fractures in dogs: A review of 123 cases. *J Small Anim Pract* 19:151–166, 1978.
5. Nakasala-Situma J: *Beckenfrakturen beim Hund in den Jahren 1970–1977.* Inaugural-Dissertation, Ludwig Maximilians-Universität Munchen, 1979.
6. Böhmer E: *Beckenfrakturen und - Luxationen bei der Katze in den Jahren 1975–1982.* Inaugural-Dissertation, Ludwig-Maximilians-Universität Munchen, 1985.
7. Betts CW: Pelvic fractures, in Slatter DH (ed): *Textbook of Small Animal Surgery.* Philadelphia, WB Saunders Co, 1985, pp 2138–2153.
8. Tarvin GB, Lenehan TM: Management of sacroiliac dislocations and ilial fractures, in Bojrab MJ (ed): *Current Techniques in Small Animal Surgery,* ed 3. Philadelphia, Lea & Febiger, 1990, pp 649–656.
9. Tarvin GB: Management of pelvic fractures, in Bojrab MJ (ed): *Current Techniques in Small Animal Surgery,* ed 2. Philadelphia, Lea & Febiger, 1983, pp 588–594.
10. Brasmer TH: *The Acutely Traumatized Small Animal Patient.* Philadelphia, WB Saunders Co, 1984.
11. Spackman CJA, Caywood DD, Feeney DA, Johnston GR: Thoracic wall and pulmonary trauma in dogs sustaining fractures as a result of motor vehicle accidents. *JAVMA* 185:975–977, 1984.
12. Tamas PM, Paddleford RR, Krahwinkel DJ: Thoracic trauma in dogs and cats presented for limb fractures. *JAAHA* 21:161–166, 1985.
13. Bjorling DE: Traumatic injuries of the urogenital system. *Vet Clin North Am [Small Anim Pract]* 14:61–76, 1984.
14. Thornhill JA, Cechner PE: Traumatic injuries to the kidney, ureter, bladder, and urethra. *Vet Clin North Am [Small Anim Pract]* 11:157–169, 1981.
15. Wingfield WE: Lower urinary tract injuries associated with pelvic trauma. *Can Pract* 1(2):25–28, 1974.
16. Selcer BA: Urinary tract trauma associated with pelvic trauma. *JAAHA* 18:785–793, 1982.
17. Rawlings CA, Wingfield WE: Urethral reconstruction in dogs and cats. *JAAHA* 12:850–860, 1976.
18. Spirnak JP: Pelvic fracture and injury to the lower urinary tract. *Surg Clin North Am* 68:1057–1096, 1988.
19. Burrows CF, Bovee KC: Metabolic changes due to experimentally induced rupture of the canine urinary bladder. *Am J Vet Res* 35:1083–1088, 1974.
20. Dorn AS, Olmstead ML: Herniation of the urinary bladder through the pubic symphysis in a dog. *JAVMA* 168:688–689, 1976.
21. Gambardella PC, Archibald J: Urinary system, in Archibald J, Catcott EJ (eds): *Canine and Feline Surgery, Vol I.* Santa Barbara, CA, American Veterinary Publications, 1984, p 416.
22. Lambrechts NE: Herniation of the bladder into the rectum in a dog. *Vet Comp Orthop Traumatol* 3:106–109, 1990.
23. Smith CW: Surgical diseases of the urethra, in Slatter DH (ed): *Textbook of Small Animal Surgery.* Philadelphia, WB Saunders Co, 1985, pp 1799–1810.
24. Jacobson A, Schrader SC: Peripheral nerve injury associated with fracture or fracture-dislocation of the pelvis in dogs and cats: 34 cases (1978–1982). *JAVMA* 190:569–572, 1987.
25. De Lahunta A: *Veterinary Neuroanatomy and Clinical Neurology,* ed 2. Philadelphia, WB Saunders Co, 1983.
26. Chambers JN, Hardie EM: Localization and management of sciatic nerve injury due to ischial or acetabular fracture. *JAAHA* 22:539–544, 1986.
27. Newton CD, Nunamaker DM: *Textbook of Small Animal Orthopedics.* Philadelphia, JB Lippincott Co, 1985, p 395.
28. Dorn AS, Hufford TJ, Anderson NV: Four cases of traumatic intestinal injuries in dogs. *JAAHA* 11:786–792, 1975.
29. Gilmore DR: Traumatic intestinal injuries associated with pelvic fractures: Two case reports. *JAAHA* 19:667–670, 1983.
30. Greiner TP, Greene RW, Archibald J: Rectum and anus, in Archibald J, Catcott EJ (eds): *Canine and Feline Surgery. Vol I.* Santa Barbara, CA, American Veterinary Publications, 1984, pp 214–215.
31. MacIntire DK, Snider TG: Cardiac arrhythmias associated with multiple trauma in dogs. *JAVMA* 184:541–545, 1984.
32. Brace JJ, Bellhorn T: The history and physical examination of the trauma patient. *Vet Clin North Am [Small Anim Pract]* 10:533–539, 1980.
33. Wingfield WE, Henik RA: Treatment priorities in cases of multiple trauma. *Semin Vet Med Surg [Small Anim]* 3:193–201, 1988.
34. Crowe DT: The first steps in handling the acute abdomen patient. *Vet Med* 83:654–674, 1988.
35. Crane SE: Evaluation and management of abdominal trauma in the dog and cat. *Vet Clin North Am [Small Anim Pract]* 10:655–689, 1980.
36. Houlton JEF: Abdominal trauma. *Vet Annu* 28:228–232, 1988.
37. Holt JC: General management of abdominal trauma. *Aust Vet Pract* 8:25–38, 1978.
38. Birchard SJ, Fingland RB: Abdominal trauma, in Bright RM (ed): *Surgical Emergencies.* New York, Churchill Livingstone, 1986, pp 111–125.
39. Crowe DT: The steps to arresting abdominal hemorrhage. *Vet Med* 83:676–681, 1988.
40. McAnena OJ, Moore EE, Marx JA: Initial evaluation of the patient with blunt abdominal trauma. *Surg Clin North Am* 70:495–515, 1990.
41. Duncan JR, Prasse KW: *Veterinary Laboratory Medicine (Clinical Pathology).* Ames, IA, Iowa State University Press, 1977, pp 3–51.
42. Amis TC, Haskins SC: Respiratory failure. *Semin Vet Med Surg [Small Anim]* 1:261–275, 1986.
43. Crowe DT: What to do with disorders of the caudal abdomen. *Vet Med* 83:700–709, 1988.
44. Spencer CP, Ackerman N: Thoracic and abdominal radiography of the trauma patient. *Vet Clin North Am [Small Anim Pract]* 10:541–559, 1980.
45. Pechman RD: Urinary trauma in dogs and cats: A review. *JAAHA* 18:33–40, 1982.
46. Crowe DT, Crane SW: Diagnostic abdominal paracentesis and lavage in the evaluation of abdominal injuries in dogs and cats: Clinical and experimental investigations. *JAVMA* 168:700–705, 1976.
47. Crowe DT: Diagnostic abdominal paracentesis techniques: Clinical evaluation in 129 dogs and cats. *JAAHA* 20:223–230, 1984.
48. Paddleford RR, Harvey RC: Critical care surgical techniques. *Vet Clin North Am [Small Anim Pract]* 19:1079–1094, 1989.
49. Henneman PL, Marx JA, Moore EE, et al: Diagnostic peritoneal lavage: Accuracy in predicting necessary laparotomy following blunt and penetrating trauma. *J Trauma* 30:1345–1355, 1990.
50. Crowe DT: Diagnostic abdominal paracentesis and peritoneal lavage, in Zaslow IM (ed): *Veterinary Trauma and Critical Care.* Philadelphia, Lea & Febiger, 1984, pp 497–506.
51. D'Amelio LF, Rhodes M: A reassessment of the peritoneal lavage leukocyte count in blunt abdominal trauma. *J Trauma* 30:1291–1293, 1990.

52. Root HD: Abdominal trauma and diagnostic peritoneal lavage revisited. *Am J Surg* 159:363–364, 1990.
53. Crowe DT: Dealing with visceral injuries of the cranial abdomen. *Vet Med* 83:682–699, 1988.
54. Allen DG, Downey RS: Exercise in electrocardiographic interpretation. *Can Vet J* 24:261, 1983.
55. McCarthy TC, McDermaid SL: Cystoscopy. *Vet Clin North Am [Small Anim Pract]* 20:1315–1339, 1990.
56. Berci G, Sackier JM, Paz-Partlow M: Emergency laparoscopy. *Am J Surg* 161:332–335, 1991.

UPDATE

OTHER DIAGNOSTIC MODALITIES

The use of computed tomography (CT) and magnetic resonance imaging (MRI) recently has become more accessible for veterinarians, especially at teaching hospitals and large referral centers. Abdominal or thoracic CT scanning is indicated for the evaluation of suspected masses. All major organs and blood vessels can be readily identified, which could augment the information obtained from standard radiographs.[1] To date, MRI has mostly been used for the evaluation of the central nervous system; however, the superior anatomic detail obtained of soft tissue structures indicates that MRI could be very helpful in the diagnosis of abdominal disorders and extravascular blood.[2] Both modalities are probably underused for abdominal and thoracic evaluation of traumatized animals.

The importance of diagnostic ultrasound for the evaluation of abdominal emergencies is borne out by the numerous recent publications on the subject.[3-5] In human medicine, focused abdominal sonogram for trauma (FAST) is advocated as a primary diagnostic modality for assessing blunt abdominal trauma cases.[6,7] One study concluded that ultrasound could be reliably used in place of diagnostic peritoneal lavage in the detection of free abdominal fluid.[7]

The technique for diagnostic laparoscopy in veterinary medicine is well described;[8] however, its potential as a modality for abdominal trauma assessment has not been explored. The value of diagnostic laparoscopy as a minimally invasive, cost-effective technique for accurately identifying human, acute abdominal patients requiring emergency or urgent surgery (where the results of traditional diagnostic modalities have been equivocal) has been described.[9,10]

REFERENCES

1. Stickle RL, Hathcock JT: Interpretation of computed tomographic images. *Vet Clin North Am [Small Anim Pract]* 23 417–435, 1993.
2. Shores A: Magnetic resonance imaging. *Vet Clin North Am [Small Anim Pract]* 23:437–459, 1993.
3. Kaplan PM, Murtaugh RJ, Ross JN: Ultrasound in emergency veterinary medicine. *Semin Vet Med Surg [Small Anim]* 3:245–254, 1988.
4. Saxon WD: The acute abdomen. *Vet Clin North Am [Small Anim Pract]* 24:1207–1223, 1994.
5. Kleine LJ, Penninck DG: Critical care imaging, in Murtaugh RJ, Kaplan PM (eds): *Veterinary Emergency and Critical Care Medicine.* St Louis, Mosby Year Book, 1992, pp 547–574.
6. Rozycki GS, Shackford SR: Ultrasound, what every trauma surgeon should know. *J Trauma* 40:1–4, 1996.
7. McKenney M, Lentz K, Nunez D, et al: Can ultrasound replace diagnostic peritoneal lavage in the assessment of blunt trauma? *J Trauma* 37:439–441, 1994.
8. Magne M: Laparoscopy: Instrumentation and Technique, in Tams TR (ed): *Small Animal Endoscopy.* St Louis, The CV Mosby Co, 1990, pp 367–375.
9. Vander Velpen GC, Shimi SM: Diagnostic yield and management benefit of laparoscopy: A prospective audit. *Gut* 35:1617–1621, 1994.
10. Carey JE, Koo R, Miller R, et al: Laparoscopy and thoracoscopy in evaluation of abdominal trauma. *Am Surg* 61:92–95, 1995.

KEY FACTS

- Proximal urinary diversion via a cystostomy catheter is recommended in complete urethral transections.
- The positive-contrast retrograde urethrogram is the preferred diagnostic test in possible cases of urethral trauma.
- Selection of appropriate treatment for urethral trauma is based on the extent, the cause, and the anatomic location of the injury.
- Potential complications of urethral trauma and urethral surgery include urethral strictures, urethral fistulas, and urinary incontinence.

Urethral Trauma and Principles of Urethral Surgery

Lawrence W. Anson, DVM
Akron/Cleveland Veterinary
 Surgical Associates
Copley, Ohio

In cases of urethral trauma, successful management depends on timely diagnosis and appropriate treatment. The decision to intervene surgically requires a knowledge of the cause and the extent of the trauma. If surgery is indicated, the success of the procedure can depend on correct application of the principles of urethral surgery. Studies of the microscopic anatomy of the urethra and investigations of urethral healing have provided the basis for these principles.

This article discusses these studies and their application to urethral surgery. The causes, diagnosis, treatment, and management of urethral trauma are presented.

Anatomy

In male dogs, the urethra can be divided into three portions.[1] The most proximal segment is the prostatic urethra. The mucosa is transitional epithelium. The submucosal layer consists of connective tissue, glands, and erectile tissue. The muscularis layer of the urethra near the bladder neck is composed of irregularly layered, circularly or obliquely oriented smooth muscle.[2] In the prostate, a circularly oriented layer of smooth muscle is present proximally and striated muscle is present distally.[2] The second segment is the membranous urethra, from the prostate to the bulb of the penis. Transitional epithelium overlies a submucosal layer. The muscularis layer is composed mainly of skeletal muscle[2] (Figure 1). The third segment, the cavernous urethra, extends from the bulb to the tip of the penis. The mucosal layer is transitional epithelium except near the external urethral sphincter, where it is stratified squamous epithelium. Cavernous tissue is present beneath the epithelium. The muscular layer is smooth muscle.[1,3,4]

The prostatic artery supplies the prostatic urethra. The membranous urethra receives branches from the internal pudendal, urethral, and prostatic arteries. The cavernous urethra is supplied by the artery of the bulb of the urethra.[1]

The urethra in female dogs is much shorter than that in males and has not been divided into segments. The mucosa is transitional epithelium with a

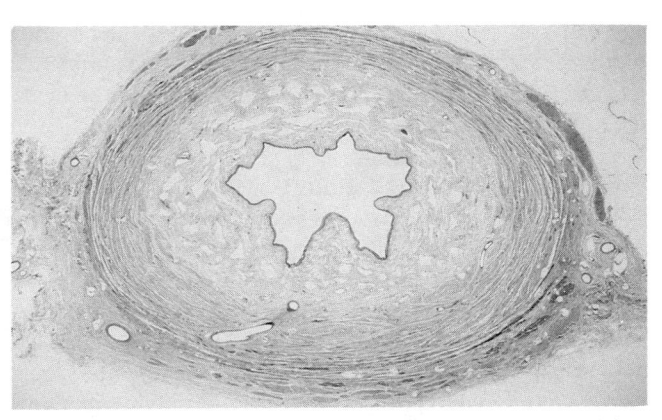

Figure 1—Cross section of canine intrapelvic urethra caudal to the prostate. From intraluminal to extraluminal, the layers are transitional epithelium, submucosa, muscularis layer (including skeletal muscle), and adventitia. (Masson's trichrome, ×4.2) (Photograph courtesy of Dr. Charles Henrikson, School of Veterinary Medicine, North Carolina State University)

vascular submucosal layer beneath. The muscular layer usually has a single layer of circularly oriented smooth muscle proximally, which changes to striated muscle distally.[5] The internal pudendal artery supplies the female urethra.[1]

Urethral Healing

After transection of the urethra, the severed urethral ends retract into the periurethral tissue. This retraction is a function of the contraction of the muscular layer. If not closed surgically, the resultant gap fills with fibrous tissue and can form a stenotic area.[6] Primary closure of complete urethral transections, rather than stenting with a catheter, reduces the incidence of posttraumatic stricture.[6]

Urethral mucosa can regenerate if a longitudinal strip of urethra remains intact. In the original experimental work, bladders in the majority of dogs were marsupialized until the urethral defect healed across a urethral stent. After seven days, the urethral mucosa had reformed but deeper layers were absent. By 21 days, vascular sinuses were observed submucosally. When there was no longitudinal strip of mucosa, the defect was filled with dense fibrous tissue.[7]

In a recent study, longitudinal incisions in healthy prescrotal urethras that were not sutured or stented healed by second intention with no strictures. Similar incisions that were sutured and stented for five days postoperatively also healed without strictures. Increased fibrosis and decreased inflammation were observed in the urethras that healed by second intention. The researchers recommended that urethrotomy incisions should not be closed primarily when mucosal and corpus spongiosum damage precludes adequate approximation. They believed that closure of these wounds could increase stricture formation.[8]

In humans, loss of the mucosal lining of the urethra results in an inflammatory response in the submucosal layer, leading to fibrosis. If the defect is not disturbed by urine passage, minimal fibrosis occurs and healing is rapid. If urine repeatedly distends the urethra, healing is delayed, with subsequent greater fibrosis and potential stricture. Proximal diversion of urine therefore is recommended in humans.[9]

Principles of Urethral Surgery

General guidelines can be given for urethral trauma surgery based on these considerations. Urine flow should be diverted by an indwelling urethral catheter and/or a cystostomy catheter.

The cystostomy technique uses a Foley catheter (8 French or smaller) introduced through a small incision in the abdominal wall and through the center of a purse-string suture on the cranioventral aspect of the bladder[10] (Figure 2). During an exploratory laparotomy, the cystostomy incision is made lateral to the midline. The omentum is wrapped around the catheter where the catheter exits the bladder and is tacked with a suture, or the omentum can be secured with the purse-string as it is tied. The bulb of the Foley catheter is inflated with sterile saline or a radiopaque contrast medium, such as meglumine iothalamate. The catheter is fixed to the skin and attached to a closed drainage system.[10-12] According to some investigators, the catheter can be removed after three days[11]; others have advocated waiting five to seven days.[12]

Gentle manipulation of tissues is an important principle of urethral surgery. Atraumatic tissue forceps should be used judiciously. Iatrogenic trauma in addition to trauma already sustained increases the possibility of fibrosis and subsequent stenosis.[12]

An anastomosis of the urethra should have minimal tension because too much tension at an anastomotic site will separate the urethral ends and cause a stricture.[6] Total transections should be debrided for 1 to 2 mm because the severed ends retract into the periurethral tissues.[6]

A 4-0 synthetic absorbable suture is recommended, such as polyglactin 910 (Vicryl™—Ethicon/Pitman-Moore), polyglycolic acid (Dexon®—Haver), or polydioxanone (PDS™—Ethicon/Pitman-Moore) suture material.[12]

Depending on the cause of the trauma and the amount of urine extravasation, copious lavage can improve the environment for healing. Drains are indicated in contaminated wounds and when extensive tissue necrosis is anticipated.[12] Placement of the drains close to the anastomosis but not in contact with it is essential because a drain touching the suture line can delay healing and lead to subsequent fistula formation.

Catheter Management

A catheter is placed in the urethra when a urethral defect is present.[11] A urethral catheter or a Foley catheter can be used. If a urethral catheter is used, it should be fixed to the tail in a female or to the abdomen in a male to help prevent premature removal. Because of the short length of Foley catheters, they are used primarily in female dogs; however, they can be used in males if placed through temporary perineal urethrostomies. The Foley bulb should be inflated and the catheter fixed to the tail. Small-gauge urethral catheters are used to allow pericatheter drainage of exudates from

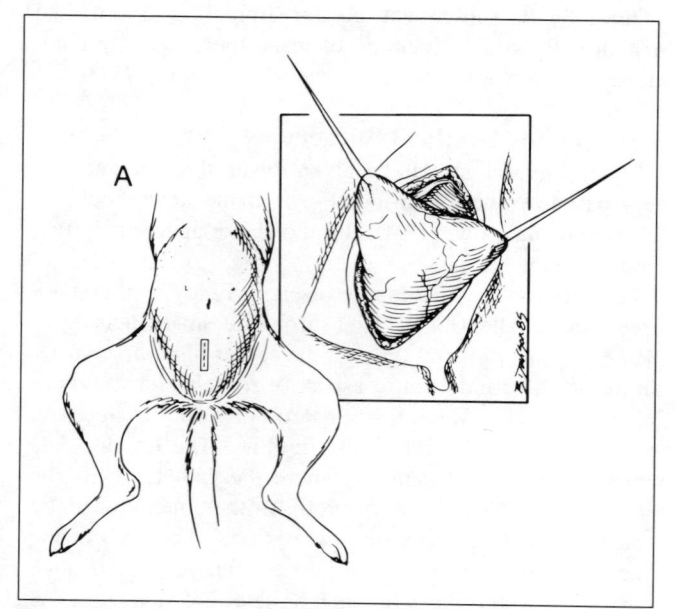

Figure 2A

the traumatized urethra.[13] Too large a catheter can promote stricture formation.[11] Cystostomy and urethral catheters can be used simultaneously. Because most urine will empty through the cystostomy catheter, a small-gauge urethral catheter can be used to splint the primary repair or defect until healing occurs.

The duration an indwelling catheter is needed is controversial. Times recommended in the literature include 5 days,[12,14] 7 to 8 days,[4] and 21 days.[4] One source asserts that catheters should be maintained for 3 to 5 days with sutured defects and as long as 21 days with unsutured ones.[15] In an experiment with urethral regeneration, noncircumferential extrapelvic defects in the canine urethra healed in 21 days with proximal urinary diversion and an indwelling catheter.[7] Appropriate duration for posttrauma catheterization is not defined. Each patient must be considered individually based on the cause and extent of the trauma.

All catheters should be maintained as a closed system incorporating the catheter, the collection tubing, and a collection bag using aseptic technique. Despite the possible difficulty associated with maintaining a closed system, the potential for preventing urinary tract infection justifies the system's use. In a study of open indwelling urethral catheters in cats, five of six (83%) had bacteriuria after three days of catheterization.[16] In a study that included 21 patients with closed systems, 52% had positive urine cultures after four days.[17] After removal of the catheter, a urine culture should be obtained and appropriate antibiotic therapy initiated.

A recent prospective study evaluating urinary tract infection resulting from indwelling bladder catheters in dogs and cats demonstrated that infections increased with catheterization for longer than four days. In some patients with prolonged catheterization and concurrent antibiotic therapy, cultures revealed the development of persistent, antibiotic-resistant infections.[17] The decision to give antibiotics when an indwelling urinary catheter is used must be made on a case-by-case basis.

Causes of Urethral Trauma

The cause of urethral trauma varies. Motor vehicle accidents account for some injuries. In a review of 600 cases involving accidents, only two cases of urethral/prostatic injury were recorded; both were associated with pubic fractures.[18] In a prospective analysis of 100 cases of pelvic trauma, five male dogs had urethral ruptures and associated fractured pubic bones. The causes of pelvic trauma in this series were not recorded.[19] In another study, urethral ruptures accounted for 11% of 281 cases of urinary tract trauma. Most were caused by automobile accidents.[20]

Dog bites and projectiles, such as bullets or arrows, can cause penetrating injury to the urethra.[12,14] Poor technique during diagnostic or therapeutic catheterization procedures can cause iatrogenic urethral trauma.[12,14] A history of previous urethral catheterization in association with signs of urinary dysfunction should suggest urethral trauma as a possible cause. Poor intraoperative technique also can cause iatrogenic urethral trauma. Urethral calculi[21,22] and urethral prolapse[4] are other causes of urethral trauma; these have been discussed in the literature.

Signalment, History, and Physical Examination

Male dogs are the animals most frequently diagnosed with urethral trauma.[11,19] The female urethra can be traumatized as a result of catheterization.[11] Animals diagnosed with urethral trauma might not have a known history of trauma. Any patient presented after motor vehicle trauma has the potential for urethral damage. The presence of pelvic fractures suggests urethral damage until such damage can be ruled out (Figures 3 and 4). Penetrating perineal wounds or caudal abdominal bruising should lead to an evaluation of the urethra. The ability to void urine does not rule out urethral trauma; a tear can be present and the patient still be able to urinate.[12]

Clinical signs associated with urethral trauma include hematuria at the beginning of urination, dysuria, or anuria.[12,14,19] Depression and anorexia might be the only signs. In some cases, perineal swelling, bruising, or a fistula might be present.[12] Palpation of a distended urinary bladder can indicate a urethral rupture. A rupture at the urethrovesical junction can allow urine to extravasate into the peritoneal cavity.[23] Clinical signs are similar to those of a ruptured urinary bladder, including abdominal distention and tenderness, vomiting, dehydration, and anorexia.[24] Physical examination might not indicate urethral trauma.[12]

Concomitant injuries must not be overlooked, especially those that are immediately life-threatening, such as hemorrhage. Associated problems that can influence the prognosis, such as neurologic dysfunction, must be critically evaluated before proceeding beyond stabilization of the patient. There are no specific laboratory tests to diagnose urethral trauma. A urethrovesical rupture with secondary extrava-

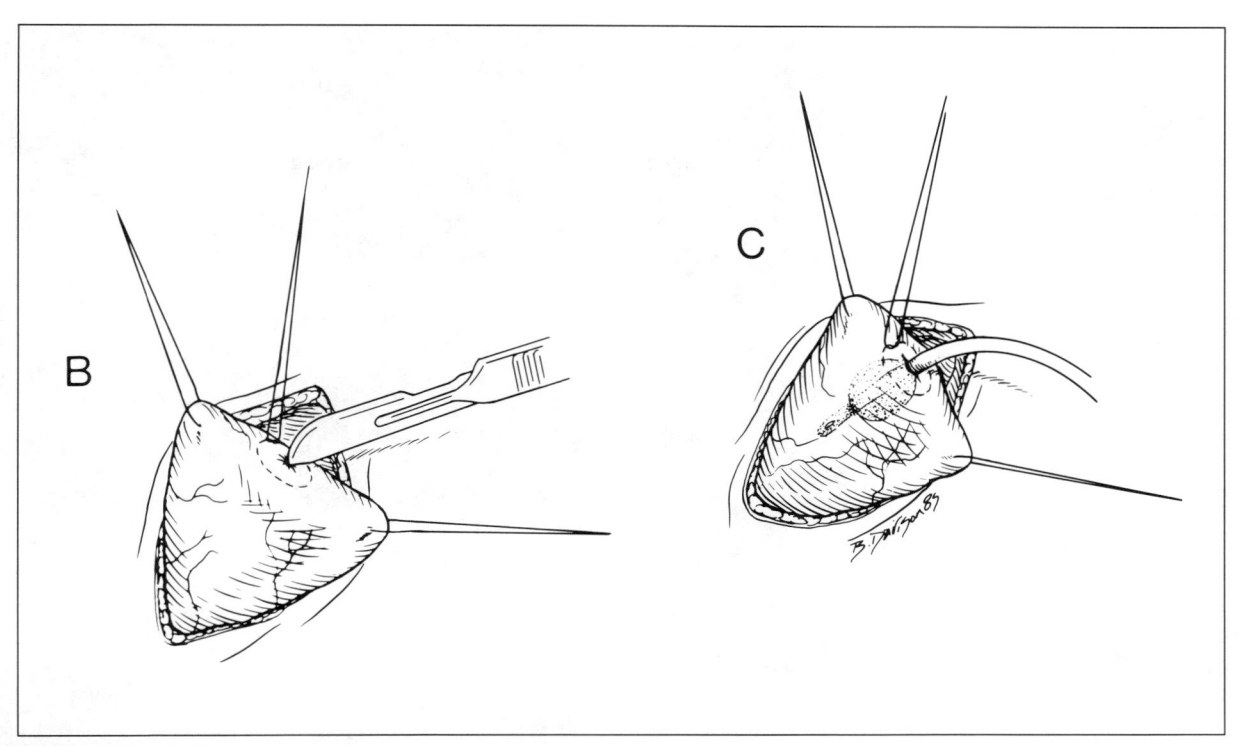

Figures 2B and 2C

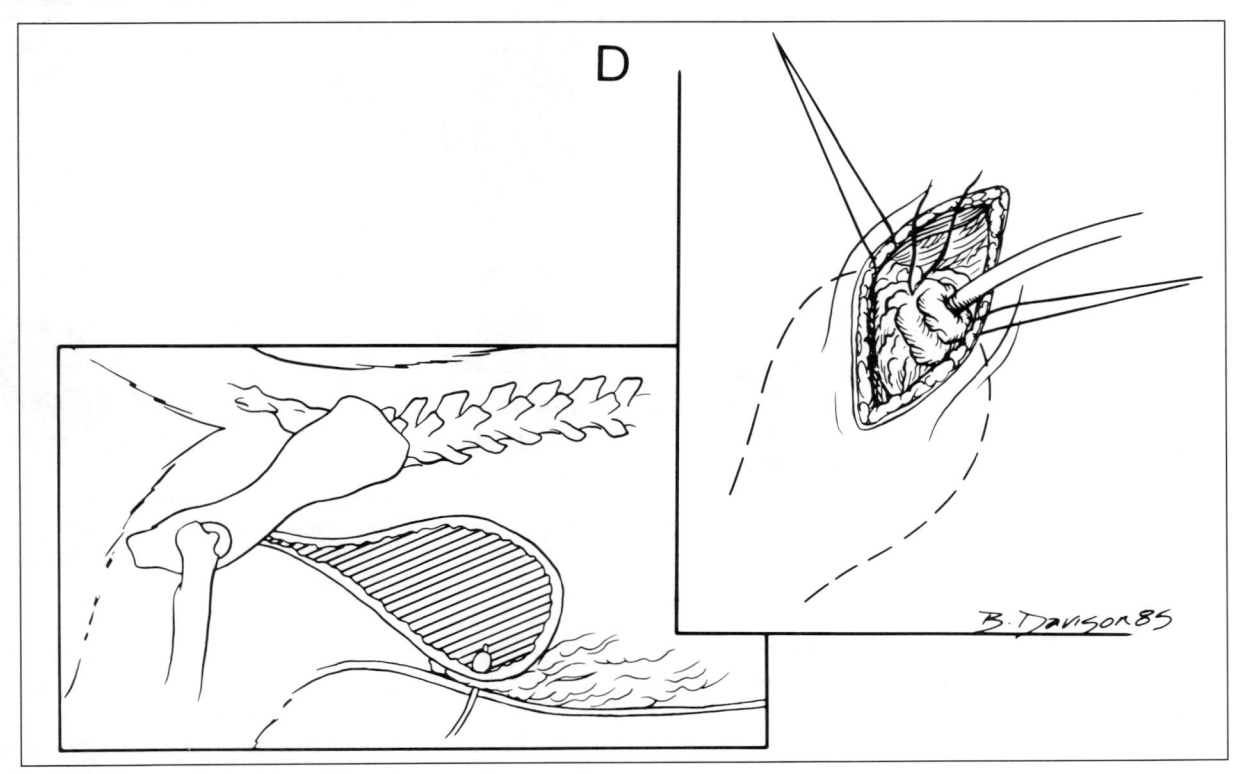

Figure 2D

Figure 2—Cystostomy catheter placement technique. (**A**) In a cat or a female dog, a 1- to 2-cm skin incision is made in the caudal third of the distance between the umbilicus and the pubic bone. In a male dog, the incision is made lateral to the prepuce. The urinary bladder is exteriorized and held with two retention sutures. (**B**) After placement of a purse-string suture through the serosa and the muscularis layers of the cranioventral bladder wall, a stab incision is made into the bladder. (**C**) The Foley catheter is inserted into the bladder and inflated with sterile saline or radiopaque contrast material. (**D**) The omentum can be incorporated into the purse-string suture as it is tied (*right*). The retention sutures are passed through the linea alba or the abdominal fascia and tied, followed by routine closure of the linea alba and the skin. The Foley catheter drains urine from the bladder into a closed drainage system (*left*). (Used by permission from Stone EA: Urologic surgery—An update, in Breitschwerdt EB [ed]: *Nephrology and Urology*. New York, Churchill Livingstone Inc, 1986.)

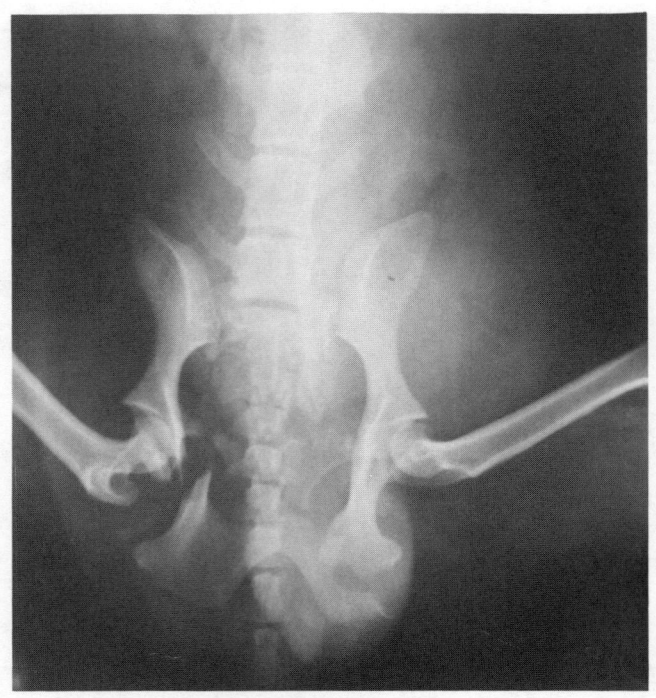

Figure 3—Ventrodorsal radiograph of an eight-year-old, male Pekingese that had been hit by a car. Pubic and ischial fractures, left sacroiliac luxation, right coxofemoral luxation, and right acetabular fracture were present.

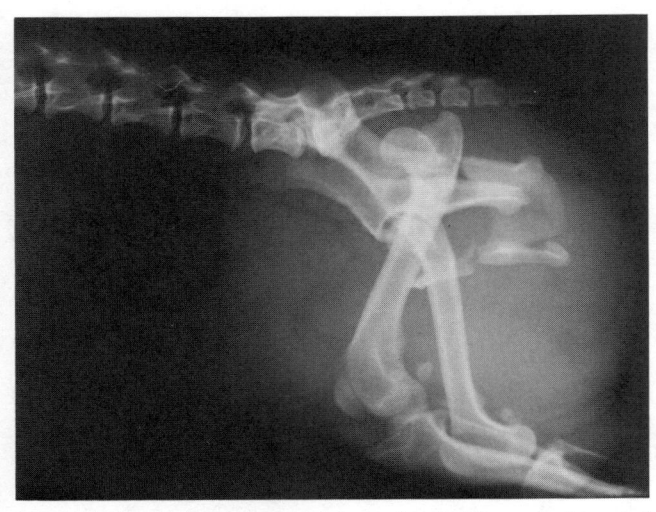

Figure 4—Lateral radiograph of the patient in Figure 3. A ventral body-wall hernia of the left side was present. An intrapelvic urethral transection was identified during surgery.

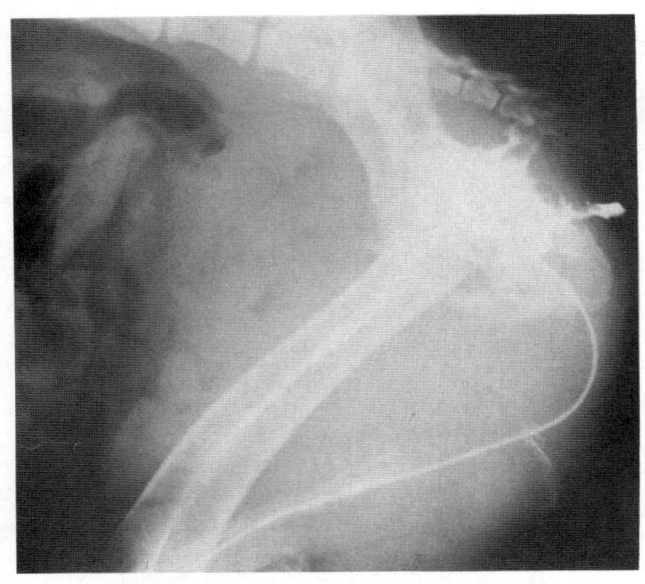

Figure 5—Positive-contrast retrograde urethrogram in a two-year-old, male weimaraner that had been shot with a hunting arrow. The urethra was totally transected in two locations, and there was a rectal laceration. Note the extravasation of contrast material from the pelvic urethra.

sation into the peritoneal cavity can cause postrenal azotemia. Associated dehydration contributes to prerenal azotemia and can be detected by elevated packed red blood cell volume and elevated plasma protein concentration.[12] Urine can be irritating to tissues and can cause severe cellulitis with associated neutrophilia.[12,14]

Radiographic Assessment

If urethral trauma is possible, urethral catheterization should not be done until after radiographic evaluation.[12,14] Survey radiographs should be obtained before proceeding to contrast studies. Critical assessment of radiographs should include evaluation of the following: perineal swelling, the presence of radiopaque foreign bodies, pelvic fractures, fractures of the os penis, changes in retroperitoneal density, and problems that might affect case management and prognosis, such as fractures of the lumbar spine and the sacrum.[19,23]

The preferred diagnostic test is the positive-contrast retrograde urethrogram[12,25,26] (Figure 5). The technique is relatively simple and requires minimal equipment and materials. A pediatric Foley catheter (6 to 12 French) or another soft, flexible catheter is recommended. A water-soluble organic iodide preparation that can be diluted to an iodide concentration of 10% to 15% is used. A commercial product containing 17.2% meglumine iothalamate (Cysto-Conray II®—Mallinckrodt) is available. Additional materials needed are 2% lidocaine solution and sterile lubricant. The descending colon and the rectum should be empty if the study is an elective procedure.

The catheter is filled with 2% lidocaine. The tip is lubricated and gently introduced into the urethra. If a Foley catheter is being used, the bulb can be inflated after insertion, avoiding overinflation and iatrogenic damage to the urethral mucosa. The lidocaine is injected first, followed by the dilute contrast material. Depending on the size of the dog, 10 to 12 ml of contrast material should be adequate. Air bubbles should not be introduced into the catheter or the urethra because bubbles can be confused with lesions. The radiograph is exposed as the last 1 to 2 ml of contrast material is injected. A lateral projection is taken first, followed by ventrodorsal and oblique views as indicated. Pulling the pelvic limbs forward helps to delineate the perineum.[25,26] In a total transection, contrast material will extravasate into the periurethral tissues and will not pass beyond the defect. With a laceration, contrast material can accumulate in the urethra proximal to the traumatized area.[25,26]

Management and Treatment

In managing a urethral trauma case, the veterinarian cannot focus efforts without first assessing the whole patient and treating more important injuries. If the patient is a surgical candidate, it should be stabilized before surgery if possible. If the animal cannot void urine, a cystostomy catheter can be placed using narcotic analgesia to temporarily remove urine until the patient is stable enough for general anesthesia and definitive surgical repair of the problem.[10,21]

Selection of appropriate treatment for urethral trauma is based on the extent, cause, and anatomic location of the injury. A urethral abrasion, as can occur with repeated catheterization, can be treated conservatively. The ideal management is to remove the catheter. If cessation of catheterization is impossible, a small-gauge catheter should be used.[9] Urethral contusion can be diagnosed with a positive-contrast retrograde urethrogram; a narrowing of the contrast material will be observed. If the urethra is intact, conservative management is again indicated. Monitoring of urination and hot packing (if the area is accessible) can be performed. If the animal is not urinating, the bladder can be expressed manually or a small-gauge urethral catheter can be placed to provide urine drainage.[4] A urethral contusion can later develop into a fistula.[12] Treatment of fistulas is discussed in the section on Complications.

A minor urethral laceration might heal spontaneously. The urethra should be stented via a small-gauge indwelling catheter.[12] Most partial urethral lacerations and all total transections require surgical correction.[11] Surgical exposure depends on the location of the laceration. The location for surgical exploration of an extrapelvic urethral laceration or a total transection can be based on urethrogram findings. A catheter is passed to the level of the defect to help identify the urethra and to act as a stent. Debridement of devitalized tissue and bacterial culture of the area, if appropriate, are indicated before repairing the defect. Drains are placed in contaminated open wounds, such as dog bites and bullet holes.[4,12]

In a dog with a fractured os penis, a urethral catheter is passed if possible. Urine is diverted through the catheter during the initial healing of the fracture, and obstruction from swelling or trauma is alleviated. If a catheter cannot be passed, repair of the fracture is attempted and a prescrotal urethrotomy is done to divert urine from the traumatized urethra while it heals. Permanent scrotal urethrostomy is performed in dogs in which repair is impossible or undesirable or in which a urethral stricture forms.[4,11,27]

An attempt to pass a urethral catheter can be made if only a laceration is present and if fluoroscopy is available.[4] The catheter remains in place until the urethra is healed. Surgical repair is required for lacerations not amenable to this approach and for total urethral transection. Traumatic injuries to the intrapelvic urethra can be approached surgically through a ventral midline incision extending to the pubis. Further exposure might require splitting of the pubic symphysis[28] or reflection of the cranial portion of the pubic bone.[29] In humans, symphysiotomy is not recommended because of stretching of the sacroiliac joints and potential back and pelvic pain.[30] Pubic fractures might need repair in conjunction with the primary urethral repair. The urethra might be anastomosed over a urethral catheter after debriding the ends; copious lavage and drainage should be considered. Prostatectomy is indicated if trauma to the prostatic urethra is extensive. A cystostomy catheter should be placed to divert the urine from the anastomotic site.[4,11,12]

If there are large defects in the urethra, some type of urinary diversion is required. For cases in which a defect in the intrapelvic urethra cannot be bridged by a primary anastomosis, extrapelvic cystourethral anastomosis can be performed in male dogs.[31] The urethra near the bladder neck is incised and then anastomosed to the penile urethra, which has been brought cranial to the pubic symphysis. It is important to salvage as much of the urethra as possible to help maintain continence. The dorsal artery to the penis should be preserved. The use of this technique in a series of cases has not been reported.

Antepubic urethrostomy can be performed when large distal defects are present in male or female dogs or cats. As much viable proximal urethra as possible is freed from its intrapelvic attachments, including the prostate gland. Vascular and nervous supply to the bladder neck must be preserved. The end of the urethra is spatulated and then brought through the ventral abdominal wall without kinking or excessive tension. The urethral mucosa is anastomosed to the skin. In females, the urethra can exit on or slightly off the midline. In males, the urethral opening will be 2 to 3 cm lateral to the prepuce. If care is taken in dissection and manipulation, the patient will retain urinary continence.[32]

Recently, a urinary bladder tube graft was used in an experimental total prostatectomy model to replace the prostatic urethra and 2 cm of membranous urethra. The clinicians believe that this is a viable technique in cases of proximal urethral loss.[33]

Postoperative Care

The patient must be restrained to prevent removal of urethral and cystostomy catheters. Judicious use of tranquilizers and incorporation of the catheters into a body bandage, an Elizabethan collar, or a side brace might be required.

If surgery is to be performed, antibiotics might be indicated before or during the operation. Antibiotics can be changed, if necessary, based on culture results obtained at surgery. Drains should be bandaged to reduce potential contamination and the risk of premature removal. They should be removed when exudation ceases. Further clinicopathologic evaluation is dictated by the patient's condition. The decision to remove the catheters is based on the condition, the extent of the injuries, and the nature of the surgical repair. A positive-contrast retrograde urethrogram can be used to accurately assess the condition of the urethra. Some clinicians believe that the pressure generated by the injection of contrast material might create or worsen urethral fistulas; these clinicians suggest that patients be evaluated postoperatively by observation of micturition.[12]

Complications

A potential complication of intrapelvic urethral trauma is urinary incontinence from the primary injury or from surgical trauma. Atraumatic technique and careful dissection is imperative because identification of vessels and nerves can be extremely difficult.[11]

Urethral fistulas can develop if a contusion becomes necrotic with subsequent extravasation of urine.[12] Failure of the primary repair of lacerated and transected urethras also can cause fistula formation. After a fistula is identified by a positive-contrast retrograde urethrogram, primary surgical repair can be performed. A urethral catheter helps to drain urine from the site until the patient is ready for surgery. If the drainage is intraperitoneal, a peritoneal catheter can be placed to drain the urine until definitive repair can be performed. Extraperitoneal leakage that is not draining to the exterior requires surgery as soon as possible.

Urethral strictures can occur after urethral trauma and are identified by a positive-contrast retrograde urethrogram.[4,12,34] In a case of urinary obstruction, an excretory urogram should be performed to evaluate the upper urinary tract.[4,34] The patient's clinical signs should be correlated with the radiographic findings because a radiographic stricture does not necessarily cause clinical problems.[34] A short stricture can be resected and anastomosed without excessive tension.[9] The treatment of longer strictures is based on the location. Prescrotal, scrotal, and perineal urethrostomies are alternatives. For an intrapelvic stricture, antepubic urethrostomy or extrapelvic cystourethral anastomosis can be performed.[4,31] In humans, internal urethrotomy via a fiber-optic scope is used extensively for urethral stricture.[35] There are no reports of internal urethrotomy being performed in dogs or cats. Posttraumatic evaluations for strictures are best performed at three to four weeks and again at three months after injury, depending on the clinical signs.[12]

Summary

Urethral trauma can be a challenging problem to treat clinically. Initial diagnosis is based on history and physical examination. Definitive diagnosis depends on the interpretation of a positive-contrast retrograde urethrogram. Treatment is based on the extent of the urethral trauma. Contusions and some lacerations can be managed conservatively; most lacerations and transections require surgery. Surgical principles—such as atraumatic technique, careful hemostasis, and knowledge of surgical anatomy—must be followed. Postoperative care is important. Potential complications include urethral fistulas, urethral strictures, and urinary incontinence.

REFERENCES

1. Evans HE, Christensen GC: *Miller's Anatomy of the Dog*, ed 2. Philadelphia, WB Saunders Co, 1979, pp 578–579, 594–595.
2. Cullen WC, Fletcher TF, Bradley WE: Histology of the canine urethra. II. Morphometry of the male pelvic urethra. *Anat Rec* 199:187–195, 1981.
3. Banks WJ: *Applied Veterinary Histology*. Baltimore, Williams & Wilkins, 1981, pp 490–491, 504.
4. Brown SG: Surgery of the canine urethra. *Vet Clin North Am [Small Anim Pract]* 5(3):457–470, 1975.
5. Cullen WC, Fletcher TF, Bradley WE: Histology of the canine urethra. I. Morphometry of the female urethra. *Anat Rec* 199:177–186, 1981.
6. McRoberts JW, Ragde H: The severed canine posterior urethra: A study of two distinct methods of repair. *J Urol* 104:724–729, 1970.
7. Weaver RG, Schulte JW: Experimental and clinical studies of urethral regeneration. *Surg Gynecol Obstet* 115:729–736, 1962.
8. Weber WJ, Boothe HW, Brassard JA, et al: Comparison of the healing of prescrotal urethrotomy incisions in the dog: Sutured versus nonsutured. *Am J Vet Res* 46(6):1309–1315, 1985.
9. Turner-Warwick RT: Urethral stricture surgery, in Glenn JF (ed): *Urologic Surgery*, ed 3. Philadelphia, JB Lippincott Co, 1983, pp 689–719.
10. Stone EA: Urologic surgery—An update, in Breitschwerdt EB (ed): *Nephrology and Urology*. New York, Churchill Livingstone Inc, 1986.
11. Bjorling DE: Traumatic injuries of the urogenital system. *Vet Clin North Am [Small Anim Pract]* 14(1):61–76, 1984.
12. Rawlings CA, Wingfield WE: Urethral reconstruction in dogs and cats. *JAAHA* 12:850–860, 1976.
13. Hackler RH: Complications of urethral and penile trauma, in Greenfield LJ (ed): *Complications of Surgery and Trauma*. Philadelphia, JB Lippincott Co, 1984, pp 741–748.
14. Wingfield WE: Lower urinary tract injuries associated with pelvic trauma. *Canine Pract* 1:25–28, 1974.
15. Smith CW: Surgical diseases of the urethra, in Slatter DH (ed): *Textbook of Small Animal Surgery*. Philadelphia, WB Saunders Co, 1985, pp 1799–1810.
16. Lee GE, Osborne CA, Stevens JB, et al: Adverse effects of open indwelling urethral catheterization in clinically normal male cats. *Am J Vet Res* 42:825–833, 1981.
17. Barsanti JA, Blue J, Edmunds J: Urinary tract infection due to indwelling bladder catheters in dogs and cats. *JAVMA* 187(4):384–388, 1985.
18. Kolata RJ, Johnston DE: Motor vehicle accidents in urban dogs: A study of 600 cases. *JAVMA* 167:938–941, 1975.
19. Selcer BA: Urinary tract trauma associated with pelvic trauma. *JAAHA* 18:785–793, 1982.
20. Kleine LJ, Thornton GW: Radiographic diagnosis of urinary tract trauma. *JAAHA* 7:318–327, 1971.
21. Stone EA: Surgical management of urolithiasis. *Compend Contin Educ Pract Vet* 3(7):627–637, 1981.
22. DiBartola SP, Chew DJ: Canine urolithiasis. *Compend Contin Educ Pract Vet* 3(3):226–238, 1981.
23. Pechman RD: Urinary trauma in dogs and cats: A review. *JAAHA* 18:33–40, 1982.
24. Burrows CF, Bovee KC: Metabolic changes due to experimentally induced rupture of the canine urinary bladder. *Am J Vet Res* 35:1083–1088, 1974.
25. Ticer JW, Spencer CP, Ackerman N: Positive contrast retrograde urethrography: A useful procedure for evaluating urethral disorders in the dog. *Vet Radiol* 21(1):2–11, 1980.
26. Watters JW: Urinary tract radiography—Bladder and urethra. *Compend Contin Educ Pract Vet* II(2):124–135, 1980.
27. Bradley RL: Complete urethral obstruction secondary to fracture of the os penis. *Compend Contin Educ Pract Vet* 7(9):759–763, 1985.
28. Knecht CD: A symphyseal approach to pelvic surgery in the dog. *JAVMA* 149(12):1729–1734, 1966.
29. Howard DR: Surgical approach to the canine prostate. *JAVMA* 155(12):2026–2031, 1969.
30. Middleton RG, Sutphin MD: Pubectomy in urological surgery. *J Urol* 133:635–637, 1985.
31. Knecht CD, Slusher R: Extrapelvic cystourethral anastomosis. *JAAHA* 6:247–251, 1970.
32. Yoshioka MM, Carb A: Antepubic urethrostomy in the dog. *JAAHA* 18:290–294, 1982.
33. Fowler JD, Holmberg DL: Proximal urethral reconstruction follow-

34. Barber DL: Postoperative radiography of the urinary system. *Vet Clin North Am [Small Anim Pract]* 14(1):31–48, 1984.
35. Kirchheim D: Internal urethrotomy, in Glenn JF (ed): *Urologic Surgery*, ed 3. Philadelphia, JB Lippincott Co, 1983, pp 749–755.

UPDATE

Since original publication of this article, several papers and review articles have been published that provide new knowledge and further clinical experience in managing patients with urethral trauma.

First and second intention healing of prescrotal urethrotomies were compared in 12 normal male dogs.[1] Urethral mucosal irregularities were observed in all 60-day postoperative urethrograms. No strictures were noted. Less postoperative hemorrhage was seen in sutured urethrotomies. This study indicates that careful primary closure of temporary urethrotomies is acceptable and will probably result in fewer postoperative complications.

Another controlled study, which involved intrapelvic urethral anastomosis in male dogs, found a lesser degree of stricture formation with urethral anastomosis using an indwelling catheter compared to suture anastomosis without an indwelling catheter, and an indwelling catheter without suture apposition of the urethra.[2] This study confirms the importance of careful, accurate suture apposition of the urethra over an indwelling catheter when complete transection has occurred.

Urethral reconstruction when there is loss of the proximal urethra is a difficult problem. This was addressed in another experimental study that used a distally–based, ventral bladder tube flap in clinically normal male dogs.[3] Over the long-term, continence was regained in all but one animal. This technique may have merit when the clinician is faced with the dilemma of how to salvage urinary tract function in a patient with proximal urethral loss.

Two case reports that discuss urethral trauma in cats have been published.[4,5] Perineal injury necessitated creation of permanent perineal urethrostomies. Two new articles that discuss urethral surgical techniques are now available for review.[6,7] Two articles about prepubic urethrostomy[8,9] confirm that this is an acceptable technique for permanently bypassing an irreparably damaged urethra. One complication of prepubic urethrostomy, urine scalding of caudal abdominal fatty skin folds, was addressed by placing the new urethral opening in a subpubic location.[10]

The basic principles of urethral healing in managing patients with urethral trauma have not changed. Success still depends on recognition of patients with urethral trauma and then, if indicated, selection of an appropriate surgical technique.

REFERENCES

1. Waldron DR, Hedlund CS, Tangner CH, et al: The canine urethra: A comparison of first and second intention healing. *Vet Surg* 14(3):213–217, 1985.
2. Layton CE, Ferguson HR, Cook JE, et al: Intrapelvic urethral anastomosis: A comparison of three techniques. *Vet Surg* 16(2):175–182, 1987.
3. Fowler JD, Holmberg DL: Proximal urethral reconstruction using a distally–based, ventral bladder tube flap: An experimental study. *Vet Surg* 16(2):139–145, 1987.
4. Goldman AL, Beckman SL: Traumatic urethral avulsion at the preputial fornix in a cat. *JAVMA* 194(1):88–90, 1989.
5. Fox SM: Surgical repair of a traumatic perineal laceration with urethral transection: A case report. *JAAHA* 26:301–304, 1990.
6. Bjorling DE, Petersen SW: Surgical techniques for urinary tract diversion and salvage in small animals. *Compend Contin Educ Pract Vet* 12(12):1699–1708, 1990.
7. Bellah JR: Problems of the urethra. Surgical approaches, in Bradley RL (ed): *Problems in Veterinary Medicine* 1(1):17–35, 1989.
8. Bradley RL: Prepubic urethrostomy. An acceptable urinary diversion technique, in Bradley RL (ed): *Problems in Veterinary Medicine* 1(1):120–127, 1989.
9. McLaren IG: Prepubic urethrostomy involving transplantation of the prepuce in the cat. *Veterinary Record* 122(15):363, 1988.
10. Ellison GW, Lewis DD, Boren FC: Subpubic urethrostomy to salvage a failed perineal urethrostomy in a cat. *Compend Contin Educ Pract Vet* 11(8):946–951, 1989.

Shock

KEY FACTS
- Shock is a multisystem disorder that affects hemodynamics of vital organs.
- Circulation failure within the cardiovascular system results in hypovolemic, distributive, or cardiogenic shock.
- The mainstay of shock management is intravenous fluid-replacement therapy.
- Successful treatment of shock depends on rapid recognition of clinical signs, quick evaluation of the patient, and immediate institution of shock management.
- Management of shock should extend beyond fluid-replacement therapy and administration of drugs.

Louisiana State University
Joseph Taboada, DVM
Johnny D. Hoskins, DVM, PhD

Rawley Memorial Animal Hospital
Springfield, Massachusetts
Rhea V. Morgan, DVM

SHOCK is defined as a decline in vital organ function as a result of maldistribution of blood flow such that delivery of oxygen and nutrients to tissue is inadequate.[1] Hemodynamic events during shock contribute to poor cardiac output, hypovolemia, and altered distribution of blood flow, which result in circulatory failure, poor tissue perfusion, cellular hypoxia, metabolic acidosis, and ultimately cell death. Most patients in shock develop systemic hypotension, a clinical hallmark of shock[1-3]; however, systemic *hyper*tension may occur when tissue perfusion is drastically reduced by peripheral vasoconstriction. Systemic hypertension is more likely to occur in patients with shock induced by sepsis or trauma.[2]

CLASSIFICATION

Shock is classified in several different ways; however, a functional classification of shock according to location of circulatory failure within the cardiovascular system is most useful to the clinician (see Causes of Shock on the following page). This classification system defines *hypovolemic shock* as circulatory failure caused by a loss of circulating blood volume, *distributive shock* as circulatory failure caused by distribution of cardiac output away from vital organs, and *cardiogenic shock* as circulatory failure caused by diminished cardiac output.[1-4]

Hypovolemic shock is the most common type of shock encountered in dogs and cats and is commonly caused by trauma. Hypovolemic shock may be associated with acute blood loss (e.g., major laceration, ruptured abdominal or thoracic organ, or surgery) or fluid loss from the extracellular space (e.g., fluid accumulation within potential spaces in the body [third-space accumulation], vomiting, diarrhea, diuresis, or plasma exudation from burns or exudative dermatopathies). Loss of as little as 15% of circulating blood volume causes tachycardia, muscle weakness, increased thirst, and altered mentation and may lead to hypovolemic shock. Loss of 15% to 35% of circulating blood volume results in hypovolemic shock that usually is corrected by systemic vasoconstriction and fluid-replacement therapy. For patients with blood loss greater than 35% to 40% of circulating blood volume, the prognosis is poor unless extensive fluid-replacement therapy is started early in the course of therapy. Acute loss of greater than 50% of circulating blood volume causes irreversible hypovolemic shock.[2]

Distributive (vasculogenic) shock occurs when maldistribution of cardiac output away from vital organs exists. Cardiac output may be low, normal, or high; the patient may have hypotension, normotension, or hypertension. Most commonly, distributive shock occurs when increased venous capacitance creates peripheral pooling of blood. This pooling may occur secondary to traumatic or surgical injury; neurologic disturbance; anaphylaxis; endotoxemia; anesthetic or sedative overdose; or metabolic, toxic, or endocrinologic depression of vasomotor tone.[3] Distributive shock also may result from arteriovenous shunting, as may occur in patients with severe sepsis.

Septic shock is a type of distributive shock that is induced by bacterial endotoxins or other bacterial or host

> **Causes of Shock**
>
> **Hypovolemic Shock**
> - Blood loss
> - Plasma loss (burns, severe exudative dermatitis, peritonitis, pancreatitis, hemorrhagic gastroenteritis)
> - Sequestration of body fluids (ascites)
> - Fluid and electrolyte loss (vomiting, diarrhea, dehydration, hypoadrenocorticism)
> - Diuresis (hypoadrenocorticism, diabetes insipidus, diabetes mellitus)
>
> **Distributive Shock**
>
> *Increased venous capacitance*
> - Trauma
> - Surgery
> - Endotoxemia
> - Anesthetic overdose
> - Metabolic causes (renal failure, hepatic failure, severe alkalosis or acidosis)
> - Endocrine disease (hypoadrenocorticism, uncontrolled diabetes mellitus)
> - Anaphylaxis
> - Neurogenic (spinal or cerebral injury)
>
> *Arteriovenous shunting*
> - Sepsis
>
> **Cardiogenic Shock**
>
> *Myocardial failure*
> - Cardiomyopathy
> - Valvular insufficiency
> - Dirofilariasis
> - Cardiac arrhythmias (bradyarrhythmias or tachyarrhythmias)
> - Congenital heart diseases
> - Overdose of cardiac drugs (vasodilators, ß-adrenergic blocking agents, calcium-channel blockers)
>
> *Obstructive disease*
> - Valvular stenosis
> - Pericardial tamponade
> - Pulmonary hypertension (dirofilariasis, pulmonary thromboembolism)
> - Intracardiac tumors
> - Hypertrophic cardiomyopathy
> - Thyrotoxic heart disease
> - Gastric dilatation/volvulus

mediators. Gram-positive and gram-negative bacteria (aerobic or anaerobic) as well as fungi may induce septic shock.[5] The type, number, and virulence of bacteria or fungi as well as host response and immune status are involved. Endotoxins and a wide array of inflammatory mediators (e.g., histamine, kinins, interleukins, eicosanoids, complement, ß-endorphins, and tumor necrosis factor) are believed to play a prominent role in the complex pathophysiologic interrelationship between invading bacteria and susceptible host.[5,6] Activation of complement and fibrinolytic and kinin systems by endotoxins and other bacterial mediators leads to maldistribution of body fluids.[6] Large volumes of fluid become sequestered in the hepatoportal system; hypotension results.[7]

Common causes of septic shock include peritonitis, pyometra, pyothorax, prostatic abscess, liver abscess, biliary tract infection, intestinal strangulation or volvulus, hemorrhagic gastroenteritis, and wound infection.[6] Sepsis-induced mortality typically is 50% to 90%; the percentage is similar in dogs, cats, and humans affected with gram-negative bacteria, gram-positive bacteria, and polymicrobial infections.[3,8,9]

NEUROGENIC SHOCK (which arises from depression of the central nervous system, primary central nervous system disease, or trauma) is a form of distributive shock that occurs infrequently in dogs and cats. Sudden loss of sympathetic tone results in peripheral vasodilation, peripheral pooling of blood, and bradycardia and is important in the mediation of neurogenic shock.[10] Deep anesthesia with such hypotensive agents as halothane or methoxyflurane may cause neurogenic shock through profound depression of the vasomotor center and loss of vascular tone.[11]

Cardiogenic shock reflects severe cardiac insufficiency and decreased cardiac output. Cardiogenic shock may result from inherent heart disease (e.g., cardiomyopathy, myocarditis, arrhythmias, myocardial injury, intracardiac neoplasia, and ruptured chordae tendineae).[3] Obstructive extracardiac conditions (e.g., cardiac tamponade, tension pneumothorax, and pulmonary hypertension) also may cause decreased cardiac output and cardiogenic shock.[3,11] In contrast to hypovolemic shock, cardiogenic shock is associated with elevated central venous pressure and peripheral venous distention.

PATHOPHYSIOLOGY

Shock is precipitated by a cascade of hemodynamic events that decrease cardiac output and cause inadequate tissue perfusion and hypotension (Figure 1). The body responds by stimulating the sympathetic nervous system and releasing catecholamines from the adrenal glands to constrict peripheral arterioles and contract the spleen.[3,7] These responses increase the heart rate and myocardial contractility and distribute blood away from the skin and intestines while maintaining circulating blood volume to the central nervous system, heart, liver, and diaphragm.[10]

Contraction of the spleen can replace up to 20% of a dog's circulating blood volume.[12] Further compensatory replacement of blood volume is mediated by increased release of renin, angiotensin, aldosterone, and antidiuretic hormone (vasopressin) with resultant sodium and water retention and decreased urine output.[3,7,12] The decrease in capillary hydrostatic pressure also alters the balance of

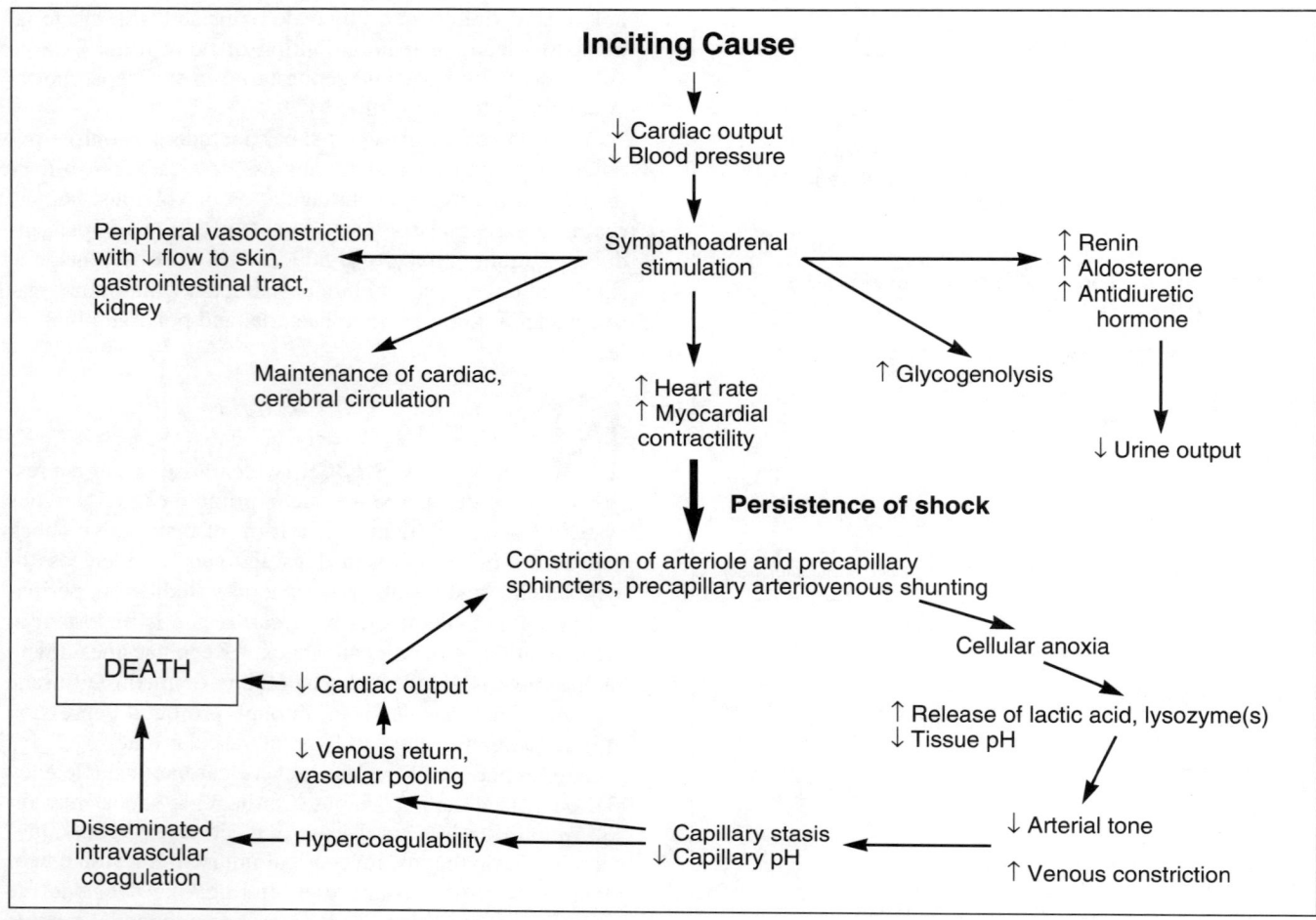

Figure 1—Pathophysiology of shock.

Starling forces so that interstitial fluid is mobilized into the circulation.

When inadequate tissue perfusion persists, hypothermia, muscle weakness, mental confusion, and hypokinetic pulses develop. Compensatory mechanisms, although initially beneficial, may worsen perfusion of peripheral tissue and later become detrimental.

An α-adrenergic sympathetic vasoconstriction occurs at the level of the arterioles and precapillary sphincters. This phenomenon, along with arteriovenous shunting, dramatically reduces total oxygen delivery to tissue. Oxidative phosphorylation is interrupted, thus allowing accumulation of lactic acid and a net lowering of tissue pH.[3,7,10] Cell permeability is affected, thus resulting in cell autolysis and release of lysozymes. Hyperglycemia may result from catecholamine-stimulated glycogenolysis as well as from insulin resistance induced by somatotropin, cortisol, and catecholamines. As carbohydrate reserves are depleted, secondary hypoglycemia develops.[3,7]

In the microvasculature, a loss of arterial tone and increased venous vasoconstriction promotes capillary stasis. Capillary pH rapidly becomes acidic, tissue ischemia worsens, and metabolites that are locally vasoactive accumulate. When capillary stasis occurs, circulation fails and shock eventually becomes irreversible.[10] Vascular pooling decreases venous return to the heart. In addition, blood pH below 7.10 diminishes ventricular contractile force.[12] Release of a depressant factor from the ischemic pancreas further depresses the myocardium.[7,12] Metabolic acidosis within the capillaries produces hypercoagulability of the blood, which in turn may cause disseminated intravascular coagulation. The terminal event in shock is cardiac failure.

EFFECTS ON ORGAN SYSTEMS

Shock is a multisystem disorder that affects the entire body. An understanding of how shock affects the function of vital organs is useful to the clinician as a prognostic tool and guide to potential complications.

The heart tolerates decreased perfusion and hypoxia poorly. Oxygen demands of myocardium are extremely high, and over 70% of the oxygen presented to myocardium is taken up. Myocardial perfusion depends on autoregulation of coronary blood flow; the autoregulation is based on oxygen demands of the myocardium. Blood flow to the heart is always maintained at the expense of other body tissue. Coronary blood flow is maintained until arterial blood pressure has decreased below the range of 60 to 70 mm Hg.[1]

Prolonged shock, which results in decreased myocardial oxygen delivery, leads to anaerobic metabolism in the myocardium. The resultant lactic acidosis, depletion of glycogen stores, and decrease in available adenosine triphosphate leads to diminished myocardial contractility. When contractility decreases, peripheral and myocardial perfusion diminish and the function of the myocardium and other vital organs declines progressively, thus eventually contributing to failure of specific organs and eventually death.

The pancreas is especially sensitive to the effects of the diminished perfusion and hypoxia. The pancreas may also play a central role in the worsening of shock once it begins. Cellular hypoxia from intense pancreatic vasoconstriction results in lysosome fragmentation and release of vasoactive and myocardial-depressant peptides. These peptides then interfere with calcium-mediated excitation–contraction coupling in the heart.

As HAPPENS in the heart, blood flow to the liver is preferentially maintained. As shock worsens, however, hepatic perfusion diminishes, thus causing hepatocellular hypoxia and necrosis. Isolated areas of centrilobular necrosis occur initially; widespread hepatocellular necrosis is an end-stage finding. In addition, the mononuclear phagocyte system of the liver is compromised, thus allowing bacteria and toxins from the intestine access to systemic circulation. Increases in liver enzyme levels may be observed; occasionally, hyperbilirubinemia and icterus occur.

The gastrointestinal tract is exquisitely sensitive to poor perfusion. The effects of shock on the gastrointestinal tract are manifested by mucosal ulceration and hemorrhage.[1] Mucosal ulceration and hemorrhage may cause substantial pooling of fluid and blood within the stomach and intestine, thus further decreasing perfusion and worsening shock. In severe cases, bowel perforation may occur. The denuded mucosal barrier, together with diminished mononuclear phagocyte function in the liver, predisposes patients to bacteremia and life-threatening sepsis.

Despite preferential circulation to the central nervous system, arterial blood pressure below 60 mm Hg results in decreased cerebral blood flow and diminished cerebral function.[1] Reduced cerebral function arises not only from lowered oxygen tension but also from depletion of the glucose supply. Hypoxic encephalopathy typically appears as transient ataxia, confusion, or stupor.[1,13] Cerebral function fortunately improves rapidly once circulatory integrity is restored.

The kidney can be dramatically affected in patients with shock. Oliguria resulting from secretion of aldosterone and antidiuretic hormone is seen as an early manifestation of shock. When shock becomes more pronounced and long-standing, ischemic injury ensues and acute renal failure results. Acute renal failure from shock has been called vasomotor nephropathy.[10] Renal failure may persist for days or weeks despite successful management of shock. Vasomotor nephropathy is usually reversible.[1]

Respiratory failure is a major problem in humans during the first 24 to 72 hours after shock has been treated.[1,14] Respiratory failure results from progressive development of pulmonary edema, thickening of alveolar walls, and ventilation–perfusion mismatching. Fatigue of muscles of respiration secondary to poor tissue perfusion is also central to the pathogenesis.[10] The terms *shock lung* or *acute* (or *adult*) *respiratory distress syndrome* (ARDS) have been used to describe this type of respiratory failure. Dogs are more resistant to shock lung than humans are. Cats, however, may be as susceptible as humans.[3]

Normal blood coagulation may be affected by shock, and disseminated intravascular coagulation often results. Disseminated intravascular coagulation is characterized by intravascular activation of blood coagulation and fibrinolytic mechanisms. Factors that incite disseminated intravascular coagulation in patients with shock include bacterial toxins, hypotension, release of thromboplastin from damaged cells, and capillary stasis.[2,15] In particular, the development of capillary metabolic acidosis contributes to disseminated intravascular coagulation. Disseminated intravascular coagulation is suspected in patients with severe, protracted bleeding or those with dysfunction of several organs—a result of tissue hypoxia that occurs secondary to microthrombi and infarcts.[12,15] The primary goal in management of disseminated intravascular coagulation is to reverse or eliminate the underlying cause.

CLINICAL MANIFESTATIONS

Clinical manifestations of shock vary greatly depending on the inciting cause and stage of shock (see Clinical Signs of Shock on the following page). Typically, patients in shock are weak, hypotensive, hypothermic, and have pale mucous membranes with poor perfusion as evidenced by prolonged capillary refill time. Tachypnea and tachycardia with weak arterial pulses are usually evident. Patients in septic shock, however, may also have fever and brick-red to muddy-red mucous membranes.[5] The skin is often cool and clammy, and the patient may be confused or nonresponsive to stimuli. Vomiting, diarrhea, depression, and anorexia may develop.

MANAGEMENT

The primary objectives in the successful management of shock are to ensure adequate respiration, control hemorrhage, and expand circulating blood volume. Initially, a patent airway should be established; endotracheal intubation may be needed. Oxygen may be delivered to patients

> **Clinical Signs of Shock**
>
> - Tachycardia
> - Hypotension
>   —Prolonged capillary refill time
>   —Weak pulses
> - Rapid respiration
> - Hypothermia
> - Muscle weakness, restlessness, and depression
> - Reduced urine output
> - Coma, dilation of pupils

> **Treatment Protocol for Shock**
>
> 1. Establish patent airway, consider oxygen therapy
> 2. Insert intravenous catheter; check packed cell volume, total solids, blood urea nitrogen
> 3. Control bleeding
> 4. Rapidly infuse crystalloid or colloid solution intravenously
> 5. Administer corticosteroids, inotropic drugs, and antimicrobial agents
> 6. Maintain body temperature
> 7. Note urine output; consider insertion of urinary catheter
> 8. Monitor color and capillary refill time of mucous membranes, pulse, respiration, central venous pressure, arterial blood pressure, and arterial or venous blood gases
> 9. Consider diuretics if patient is overhydrated and sodium bicarbonate if metabolic acidosis is present

via mask, nasal catheter, transtracheal catheter, closed-environment oxygen cage, or endotracheal or tracheostomy tube. Bleeding is controlled by application of direct pressure, bandages, tourniquet, or ligation. Restoration of arterial blood pressure, circulating blood volume, and cardiac output is of paramount importance in ensuring adequate tissue perfusion and oxygenation. The mainstay of shock management is intravenous fluid-replacement therapy (see the treatment protocol on this page).

Fluid-Replacement Therapy

Several fluid-replacement solutions may be used in shock management; fluid-replacement solutions include crystalloids, whole blood, and colloids (i.e., dextrans, hetastarch, and plasma). Isotonic crystalloid solutions are the most commonly used blood-volume expanders (except in the presence of cardiogenic shock). Large volumes (60 ml/kg for dogs; 40 ml/kg for cats) are infused intravenously as fast as possible. Ideally, central venous pressure should be monitored and fluid administration rate decreased as central venous pressure exceeds 15 cm H_2O.[2] Most dogs can be given one blood volume (e.g., 90 ml/kg) per hour without adverse circulatory effects. Rapid volume replacement can produce hemodilution, which may, in turn, decrease oxygen delivery to tissue.

Recently, small-volume resuscitation using hypertonic saline solution has been advocated for initial management of hypovolemic and distributive shock.[16] Hypertonic saline solution increases systemic arterial pressure, cardiac output, cardiac contractility, and stroke volume; whereas total peripheral vascular resistance and pulmonary vascular resistance decrease and circulatory filling pressure increases.[16] Restored tissue perfusion results in improved acid–base status and increased urine output. Benefits derived from administration of hypertonic saline solution are increased plasma tonicity and decreased hydrostatic pressure. Increased plasma osmolality promotes transcompartmental and transcellular shift of fluid into the vascular compartment. Administration of 4 to 5 ml/kg of 7.0% to 7.5% saline solution is recommended, but commercial solutions are not yet widely available.

Potential problems with administration of hypertonic saline include hypernatremia, hyperosmolality, and hypokalemia. Hemorrhage may worsen in patients with active bleeding; thus, hypertonic saline should not be used in these patients. Hypertonic saline is contraindicated in cases of heart failure, and care should be taken if the animal's renal function is compromised.

WHOLE BLOOD (15 ml/kg) should be administered when the initial packed-cell volume (PCV) is less than 25%.[2] Packed-cell volume should be maintained between 25% and 50%. Dextrose solution (50%) is added to each liter of multiple-electrolyte solution and administered at a rate of 0.5 to 1 ml/kg/hr if the patient is hypoglycemic. Glucose reduces peripheral resistance, improves myocardial oxygen availability and contractility, and minimizes the hypoglycemia that is often present in patients with shock.[13]

Colloid solutions are hypertonic fluids that can osmotically expand circulating blood volume. Commercially available colloid solutions include dextrans, mannitol, gelatin, and hydroxyethyl starch (hetastarch). Dextrans are branched polysaccharides.[17] Dextran 70 or 75 (i.e., molecular weight 70,000 or 75,000) as well as the low-molecular-weight dextran 40 (i.e., molecular weight 40,000) are available in 5% dextrose or saline solution. Dextran 40 retards erythrocyte sludging and is excreted by the kidneys. Thrombocytopathy and renal failure are reported side effects from administration of dextrans.[5,17] Hetastarch is a mixture of polysaccharides derived from amylopectin, with an average molecular weight of 450,000. Hetastarch use has gained popularity owing to its much longer half-life and few side effects. In most situations, however, crystalloid solutions are still preferred for use in shock patients.

Fresh frozen plasma may also be used in shock management; however, use of fresh frozen plasma has greatest value in management of severe chronic protein loss. Hypoproteinemia that arises with abdominal effusion, burns, and chronic bleeding can be successfully treated with transfusion of fresh plasma. Fresh frozen plasma is available from small animal blood banks, such as the Animal Blood Bank (Dixon, CA).

Corticosteroids

The use of corticosteroids in shock management is generally accepted, although whether they should be used in patients with septic shock is still controversial.[2,5,18,19] Despite the acceptance of corticosteroid use, the mechanisms of action of corticosteroids remain debatable. Documented corticosteroid effects that may be beneficial in the reversal of shock include (1) an increase in cardiac output, (2) a decrease in peripheral resistance, (3) an increase in metabolism of lactic acid, (4) stabilization of lysosomal membranes, (5) interference with endotoxin-induced immune reactions, (6) inhibition of complement-induced granulocyte aggregation, (7) modulation of the release of endogenous opiates, (8) decrease in production of arachidonic-acid metabolites, (9) a right shift in the oxyhemoglobin dissociation curve, (10) the prevention of platelet aggregation, and (11) disinhibition of gluconeogenesis with elevation in blood glucose concentrations.[3,5,12,13,20] Detrimental effects may include immunosuppression, increased risk of secondary infection, and gastrointestinal ulceration and hemorrhage.[21]

WHEN CORTICOSTEROIDS are used in shock management, an aqueous salt of the selected corticosteroid should be used. Corticosteroids are given in high doses and should be used as early as possible. In experiments, synthetic analogues of hydrocortisone have been shown to be most effective.[12] The aqueous corticosteroids, such as hydrocortisone sodium succinate (20 to 30 mg/kg intravenously [Solu-Cortef®—Upjohn]) and prednisolone sodium succinate (10 to 30 mg/kg intravenously [Solu-Delta-Cortef®—Upjohn]) have an onset of action of about four minutes. Their sustained effect is short, and the dose may be repeated in three to four hours.[12,22] Another popular product is methylprednisolone sodium succinate (one 30-mg/kg intravenous dose). Dexamethasone sodium phosphate (3 to 8 mg/kg intravenously) has a slightly slower onset of action and a longer effect and is considered effective when used every 12 hours.[3] Despite their positive effects, corticosteroids should never be used as a substitute for adequate fluid-replacement therapy.

Vasoactive and Inotropic Drugs

Vasoactive and positive inotropic drugs are used in shock management to modify sympathetic and adrenal-gland responses. Vasoactive drugs stimulate dopaminergic receptors or stimulate or block α-adrenergic or ß-adrenergic receptors. Blockade of α-adrenergic receptors is generally not indicated in management of shock because most α-adrenergic agonist vasoactive drugs have powerful vasoconstrictive effects. Blockade of ß-adrenergic receptors, however, results in increased myocardial contractility, vasodilation, and improved tissue perfusion. Vasoactive drugs are best used when elevated central venous pressure but poor peripheral tissue perfusion are evident and cardiac output is low despite aggressive fluid-replacement therapy. Vasoactive drugs are useful in the management of cardiogenic shock.

DOPAMINE and dobutamine are the most commonly used vasoactive drugs in the management of shock patients.[3,4] Dopamine is the precursor of norepinephrine and increases myocardial contractility by direct stimulation of cardiac ß-adrenergic receptors. Stimulation of specific dopaminergic receptors in the renal, mesenteric, coronary, and intracerebral arterial beds results in vasodilation.[23] Dopamine increases myocardial contractility with little effect on heart rate at 2 to 5 µg/kg/min intravenously. Higher doses may cause tachycardia and vasoconstriction and should be avoided.

Dobutamine is an analogue of isoproterenol and primarily affects the cardiac $ß_1$-adrenergic receptors with minimal effect on the vascular α- and $ß_2$-adrenergic receptors.[23] Dobutamine may be used at doses of 3 to 10 µg/kg/min. Dobutamine increases myocardial contractility but does not have the renal vasodilative effects of dopamine.

Dopamine and dobutamine are commonly used for inotropic support after volume loading. Whenever possible, arterial blood pressure is monitored during their administration. Vasoactive drugs should be administered with extreme care because small changes in infusion rate may dramatically change the properties of the drug.[23]

Nonsteroidal Antiinflammatory Drugs

Cyclooxygenase prostanoids clearly play a role in the pathogenesis of shock.[4] Cyclooxygenase inhibitors would, therefore, seem to be indicated. Nonsteroidal antiinflam-

TABLE I
Common Drug Doses Used in Patients with Shock

Multiple-electrolyte solution	*Dogs*: 50–150 ml/kg over several hours *Cats*: 100–200 ml/aliquot
Hetastarch	20 ml/kg/day intravenously
Hypertonic saline (7%)	4–5 ml/kg slowly intravenously
Dextran 40	10–20 ml/kg/day intravenously in 5% dextrose in water solution at infusion rate of 2 ml/kg/hr
Hydrocortisone sodium succinate	20–30 mg/kg intravenously
Prednisolone sodium succinate	10–30 mg/kg intravenously
Dexamethasone sodium phosphate	3–8 mg/kg intravenously or subcutaneously
Sodium bicarbonate	1–2 mEq/kg in intravenous fluids
Dopamine	2–5 µg/kg min intravenously in 250 ml of 5% dextrose in water
Dobutamine	3–10 µg/kg/min intravenously in 5% dextrose in water
Heparin	200 IU/kg intravenously, followed by 50–100 IU/kg subcutaneously every six to eight hours
Furosemide	2–4 mg/kg intravenously or subcutaneously

matory drugs are cyclooxygenase inhibitors that prevent the formation of prostaglandins. They are more commonly used in the management of septic shock.[4,5] Although positive hemodynamic effects have been noted in experiments, controversy concerning their recommended use in septic shock remains.[4,5,6,24,25] Flunixin meglumine (1 mg/kg given once for dogs) has been used most commonly for this purpose.[24,25] Flunixin meglumine is most effective when used during the first two hours of the onset of sepsis[10]; however, animals are rarely presented to the clinician within this time. Nonsteroidal antiinflammatory drugs also have pronounced gastrointestinal ulcerogenic properties in dogs and cats. Thus, their use is rarely indicated in veterinary management of shock.

Narcotic Antagonists

The ß-endorphins are powerful hypotensive substances that are antagonized by such drugs as naloxone hydrochloride. Such narcotic antagonists as naloxone hydrochloride have been used with mixed results in the management of septic shock.[5,20] Reported benefits include improved arterial blood pressure, left ventricular contractility, stroke volume, and cardiac output. Large doses of naloxone hydrochloride are needed (2 mg/kg/hr intravenously), and the effectiveness is controversial.

Supportive Care

Sodium bicarbonate may be included in shock management. Cellular hypoxia with accumulation of lactic acid leads to generalized metabolic acidosis. If arterial blood gases are measured, the base deficit can be determined and corrected (0.3 × body weight [kg] × base deficit [mEq/L]). Severe acidemia (pH below 7.1) warrants the use of sodium bicarbonate; higher pH probably does not warrant its use. Empirical sodium bicarbonate therapy is not advised; if the clinician uses it, however, approximately 1 to 2 mEq/kg can be given in a single intravenous injection, with 1 to 4 mEq/kg added to each liter of intravenous fluid-replacement solution. Caution must be used with the administration of sodium bicarbonate because paradoxical acidosis of the central nervous system or cerebral edema may occur shortly after its administration.

ANTIMICROBIAL AGENTS are important if septic shock is suspected. Broad-spectrum, bactericidal agents are ideal. Early use of broad-spectrum antimicrobial agents can diminish the bacteremia and endotoxin release. Because of hypotension, most tranquilizers are contraindicated in management of most shock patients (Table I).

Arrhythmias are common sequelae of shock, particularly shock resulting from trauma. Arrhythmias can range from benign occasional premature ventricular contractions to ventricular tachyarrhythmias that markedly compromise cardiac function. Early detection and treatment of cardiac arrhythmias are an important part of shock management. Lidocaine is generally indicated for ventricular extrasystoles or tachyarrhythmias and can be given in bolus form (1 to 2 mg/kg intravenously for dogs, 0.25 to 0.75 mg/kg intravenously for cats) or as a continuous infusion (40 to 80 µg/kg/min for dogs, 10 to 40 µg/kg/min for cats).

PATIENT MONITORING

Management of shock extends beyond fluid-replacement therapy and administration of drugs. Each patient must be closely monitored for clinical responsiveness to fluid-replacement therapy, deterioration of vital signs, and development of complications. In addition to vital signs (e.g., body temperature, pulse rate, respiration rate, color of mucous membranes, and capillary refill time), other parameters should also be monitored (see Patient Monitoring on this page).

Perhaps the most accurate measurement of the hemodynamics of shock is blood pressure. Normal systolic arterial blood pressure in canine patients is 110 to 190 mm Hg and in feline patients is 117 to 149 mm Hg.[26] Mean blood pressure below 80 mm Hg usually denotes shock. Direct measurement of arterial blood pressure provides accurate information about left-ventricle contractility; but it requires arterial puncture, which may require sedation. Access to the femoral artery is obtained with a small-gauge (23- to 25-gauge) needle attached with stiff polyethylene tubing to pressure-recording equipment.

Indirect measurements of arterial blood pressure can be accomplished by palpating the pulses or using oscillometric or Doppler techniques. Pulses are usually palpable at pressures of 70 mm Hg or greater.[12,27] With a Doppler technique, an inflatable cuff is used to occlude arterial blood flow. With gradual release, the cuff pressure obtained at the time blood flow recommences (first sound obtained with Doppler-sensed flow) is recorded as the systolic pressure. Diastolic pressure is recorded when the sounds are lost. Diastolic pressure may be difficult to determine with the Doppler technique in some patients because the sounds may persist, with only muffling of the sounds noted as the diastolic pressure. The size of the cuff and its placement are critical to accurate blood-pressure measurement. Care in selection and placement of the cuff is necessary to obtain consistent and reproducible results. Oscillometric methods reliably detect arterial pressures in animals larger than 5 kg but have difficulty in detecting blood pressure in smaller animals.

New devices for measuring various gas-analysis variables, including transcutaneous oxygen and carbon dioxide tension, pulse oximetry, and transconjunctival oxygen tension, are available and provide quantitative information dependent on blood flow and oxygen content. Potentially the most accurate method for the serial assessment of the cardiovascular system of shock patients is two-dimensional echocardiography with Doppler capabilities.

Central venous pressure is a measurement of the fluid pressure in the anterior vena cava or right atrium. This

---

Patient Monitoring

Blood pressure (mm Hg)
  Systolic: 110 to 190
  Diastolic: 60 to 100

Central venous pressure (cm H_2O)
  Normal: 0 to 10
  Shock: 0
  Overhydration: 8 to 12
  Heart failure: 20
  Cardiac tamponade: 22 to 25

Packed-cell volume
  Normal dogs: 45% to 55%
  Normal cats: 40%

Total solids (g/dl)
  Normal dogs: 7.0
  Normal cats: 6.0

Urine output
  Normal: 1–2 ml/kg/hr

Electrocardiography

Blood gases
  Arterial
    pH: 7.35 to 7.45
    Pco_2: 40 mm Hg
    Po_2: 90 mm Hg
    Bicarbonate: 25 mEq/L
  Venous
    pH: 7.35 to 7.45
    Pco_2: 45 mm Hg
    Po_2: 40 mm Hg
    Bicarbonate: 25 mEq/L

---

pressure is a dynamic function of cardiac output and venous return to the heart. Any increase in fluid volume entering the heart or any decrease in outflow from the heart increases central venous pressure. Conversely, any decrease in volume returned to the heart lowers the central venous pressure.

Central venous pressure is measured by inserting an indwelling catheter into the patient's external jugular vein. The tip of the catheter is brought to rest in or near the right atrium. The catheter is connected by extension tubing to the male end of a three-way stopcock. A manometer calibrated in centimeters of water is attached to the stopcock, perpendicular to the catheter line. The third portal of the stopcock is attached to an intravenous fluid solution. The entire length of tubing, as well as the manometer, is filled with the intravenous fluid or heparinized saline solution.

Central venous pressure is read as centimeters of water. Measurements are taken with the zero mark of the manometer held level to right atrium of the heart. With the patient in sternal recumbency, the zero point is positioned at the fourth intercostal space approximately two or three inches above the sternum. If the patient is in lateral recumbency, the measurement is taken parallel to the sternum.

The stopcock is turned so that the manometer and jugular catheter lines are free flowing, and the infusion set is turned off. The column of liquid in the manometer is allowed to equilibrate over a short time. Once the fluid pressure in the right atrium equals that in the manometer, the meniscus will stop descending. Small fluctuations of the meniscus occur with each respiration. If the meniscus falls below zero, then the manometer can be lowered. The new zero point should be taken at the 5-cm H_2O mark, with all values between 0 and 5 cm H_2O denoting negative measurements of central venous pressure.

Normal central venous pressure in dogs and cats ranges from 0 to 10 cm H_2O. Patients that are in hypovolemic shock may have measurements below zero. During intravenous fluid-replacement therapy, recordings of 8 to 12 cm H_2O denote overhydration. The clinician should suspect right-sided heart failure when measurements approach 15 to 20 cm H_2O. Values greater than 22 to 25 cm H_2O may reflect impending cardiac tamponade (see Patient Monitoring on previous page).

WHEN USED CORRECTLY, central venous pressure can be a diagnostic as well as a monitoring tool. It is particularly helpful in assessing the adequacy of fluid-replacement therapy in shock patients and the hemodynamic effects of intravenous fluids in patients with life-threatening cardiac conditions. With elevations of central venous pressure and development of pulmonary edema in overhydrated patients, fluid-replacement therapy should be stopped and loop (furosemide) or osmotic (mannitol) diuretics given.

There are several potential sources of error in measuring central venous pressure. Correct positioning of the manometer in relation to the patient is imperative. Rapid or labored breathing can cause continuous movement of the meniscus, thus making reading of the manometer difficult. Technical problems, such as kinking of the jugular catheter (the position of the patient's head should be watched), clots within the catheter, or malfunctioning of the stopcock, can all produce errors. Complete patency of the intravenous lines must be maintained.

Measurements of central venous pressure are relatively insensitive, with a margin of error of approximately 2 cm H_2O. Despite this insensitivity, however, central venous pressure can be vital in patient monitoring. Sensitivity can be increased by using minimal lengths of connecting tubing and by removing all extraneous catheter adapters. The clinician should realize that the trends that develop with sequential recordings of central venous pressure are more significant than isolated or individual measurements.

Another parameter to monitor is urine output. As successful fluid-replacement therapy restores normal glomerular filtration rate, urine output will resume. Normal urine production is 1 to 2 ml/kg/hr.[13] If urine output is less than 1 ml/kg/hr despite aggressive volume replacement, loop (furosemide) or osmotic (mannitol) diuretics can be used to improve renal blood flow and enhance urine production. Dopamine may also be effective in restoring urine output because of its renal vasodilative properties.

The hematocrit and the packed cell volume (PCV) are unreliable during the early stages of shock. Splenic contraction from sympathoadrenal stimulation may allow the packed cell volume to remain normal despite significant blood loss. The packed cell volume will equilibrate over several hours, however, and can become more reliable. Slow, constant bleeding may be reflected by a continuous drop in packed cell volume. Inadequate fluid-replacement therapy should be suspected if the hematocrit remains above 50%.

Along with the hematocrit, refractometer measurements of total solids aid in assessment of fluid-replacement therapy. A serial decrease in total solids accompanies overzealous fluid-replacement therapy and persistent protein loss. Persistently high values for total solids occur in patients with dehydration (inadequate fluid replacement) or hyperglobulinemia.

Blood chemistry profiles are important in evaluation of shock patients. Screening tests that are important for detecting organ function and/or tissue damage include determination of serum blood urea nitrogen, creatinine, and electrolyte concentrations (sodium, potassium, and chloride). Determinations of arterial blood gases allow exact evaluation of the respiratory status, presence of metabolic acidosis, and compensatory mechanisms in shock patients.

SUMMARY

Shock results from various pathophysiologic mechanisms. Mortality is highest among patients with septic and cardiogenic shock, approaching 70% to 80%. Other forms of distributive or hypovolemic shock may be treated more successfully. Successful reversal of shock depends on rapid recognition of the clinical signs, quick evaluation of the patient, and immediate institution of shock management. Once medical therapy is under way, diligent monitoring is required to ensure the maximal chance for patient survival.

About the Authors

Dr. Taboada and Dr. Hoskins are affiliated with the Department of Veterinary Clinical Sciences of the School of Veterinary Medicine, Louisiana State University in Baton Rouge, Louisiana. Dr. Morgan is affiliated with the Rawley Memorial Animal Hospital in Springfield, Massachusetts. Drs. Taboada, Hoskins, and Morgan are Diplomates of the American College of Veterinary Internal Medicine. Dr. Morgan is a Diplomate of the American College of Veterinary Ophthalmologists.

REFERENCES

1. Billhardt RA, Rosenbush SW: Cardiogenic and hypovolemic shock. *Med Clin North Am* 70:853-876, 1986.
2. Schertel ER, Muir WW: Shock: Pathophysiology, monitoring, and therapy, in Kirk RW (ed): *Current Veterinary Therapy X.* Philadelphia, WB Saunders Co, 1989, pp 316-330.
3. Ware WA: Shock, in Murtaugh RJ, Kaplan PM (eds): *Veterinary Emergency and Critical Care Medicine.* Chicago, Mosby–Year Book, 1992, pp 163-175.
4. Haskins SC: Shock, in Fox PR (ed): *Canine and Feline Cardiology.* New York, Churchill Livingstone, 1988, pp 229-254.
5. Goodwin JK, Schaer M: Septic shock. *Vet Clin North Am* 19:1239-1258, 1989.
6. Hardie EM: Sepsis versus septic shock, in Murtaugh RJ, Kaplan PM (eds): *Veterinary Emergency and Critical Care Medicine.* Chicago, Mosby–Year Book, 1992, pp 176-193.
7. Clark DR: Circulatory shock: Etiology and pathophysiology. *JAVMA* 175:77-81, 1979.
8. Natanson C: A canine model of septic shock. *Ann Intern Med* 113:227-242, 1990.
9. Dow SW, Curtis CR, Jones RL, et al: Bacterial culture of blood from critically ill dogs and cats: 100 cases (1985-1987). *JAVMA* 195:113-117, 1989.
10. Skowronski GA: The pathophysiology of shock. *Med J Aust* 148:576-583, 1988.
11. Ross JN: Current concepts in the pathophysiology of shock. *ACVIM Sci Proc*:9-46, 1980.
12. Brasmer TH (ed): Symposium on shock. *Vet Clin North Am* 6(2):173-308, 1976.
13. Kolata RJ, Burrows CF, Soma LR: Shock pathophysiology and management, in Kirk RW (ed): *Current Veterinary Therapy VII.* Philadelphia, WB Saunders Co, 1980, pp 32-48.
14. Rinaldo JE, Rogers RM: Adult respiratory distress syndrome: Changing concepts of lung injury and repair. *N Engl J Med* 306:900-909, 1982.
15. Hardaway RM III: Cellular and metabolic effects of shock. *JAVMA* 175:81-86, 1979.
16. Muir WW: Small volume resuscitation using hypertonic saline. *Cornell Vet* 80:7-12, 1990.
17. Wolfsheimer KJ: Fluid therapy in the critically ill patient. *Vet Clin North Am* 19:361-378, 1989.
18. Sprung CL, Caralis PV, Marcial EH, et al: The effects of high-dose corticosteroids in patients with septic shock. *N Engl J Med* 311:1137-1143, 1984.
19. White GL, White GS, Kosanke SD, et al: Therapeutic effects of prednisolone sodium succinate versus dexamethasone in dogs subjected to *E. coli* septic shock. *JAAHA* 18:639-648, 1982.
20. Karakusis PH: Considerations in the therapy of septic shock. *Med Clin North Am* 70:933-944, 1986.
21. Bone RC, Fisher CJ, Clemmer TP, et al: A controlled clinical trial of high-dose methylprednisolone in the treatment of severe sepsis and septic shock. *N Engl J Med* 317:653-658, 1987.
22. Adams HR, Parker JL: Pharmacologic management of circulatory shock: Cardiovascular drugs and corticosteroids. *JAVMA* 175:86-92, 1979.
23. Ruggie N: Congestive heart failure. *Med Clin North Am* 70:829-851, 1986.
24. Hardie EM, Kolata RJ, Rawlings CA: Canine septic peritonitis: Treatment with flunixin meglumine. *Circ Shock* 11:159-173, 1983.
25. Hardie EM, Rawlings CA, Collins LG: Canine *Escherichia coli* peritonitis: Long-term survival with fluid, gentamicin sulfate and flunixin meglumine treatment. *JAAHA* 21:691-699, 1985.
26. Ross LA: Hypertension, in Murtaugh RJ, Kaplan PM (eds): *Veterinary Emergency and Critical Care Medicine.* Chicago, Mosby–Year Book, 1992, pp 648-656.
27. Guyton AC: *Basic Human Physiology.* Philadelphia, WB Saunders Co, 1977, pp 258-266.

BIBLIOGRAPHY

Ross JN: Comprehensive patient management in shock. *JAVMA* 175:92-96, 1979.

Shock Syndrome in Cats

Gulf Coast Veterinary Specialists
Houston, Texas
Susan L. Ford, DVM

University of Florida
Michael Schaer, DVM

KEY FACTS

❏ **The basic pathophysiologic abnormality that is involved in the complex clinical syndrome of shock is inadequate delivery of nutrients and oxygen to the tissues.**

❏ **The functional categorization of shock is based on hemodynamic effects.**

❏ **Optimum physiologic function is the aim of treatment of patients in shock.**

❏ **Restoring effective blood volume and optimizing tissue oxygenation are the primary therapeutic goals.**

Shock is a complex clinical syndrome with multiorgan involvement. Regardless of the cause, the eventual result involves a maldistribution of systemic blood flow, which causes inadequate delivery of oxygen and nutrients to the tissue. Impaired tissue perfusion leads to local ischemia, hypoxia, acidosis, and alteration of cell function; if untreated, these conditions can cause death.

The classification of shock by cause includes hemorrhagic, cardiogenic, traumatic, septic, and anaphylactic syndromes.[1] This implies that each type of shock has a characteristic clinical pattern and a specific therapeutic approach to the particular underlying mechanism. A more functional classification has been developed to address the diverse neurohumoral and immunologic mechanisms that lead to circulatory compromise. This functional categorization of shock is based on hemodynamic defects: hypovolemic, cardiogenic, vasogenic (distributive), and obstructive.[2]

Hypovolemic shock is caused by loss of circulating blood volume and is the most common form in veterinary medicine. Such shock may result from internal or external hemorrhage; fluid losses from vomiting, diarrhea, or polyuria; plasma depletion associated with large degloving injuries or burns; or fluid sequestration, as is evident in crushing injuries and in such third-space phenomena as peritonitis or ileus.

Cardiogenic shock is the result of markedly impaired cardiac function. Cardiomyopathy and valvular disease are frequent causes of acute cardiac insufficiency and decreased cardiac output. Pericardial effusion with cardiac tamponade, arrhythmias, and certain drugs (i.e., anesthetics and tranquilizers) can also contribute to cardiogenic shock.

Vasogenic shock is most often associated with sepsis and endotoxemia. Anaphylaxis, neurogenic injury, and vasodilator drug overdose also produce this type of shock.

Obstructive shock is considered by some to be a type of cardiogenic shock[3,4]; others classify it as a separate functional entity.[2-4] Obstruction to blood flow is the primary mechanism in the development of this form of shock and may be caused by pericardial tamponade, heartworm disease, intracardiac tumors, aortic emboli, or pulmonary thromboembolism.

PATHOPHYSIOLOGY

The body responds to the acute stress of circulatory failure by activating diverse neurohumoral and immunologic mechanisms in an attempt to maintain tissue perfusion and oxygenation (Figure 1). Autonomic sympa-

```
                        Causes
                        - Trauma
                        - Fluid losses
                        - Anaphylaxis
                        - Heart failure
                        - Drugs, toxins
                        - Environmental
                              ↓
                      Circulatory Failure
                       ↙              ↘
                Neural Responses      Humoral Responses
```

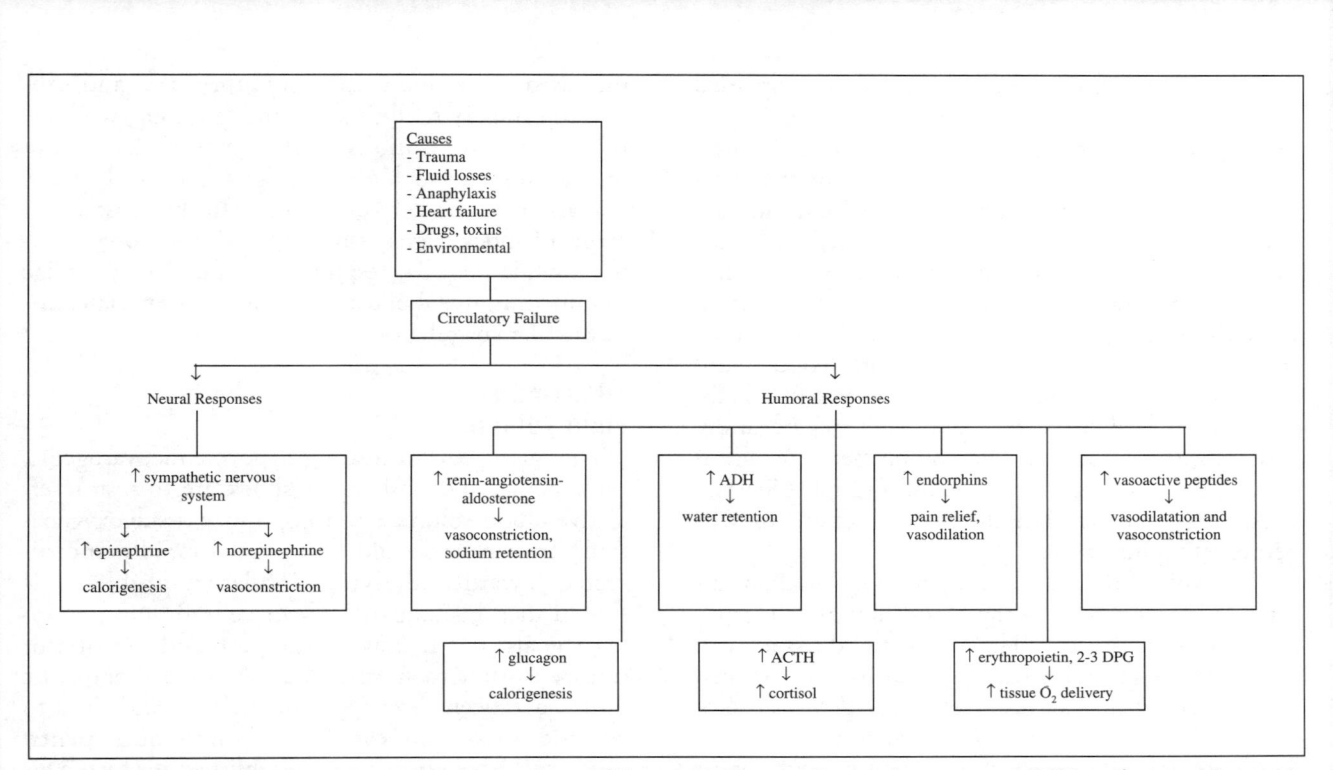

Figure 1—Neural and humoral responses to circulatory failure. *ADH* = antidiuretic hormone, *ACTH* = adrenocorticotropic hormone, and *DPG* = diphosphoglyceraldehyde.

Boxes under Neural Responses:
- ↑ sympathetic nervous system → ↑ epinephrine → calorigenesis; ↑ norepinephrine → vasoconstriction

Boxes under Humoral Responses:
- ↑ renin-angiotensin-aldosterone ↓ vasoconstriction, sodium retention
- ↑ ADH ↓ water retention
- ↑ endorphins ↓ pain relief, vasodilation
- ↑ vasoactive peptides ↓ vasodilatation and vasoconstriction
- ↑ glucagon ↓ calorigenesis
- ↑ ACTH ↓ ↑ cortisol
- ↑ erythropoietin, 2-3 DPG ↓ ↑ tissue O$_2$ delivery

thetic nervous activity is an immediate response to hypovolemia; afferent stimuli come from baroreceptors and chemoreceptors, anxiety and pain, and widespread arteriolar and venous constriction. The consequences of these reactions include increased cardiac inotropic and chronotropic activity as well as the diversion of central splanchnic blood flow to the heart, brain, and lungs.

Circulating catecholamine concentrations increase quickly to stimulate glycogenolysis and the release of plasma free fatty acids as energy sources. Glucagon is secreted by pancreatic α cells in response to stress, catecholamines, and hypoglycemia. Glucagon primarily stimulates hepatic gluconeogenesis and glycogenolysis and (to a lesser extent) free fatty acid and glycerol production from adipose tissue.

The renin–angiotensin system is activated by reduced glomerular blood flow, stimulation of the macula densa, reduced renal afferent arteriolar pressure, and increased sympathetic activity. Renin catalyzes the conversion of hepatic angiotensinogen to angiotensin I, which is converted to angiotensin II in the lung and other tissues. Angiotensin II is a potent vasoconstrictor that acts at the adrenal cortex to stimulate aldosterone release. Angiotensin III, another metabolite, has only 25% of the vasoconstrictor activity of angiotensin II but is a potent stimulant of aldosterone synthesis.[5] Aldosterone increases renal distal tubular sodium reabsorption and thus contributes to attempts to increase blood pressure.

In shock, antidiuretic hormone (ADH) is released by the neurohypophysis in response to decreased input from the arterial and atrial baroreceptors. Antidiuretic hormone contributes to splanchnic vasoconstriction and permits increased distal renal tubular and collecting duct water reabsorption.

Adrenocorticotropic hormone (ACTH) and β endorphins are released from the hypophysis in response to sudden blood loss, corticotropic-releasing hormone, antidiuretic hormone, and epinephrine. Adrenocorticotropic hormone stimulates the production and release of glucocorticoids from the adrenal cortex. The glucocorticoids may dampen the endogenous defense reactions originally activated by the stressors and may facilitate an adequate cardiovascular response mediated by permissive support for the vascular effects of catecholamines and other hormones. Increased cortisol concentrations apparently play a role in restricting blood volume after hemorrhage by rapidly increasing plasma osmolality.[6] Endorphins relieve pain and counteract some of the vasoconstrictive properties of the other hormones, thereby helping to maintain tissue perfusion but possibly helping to perpetuate hypotension.

Erythropoietin and 2-3 diphosphoglycerate (2-3 DPG) concentrations increase after acute blood loss. Hypoxia and shock also stimulate increased 2-3 diphosphoglycerate; this increase facilitates the downloading of oxygen from hemoglobin in the shock tissue.[6]

These homeostatic mechanisms are accompanied by various local reactions that may play a role in preserving organ function but may cause deleterious effects if they occur on a large scale or without inhibition. Vasoactive peptides and lysosomal enzymes are released, increasing capillary permeability and causing leukocytes to accumulate and destroy cell membranes. The arachidonic acid cascade is activated, with the subsequent production of the autacoids (prostaglandins, prostacyclin, thromboxanes, and leukotrienes), which relax or constrict vascular beds, release lysosomal enzymes, cause platelet aggregation, and activate leukocytes. The complement cascade is activated and leads to the release of multiple bioactive substances that may initiate chain reactions or self-perpetuating inflammatory processes.

The result of the body's compensatory mechanisms often is inadequate, and the blood flow to the capillary beds is insufficient. The less-perfused tissue, such as that of the gastrointestinal system, is affected first. Poor oxygen delivery causes cellular hypoxia, anaerobic metabolism, lactic acidosis, ischemic injury, and continued release of such potentially toxic substances as myocardial depressant and tumor necrosis factors. The capillary beds are adversely influenced by local vasodilating factors, hypoxia, decreased pH, arteriolar vasodilation, and venular constriction; the beds will continue to lose absolute and relative intravascular volume.

Anaphylaxis, or type I hypersensitivity, is characterized as an allergic reaction immediately after contact with an antigen to which the animal has been sensitized. The antigen encounters immunoglobulin E bound to a mast cell or basophil. Binding initiates a chain of intracellular biochemical reactions that lead to the systemic release of mediators, including histamine, eosinophil chemotactic factor of anaphylaxis, arachidonic acid metabolites, and leukotrienes.[7,8] Anaphylaxis is best managed by establishing a patent airway, administering epinephrine, and rapidly correcting hypovolemia via intravenous fluids. Antihistamines and corticosteroids may be helpful.

The continued activation of the neurohumoral mechanisms and the maldistribution of blood flow perpetuate the continued loss of plasma volume and eventual tissue death. The ability of the macrophage–monocyte system to destroy and clear invading microorganisms is impaired during states of low blood flow; the host is thus predisposed to secondary infections. With continued decompensation, disseminated intravascular coagulation may ensue.

CLINICAL SIGNS

The earliest signs of shock are subtle and may include mild mentation changes in conjunction with increased pulse, increased respiratory rate, and prolonged capillary refill time. As the syndrome worsens, the patient also exhibits marked mental depression, prostration, and such obvious signs of vasocollapse as a weak pulse and cool extremities. In the most severe forms of shock, signs associated with multiorgan failure include oliguria, respiratory insufficiency, cardiac dysfunction, metabolic acidosis, and disseminated intravascular coagulation.

TREATMENT
Fluid Volume

The main goals in treating hypovolemic, vasogenic, cardiogenic, and obstructive shock are to restore effective blood volume and to optimize tissue oxygenation. Treatment should be initiated rapidly and directed toward underlying circulatory problems. It should then be adjusted to achieve optimum physiologic goals, not merely to restore blood pressure or cardiac output to normal. Supranormal therapeutic goals have been developed for humans and dogs to provide for the increased metabolic requirements; such goals have not yet been established for cats. This discussion of treatment pertains to hypovolemic shock because of its high rate of occurrence. The essential therapeutic steps are listed in the box.

Because of the dependence of the cardiovascular system on blood volume, aggressive fluid therapy is the foundation of treatment for patients with noncardiogenic shock. Baseline packed cell volume and total plasma protein levels are reference values to be considered before initiating fluid therapy. Adjustments in treatment are guided by subsequent laboratory test results and patient reevaluation. The fluid volume required varies among individuals and is difficult to determine with standard noninvasive monitoring techniques. A general rule for cats with hypovolemic shock is to deliver one blood volume of an isotonic electrolyte solution in one hour.[9] In severe hypotension, cats may require as much as 30 to 60 ml/kg of crystalloid solution within the first hour.[10–13]

Intravenous access is important for optimum fluid delivery. Jugular catheters facilitate rapid vascular volume expansion because (1) they are less prone to interruptions in flow caused by kinking or positional changes and (2) the large internal diameter allows rapid flow rates (Figure 2). The catheters also can be used to monitor central venous pressure (CVP). This measurement is an easy, often-overlooked monitoring method that can facilitate fluid management. Normal central venous pressure ranges from 0 to 10 centimeters of water; the pressure of an animal in noncardiogenic shock is often 0 or less centimeters of water.[3] The goal of fluid therapy is to raise central venous pressure to 5 to 12 centimeters of water.[14]

> **Recommended Steps for Treating Patients with Hypovolemic Shock**
>
> 1. Diagnose shock; note pulse, mucous membrane color, and capillary refill time.
> 2. Place an intravenous or intraosseous catheter.
> 3. Take a baseline blood sample for packed cell volume, plasma total protein, and glucose.
> 4. Measure central venous pressure if possible.
> 5. Start intravenous lactated Ringer's solution at 60 ml/kg/hour.
> 6. Monitor central venous pressure:
>   If greater than 15 cm H_2O, stop fluids.
>   If greater than 12 cm H_2O, decrease fluid administration to 10 to 20 ml/kg/hour.
>   If 5 to 12 cm H_2O, slow fluid rate and continue to monitor pressure to ensure cardiovascular stability.
>   If less than 5 cm H_2O, continue fluids at 60 ml/kg/hour.
> 7. Monitor packed cell volume:
>   If less than 20, perform crossmatch and whole blood transfusion.
> 8. Monitor plasma total protein:
>   If less than 4.0 g/dl, prepare plasma or synthetic colloids for intravenous administration.
> 9. Monitor pulse, mucous membrane color, and capillary refill time:
>   If pulse is strong, color is pink, and capillary refill time is less than 2 seconds, proceed to Step 10.
>   If pulse is weak, color is pale, and capillary refill time is greater than 2 seconds, repeat Steps 5 through 9.
> 10. Obtain a complete history, and initiate diagnostic testing.
> 11. Begin maintenance fluids.
> 12. Monitor urine output:
>   If less than 1 ml/kg/hour, consider diuretic therapy.

Occasionally, the central venous pressure is high at the onset of treatment, especially in cases of septic shock in which hyperdynamic circulation characterizes the early phase[14]; this warrants reevaluation of the patient to ensure that fluid therapy is being used appropriately. A test bolus of intravenous fluid (5 ml/kg)[14] is given, and the central venous pressure is monitored; if the pressure does not rise, fluid therapy can proceed at a more aggressive rate. The patient should be monitored frequently. If intravenous access is impossible in cats or kittens, placement of an intraosseous catheter is a good alternative.[15-18] After a 20-gauge needle is introduced through the trochanteric fossa and into the medullary cavity of the femur or tibial tuberosity, a blood sample can be obtained for packed cell volume, plasma total protein, and glucose. Fluids or whole blood can then be administered. This route might not allow rapid rates of volume expansion and thus might require supplemental treatment with hypertonic saline or colloids. Subcutaneous and intraperitoneal fluids are useless in hypovolemic shock because they tend to remain at the site of deposit as a result of peripheral vasocollapse.

Pneumatic garments or body wraps can be applied to the pelvic limbs and caudal abdomen of patients in hypovolemic shock in an attempt to improve central cardiovascular function and to slow active hemorrhage.[19,20] Close patient monitoring is essential to avoid marked interruptions in venous return and impaired ventilation associated with overly tight body compression. In order to avoid vasocollapse caused by maldistribution of blood flow, a wrap should be removed by starting slowly at the cranial aspect and moving caudally.

Crystalloids

Crystalloids are the preferred initial fluids because they are proven to be effective, easy to administer, readily available, and relatively inexpensive. The fluids should be a solution with adequate sodium concentration because of the relatively high sodium level in the extracellular fluid space. Such isotonic fluids as lactated Ringer's solution and 0.9% saline solution tend to stay in the interstitial and vascular compartments, where they are most needed in treating hypovolemia. Mild dilutional acidosis can be caused by 0.9% saline solution. In cases of shock, the lactate in lactated Ringer's solution might not be converted to bicarbonate until hepatic perfusion improves. A large volume of fluid replacement is needed because only 25% to 30% of a crystalloid solution remains in the vascular space after 30 minutes. This phenomenon is caused by the rapid diffusion of fluid from the vascular space to the interstitium.[10]

Intravenous administration of a small volume of hypertonic (7.5%) saline solution to hypovolemic cats induces an immediate improvement in cardiovascular parameters and tissue perfusion; the duration of this effect is 15 to 60 minutes.[21,22] Hypertonic solutions should be used as adjunctive therapy only (for

Figure 2A

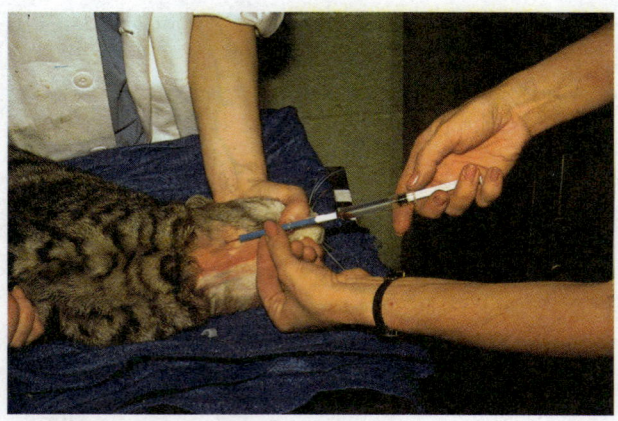

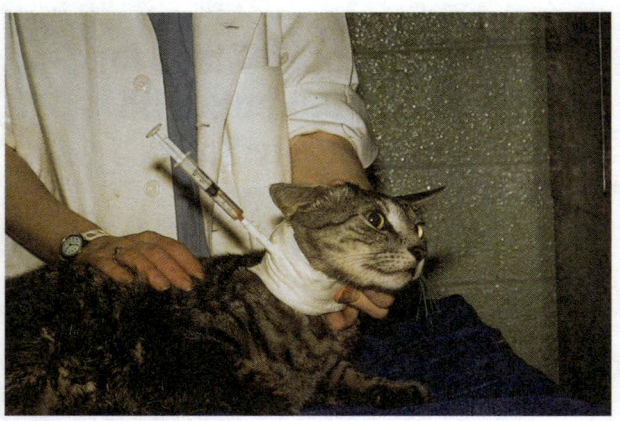

Figure 2B

Figure 2—(**A**) Initial and (**B**) final stages of the insertion of an 18-gauge, through-the-needle, indwelling jugular venous catheter.

rapid reestablishment of circulatory function) and followed by the administration of conventional crystalloid fluids. Hypertonic saline combined with dextrans produces a prolonged effect and may be used clinically in situations in which rapid delivery of a large volume of fluid is difficult. Constant care should be exercised to avoid intravascular fluid overload.

Hypertonic saline is contraindicated in hypernatremic or hyperosmotic conditions, such as dehydration, ketoacidotic diabetes, cardiogenic shock, and renal failure.[14] The infusion must be given slowly for three to five minutes to avoid causing hypotension, bronchoconstriction, and bradyarrhythmias. Hypertonic saline, alone or in combination with 6% dextran 70, is given slowly at a dose of 3 to 5 ml/kg.

Because urine output is an indirect reflection of restored blood volume, arterial pressure, and renal perfusion, it should be monitored closely in shock patients. Diuretic therapy is indicated at urine production levels less than 1 ml/kg/hour despite a large amount of volume replacement; such therapy should be used only after vascular volume and pressure have been normalized. Intravenous furosemide (2 to 5 mg/kg) can be given and followed by a second dose if there is no effect after 20 minutes. Mannitol (1 g/kg) and dopamine (1 to 2 µg/kg/min) also may be considered.

Anemia and hypoproteinemia can be life-threatening sequelae of shock and aggressive fluid therapy. If the packed cell volume falls to less than 20%, whole blood is required. Because cats can have nearly fatal transfusion reactions, a simple in-house crossmatch can be performed.[23] The amount of blood volume needed to raise a cat's packed cell volume 1% is approximately 2.2 ml/kg (e.g., a four-kilogram cat needs 44 milliliters of blood to increase its packed cell volume 5%). The following formula[24] can be used to determine more accurately the volume of blood required (BW = body weight, and PCV = packed cell volume):

Blood volume needed =

$$2.2 \times BW\ (kg) \times 30 \times \frac{\text{Desired PCV} - \text{Patient PCV}}{\text{Donor PCV}}$$

If the total protein falls below 4.0 g/dl or the albumin level is less than 1.5 g/dl, the decreased plasma colloid oncotic pressure will allow fluids to flow more rapidly into the interstitial space. Edema and compromised organ function can result. At this point, the effectiveness of crystalloid treatment is minimal until colloid replacement occurs.

Colloids

Fresh plasma is the ideal source of colloids because it supplies such important substances as albumin and clotting factors. Plasma can be administered at a dose of 10 to 20 ml/kg. Fresh frozen or frozen plasma may be used as a source of albumin. Synthetic colloids (hetastarch and dextrans) are used in many veterinary practices because of the difficulty in obtaining feline plasma. Hydroxyethyl substituted branched-chain amylopectins are produced in a 6% hetastarch solution and a 10% pentastarch solution. After 24 hours, 40% of the maximum plasma expansion capability persists.[25]

Dextrans are polysaccharides of high molecular weight that are available in two forms. Dextran 70 (the preferred product) is prepared in a 6% solution with a particle size similar to that of albumin and a half-life of approximately 24 hours. The dosage for the colloids is 10 to 20 ml/kg/day, and infusion rates should be limited to 2 to 5 ml/kg/hour. The main adverse effects of synthetic colloids include hypervolemia, hyperviscosity, hemorrhagic diathesis, and anaphylaxis. These effects generally result from too rapid or excessive administration and are rare in veterinary patients.[26]

Increased oxygen demands can be met by increasing the effective circulating blood volume, adding red blood cells (if required), and providing a supplemental source of oxygen. Most conscious animals do not tolerate intubation or a face mask but do accept oxygen delivery through a nasal catheter. A soft, red-rubber feeding tube can be passed intranasally and secured with cyanoacrylate glue at the meatus and over the frontal sinus area. The oxygen flow rate should be 0.5 to 2.0 L/min.[27,28]

Vasoactive Drugs

In most cases of hypovolemic shock, cardiac output and myocardial perfusion respond well to fluid therapy and improved venous return. In the later stages of shock, when the heart and vessels are unresponsive to fluid therapy, vasoactive drugs can be useful. Inotropic support is indicated if the central venous pressure is greater than 12 centimeters of water after adequate fluid therapy and there is still evidence of poor peripheral perfusion and low cardiac output.

Dopamine is an adrenergic agonist that exerts positive inotropic effects and may provide improved renal and splanchnic blood flow if used at a rate of 2 to 5 µg/kg/min. Higher doses cause tachycardia and vasoconstriction and are avoided unless poor cardiac function is combined with low peripheral vascular resistance. Dobutamine is primarily a β-adrenergic agonist and acts mainly to increase cardiac contractility. It is used at a rate of 3 to 10 µg/kg/min if inadequate cardiac function is believed to be contributing to poor peripheral perfusion.

Antiarrhythmic therapy may be indicated in cats with severe arrhythmias resulting in hemodynamic compromise. Lidocaine is the preferred drug for ventricular tachycardia because it is short acting and has minimal cardiodepressant and hypotensive effects. Cats are sensitive to the drug and thus require a reduced dose of 0.25 to 1.0 mg/kg given slowly intravenously.[27,29]

Bicarbonate

Metabolic acidosis is common in shock and is associated with poor tissue oxygen delivery, which produces a shift toward anaerobic metabolism and an accumulation of lactic acid. If the acidosis is presumed to be severe in the absence of blood acid-base measurements, intravenous sodium bicarbonate may be given empirically at a dose of 1 to 2 mEq/kg slowly. Sodium bicarbonate treatment may not be very effective in patients with lactic acidosis. The adverse side effects include shifting the oxygen saturation curve to the left (Bohr effect), metabolic alkalosis, hypokalemia, cerebrospinal fluid acidosis, plasma hypertonicity, and cellular acidosis.

Antibacterial Therapy

If sepsis exists in a patient with shock, appropriate samples for bacterial culture and sensitivity should be taken and broad-spectrum antimicrobial drugs should be started. Satisfactory initial therapy usually involves administering a bactericidal combination, such as a cephalosporin and an aminoglycoside. The latter drug should not be administered until urine output and renal function are deemed to be adequate.

Glucocorticoids

The use of glucocorticoid drugs for treating patients with hypovolemic shock has been controversial for decades.[2,3,10,30–39] The beneficial effects include inhibition of acidosis and granulocyte aggregation, stabilization of cell organelles and membranes, improved cellular metabolism and gluconeogenesis, improved microcirculation and oxygen transport, inhibition of the release of vasoactive peptides, and inhibition of phospholipase A_2 (a critical step in the arachidonic acid cascade).

According to one source, "most data suggest that if corticosteroids are going to be used they should be administered early and in large doses and that although they may not produce a beneficial effect on long-term survival, the patient feels better while recovering or until death occurs."[3] Other studies, however, have indicated that glucocorticoid use in hypovolemic shock is not beneficial and may predispose patients to life-threatening infection.[34]

Maintenance

Intravenous fluid support should initially be reduced to 10 to 20 ml/kg/hour[14] until the patient is stable and should then be continued at a rate of 40 to 80 ml/kg/day.[12,13] Potassium chloride supplementation is generally required (10 to 20 mEq/L of potassium). When hemodynamic stability is reestablished, further assessment should be made in order to meet the patient's changing needs.

SUMMARY

An effective approach to shock is based on early diagnosis, a fundamental knowledge of the pathophysiology and predisposing factors of shock, an early and effective treatment plan, and the correction of known causes. Treatment should be adjusted to achieve supranormal physiologic goals. Isotonic crystalloid fluid therapy remains the foundation for increasing effective blood volume; hypertonic saline and synthetic colloids serve as useful adjuvants. Glucocorticoid drug use remains controversial. The knowledge derived from continued research involving the pathophysiology of shock should lead to further advances in treatment and improved patient outcome.

About the Authors

Dr. Ford is a board-certified internist affiliated with Gulf Coast Veterinary Specialists in Houston. Dr. Schaer is affiliated with the Department of Small Animal Clinical Sciences, College of Veterinary Medicine, University of Florida, Gainesville, Florida.

REFERENCES

1. Shoemaker WC: Shock states: Pathophysiology, monitoring, outcome, prediction, and therapy, in Shoemaker WC, Ayres S, Grenvik A, et al (eds): *Textbook of Critical Care*, ed 2. Philadelphia, WB Saunders Co, 1989, pp 977–993.
2. Ware WA: Shock, in Murtaugh RJ, Kaplan RM (eds): *Veterinary Emergency and Critical Care Medicine*, ed 1. St Louis, CV Mosby Co, 1992, pp 163–175.
3. Schertel ER, Muir WW: Shock: Pathophysiology, monitoring and therapy, in Kirk RW (ed): *Current Veterinary Therapy. X*. Philadelphia, WB Saunders Co, 1989, pp 316–330.
4. Teba L, Banks DE, Balaan MR: Understanding circulatory shock: Is it hypovolemic, cardiogenic, or vasogenic? *Postgrad Med* 91(7):121–129, 1992.
5. Thompson WL: Hypertensive urgencies and emergencies, in Shoemaker WC, Ayres S, Grenvik A, et al (eds): *Textbook of Critical Care*. Philadelphia, WB Saunders Co, 1989, pp 391–411.
6. Kemppainen RJ: Pituitary adrenal responses to hemorrhage. *Proc 5th ACVIM Forum*:84–87, 1987.
7. Runciman WB, Skowronski GA: Pathophysiology of haemorrhagic shock. *Anesth Intensive Care* 12(3):193–205, 1984.
8. Haupt MT, Carlson RW: Anaphylactic and anaphylactoid reactions, in Shoemaker WC, Ayres S, Grenvik A, et al (eds): *Textbook of Critical Care*. Philadelphia, WB Saunders Co, 1989, pp 993–1002.
9. Garvey MS: Fluid and electrolyte balance in critical patients. *Vet Clin North Am Small Anim Pract* 19(6):1021–1057, 1989.
10. Haskins SC: Shock, in Fox PR (ed): *Canine and Feline Cardiology*. New York, Churchill Livingstone, 1988, pp 229–254.
11. Willard M: General therapeutic principles, in Nelson RW, Couto CG (eds): *Essentials of Small Animal Internal Medicine*. St Louis, CV Mosby Co, 1992, pp 302–304.
12. Haskins SC: A simple fluid therapy planning guide. *Semin Vet Med Surg (Small Anim)* 3(3):227–236, 1988.
13. DiBartola SP: Planning fluid therapy. *Proc 9th ACVIM Forum*:9–11, 1991.
14. Schertel ER: Fluid therapy for noncardiogenic shock. *14th Kal Kan Waltham Symp*:27–31, 1990.
15. Okrasinski EB, Krahwinkel DJ: Treatment of hemorrhagic shock with hypertonic intraosseous fluid. *Proc 2d Int Vet Emerg Crit Care Symp*:646, 1990.
16. Fiser DF: Intraosseous infusion. *N Engl J Med* 322(22):1579–1581, 1990.
17. Orlowski JP, Julius CJ, Petras RE, et al: The safety of intraosseous infusions. Risks of fat and bone marrow emboli to the lungs. *Ann Emerg Med* 18(10):1062–1067, 1989.
18. Otto CM, Kaufman GM, Crowe DT: Intraosseous infusion of fluids and therapeutics. *Compend Contin Educ Pract Vet* 11(4):421–431, 1989.
19. Crowe DT, McDonald M, Gaston J: The use of a pneumatic garment in the management of hemorrhage and hypovolemic shock in dogs and cats: A prospective clinical investigation. *Proc 2d Int Vet Emerg Crit Care Symp*:650, 1990.
20. Kirby R: Approach to the trauma patient. *14th Kal Kan Waltham Symp*:15–25, 1990.
21. Muir MW, Sally J: Small volume resuscitation with hypertonic saline solution in hypovolemic cats. *Am J Vet Res* 50(11):1883–1888, 1989.
22. Gibbons G: Hypertonic solutions in the treatment of shock. *Proc 8th ACVIM Forum*:69–71, 1990.
23. Aver LA, Bell K: Feline blood transfusion reactions, in Kirk RW (ed): *Current Veterinary Therapy. IX*. Philadelphia, WB Saunders Co, 1986, pp 515–521.
24. Wolfsheimer KJ: Fluid therapy in the critically ill patient, in Schaer M (ed): *Vet Clin North Am Small Anim Pract* 19(2):361–378, 1989.
25. Kirby R: Clinical advantages of 6% hetastarch during fluid resuscitation. *Proc 2d Int Vet Emerg Crit Care Symp*:331–332, 1990.
26. Zoran DL, Jergens AE, Riedesel DH, et al: Evaluation of hemostatic analytes after use of hypertonic saline solution combined with colloids for resuscitation of dogs with hypovolemia. *Am J Vet Res* 53(10):1791–1796, 1992.
27. Haskins SC: Shock, in Kirk RW, Bistner SI, Ford RB (eds): *Handbook of Veterinary Procedures and Emergency Treatment*, ed 5. Philadelphia, WB Saunders Co, 1990, pp 33–52.
28. Fitzpatrick RK, Crowe DT: Nasal oxygen administration in dogs and cats: Experimental and clinical investigations. *JAAHA* 22:293–300, 1986.
29. Fox PR: Critical care cardiology. *Vet Clin North Am Small Anim Pract* 19(6):1095–1126, 1989.
30. Dillon R, Hankes GH, Nachreiner RF, et al: Experimental hemorrhage in dogs: Effects of prednisolone sodium succinate. *JAAHA* 14:673–682, 1978.
31. Abboud FM: Shock, in Wyngaarden JB, Smith LH (eds): *Cecil—Textbook of Medicine*, ed 18. Philadelphia, WB Saunders Co, 1988, pp 236–250.
32. Shoemaker WC: Effects of steroids and prostaglandin E_1 in shock and shock lung. *Proc 2d Int Vet Emerg Crit Care Symp*:325, 1990.
33. Bone RC, Fisher CJ, Clemmer TP, et al: A controlled clinical trial of high-dose methylprednisolone in the treatment of severe sepsis and septic shock. *N Engl J Med* 317(11):653–658, 1987.
34. Hinshaw L, Peduzzi P, Young E, et al: Effect of high-dose glucocorticoid therapy on mortality in patients with clinical signs of systemic sepsis. *N Engl J Med* 317(11):659–665, 1987.
35. Sprung CL, Caralis PV, Moncial EH, et al: The effects of high-dose corticosteroids in patients with septic shock. *N Engl J Med* 311(18):1137–1143, 1984.
36. Haskins SC: Management of septic shock. *JAVMA* 200(12):1915–1924, 1992.
37. Weeren FR, Muir WW: Clinical aspects of septic shock and comprehensive approaches to treatment in dogs and cats. *JAVMA* 200(12):1859–1869, 1992.
38. Haskins SC: Fluid, electrolyte, and acid-base therapy. *Proc 2d Int Vet Emerg Crit Care Symp*:375–380, 1990.
39. Garvey MS: The use of sodium bicarbonate in cardiopulmonary arrest—The controversy. *Proc 2d Int Vet Emerg Crit Care Symp*:87–88, 1990.

Use of Hypertonic Saline Solutions in Hypovolemic Shock

From the *Therapeutics in Practice* series

Derek Duval, VMD*
Department of Small Animal Medicine
College of Veterinary Medicine
University of Georgia
Athens, Georgia

Hypertonic saline solutions (HTSs) have been described for treatment of hypovolemic shock for more than 70 years, and the benefits of these solutions have been demonstrated in many species. In the past few years, the mechanism of action has been better elucidated[1-3] and hypertonic saline solutions have entered widespread use in university and referral practices. These solutions are inexpensive, effective, and relatively safe as a treatment option for private practitioners.

Saline solutions of various tonicities are manufactured by many companies. Normal saline, or 0.9% NaCl (sodium chloride) solution, is an acid solution (pH 5.6) of normal osmolarity (308 mOsm). Hypertonic saline is a solution that is more concentrated than 0.9%. The most common concentrations of hypertonic saline solutions are 3%, 5%, and 7%. Most of the experimental and clinical protocols use 7% hypertonic saline solutions. This type of hypertonic saline solution is an acid solution (pH 5 to 6) of high osmolarity (2400 mOsm). Solutions more concentrated than 7% are available primarily for use as fluid additives. In order to increase the sodium load and tonicity, 23.4% NaCl can be added to other solutions, such as dextran or hetastarch.

Mechanisms of Action

Hypertonic saline solutions have a number of beneficial actions in hypovolemic shock. In induced states of hypovolemia in dogs, cats, calves, sheep, and horses, low volumes of hypertonic saline solutions reverse signs of shock.[3,4] Three mechanisms are proposed for the action of hypertonic saline solutions. First, hypertonic saline induces plasma volume expansion.[1,3-5] The high sodium load pulls fluid from the extravascular compartment (interstitial and cellular spaces) to expand the vascular volume. This action is almost immediate and of short duration. Plasma volume expansion decreases rapidly and is negligible in 30 to

---
*Dr. Duval is currently with the Department of Clinical Studies, School of Veterinary Medicine, University of Pennsylvania, Philadelphia, Pennsylvania.

TABLE I
Indications and Contraindications of Hypertonic Saline

Indications	Contraindications
Hypovolemia	Severe dehydration
Head trauma	Hyperosmolar conditions Severe hypernatremia

60 minutes.[3] Plasma volume expansion results in increased cardiac output, oxygen delivery, and oxygen consumption to the internal organs.[2] This expansion depends on the availability of extravascular fluid. Many experiments have demonstrated plasma volume expansion with hypertonic saline solutions, and this expansion is perhaps the most important action of such solutions.

The second proposed mechanism is the so-called direct effect of hypertonic saline solutions. These solutions have been shown to increase cardiac output, increase stroke work, cause precapillary dilatation, and decrease systemic vascular resistance.[5]

The last and most poorly validated effect of hypertonic saline solutions is known as the pulmonary reflex arc. The proposed mechanism begins with high sodium concentrations that stimulate pulmonary receptors after intravenous injection.[8] The impulse is carried to the brain via the vagus nerve. Efferent nerves carry signals to the vasculature and organs, resulting in shunting of blood from the skin and muscles to the internal organs.[9] Recently, investigators have demonstrated that intact pulmonary innervation is not necessary for hypertonic saline solutions to act, making the pulmonary reflex arc effect suspect.[1,2] These combined effects of hypertonic saline solutions given in hypovolemic shock result in increased survival.

Contraindications and Physiologic Effects

The major contraindications of hypertonic saline solutions (Table I) are severe dehydration and hyperosmolar conditions. In cases of severe dehydration, the necessary extravascular fluid stores are markedly depleted, and hypertonic saline solutions cannot cause volume expansion to the same extent that they would under normal circumstances; as a result, tissue may dehydrate further.[10] In hyperosmolar conditions, such as with a hyperosmolar diabetic crisis, hypertonic saline solutions further increase blood osmolarity and may exacerbate clinical signs.

Recurrence or exacerbation of hemorrhage is a reported complication of hypertonic saline solutions. After the solutions are administered, bleeding may recur at sites where it had stopped or elevate to the level of uncontrolled hemorrhage.[11,12] This response is due to improved cardiac output and blood pressure. The clinician must be alert and prepared to intervene because patients with trauma may begin to hemorrhage again, as resuscitation (by any means) increases cardiac output.

Hypertonic saline solutions increase serum sodium concentration. A standard shock dose (4 ml/kg of 7% hypertonic saline solution) increases sodium serum concentration to 150 to 160 mEq/l and increases the serum osmolarity by 20 to 30 mOsm in patients with normal hydration status. These effects diminish quickly, and serum sodium concentration and osmolarity return to normal limits in three to four hours.[5] Some investigators suggest that larger volumes of hypertonic saline solutions can cause coagulopathies. Low volumes, such as those used for treating hypovolemic shock, have not been demonstrated to cause clotting abnormalities.[13]

Use in Shock Therapy

Hypertonic saline solutions are given as part of standard hypovolemic shock therapy (Table II). Use of hypertonic saline solutions decreases crystalloid requirements and improves cardiac output, oxygen delivery, and oxygen consumption.[2] *The dose of hypertonic saline solutions is a 4 ml/kg intravenous bolus of 7% NaCl solution.* The solution can be given via a peripheral vein, central vein, or intraosseous line. Crystalloid solutions, such as lactated Ringer's, should also be given to effect. If the hydration status of the patient is questionable, standard shock therapy with crystalloid fluids should be given concurrently to increase the intravascular space.

Large-volume crystalloid fluid therapy may result in expansion of both the extravascular and the intravascular space. Because sodium ions can freely transverse the vessel wall, large volumes of crystalloids cause accumulation of sodium ions and the accompanying water outside the vessels. This occurrence can lead to impaired cellular oxygenation and peripheral edema. Expansion of the extravascular space can occur with any fluid type and depends on rate and volume. Hypertonic saline solutions act to expand the intravascular space. Nonetheless, patients with preexisting poor oncotic pressure or those that require large volumes of crystalloid substances despite hypertonic saline therapy also require oncotic agents to prevent impaired oxygen delivery due to extravascular fluid extravasation.

Pentastarch, hetastarch, and dextran are synthetic colloid agents that help to hold fluid in the vascular space by increasing the oncotic pull of the blood. Hypertonic saline solutions can be added to the colloid agents for use in shock therapy. Investigators have

TABLE II
Hypovolemic Shock Therapy

Severity	Treatment Options
Mild to moderate	Crystalloids (90 ml/kg) ± glucocorticoids
Moderate to severe	Crystalloids (90 ml/kg) Hypertonic saline (4 ml/kg) ± glucocorticoids
Severe ± decreased oncotic pressure	Crystalloids (90 ml/kg) Hypertonic saline in colloid (4 ml/kg) ± glucocorticoids

demonstrated improved survival from hypovolemic shock with the combination therapy and increased duration of action when compared with hypertonic saline solutions alone.[14-16]

Because there are no commercially prepared colloid–hypertonic saline solution products available, such solutions must be prepared as needed. Two parts of a colloid substance can be mixed with one part 23.4% hypertonic saline solution to yield approximately 7.8% hypertonic saline solution in colloid. This mixture is given at the standard 4 ml/kg shock dose.

> For example, a 30-kg patient requires 120 milliliters (4 ml/kg) of hypertonic saline solution in colloid. Two thirds (or 80 ml) of hetastarch are mixed with one third (or 40 ml) of 23.4% hypertonic saline solution to achieve 120 milliliters of 7.8% hypertonic saline solution in hetastarch. The mixture is given as an intravenous bolus.

If a shock patient requires additional colloid support, the amount used for shock therapy is subtracted from the total daily colloid dose.

During shock accompanied by head trauma, a major concern is increasing intracranial pressure. Hypertonic saline solutions provide an excellent fluid choice for resuscitation of head trauma patients.[17] These solutions allow low-volume resuscitation and have been demonstrated not to increase intracranial pressure and cerebral edema as much as crystalloid or colloid resuscitation.[18,19]

Because resuscitation by any means during active intracranial hemorrhaging increases cardiac output and blood pressure and may exacerbate neurologic signs, the treatment of choice for persistent intracranial hemorrhage is surgical decompression. Seizures following head trauma may indicate diffuse damage or concurrent metabolic disturbances. In this situation, hypertonic saline solutions may be contraindicated.

Severe pulmonary injury accompanying hypovolemic shock is another indication for hypertonic saline solutions. Because large volumes of crystalloid fluids may increase pulmonary edema and impair ventilation and oxygenation, conservative fluid therapy is recommended. Hypertonic saline solutions have been demonstrated to allow effective low-volume resuscitation from pulmonary injury and have not been demonstrated to increase pulmonary edema.[20]

Summary

Hypertonic saline solutions are inexpensive, effective, and readily available to treat hypovolemic shock. They can be used for shock alone or when it is accompanied by head trauma or pulmonary injury. The low volume of hypertonic saline solutions needed for resuscitation rapidly increases cardiac output, blood pressure, oxygen delivery, and tissue oxygen consumption and decreases the requirement for crystalloid fluid therapy. Hypertonic saline solutions in such colloids as dextran or hetastarch may have improved efficacy and prolonged duration versus hypertonic saline solutions used alone. Hypertonic saline solutions can be a powerful tool in hypovolemic shock therapy.

REFERENCES

1. Allen DA, Schertel ER, Schmall LM, Muir WW: Lung innervation and the hemodynamic response to 7% sodium chloride in hypovolemic dogs. *Circulatory Shock* 38:189–194, 1992.
2. Tobias TA, Schertel ER, Schmall LM, et al: Comparative effects of 7.5% NaCl in 6% dextran 70 and 0.9% NaCl on cardiorespiratory parameters after cardiac output-controlled resuscitation from canine hemorrhagic shock. *Circulatory Shock* 398:139–146, 1993.
3. Velasco IT, Pontieri V, Rocha e Silva M, Lopes OU: Hyperosmotic NaCl and severe hemorrhagic shock. *Am J Physiol* 239 (Heart Circ Physiol 8): H664–H673, 1980.
4. Muir WW, Sally J: Small-volume resuscitation with hypertonic saline solution in hypovolemic cats. *Am J Vet Res* 50:1883–1888, 1989.
5. Rocha e Silva M, Velasco IT, Nogueira da Silva RI, et al: Hyperosmotic sodium salts reverse severe hemorrhagic shock: Other solutes do not. *Am J Physiol* 253 (Heart Circ Physiol 22): H751–H762, 1987.
6. Hellyer PW, Meyer RE: Effects of hypertonic saline on myocardial contractility in anesthetized pigs. *J Vet Pharm Ther* 17:211–217, 1994.
7. Constable PD, Muir WW, Binkley PF: Hypertonic saline is a negative inotropic agent in normovolemic dogs. *Am J Physiol* 241:H883–H890, 1994.
8. Lopes OU, Pontieri V, Rocha e Silva M, Velasco IT: Hyperosmotic NaCl and severe hemorrhagic shock: Role of the innervated lung. *Am J Physiol* 241 (Heart Circ Physiol 10): H883–H890, 1981.
9. Rocha e Silva M, Negraes GA, Soares AM, et al: Hypertonic

resuscitation from severe hemorrhagic shock: Patterns of regional circulation. *Circulatory Shock* 19:165–175, 1986.
10. Malcolm DS, Friedland M, Moore T, et al: Hypertonic saline resuscitation detrimentally affects renal function and survival in dehydrated rats. *Circulatory Shock* 40:69–71, 1993.
11. Krausz MM, Landau EH, Klin B, Gross D: Hypertonic saline treatment of uncontrolled hemorrhagic shock at different periods from bleeding. *Arch Surg* 127:93–96, 1992.
12. Krausz MM, Bar-Ziv M, Rabinovici R, Gross D: "Scoop and Run" or stabilize hemorrhagic shock with normal saline or small-volume hypertonic saline? *J Trauma* 33(1):6–10, 1992.
13. Zoran DL, Jergens AE, Riedesel DH, et al: Evaluation of hemostatic analytes after use of hypertonic saline solution combined with colloids for resuscitation of dogs with hypovolemia. *Am J Vet Res* 53(10):1791–1796, 1992.
14. Kramer GC, Perron PR, Lindsey DC, Ho HS, et al: Small-volume resuscitation with hypertonic saline dextran solution. *Surgery* 100(2) 239–245, 1986.
15. Allen DA, Schertel ER, Muir WW, Valentine AK: Hypertonic saline/dextran resuscitation of dogs with experimentally induced gastric dilatation–volvulus shock. *Am J Vet Res* 52(1):92–96, 1991.
16. Prough DS, Whitley JM, Taylor CL, et al: Small-volume resuscitation from hemorrhagic shock in dogs: Effects of systemic hemodynamics and systemic blood flow. *Crit Care Med* 19(3):365–372, 1991.
17. Dewey CW, Budsberg SC, Oliver JE: Principles of head trauma management in dogs and cats—Part II. *Compend Contin Educ Pract Vet* 15(2):177–193, 1993.
18. Gunnar W, Jonasson O, Merlotti G, et al: Head injury and hemorrhagic shock: Studies of the blood–brain barrier and intracranial pressure after resuscitation with normal saline solution, 3% saline solution, and dextran-40. *Surgery* 103(4) 398–407, 1988.
19. Gunnar W, Merlotti G, Jonasson O, Barrett J: Resuscitation from hemorrhagic shock—Alterations of the intracranial pressure after normal saline, 3% saline and dextran-40. *Ann Surgery* 204(6):686–692, 1986.
20. Johnston WE, Alford PT, Prough DS, et al: Cardiopulmonary effects of hypertonic saline in canine oleic acid-induced pulmonary edema. *Crit Care Med* 13(10):814–817, 1985.

Acute Hemorrhage: A Hematologic Emergency in Dogs

KEY FACTS

- Common causes of acute blood loss include trauma, hemostatic disorders, splenic rupture, gastrointestinal hemorrhage, and epistaxis.
- Dogs that are presented with acute loss of 30% to 40% of their blood volume exhibit signs of shock; a loss of 50% or more usually results in death if the patient is untreated.
- Blood products that are available for transfusion include fresh whole blood, packed red blood cells, fresh plasma, fresh-frozen plasma, cryoprecipitate, platelet-rich plasma, and platelet concentrates.
- Signs of acute hemolytic reaction are fever, tachycardia, tachypnea, weakness, tremors, vomiting, urticaria, pruritus, renal failure, urinary and fecal incontinence, and collapse.

Oklahoma State University
Mitchell A. Crystal, DVM

Tufts University
Susan M. Cotter, DVM

HEMATOLOGIC emergencies are life-threatening conditions that are frequently presented to veterinary practitioners. Such emergencies are characterized by marked increases or decreases in circulating blood cells. Hemorrhage is a common hematologic emergency in dogs. The site of hemorrhage may be focal (e.g., from a laceration, ruptured spleen, or gastric ulcer) or systemic (e.g., at various sites secondary to a hemostatic disorder). Such patients pose a diagnostic challenge yet require immediate attention to preserve life.

This article considers the common causes of acute hemorrhage in dogs and describes appropriate diagnostic and therapeutic management. The important role of transfusion and transfusion reactions is discussed.

FACTS ABOUT HEMORRHAGE

Acute blood loss anemia usually results from trauma but may be related to gastrointestinal, genitourinary, oronasal, or surgical bleeding. Hemorrhage may be obvious if it occurs outside the body or less detectable if it occurs in less visible areas inside the body, such as the thoracic or abdominal cavity or the gastrointestinal tract.

Dogs presented with acute loss of 30% to 40% of their blood volume exhibit such signs of hypovolemic shock as tachycardia, hypotension, prolonged capillary refill time, and tachypnea[1]; a loss of 50% or more usually results in death if treatment is not instituted.[2] Clinical signs of blood loss (shock) may be apparent before the onset of decreased packed cell volume (PCV). This decrease occurs because plasma and red blood cell components are lost simultaneously[3] and because of splenic contraction.[4] The true packed cell volume may not be evident for as long as three days after blood loss; some degree of anemia will be apparent within 24 hours, especially if fluids are administered.[1]

INITIAL TREATMENT

Initial treatment of patients with acute blood loss includes managing shock, preventing further bleeding, and deciding whether transfusion is necessary. If the inciting cause of the hemorrhage is unknown, samples for laboratory analysis should be taken before therapy is instituted. Causes of acute blood loss other than trauma should be considered when the patient is stable (see Causes of Blood Loss Anemia in Dogs).

Hypovolemic Shock

Balanced electrolyte or colloid solutions are the preferred fluids in the initial management of acute blood loss.

> **Causes of Blood Loss Anemia in Dogs**
>
> **Trauma**
>
> **Coagulopathies**
> - Congenital
> - Acquired (anticoagulants, hepatic disease)
>
> **Platelet disorders**
> - Thrombocytopenia (immune, drugs, rickettsial diseases)
> - von Willebrand's disease
> - Functional disorders (drugs, dysproteinemias, thrombopathias)
>
> **Splenic rupture**
> - Neoplasia
> - Trauma
> - Torsion
>
> **Gastrointestinal hemorrhage**
> - Ulceration
> - Neoplasia
> - Parasites
> - Foreign bodies
> - Hemostatic disorders
>
> **Epistaxis**
> - Neoplasia
> - Infection
> - Hemostatic disorders

These solutions are effective in managing hypovolemic shock, are readily available, and do not expose previously transfused patients to risks.[5] In one study, all patients survived loss of 30% of their blood volume when treated with lactated Ringer's solution alone. All patients initially survived loss of 50% of their blood volume when treated with lactated Ringer's solution alone, but 38% of the patients died within three days.[2] Balanced electrolyte solutions alone are unable to maintain adequate blood pressure or oxygenation if blood loss is severe; the use of colloids or blood products thus is also required.[5]

Colloids (dextran, hydroxylethyl starch, or plasma) provide better blood pressure support and better prevention of hypoxemia than balanced electrolyte solutions do.[5] Colloids contain large particles, which remain in the vascular space for as long as 48 hours and maintain vascular volume and blood pressure. All colloids can cause allergic reactions and anaphylactic shock; synthetic colloids can interfere with platelet function and coagulation, although clinically significant allergic reactions and coagulopathies have not been reported in animals and are rare in humans.[6]

Other possible side effects include pulmonary edema, renal failure, and immunosuppression.[6-8] The dosage of dextran and hydroxylethyl starch (6% solutions in normal saline) is 10 to 20 ml/kg/day given for two to four hours. Treatment with colloids alone in patients that lost 64% of their blood volume resulted in 86% survival at the end of a three-hour study; long-term survival was not assessed.[5] In patients with acute blood loss, colloids apparently are a reasonable choice in the initial restoration of vascular volume until appropriate blood products are available.

HYPERTONIC SALINE is useful in restoring effective circulating vascular volume during hemorrhagic shock. Two studies using hypertonic saline demonstrated nearly 100% survival in patients that had 50% blood loss. Doses of 5 ml/kg of 7.5% saline solution (with or without dextran) are currently recommended in managing severe hypovolemic shock.[9-11]

In summary, initial management of patients with acute hemorrhage involves balanced electrolyte solutions at shock dosages (as high as 90 ml/kg/hour) or hypertonic saline. If hemorrhage is severe or the patient does not respond to initial fluid therapy, colloids can be added. Hemodilution as a result of fluid therapy is not a concern because appropriate volume is necessary to overcome shock. If the packed cell volume drops below acceptable levels or if the patient does not respond, the decision to transfuse should be made.

Preventing Further Bleeding

Bleeding from visible sites should be controlled with direct pressure or blood vessel ligation. Pressure bandages can be applied and left in place until shock has subsided. If there is internal hemorrhage, the practitioner must decide whether to perform emergency exploratory surgery. Stabilization can be attempted via shock therapy and blood transfusion as well as pressure wraps for abdominal hemorrhage. Thoracocentesis may help to relieve dyspnea caused by pleural hemorrhage but also creates space for further hemorrhage. Exploration is necessary if stabilization is unsuccessful.[12,13]

Deciding to Transfuse

Transfusion with red blood cells is required if reduction in the number of red blood cells results in inadequate oxygen-carrying capacity. If blood pressure and circulatory volume are adequate, myocardial oxygenation is maintained until the hematocrit drops to less than 15%.

Transfusion is not indicated until the packed cell volume drops below 20%. Because the packed cell volume may not drop initially after blood loss, other parameters should

Parameters That Suggest the Need for Blood Transfusion in Dogs with Acute Blood Loss[a]

- Acute loss of more than 30% of blood volume (approximately 30 ml/kg)
- Packed cell volume less than 20%[b]
- Ongoing hemorrhage
- Poor response to shock therapy
- Collapse associated with severe blood loss
- Pale mucous membranes[c]
- Poor capillary refill time (greater than 2.0 seconds)[c]
- Elevated heart rate (greater than 180 beats/min)[c]
- Elevated respiratory rate (greater than 60 breaths/min)[c]
- Depressed arterial blood pressure (mean less than 80 mm Hg)[c]
- Depressed central venous pressure (0 centimeters of water)[c]

[a]More than one parameter should be considered in determining the need for transfusion.
[b]Percentages may not be significant in acutely bleeding dogs, especially those being treated with fluids. Patients may have low packed cell volumes and not need transfusion if the blood loss occurred more than 24 hours before evaluation and if other parameters are stable.
[c]These conditions may be caused by hypovolemic shock without loss of oxygen-carryng capacity. Persistence despite shock therapy increases the significance.

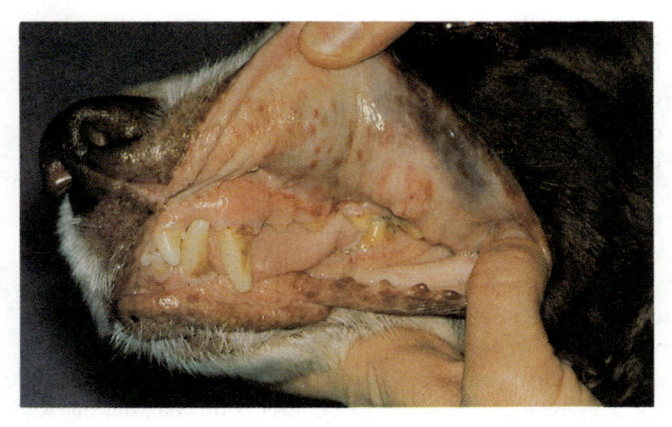

Figure 1—Petechial hemorrhage in a patient with thrombocytopenia.

be considered in assessing the need for transfusion (see the list on this page). The parameters include depth and rate of respiration, mucous membrane color, capillary refill time, ongoing hemorrhage, central venous pressure, and arterial blood pressure.[4,14,15] Plasma replacement is not routinely necessary because adequate concentrations of coagulation factors remain and movement of albumin from the interstitium to the plasma occurs after hemorrhage.

CAUSES OF BLOOD LOSS
Trauma

Trauma is one of the most common causes of acute hemorrhage in animals. If history or physical evidence of trauma is consistent with the severity of blood loss, therapy can be instituted without further investigation of less common causes of bleeding. If such evidence of trauma is lacking or if the degree of trauma is inconsistent with the severity of blood loss, further diagnostic evaluation is indicated.

Coagulopathies and Platelet Disorders

Bleeding with slight trauma warrants evaluation for abnormal coagulation or defects in platelet number or function. Coagulation factor abnormalities result in bleeding into body cavities, isolated hematomas, and hemarthroses; platelet defects result in petechial and ecchymotic hemorrhages, hematuria, melena, and epistaxis[16,17] (Figure 1).

Common causes of abnormal coagulation include anticoagulant rodenticide (warfarin) intoxication, inherited clotting disorders, liver disease, and disseminated intravascular coagulation (DIC). Common causes of platelet disorders include thrombocytopenia (caused by immune-mediated thrombocytopenia [ITP]), rickettsial diseases (Rocky Mountain spotted fever and ehrlichiosis), drug reactions (sulfonamides, modified live distemper virus vaccines, estrogens, chemotherapeutic agents), and disseminated intravascular coagulation as well as decreased platelet function caused by drugs (aspirin, phenylbutazone, phenothiazines, and dextrans), von Willebrand's disease, inherited thrombopathias, and dysproteinemias (multiple myeloma and ehrlichiosis).[18-21] To determine possible causes of abnormal hemostasis, owners should be questioned thoroughly regarding travel, ticks, toxins, and whether other related animals are affected.

Tables I and II outline the common tests for disorders of hemostasis and the normal values as well as the diseases expected when these tests are abnormal. Specific assays for coagulation factors are available.

ELEVATION of activated clotting time (ACT) and activated partial thromboplastin time (APTT) indicates an abnormality in the intrinsic coagulation pathway, such as factor VIII deficiency (hemophilia A) or factor IX deficiency (hemophilia B). Elevation of one-stage prothrombin time (OSPT) indicates an abnormality in the extrinsic coagulation pathway (factor VII deficiency); this is uncommon and usually not associated with hemorrhage. Elevation of activated clotting time, activated partial thromboplastin time, and one-stage prothrombin time indicates an abnormality in both intrinsic and extrinsic pathways or in the common coagulation pathway. Examples include warfarin (or other anticoagulant rodenticide) intoxication, liver disease, and disseminated intravascular coagulation.

Elevation of fibrin degradation products (FDP) indicates disseminated intravascular coagulation or severe liver disease but also may occur with internal bleeding. Elevation of buccal bleeding time (BT) indicates von Willebrand's disease or a functional platelet disorder but may also occur with thrombocytopenia.[16,22-24]

Hemostatic disorders require treatment of the disorder itself as well as the acute blood loss. For coagulation defects, plasma (fresh, fresh-frozen, or as part of fresh whole blood) or cryoprecipitate is indicated depending on the deficiency.[25,26] Platelets can be supplied via fresh whole blood, platelet-rich plasma, or platelet concentrates.[27]

Splenic Rupture

Splenic rupture, which is usually caused by splenic hemangiosarcoma, is a common cause of intraabdominal hemorrhage in dogs[28-30] (Figure 2). Other causes of hemoperitoneum (trauma and coagulopathy) are far less common. Intraabdominal hemorrhage can be confirmed via abdominocentesis, radiography, and ultrasonography. Abdominocentesis with a small needle (25- or 22-gauge) is fast and easy but does not indicate the source of bleeding; cytologic evaluation of fluid is usually nondiagnostic.[31]

Abdominal radiography and ultrasonography demonstrate splenic lesions and effusion. Lack of clotting of blood withdrawn from the abdomen does not distinguish coagulopathies from other causes of abdominal hemorrhage because blood in the abdominal cavity becomes defibrinated within 45 to 60 minutes. Thoracic radiography and abdominal ultrasonography may detect pulmonary or hepatic metastases; hepatic metastases may be hard to distinguish from benign hepatic nodular hyperplasia via ultrasonography.[32] When the patient is stabilized, exploratory laparotomy for splenectomy should be performed. Hepatic biopsies should be taken if lesions are noted.

Gastrointestinal Hemorrhage

Patients with gastrointestinal hemorrhage may be acutely anemic at presentation. A history of melena or hematochezia helps to localize bleeding to the intestine but may be absent if the hemorrhage is recent (Figure 3). Oronasal bleeding may present as melena. Causes of acute gastrointestinal hemorrhage include ulceration, neoplasia, sharp foreign bodies, intestinal parasites (in young dogs), and hemostatic (especially platelet) disorders.[33]

Definition of the inciting cause and direct local therapy may be facilitated by a history of ulcerogenic drug administration (aspirin and other nonsteroidal antiinflammatory drugs or glucocorticoids) or foreign body ingestion coupled with abdominal and thoracic radiographs and fecal ex-

TABLE I
Laboratory Tests Used to Screen for Hemostatic Disorders

Test	Reference Range
One-stage prothrombin time	7 to 10 seconds
Activated partial thromboplastin time	14 to 20 seconds
Activated clotting time	60 to 120 seconds
Platelet count	200,000 to 500,000/μl
Buccal bleeding time[a]	4 to 5 minutes
Fibrin degradation products	Less than 10 μg/dl

[a]Bleeding time is contraindicated in patients that are known to be thrombocytopenic.

amination.[34] Hemostatic evaluation should be performed, especially if there is bleeding from multiple sites or if the initial tests and history are inconclusive.

PATIENTS with chronic gastrointestinal hemorrhage may present acutely as anemia becomes severe. In addition to determining and correcting the underlying cause, oral iron therapy is indicated. The presence of microcytic, hypochromic anemia differentiates chronic from acute gastrointestinal hemorrhage (Figure 4).

Epistaxis

Epistaxis can be caused by trauma, bacterial or fungal infection, neoplasia, or hemostatic disorders. Most cases of recurrent or prolonged epistaxis are related to hemostatic defects, especially platelet disorders. If trauma is unlikely, platelet number and function as well as coagulation should be assessed before invasive diagnostic procedures (e.g., biopsy) are performed.[23]

TRANSFUSION

Products that are available for transfusion include fresh whole blood, packed red blood cells, fresh plasma, fresh-frozen plasma, cryoprecipitate, platelet-rich plasma, and platelet concentrate. Preparation of these products has been described in the literature.[25,26,35] Blood substitutes, such as hemoglobin solutions and perfluorocarbon compounds, may be useful in the future but are not currently available commercially.[36,37]

Fresh whole blood and packed red blood cells are sources of red blood cells. Blood should be typed before transfusion and crossmatched if previous transfusions have been received. If this is impossible, donor blood should be negative for alleles at the DEA-1 locus (A negative). There are many formulas for estimating the amount of blood

TABLE II
Diseases Expected with Abnormal Hemostatic Screening Test Results

Disease	Buccal Bleeding Time	Platelet Count	One-Stage Prothrombin Time	Activated Partial Thromboplastin Time	Activated Clotting Time	Fibrin Degradation Products
Thrombocytopenia	Increased	Decreased	Normal	Normal	Normal or decreased	Normal
Platelet function disorder (including von Willebrand's disease)	Increased	Normal	Normal	Normal	Normal	Normal
Intrinsic clotting system disorder	Normal	Normal	Normal	Increased	Increased	Normal or increased
Extrinsic clotting system disorder	Normal	Normal	Increased	Normal	Normal	Normal or increased
Intrinsic and extrinsic or common clotting system disorder	Normal	Normal	Increased	Increased	Increased	Normal or increased
Disseminated intravascular coagulation	Increased	Decreased	Increased	Increased	Increased	Increased

needed for transfusion; a simple estimation is that a transfusion of 20 ml/kg of fresh whole blood or 10 ml/kg of packed red blood cells will raise the hematocrit 10 points. The transfusion is given warm at a rate of approximately 22 ml/kg/hour. The transfusion should be completed within four hours but can be given faster in cases of severe blood loss.[25,38]

Blood from intraabdominal or intrathoracic hemorrhage can be autotransfused as a source of red blood cells. The blood must be filtered of debris and free from such contaminants as urine, neoplastic cells, or intestinal contents. Anticoagulation is only necessary if blood defibrination has not occurred. Sixty-three milliliters of citrate phosphate dextrose adenine (CPDA), citrate phosphate dextrose (CPD), or acid citrate dextrose (ACD) per 500 milliliters of blood (or just enough heparin [1000 units per milliliter] to coat a 60-milliliter syringe) is used if needed.[39]

Fresh plasma, fresh-frozen plasma, cryoprecipitate, and fresh whole blood are sources of clotting factors. All clotting factors and von Willebrand's factor are available in fresh plasma, fresh-frozen plasma, and fresh whole blood. Fibrinogen, factor VIII, von Willebrand's factor, and fibronectin are present in higher concentration in cryoprecipitate. Fresh plasma and fresh-frozen plasma should be administered at a rate of 6 to 10 ml/kg two to three times daily for three to five days or until bleeding stops. Cryoprecipitate is administered at one unit (containing 10 to 15 milliliters prepared from one unit of fresh-frozen plasma) per 10 kilograms every eight hours until bleeding stops.[25,40]

Fresh whole blood, platelet-rich plasma, and platelet concentrates are sources of platelets. The method of preparation and short half-life (less than 72 hours) of platelet-rich plasma and platelet concentrates preclude their general use in practice. Fresh whole blood administered within 12 hours is more commonly used; 250 milliliters of fresh whole blood with a platelet count of 200,000/μl will raise the platelet count of 20-kilogram dog approximately 13,000/μl.[41] The increment may be less than expected if there is fever, sepsis, disseminated intravascular coagulation, bleeding, splenomegaly, or immune-mediated thrombocytopenia.[42]

TRANSFUSION REACTIONS

In human medicine, 20% of blood transfusions result in some type of adverse reaction.[43] Reactions may be immunologic or nonimmunologic, hemolytic or nonhemolytic, and acute or delayed (Table III).

Because of the low incidence of naturally occurring isoantibodies, acute hemolytic reactions are rare in dogs that have not been transfused.[38] Signs of acute hemolytic reaction include fever, tachycardia, tachypnea, weakness, tremors, vomiting, urticaria, pruritus, renal failure, urinary and fecal incontinence, and collapse.[26,38] If there are signs of an acute hemolytic reaction, the transfusion should be stopped and the patient should be treated for hypotensive shock with intravenous fluids and (if necessary) such pressor agents as dopamine hydrochloride.[38] With appropriate therapy, most patients recover within 12 to 24 hours.[44]

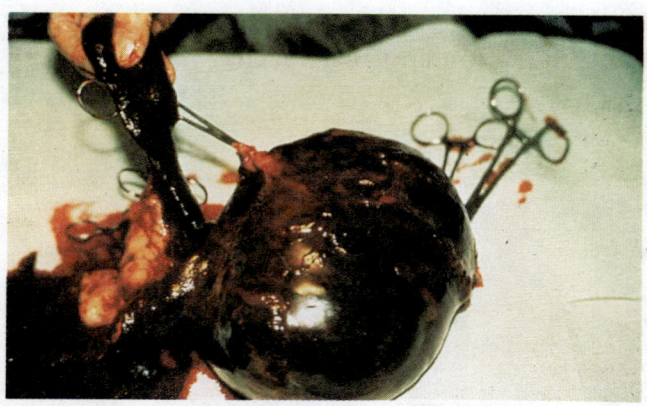

Figure 2—Splenic hemangiosarcoma in a patient with hemoperitoneum.

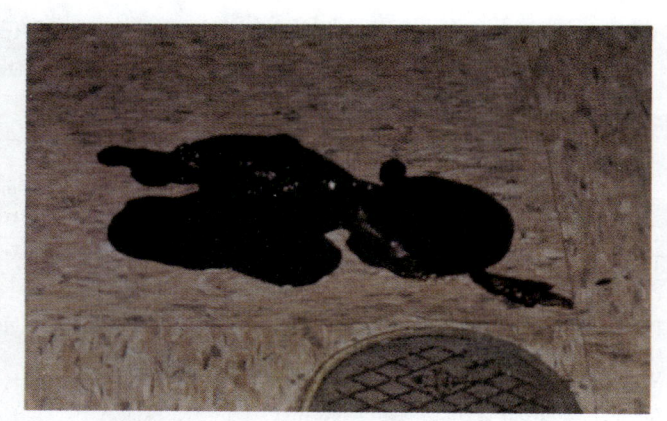

Figure 3—Melena from a patient with gastric ulceration.

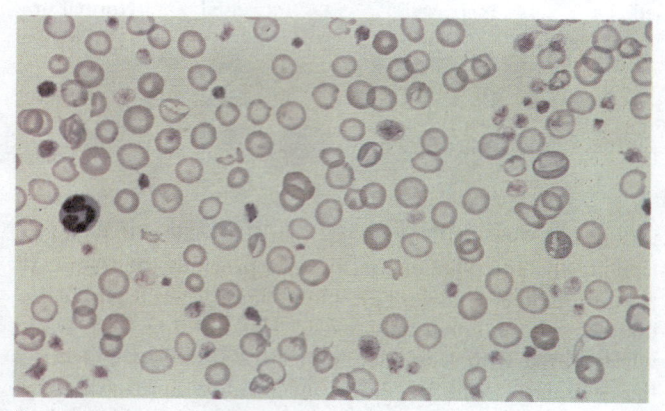

Figure 4—Hypochromic, microcytic red blood cells from a patient with chronic gastrointestinal hemorrhage. (Courtesy of Sonjia M. Shelly, DVM, California Veterinary Diagnostics, Inc., West Sacramento, CA)

Delayed hemolysis is more common than acute hemolysis. The delayed condition occasionally occurs in sensitized individuals after blood transfusion. Clinical signs include an unexpected decline in the packed cell volume and a positive direct Coombs' test 2 to 21 days after transfusion.[4] Other clinical signs are fever, anorexia, and mild icterus.[44]

Transfusion with hemolyzed blood may mimic an acute hemolytic reaction. Causes of hemolyzed donor cells include heating of the blood to temperatures above 50°C; freezing; mechanical trauma to red blood cells during collection, preparation of components, or administration; mixing with hypotonic solutions; and contamination with hemolytic bacteria.[38] Saline is the only solution that may contact blood during administration. Blood can be checked for hemolysis by centrifuging a microhematocrit tube of blood from the donor bag and examining the supernatant.

The foremost treatment for hemolytic reactions is prevention. This is best accomplished by pretransfusion compatibility testing and avoiding hemolyzed donor cells. The use of intramuscular diphenhydramine (2 to 4 mg/kg) has been advocated to prevent or treat immunologic transfusion reactions[4,25]; no evidence supports the effectiveness of this approach.[38]

Other immunologic transfusion reactions can occur in addition to hemolysis. Leukocyte, platelet, and plasma protein incompatibility can lead to fever, petechiation, neurologic signs, vomiting, and urticaria.[25,26] If these signs occur, the transfusion is slowed or stopped and supportive care is given as needed.

Circulatory overload occurs if large volumes are delivered to normovolemic patients or to patients with underlying cardiac failure.[4,25,38] Clinical signs include coughing, dyspnea, and vomiting.[4,26,45] Therapy involves discontinuing the transfusion until clinical signs resolve and then resuming the transfusion at a slower rate. Furosemide (1 to 2 mg/kg) and oxygen may be required. Circulatory overload can be prevented by using packed red blood cells in place of whole blood.[4]

Citrate intoxication is a rare problem caused by calcium chelation and subsequent hypocalcemia. Clinical signs include tremors, arrhythmias, and such electrocardiographic changes as prolongation of the QT interval and depression of the P and T waves. Citrate is rapidly metabolized by the liver. Patients with hepatic insufficiency might experience toxicity if given large amounts of whole blood or plasma stored in citrate anticoagulant.[25,38] Treatment involves stopping the transfusion for 5 to 10 minutes and then resuming at a slower rate. Calcium administration is seldom needed.[25,28]

AMMONIA LEVELS slowly increase in stored blood. This is usually not a problem except in patients with hepatic insufficiency.[38] Hemosiderosis, a condition of excessive iron storage, causes hepatic damage after repeated

TABLE III
Transfusion Reactions

Hemolytic or Nonhemolytic	Acute	Delayed
Immunologic		
Hemolytic	Acute hemolysis	Delayed hemolysis
Nonhemolytic	Pyrexia	Red blood cell antibody production
	Urticaria	Platelet antibody production
	Anaphylaxis	White blood cell antibody production
Nonimmunologic		
Hemolytic	Donor cell hemolysis before transfusion	—
Nonhemolytic	Circulatory overload	Infectious diseases
	Contaminated blood	Hemosiderosis
	Citrate toxicity	
	Hyperammonemia	
	Disseminated intravascular coagulation	

transfusions. Unless the cause of anemia is chronic blood loss, iron supplementation should be avoided in patients that are receiving transfusions.[38]

Recipients of transfusions are at risk of contracting such infectious diseases as babesiosis, hemobartonellosis, ehrlichiosis, Rocky Mountain spotted fever, brucellosis, borreliosis, trypanosomiasis, and microfilariasis.[15,35] The potential for disease transmission is minimized by appropriately screening donors for diseases that are present in their geographic areas.

Transfusion reactions are infrequent and usually preventable. With appropriate therapy, most patients recover within 12 to 24 hours.

About the Authors
Dr. Crystal is a Diplomate of the American College of Veterinary Internal Medicine (Internal Medicine) and is affiliated with the Department of Medicine and Surgery, College of Veterinary Medicine, Oklahoma State University, Stillwater, Oklahoma. Dr. Cotter is a Diplomate of the American College of Veterinary Internal Medicine (Internal Medicine, Oncology) and is affiliated with the Department of Medicine, School of Veterinary Medicine, Tufts University, North Grafton, Massachusetts.

REFERENCES

1. Feldman BF: Anemias associated with blood loss and hemolysis. *Vet Clin North Am [Small Anim Pract]* 11(2):265-275, 1981.
2. Rush B, Eiseman B: Limits of non-colloid solution replacement in experimental hemorrhagic shock. *Ann Surg* 165(6):977-984, 1967.
3. Schaer M: The internist's assessment of the anemic dog and cat. *Proc East States Vet Conf* 4:39-40, 1990.
4. Tanger CH: Transfusion therapy for the dog and cat. *Compend Contin Educ Pract Vet* 4(6):521-527, 1982.
5. Kirimli B, Kampschulte S, Safar P: Resuscitation from cardiac arrest due to exsanguination. *Surg Gynecol Obstet* 129:89-97, 1968.
6. Stehling LC: Volume replacement in the surgical patient, in Rossi E, Simon T, Moss G (eds): *Principles of Transfusion Medicine.* Baltimore, Williams & Wilkins, 1991, pp 429-434.
7. Garvey MS: Fluid and electrolyte balance in critical patients. *Vet Clin North Am [Small Anim Pract]* 19(6):1021-1057, 1989.
8. Smiley LE, Garvey MS: The use of hetastarch in hypoalbuminemic dogs and cats. *Proc 9th ACVIM Forum*:890, 1991.
9. Lopes OU, Pontieri V, Rocha de Silva M, Velasco IT: Hyperosmotic NaCl and severe hemorrhagic shock: Role of the innervated lung. *Am J Physiol* 241:H883-H890, 1981.
10. Rocha de Silva M, Velasco IT, Nogueira da Silva RI, et al: Hyperosmotic sodium salts reverse severe hemorrhagic shock: Other solutes do not. *Am J Physiol* 253:H751-H762, 1987.
11. Muir WW: Small volume resuscitation using hypertonic saline. *Cornell Vet* 80(1):7-12, 1990.
12. Haskins SC: Monitoring the critically ill patient. *Vet Clin North Am [Small Anim Pract]* 19(6):1059-1078, 1989.
13. Jennings PB, Whitten NJ, Sleeman HK: The diagnosis and treatment of shock in the critical care patient, in Slatter FP, Knowles RP, Whittick WG (eds): *Veterinary Critical Care.* Philadelphia, Lea & Febiger, 1981, pp 486-523.
14. Katz AJ: Transfusion therapy: Its role in the anemias. *Hosp Pract* 15:77-84, 1980.
15. Pichler ME, Turnwald GH: Blood transfusion in the dog and cat. Part I. Physiology, collection, storage, and indications for whole blood therapy. *Compend Contin Educ Pract Vet* 7(1):64-72, 1985.
16. Dodds WG: Hemostasis, in Kaneko JJ (ed): *Clinical Biochemistry of Domestic Animals,* ed 4. San Diego, Academic Press, 1989, pp 274-315.
17. Johnstone IB: Clinical and laboratory diagnosis of bleeding disorders. *Vet Clin North Am [Small Anim Pract]* 18(1):21-33, 1988.
18. Davenport DJ: Platelet disorders in the dog and cat. Part I: Physiology and pathogenesis. *Compend Contin Educ Pract Vet* 4(9):762-776, 1982.
19. Dodds WG: Sulfonamides and blood dyscrasias (letter). *JAVMA* 196(5):681-682, 1990.
20. McAnulty JF, Rudd RG: Thrombocytopenia associated with vaccination of a dog with a modified-live paramyxovirus vaccine. *JAVMA* 186(11):1217-1219, 1985.
21. Catalfamo JL, Dodds WJ: Hereditary and acquired thrombopathies. *Vet Clin North Am [Small Anim Pract]* 18(1):185-193, 1988.
22. Troy GC: Clinical approach to hemostatic disorders. *VM SAC* 79:917-930, 1984.
23. Littlewood JD: A practical approach to bleeding disorders in the dog.

J Small Anim Pract 27:397–409, 1986.
24. Slappendel RJ: Disseminated intravascular coagulation. *Vet Clin North Am [Small Anim Pract]* 18(1):169–184, 1988.
25. Authement JM, Wolfsheimer KJ, Catchings S: Canine blood component therapy: Product preparation, storage, and administration. *JAAHA* 23:483–493, 1987.
26. Killingsworth CR: Use of blood and blood components for the feline and canine patient. *J Vet Crit Care* 7(1):6–10, 1984.
27. Thomason KJ, Feldman BF: Immune-mediated thrombocytopenia: Diagnosis and treatment. *Compend Contin Educ Pract Vet* 7(7):569–576, 1985.
28. Macintire DK: Hematologic emergencies. *Proc East States Vet Conf* 4:59–60, 1990.
29. Prymak C, McKee LJ, Goldschmidt MH, Glickman LT: Epidemiologic, clinical, pathologic, and prognostic characteristics of splenic hemangiosarcoma and splenic hematoma in dogs: 217 cases (1985). *JAVMA* 193(6):706–712, 1988.
30. Hosgood G: Canine hemangiosarcoma. *Compend Contin Educ Pract Vet* 13(7):1065–1075, 1991.
31. Johnson KA, Powers BE, Withrow SJ, et al: Splenomegaly in dogs. *J Vet Intern Med* 3:160–166, 1989.
32. Feeney DA, Johnston GR, Hardy RM: Two-dimensional, grey-scale ultrasonography for assessment of hepatic and splenic neoplasia in the dog and cat. *JAVMA* 184:68–81, 1984.
33. Strombeck DR, Guilford WG: Approach to clinical problems in gastroenterology, in *Small Animal Gastroenterology*. Davis, CA, Stonegate Publishing Co, 1990, pp 56–89.
34. Wallace MS, Zawie DA, Garvey MS: Gastric ulceration in the dog secondary to the use of nonsteroidal antiinflammatory drugs. *JAAHA* 26:467–472, 1990.
35. Feldman BF: Practical transfusion medicine for the small animal practice. *VA-MD Coll Vet Med Newsl*:2–4, 1991.
36. Greene CE: Blood substitute therapy, in Kirk RW (ed): *Current Veterinary Therapy. IX.* Philadelphia, WB Saunders Co, 1986, pp 107–109.
37. Rentko VT, Cotter SM: Transfusion therapy: Blood substitutes and autotransfusion, in Kirk RW (ed): *Current Veterinary Therapy. XI.* Philadelphia, WB Saunders Co, 1992.
38. Cotter SM: Clinical transfusion medicine, in *Comparative Transfusion Medicine*. San Diego, Academic Press, 1991, pp 188–223.
39. Crow DT: Autotransfusion in the trauma patient. *Vet Clin North Am [Small Anim Pract]* 10(3):581–597, 1980.
40. Mollison PC, Engelfret CP, Contreras M: Blood transfusion, in *Clinical Medicine*, ed 8. Oxford, Blackwell Scientific Publications, 1987, p 187.
41. Feldman BF, Thomason KJ, Jain NC: Quantitative platelet disorders. *Vet Clin North Am [Small Anim Pract]* 18(1):35–49, 1988.
42. Simon T: Platelet transfusion therapy, in Rossi E, Simon T, Moss G (eds): *Principles of Transfusion Medicine*. Baltimore, Williams & Wilkins, 1991, pp 219–222.
43. Capon SM, Sacher RA: Hemolytic transfusion reactions: A review of mechanisms, sequelae, and management. *J Intens Care Med* 4:100–111, 1989.
44. Turnwald GH, Pichler ME: Blood transfusion in dogs and cats. Part II. Administration, adverse affects, and component therapy. *Compend Contin Educ Pract Vet* 7(2):115–126, 1985.
45. Killingsworth CR: Use of blood and blood components for feline and canine patients. *JAVMA* 185(11):1452–1454, 1984.

An Introduction to Reperfusion Injury

KEY FACTS

- Hypoxia allows the oxygenase system to predominate in cell metabolism and subsequently produces free radicals.
- Superoxide ions, hydrogen peroxide ions, and hydroxyl ions are free radicals that are responsible for the destructive processes of reperfusion injury. Hydroxyl ions are the most destructive ions of this group.
- The presence of iron greatly increases the degree of destruction that occurs during reperfusion injury.
- The interaction of free radicals with unsaturated free fatty acids produces lipid peroxidation products that damage cell and organelle membranes. The degree of damage often is measured by levels of malondialdehyde, which is an innocuous by-product of lipid peroxidation.
- Neutrophils contribute to the perpetuation of cellular destruction by producing free radicals, oxidants, and enzymes.
- Such drugs as dimethyl sulfoxide (DMSO), deferoxamine, superoxide dismutase, allopurinol, and nonglucocorticoid aminosteroids are being evaluated in preventing and treating reperfusion injury.

Oklahoma State University
Mark C. Rochat, DVM

ISCHEMIA and associated pathologic consequences are common in various disease processes. Equally important are the alterations that occur when ischemic tissue is reperfused with oxygen. Biochemical processes after reperfusion of ischemic tissue may result in ultrastructural changes and, ultimately, cell death; this process has been termed *reperfusion injury* or *the oxygen paradox*. Various theories attempt to explain the cellular events that occur after reoxygenation. Products of anaerobic metabolism (e.g., unbuffered acids, potassium, and lysosomal enzymes from injured cells as well as embolism of platelet microaggregates) during ischemia represent more traditional explanations; however, a growing body of evidence suggests that generation of oxygen-derived free radicals is responsible for cytotoxic effects observed after ischemia and reperfusion.[1] Although these effects are evident at a local level, they also may contribute to systemic complications, such as pulmonary edema and respiratory failure.[2] Metabolic changes that occur during ischemia often cause less destruction than does the addition of oxygen to ischemic tissue. In the past decade, veterinarians have dramatically increased their understanding of the mechanisms by which reoxygenation further damages ischemic tissue.

Current knowledge of the mechanisms of reperfusion injury has presented new opportunities for treating and preventing cellular injury in various diseases that affect both humans and animals.

Veterinarians often are challenged with the complexities of reperfusion injury. Common disease processes that are influenced by reperfusion injury include shock and gastric dilatation volvulus. Animals that undergo severe ischemic episodes (regardless of the degree of severity) occasionally fail to improve with current therapeutic approaches. For successful treatment of reperfusion injury patients, veterinarians must recognize that reperfusion can be harmful. This article discusses current understanding of the basic mechanisms of reperfusion injury. Drugs that are commonly used to treat or prevent reperfusion injury also are discussed.

MECHANISM OF ACTION

An understanding of free radicals and biochemical pathways that produce these free radicals is fundamental to the concept of reperfusion injury. A normal chemical bond is composed of a pair of electrons that spin in opposite directions and share a single molecular orbit.[3,4] A molecule with an odd number of electrons is a free radical.[4-6] This single electron often is denoted as a dot (Figure 1). Because of the open (or half) bond, this molecule is highly receptive to participation in chemical reactions.[3,4] When two radicals react with each other, both radicals are eliminated. If a radical reacts with a nonradical, another radical is produced, thereby potentially allowing a chain reaction that may be thousands of events long.[3,7] The half-life of free radicals is extremely short (ranging from nanoseconds to milliseconds).[4] Radicals may function as oxidants or as reductants.[8] Oxidants are compounds that may receive an electron; reductants are compounds that may donate an electron. The radicals that are important in reperfusion injury are derived from molecular oxygen.

Oxygen use by tissue occurs at the cellular level in one of two ways. The oxidase pathway oxidizes energy substrates using cytochrome oxidase (Figure 2). Oxygen accepts four electrons and is reduced to water.[4,9-12] The oxygen molecule is not incorporated into the oxidizing substrate molecule but is coupled with adenosine triphosphate (ATP) synthesis and serves as an energy source.[3,8,11] Under normal circumstances, approximately 1% to 5% of available oxygen leaks into the second less common pathway, which is called the oxygenase pathway.[8,11-14] In this pathway, mitochondria produce superoxide (O_2) and hydrogen peroxide (H_2O_2) but the levels of these substances are minimized by the rapid action of natural intracellular free radical scavengers, such as glutathione peroxidase, superoxide dismutase (SOD), and catalase.[5,9,11,12,15]

UBISEMIQUINONE, an intermediate of electron transport reactions, is the parent compound from which peroxide is produced in mitochondria.[5,12] Peroxide production occurs at the mitochondrial level, and these peroxides can then serve as substrates for the production of superoxide and hydrogen peroxide radicals. This oxygenase pathway predominates under conditions of hypoxia. During hypoxia, the oxygenase pathway results in the stepwise formation of the activated oxygen species, O_2 and H_2O_2, by the acceptance of one and two electrons, respectively.[4,5,9,10,14] Hydroxyl ions (OH^-) are then formed from these ions by the addition of a third electron and are much more destructive than is superoxide or hydrogen peroxide.[4,5,9,14] Hypoxia results in two concurrent processes that facilitate the oxygenase pathway: the production of adenylate (AMP) from adenosine triphosphate and the conversion of xanthine dehydrogenase (XD) to xanthine oxidase (XO).[3,12,16,17] Oxygen serves as an electron acceptor, and the limitation of oxygen results in depletion of adenosine triphosphate and concurrent elevated levels of adenylate.[18-20] Adenylate is converted to adenosine and then to inosine and finally to hypoxanthine.[6] Hypoxanthine cannot be further metabolized and accumulates intracellularly.[16,21] Hypoxanthine then serves as a metabolizable purine substrate for xanthine oxidase after reperfusion.[4,22]

The loss of cellular energy in the form of adenosine triphosphate results in the inability of the cell to maintain appropriate ion gradients across its membranes.[19] Free calcium concentrations may increase as a result of calcium loss from mitochondria and endoplasmic reticulum. Mitochondrial function is depressed by ischemia and mitochondrial buffering of increased cytosolic calcium is hampered, thereby leading to a further increase in intracellular calcium concentrations.[4,19,23,24] Calcium ion redistribution to the cytosol is believed to activate a proteinase enzyme that converts xanthine dehydrogenase to xanthine oxidase. The conversion rate of xanthine dehydrogenase to xanthine oxidase depends on involved tissue.[3,18,25] Conversion occurs within 10 seconds in the intestines. Xanthine oxidase levels double in concentration in the heart within 8 to 10 minutes, and the amount of the substance converted in lungs, liver, spleen, and kidneys doubles in approximately 30 minutes.

The major pathway by which the previously mentioned oxygen-free radicals are formed by the oxygenase pathway begins with xanthine oxidase.[3,14,20,21] Xanthine oxidase normally converts xanthine to uric acid.[16,19] Uric acid is present in most tissue and is particularly abundant in the intestines, lungs, and liver.[3,26] Xanthine oxidase is absent or diminished in the blood of humans, cats, sheep, and pigs but is present in large quantities in the blood of dogs and horses.[26] Xanthine oxidase is synthesized under normal conditions as xanthine dehydrogenase, which accounts for approximately 90% of total activity. Xanthine dehydrogenase cannot transfer electrons to oxygen but instead is able to reduce nicotinamide adenine dinucleotide (NAD)[16] (Figure 3A). Under hypoxic conditions, xanthine dehydrogenase is converted to xanthine oxidase, which can use oxygen instead of nicotinamide adenine dinucleotide after reperfusion but produces destructive free radicals in the process[19] (Figure 3B). Xanthine dehydrogenase can be converted rapidly to xanthine oxidase by sulfhydryl oxidation (reversible) or limited proteolysis (irreversible).[6,12,16,18,27]

Rapid oxidation during reperfusion causes a dramatic increase in free radical levels to the extent that levels of superoxide dismutase and catalase enzymes are overwhelmed. This excessive production of superoxide and hydrogen peroxide radicals is enhanced by the presence of reduced flavoproteins.[12,17,28] Flavoproteins are enzymes that depend on flavins, which are compounds with an isoalloxazine nucleus. This reaction is catalyzed by cytochrome P-450 reductase.[7,25,28,29] The reduction of nicotinamide adenine dinucleotide also produces free radicals.[12,30] Superoxide and hydrogen peroxide are converted to hydroxyl ions by an iron-catalyzed reaction known as the Haber-Weiss reaction (also called the superoxide-driven Fenton reaction)[4-6,9,14,17,29,31] (Figure 4). The Haber-Weiss reaction is further assisted by the presence of phosphorus and the

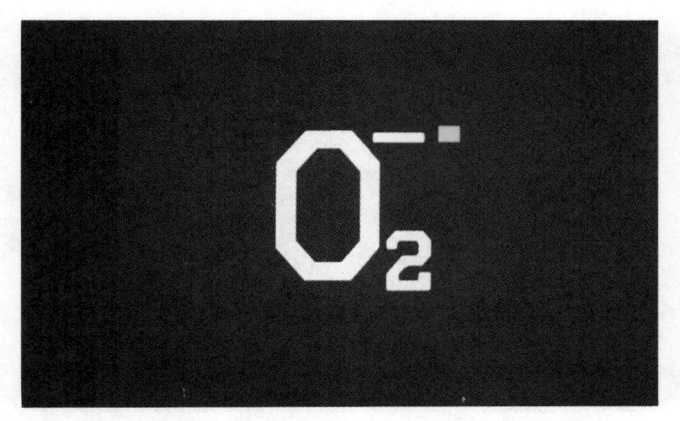

Figure 1—Typical representation of a free radical oxygen molecule. The extra electron is indicated by the red square.

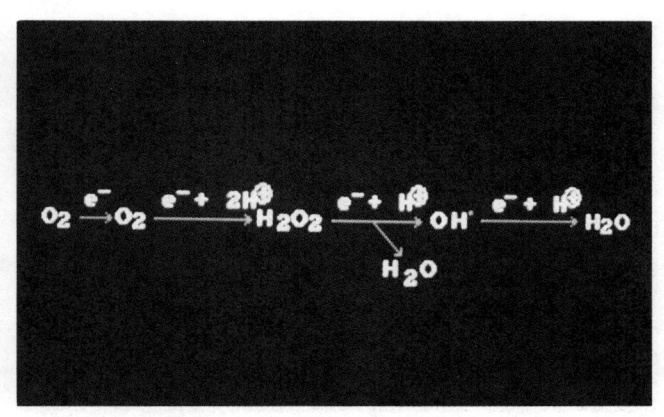

Figure 2—Stepwise reduction of molecular oxygen to water by the addition of four electrons. This reduction is typical of the oxidase pathway, which is the route of energy metabolism under normal aerobic conditions.

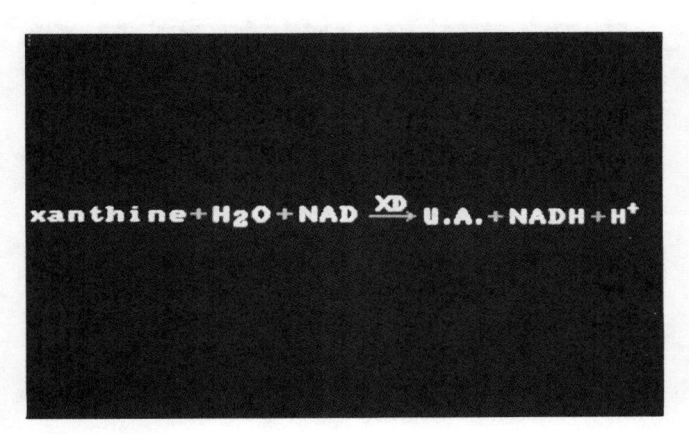

Figure 3A

Figure 3B

Figure 3—(**A**) Reduction of nicotinamide adenine dinucleotide by xanthine dehydrogenase. Oxygen is not used by xanthine dehydrogenase. (**B**) Xanthine oxidase uses oxygen after reperfusion. Xanthine is converted to uric acid in this process; damaging free radicals also are produced.

Figure 4—Conversion of superoxide and hydrogen peroxide ions to hydroxyl ions occurs by the Haber-Weiss reaction. Iron is a vital catalyst that greatly increases the rate, intensity, and longevity of the reaction.

abundance of hydrogen ions that accumulate as ischemia forces the cell to change to anaerobic metabolic pathways. Lactic acid and other acids are produced as end products of these pathways, thereby yielding abundant hydrogen ions.[4]

IRON CATALYZATION of the Haber-Weiss reaction is vital; and iron availability determines the speed, intensity, and longevity of the ensuing reaction.[32] Iron is extracellularly carried by transferrin with 1000 to 2000 atoms of iron being carried by each transferrin molecule. Iron is intracellularly provided by ferritin, cytochromes in the mitochondria, and iron-containing enzymes.[29,33] Ferritin, which is a protein with a molecular weight of 440,000, supplies most of the iron. Ferritin is present in virtually every mammalian cell and is especially abundant in bone marrow as well

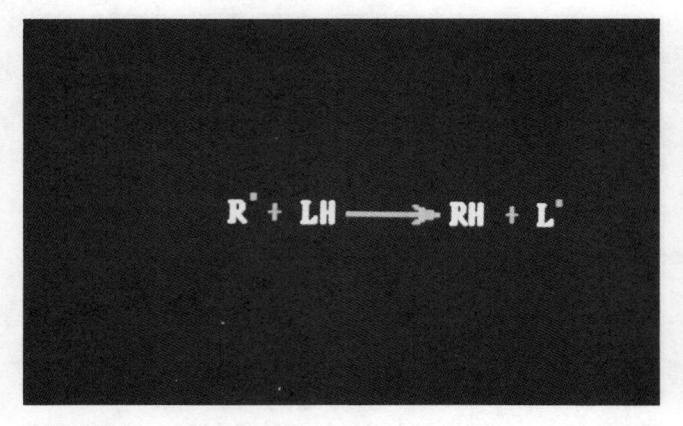

Figure 5A

$$R^\cdot + LH \longrightarrow RH + L^\cdot$$

Figure 5B

$$L^\cdot + O_2 \longrightarrow LOO^\cdot$$

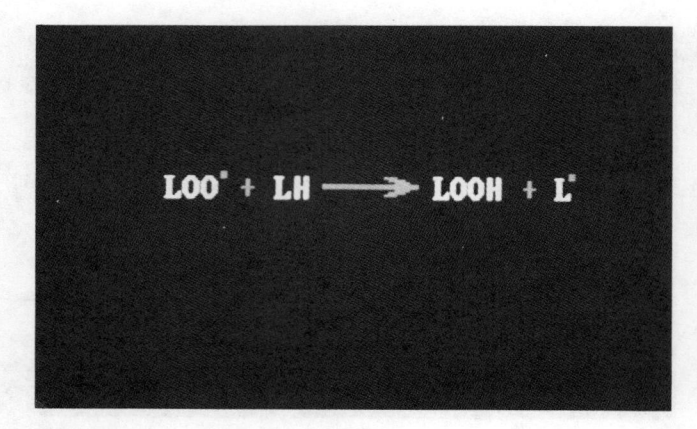

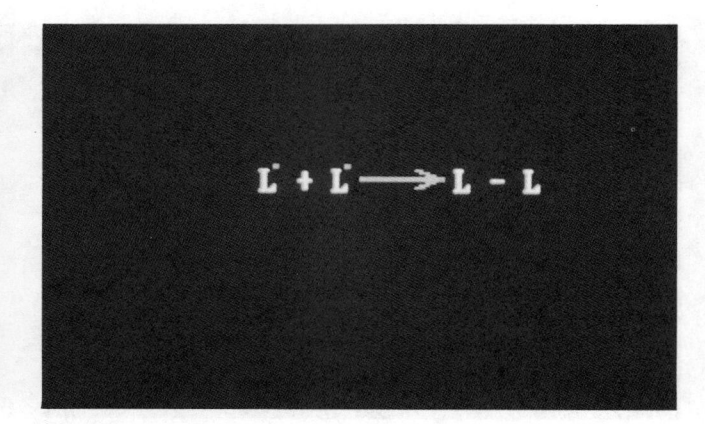

Figure 5C

$$LOO^\cdot + LH \longrightarrow LOOH + L^\cdot$$

Figure 5D

$$L^\cdot + L^\cdot \longrightarrow L-L$$

Figure 5—(**A**) The first step in the lipid peroxidation process involves abstraction of a methylene hydrogen atom by a free radical (*R*) from an unsaturated fatty acid (*LH*) to form a lipid alkyl radical. (**B**) The second step of lipid peroxidation involves alteration of double bonds of the lipid alkyl radical and the presence of oxygen to form peroxy- or alkoxyradicals (*LOO*). (**C**) Lipid hydroperoxides (*LOOH*) can be formed by the addition of hydrogen to lipid peroxyradicals. Iron is a necessary element of this reaction. (**D**) Interaction of free radicals can lead to production of nonreactive species (*L-L*), thereby terminating the reaction.

as the liver and spleen.[33] This protein structurally is a hollow, spheroidal shell that can contain as many as 4500 iron atoms. Six windows for exchange of iron are present on the ferritin molecule. The release of iron is most rapid during anaerobic conditions.[14] The reduction of Fe^{3+} to Fe^{2+} by superoxide radicals can serve as an alternate pathway for iron acquisition to perpetuate the Haber-Weiss reaction.[18]

Hydroxyl ions attack structural protein, enzymes, and lipid cell components, such as mitochondrial, lysosomal, nuclear, and plasma membranes, and damage them so that more free iron is released from ferritin.[14] Lysosomal membrane damage results in leakage of proteolytic enzymes that cause further cellular destruction. Reaction of hydroxyl ions with water in organelle membranes results in the production of more hydroxyl ions, thereby perpetuating the cycle without large numbers of initiating substances. The sequence is continued and results in loss of selective permeability, membrane dysfunction, and cellular destruction.[7] Hydroxyl ions are highly electrophilic and can react with sulfhydryl groups and the sugar groups of deoxyribonucleic acid (DNA), thereby resulting in deoxyribonucleic acid destruction, enzyme inactivation, and altered protein structure.[4]

Another source of cellular destruction is the lipid peroxidation (LPO) pathway.[34,35] Lipid peroxidation is a normal cellular process that, at physiologic levels, is vital to the synthesis of prostaglandins and leukotrienes, pinocytosis, and controlled disassembly of intracellular membranes.[35] Lipid peroxidation also is responsible for lysis of bacteria in phagosomes.[8] Lipid peroxidation can be induced by administration of hyperbaric oxygen and x-radiation and by vitamin E deficiencies and ischemia.[35] When hypoxia prevails, efficient use of available oxygen can be accomplished if the cell switches from the oxidase pathway to the oxygenase pathway. This switch allows formation of lipid peroxidation products.[14] Lipid peroxidation occurs when any free radical abstracts a methylene hydrogen atom from an unsaturated fatty acid and forms a lipid alkyl radical[14,18,31,34] (Figure 5A). Rearrangement of the double bonds forms a conjugated diene that when attacked by molecular oxygen, produces lipid peroxy- and alkoxyradicals[4,5,11,14,34] (Figure 5B). When combined with iron, lipid peroxyradicals can form lipid endoperoxides; if another hydrogen atom is accepted, lipid hydroperoxides are formed[14] (Figure 5C).

IF ENDOPEROXIDES are formed in the presence of iron and unsaturated fatty acids that contain at least three methylene interrupted double bonds, malondialdehyde may be formed as a breakdown product.[34] Malondialdehyde, lipid hydroperoxides, and lipid-containing conjugated dienes often are assayed as indicators of reperfusion injury.[4,18,28,33,34,36,37] After reoxygenation, the oxygenase system can further be activated by the interaction of large amounts of oxygen with the small numbers of reduced electron carriers. Reaction of oxygen radicals with intracellular unsaturated fatty acids present in the cell produces unstable lipid peroxidation products that decompose into secondary end products, such as conjugated dienes, Schiff bases, lipid alkoxyradicals, and lipid peroxyradicals.[8,11,13,26] Generated lipid radicals propagate through cellular and organelle membranes in an end-to-end fashion. When oxygen is added, a self-perpetuating sequence of lipid peroxidation ensues. Changes in the lipid microenvironment occur with lipid peroxidation or carboxylation by reorientation of hydrophilic groups attached to alkyl chains of membrane fatty acids into an aqueous phase. This change produces a defect in the membrane, thereby allowing further disruption of ion gradients and continued cellular destruction.[7,11,28]

Formation of new permeability channels by the generation of transmembrane peroxyclusters is among the effects of lipid peroxidation products on biomembranes.[28] The peroxyclusters serve as ion permeability channels, especially for calcium, which may explain the loss of calcium from mitochondria and endoplasmic reticulum and subsequent accumulation of calcium in the cytosol.[38] Further cluster elevations may lead to fragmentation and destruction of sarcolemmal and sarcoplasmic reticulum membranes as a result of high calcium levels. Disruption of the calcium-magnesium–adenosine triphosphatase pump in the sarcoplasmic reticulum by these clusters disrupts adenosine triphosphate metabolism.[35,39]

Computer simulation of lipid peroxidation reactions suggest that cell destruction can continue for hours to days after the hypoxic episode.[40] These simulations reinforce clinical observations of organ systems subjected to hypoxia and reperfusion.

These reactions eventually terminate as a result of substrate consumption, interaction of free radicals to produce nonreactive species, or reaction of radicals with radical scavengers (Figure 5D).

Neutrophils also play a role in reperfusion and tissue injury.[6,41] Neutrophils normally generate free radicals during destruction of bacteria.[11] Neutrophil infiltration into damaged tissue occurs in the later stages of the cascade of reperfusion injury and is mediated by intracellular pH and preexisting products of reperfusion.[12,23,41,42] There is much debate regarding the full extent of neutrophilic participation in the reperfusion process; but current theory holds that neutrophils are attracted to reperfused areas by proinflammatory agents, such as leukotrienes. The production and release of these agents are initiated by oxygen radicals.[4,12,18] Superoxide ions also are produced by neutrophils, thereby producing hydrogen peroxide and hydroxyl ions and perpetuating the destructive cycle.[4,11] Oxidants and enzymes, such as myeloperoxidase and elastase, are released by neutrophils by means of NADPH oxidase; surrounding cells are subsequently destroyed.[5,14] Adherence of the neutrophil to the endothelium also is important in the pathogenesis of cellular destruction and may be a rate-limiting factor.[4,18]

FREE RADICAL SCAVENGERS USED IN TREATING REPERFUSION INJURY

Numerous compounds are proven to be beneficial in the prevention or treatment of reperfusion injury. These compounds may disrupt the cycle by chelation of free iron; by reduction of free radicals; or by interference with major enzyme pathways, such as xanthine oxidase. Many of these agents have other properties that make them useful in controlling reperfusion injury, but the agents do not contribute directly to limiting free radical production.

Antioxidative enzymes, such as superoxide dismutase and catalase, catalyze the superoxide radical by dismutation to hydrogen peroxide and oxygen[4] (Figure 6A). In one study, superoxide dismutase and catalase restricted the activation of oxygen radicals by 16% to 18%.[8,35] Superoxide dismutase is only present intracellularly and minimizes the level of oxygen-derived free radicals that occur during normal cellular oxygen metabolism. Two types of superoxide dismutase exist in mitochondria: manganese enzyme in the mitochondria and a copper-zinc enzyme in the cytoplasm.[4,5,13] Catalase is a hemoprotein present only in subcellular organelles called peroxisomes. Catalase specifically destroys hydrogen peroxide (Figure 6B).

Glutathione peroxidase is a selenium-containing enzyme that catalyzes peroxide and hydrogen peroxide decomposition, thereby forming organic alcohols, water, and oxi-

$$2O_2^{-\cdot} + 2H^+ \longrightarrow H_2O_2 + O_2$$

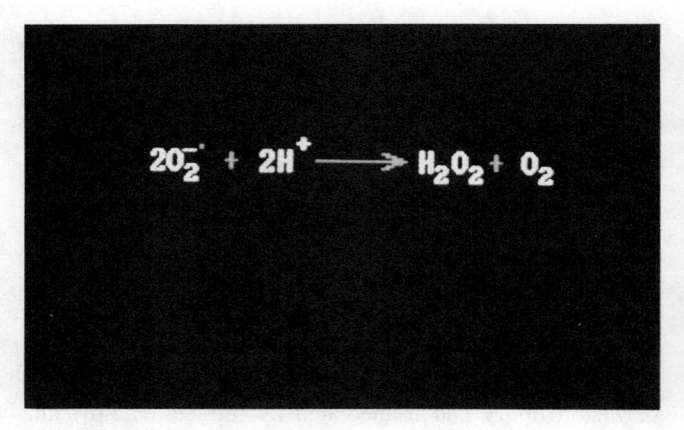

Figure 6A

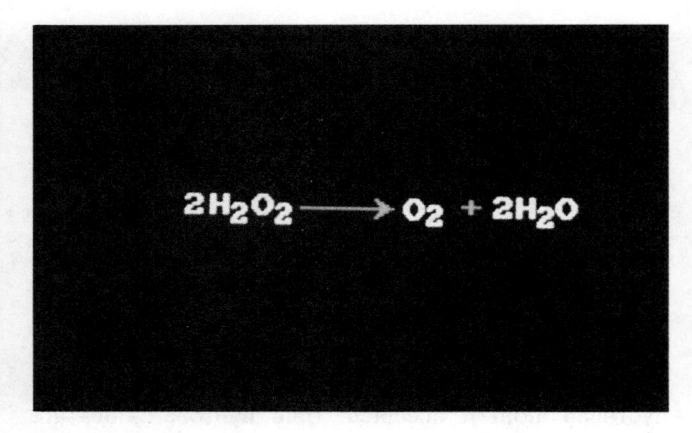

$$2H_2O_2 \longrightarrow O_2 + 2H_2O$$

Figure 6B

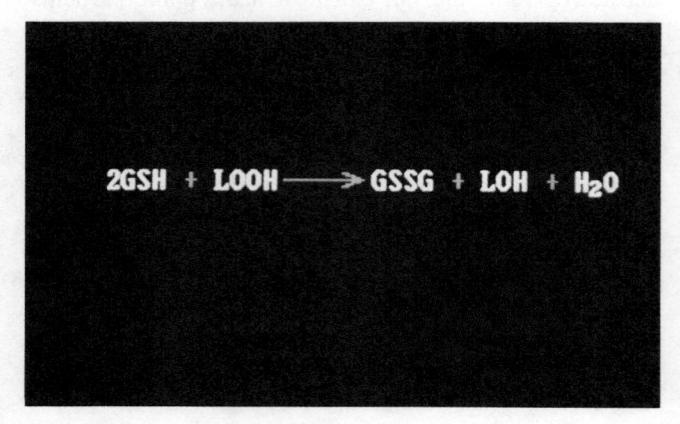

$$2GSH + LOOH \longrightarrow GSSG + LOH + H_2O$$

Figure 6C

Figure 6—(**A**) Superoxide is changed to hydrogen peroxide and water by dismutation. Superoxide dismutase is an antioxidative enzyme that catalyzes this reaction. (**B**) Catalase, which is a hemoprotein present in organelles, reduces hydrogen peroxide to oxygen and water. (**C**) Glutathione peroxidase catalyzes reduced glutathione (*GSH*) and lipid peroxidation products to produce oxidized glutathione (*GSSG*), organic alcohols (*LOH*), and water.

dized glutathione (GSSG).[4,30,43] Glutathione peroxidase is present in most mitochondrial cells and in the cytosol.[4] Vitamin E, an antioxidant, is present in large amounts in the body and lessens the effects of lipid peroxidation by interrupting the lipid peroxidation chain reaction and intercepting radicals by binding to the cell membrane[5,28] (Figure 6C).

Deferoxamine inhibits the iron-catalyzed formation of hydroxyl radicals (Haber-Weiss reaction) by chelating iron.[4] The resultant coupler, ferrioxamine, is chemically inert.[22] Deferoxamine is water soluble, is well tolerated, has minimal toxicity, and does not interfere with the oxygen transport function of hemoglobin.[44] Recent investigation suggests that deferoxamine may be clinically valuable.[7,10] Deferoxamine has been used to treat iron poisoning and iron storage diseases.[44] Apotransferrin is another iron-binding protein that acts in the same manner as deferoxamine.[18]

Allopurinol inhibits the formation of superoxide radicals formed by the xanthine oxidase pathway.[30] Xanthine oxidase is the major pathway that is responsible for producing free radicals, as is evidenced to a large degree by the ability of allopurinol to lessen histologic destruction in experimental models. Allopurinol and oxypurinol also have some oxygen radical scavenging capabilities and enhance purine salvage at much greater concentrations than are normally encountered in extracellular fluid (10 to 20 μM).[5,10,18]

Dimethyl sulfoxide (DMSO) is a hydroxyl radical scavenger[45,46] that inhibits prostaglandins, reduces platelet aggregation, and interferes with neutrophil chemotaxis and arachidonate metabolism.[18,45] Its reduction metabolite, dimethyl sulfide (DMS), also can trap superoxide radicals.[4] Dimethyl sulfoxide is relatively effective as a radical scavenger; however, some side effects are noted with its use. Dimethyl sulfoxide readily reacts with radicals to produce the methyl radical CH_3^-. This methyl radical is able to abstract hydrogen atoms from unsaturated fatty acids and other biomolecules and subsequently produces methane gas and harmful chain reactions.[46] This methyl radical also can react with oxygen to yield methyl peroxyradicals (CH_3OO^-), which either continue to oxidize unsaturated fatty acids or react with themselves to form formaldehyde and methanol by a Russell reaction mechanism.[30,46]

Another class of drugs used to combat reperfusion injury are nonglucocorticoid aminosteroids, which are known commonly as lazaroids.[47-50] Lazaroids are potent inhibitors of lipid peroxidation and may scavenge free radicals in the same manner as superoxide dismutase and vitamin E. Use of lazaroids has been focused on the central nervous system where the drugs have shown much potential in dampening or alleviating the effects of reperfusion injury after stroke, trauma, and vascular accidents.

SUMMARY

Reperfusion injury results from a complex series of biochemical reactions that occur at the cellular level after reperfusion of ischemic tissue. Effects may be both local and systemic. Cellular destruction may be severe and may persist long after correction of ischemia. Understanding the basic mechanisms of reperfusion injury gives the practitioner new insight into acute ischemic diseases and their treatment.

About the Author
Dr. Rochat, who is a Diplomate of the American College of Veterinary Surgeons, is an Assistant Professor of Surgery, with the Veterinary Teaching Hospital, Oklahoma State University.

REFERENCES

1. Beyersdorf F, Mathies G, Kruger S, et al: Avoiding reperfusion injury after limb revascularization: Experimental observations and recommendations for clinical application. *J Vasc Surg* 9:757-766, 1989.
2. Klausner JM, Paterson IS, Mannick JA, et al: Reperfusion pulmonary edema. *JAMA* 261:1030-1035, 1989.
3. McCord JM: Oxygen-derived free radicals in postischemic tissue injury. *New Engl J Med* 312: 159-163, 1985.
4. Flaherty JT, Weisfeldt ML: Reperfusion injury. *Free Radic Biol Med* 5:409-419, 1988.
5. Bostek CC: Oxygen toxicity: An introduction. *Amer Assoc Nurse Anesth J* 57:231-237, 1989.
6. Kloner RA, Przyklenk K, Whittaker P: Deleterious effects of oxygen radicals in ischemia/reperfusion. *Circ Res* 80:1115-1127, 1989.
7. Babbs CF: Role of iron ions in the genesis of reperfusion injury following successful cardiopulmonary resuscitation: Preliminary data and a biochemical hypothesis. *Ann Emerg Med* 14:777-783, 1985.
8. Bulkley GB: The role of oxygen free radicals in human disease processes. *Surg* 94:407-411, 1983.
9. McCord IM: The superoxide free radical: Its biochemistry and pathophysiology. *Surg* 94:412-414, 1983.
10. Darley-Usmar VM, Stone D, Smith DR: Oxygen and reperfusion damage: An overview. *Free Radic Res Commun* 7:247-254, 1989.
11. Hess ML, Manson NH: Molecular oxygen: Friend or foe. Part I. *Mol Cell Cardiol* 16:969-985, 1984.
12. Grisham MB, Granger DN: Metabolic sources of reactive oxygen metabolites during oxidant stress and ischemia with reperfusion. *Clin Chest Med* 10:71-81, 1989.
13. Boveris A: Mitochondrial production of superoxide radical and hydrogen peroxide. *Adv Exp Med Bio* 78:67-82, 1977.
14. Babbs CF: Reperfusion injury of postischemic tissues. *Ann Emerg Med* 17:1148-1157, 1988.
15. Fridovich I: Superoxide dismutases: Defence against endogenous superoxide radical, in *Oxygen Free Radicals and Tissue Damage*. New York, Excerpta Medica, 1979, pp 77-93.
16. Greenwald RA, Cohen G: Superoxide and ischemia: Conversion of xanthine dehydrogenase to xanthine oxidase, in *Proceedings of the Third International Conference on Superoxide and Superoxide Dismutase*. New York, Elsevier Science Publishing Co, 1982, pp 145-153.
17. Hill HAO: The chemistry of dioxygen and its reduction products, in *Oxygen Free Radicals and Tissue Damage*. New York, Excerpta Medica, 1979, pp 5-17.
18. Granger DN: Role of xanthine oxidase and granulocytes in ischemia-reperfusion injury. *Am J Physiol* 255:H1269-H1275, 1988.
19. Burnier M, Schrier RW: Pathogenesis of acute renal failure. *Adv Exp Med Biol*:212-213, 1987.
20. Granger DN, Rutili G, McCord IM: Superoxide radicals in feline intestinal ischemia. *Gastroenterology* 81:22-29, 1981.
21. Younes M, Mohr A, Schoenberg MH, et al: Inhibition of lipid peroxidation by superoxide dismutase following regional intestinal ischemia and reperfusion. *Res Exp Med* 187:9-17, 1987.
22. Badylak SF, Simmons A, Turek J, et al: Protection from reperfusion injury in the isolated rat heart by postischaemic deferoxamine and oxypurinol administration. *Cardiovasc Res* 21:500-506, 1987.
23. Granger DN, Hollwarth ME, Parks DA: Ischemia-reperfusion injury: Role of oxygen-derived free radicals. *Acta Physiol Scand* 548:47-63, 1986.
24. Opie LH: Proposed role of calcium in reperfusion injury. *Int J Cardiol* 23:159-164, 1989.
25. Parks DA: Ischemia-reperfusion injury: A radical view. *Hepatology* 8:680-682, 1988.
26. Al-Khalidi UAS, Chaglassian TH: The species distribution of xanthine oxidase. *Biochem J* 97:318-320, 1965.
27. Batteli MG, Corte ED, Stirpe F: Xanthine oxidase type D (dehydrogenase) in the intestine and other organs of the rat. *Biochem J* 126:747-749, 1972.
28. Bindoli A: Lipid peroxidation in mitochondria. *Free Radic Biol Med* 5:247-261, 1988.
29. Aust SD, Svingen BA: *Free Radicals in Biology*, vol 5, ed 1. New York, Academic Press, 1982, pp 1-27.
30. Badylak SF, Babbs CF, Kougias C, et al: Effect of allopurinol and dimethysulfoxide on long-term survival in rats after cardiopulmonary arrest and resuscitation. *Am J Emerg Med* 4:313-318, 1986.
31. Wilson RL: Hydroxyl radicals and biological damage in vitro: What relevance in vivo?, in *Oxygen Free Radicals and Tissue Damage*. New York, Excerpta Medica, 1979, pp 19-42.
32. Ward PA, Warren JS, Till J, et al: Modification of disease by preventing free radical formation: A new concept in pharmacological intervention, in *Bailliere's Clinical Haematology*. Philadelphia, WB Saunders Co, 1989, pp 391-403.
33. Crichton RR: Interactions between iron metabolism and oxygen activation, in *Oxygen Free Radicals and Tissue Damage*. New York, Excerpta Medica, 1979, pp 57-76.
34. Buege JA, Aust SD: Microsomal lipid peroxidation, in Fleischer S, Packer L (eds): *Biomembranes*. New York, Academic Press, 1978, pp 302-310.
35. Meerson FX, Kagan VE, Kozlov YP, et al: The role of lipid peroxidation in pathogenesis of ischemic damage and the antioxidant protection of the heart. *Basic Res Cardiol* 77:465-485, 1982.
36. Opie LH: Reperfusion injury and its pharmacologic modification. *Circ Res* 80:1049-1062, 1989.
37. Slater TF: Mechanisms of protection against the damage produced in biological systems by oxygen-derived radicals, in *Oxygen Free Radicals and Tissue Damage*. New York, Excerpta Medica, 1979, pp 143-176.
38. Hearse DJ, Humphrey SM, Nayler WG, et al: Ultrastructural damage associated with reoxygenation of the anoxic myocardium. *J Mol Cell Cardiol* 7:315-324, 1975.
39. Del Nido PH, Nakamura H, Mickle DAG, et al: Maturational difference in functional/metabolic sequellae of free radical formation on reperfusion. *J Surg Res* 46:532-536, 1989.
40. Kompala SD, Babbs CF, Blaho KE: Effect of deferoxamine on late deaths following CPR in rats. *Ann Emerg Med* 15:405-407, 1986.
41. Klebanoff SJ, Rosen H: The role of myeloperoxidase in PMN microbicidal activity, in *Oxygen Free Radicals and Tissue Damage*. New York, Excerpta Medica, 1979, pp 269-284.
42. Simchowitz IL: Intracellular pH modulates the generation of superoxide radicals by human neutrophils. *J Clin Invest* 76:1079-1089, 1985.
43. Reeves MH, VanSteenhouse J, Stashak TS, et al: Evaluation of the significance of reperfusion injury after ischemia of the equine large colon. *Vet Surg* 18:67, 1989.
44. Keberle H: The biochemistry of desferrioxamine and its relation to iron metabolism. *Ann NY Acad Sci* 119:758-768, 1974.
45. Brayton CF: Dimethyl sulfoxide (DMSO): A review. *Cornell Vet* 76:61-90, 1986.
46. Klein SM, Cohen G, Cederbaum AI: Production of formaldehyde during metabolism of dimethyl sulfoxide by hydroxyl radical generating systems. *Biochem* 20:6006-6012, 1981.
47. Badylak SF, Lantz GC, Jeffries M: Prevention of reperfusion injury in surgically induced gastric dilatation-volvulus in dogs. *Am J Vet Res* 51:294-299, 1990.
48. Hall ED: Beneficial effects of the 21-aminosteroid U74006F in acute CNS trauma and hypovolemic shock. *Acta Anaesth Belgica* 38:421-425, 1987.
49. Hall ED, Yonkers PA: Attenuation of postischemic cerebral hypoperfusion by the 21-aminosteroid U74006F. *Stroke* 19:340-344, 1988.
50. Hall HD: Effects of the 21-aminosteroid U74006F on posttraumatic spinal cord ischemia in cats. *J Neurosurg* 68:462-465, 1988.

UPDATE

FUTURE DIRECTIONS AND CLINICAL APPLICATIONS

Despite a greatly improved understanding of the mechanisms responsible for reperfusion injury, distinct recommendations for prevention and treatment of reperfusion injury in small animal clinical practice remain elusive. While control or prevention of the cascade of events associated with the classic pathways of reperfusion injury has been demonstrated in research models, clinical trials either have failed to confirm the effectiveness of drugs intended to prevent or reduce the severity of reperfusion injury, or have produced inconclusive or incomplete results.[51-53]

One explanation for this apparent conflict is that, like many other disease processes, the best treatment often results from combined chemotherapy and proper timing of administration of therapeutic agents. Uncovering these combinations and timing is a significant task. Another important reason why research models fail to yield solutions to clinical reperfusion injury scenarios is that multiple mechanisms and pathways often contribute to the production of a clinical disease or syndrome. The complicated pathogenesis of many clinical examples of ischemic disease makes evaluation of isolated components and possible treatment modalities difficult at best. Successfully preventing one particular pathway from progressing may not result in significant alteration of the disease's overall progression. Single agents may have only a partial effect that may be difficult to measure under clinical conditions.

A prime example of the difficulties encountered in unraveling the interrelation of reperfusion injury and other pathogenic pathways is the emerging concept of the systemic inflammatory response syndrome (SIRS). Reperfusion injury certainly plays an important role in the sequence of events resulting in SIRS. However, other avenues of inflammation, cellular destruction, and, ultimately, organ failure, are unaffected by drugs aimed at preventing reperfusion injury and must be addressed simultaneously with the reperfusion aspects of SIRS.

As our understanding of the mechanisms of reperfusion injury advances, so does our enlightenment as to the clinical manifestations of reperfusion injury. Evidence of the far-reaching effects of reperfusion injury can be seen in human medicine. Reperfusion injury is currently being investigated as a contributor to cardiovascular disease, stroke, organ transplantation, reconstructive surgery, arthritis, gastrointestinal disease, trauma, shock, multi-system organ failure, oncology, and a host of other areas. As our ability to detect the products and effects of reperfusion injury in clinical practice increases, so will our ability to evaluate the effects of single or, more likely, combined therapies to prevent or ameliorate the effects of reperfusion injury. It may not be in the too distant future when standard protocols for the treatment of common animal diseases include drugs designed to combat reperfusion injury.

REFERENCES

1. Lantz GC, Badylak SF, Hiles MC, et al: Treatment of reperfusion injury in dogs with experimentally induced gastric dilatation volvulus. *Am J Vet Res* 1992, 53:1594–1598.
2. Badylak SF, Lantz GC, Jeffries M: Prevention of reperfusion injury in surgically induced gastric dilatation-volvulus in dogs. *Am J Vet Res* 1990, 51:294–299.
3. Abood SK, McLoughlin MA, Bailey MQ, et al: Effect of glutamine on mucosal permeability in a canine model of ischemia and reperfusion injury. *Vet Surg* 1994, 23:421.

Intraosseous Infusion of Fluids and Therapeutics

KEY FACTS

- Intraosseous infusion is indicated whenever rapid access to the circulatory system (particularly of small patients) is required and peripheral or central access is impossible or too time-consuming.
- Many drugs and large volumes of fluid can be infused through bone.
- No special equipment is required for intraosseous infusion.
- Indications include hemodynamic failure, severe burns, edematous states, morbid obesity, and peripheral thrombosis.
- Intraosseous infusion should not be used in bones that have recently been fractured or in pneumatic bones of birds; in patients with sepsis, the benefits of intraosseous infusion must be weighed against the risk of initiating osteomyelitis.

University of Pennsylvania
Cynthia M. Otto, DVM   Geraldine McCall Kaufman, DVM

University of Georgia
Dennis T. Crowe, Jr., DVM

RAPID ACCESS to the circulation can save the life of an emergency patient. If the patient is in shock and particularly if the patient is small, however, such access is often difficult or impossible for even the most experienced personnel to attain. According to one study, establishing access to the veins during cardiac arrest took longer than 10 minutes in 24% of human pediatric patients. In 6% of these cases, venous access was never achieved.[1] No comparable studies have been published in the veterinary literature, although a similarly high incidence of failure to establish access to the circulation would be expected.

Alternative routes of drug administration for cases in which direct venous access is unavailable, particularly during cardiac arrest, have been described. For example, a small quantity of epinephrine can rapidly be administered through the trachea.[2] The alternative routes preclude the use of large fluid volumes and many other drugs that are critical in resuscitation (e.g., calcium, sodium bicarbonate, and dopamine infusions).[3] When vascular collapse and poor peripheral circulation are encountered, such as in cases of shock, substances administered into the peritoneal cavity or subcutaneously are not absorbed rapidly enough (if at all) and therefore may be inadequate to support appropriate large-volume resuscitation.[3-5]

Intraosseous administration (Figure 1) can be performed without special equipment and is thus relatively inexpensive. This route of infusion for drugs and fluids has been described several times during the past 60 years, but its usefulness has been underestimated. Intraosseous administration provides rapid access to the central circulatory system through the capillary-rich bone marrow. The bone surrounding the marrow prevents the collapse of vascular space that occurs in peripheral veins during shock. Bone provides stability and allows easy administration and rapid delivery of blood, colloids, crystalloids, and drugs.[6-16] For a practitioner with minimal experience, the establishment of an intraosseous catheter takes only approximately three minutes from the time the skin is prepared to the time fluid can be delivered.[7,8]

PHYSIOLOGY

The blood circulation in bone marrow was described as early as 1922.[17] Substances injected into the marrow flow via sinusoids into the large medullary venous channels and finally through the nutrient and emissary veins into the central systemic circulation[4,10,14,18] (Figure 2). The rate of absorption of a substance injected into bone marrow is equal to that of the same substance injected into a peripheral vein.[5]

Clinical and pharmacokinetic trials have shown that the intraosseous route has no significant effect on drug efficacy or on the time to peak activity even in patients with

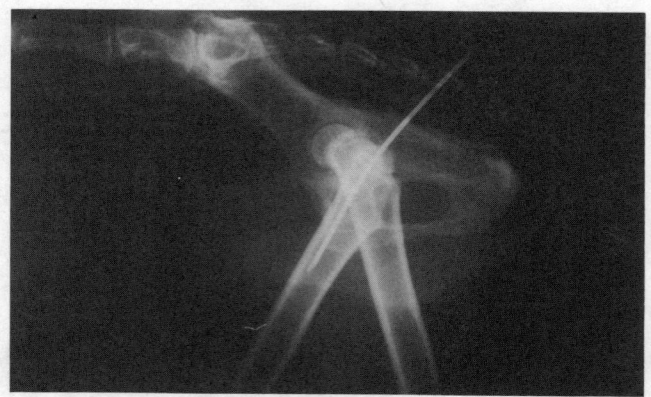

Figure 1—A radiograph of a 20-gauge spinal needle placed in the greater trochanter of a cat for delivery of fluids and drugs.

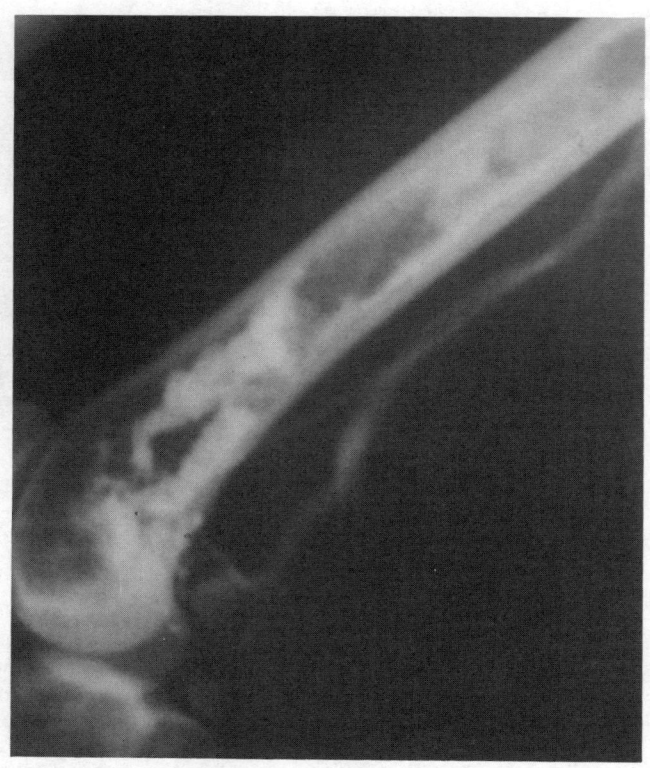

Figure 2—A radiograph taken during injection of radiopaque dye through a 20-gauge intraosseous catheter.

hypovolemia.[5,6,10,15,18,19] Because of the rigid support that bone provides to the medullary vascular system,[7] the intraosseous route is preferred over access to peripheral veins in patients with complete peripheral circulatory collapse. In patients with circulatory collapse, decreased blood flow, lowered blood pressure, and pooling of blood in veins result in collapsed peripheral veins and poor venous return. Even if the collapsed peripheral vein is cannulated by cut-down, rapid fluid administration is hampered by the fragility of the vein and by the sluggish column of blood between the access site and the heart.[6,7] In terms of the rate of fluid uptake, the intraosseous route is second only to a central venous route with the tip of the catheter resting within the large thoracic vena cava.[6]

INFUSED SUBSTANCES

Intraosseous infusion is an alternative route for rapid administration of large volumes of fluid and can be used for many drugs. The following substances have successfully been infused into bone[1,3–16,18–22]:

Fluids
- Blood and blood components
- Colloids
- Crystalloids

Electrolytes
- Sodium bicarbonate

Drugs
- Aminophylline
- Antisera
- Antitoxins
- Atropine
- Aureomycin
- Calcium gluconate
- Cefoxitin
- Dexamethasone
- Diazepam
- Digitalis
- Diphenhydramine hydrochloride
- Dobutamine
- Dopamine hydrochloride
- Epinephrine
- Insulin
- Morphine
- Penicillin
- Procaine hydrochloride
- Radiopaque dyes
- Streptomycin
- Sulfadiazine
- Sulfathiazole
- Thiopental sodium 5%

Nutrients
- Amino acids
- Dextrose
- Vitamins

Other agents
- Bone marrow
- Liver extracts.

Pharmacokinetic studies on intraosseous administration of the following have been performed[5,6,18,19]:

- Atropine
- Diazepam
- Epinephrine
- Sodium bicarbonate.

INDICATIONS

Intraosseous administration of fluids is indicated when-

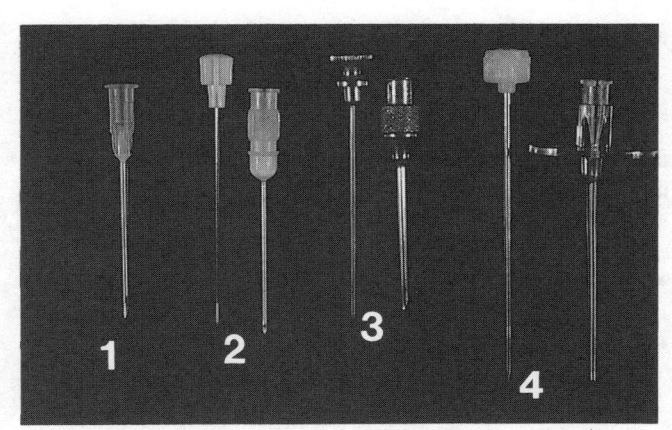

Figure 3—Intraosseous catheters: (1) 18-gauge hypodermic needle, (2) 20-gauge spinal needle and stylet, (3) Illinois sternal bone marrow needle and stylet, and (4) Cooke® intraosseous catheter and stylet.

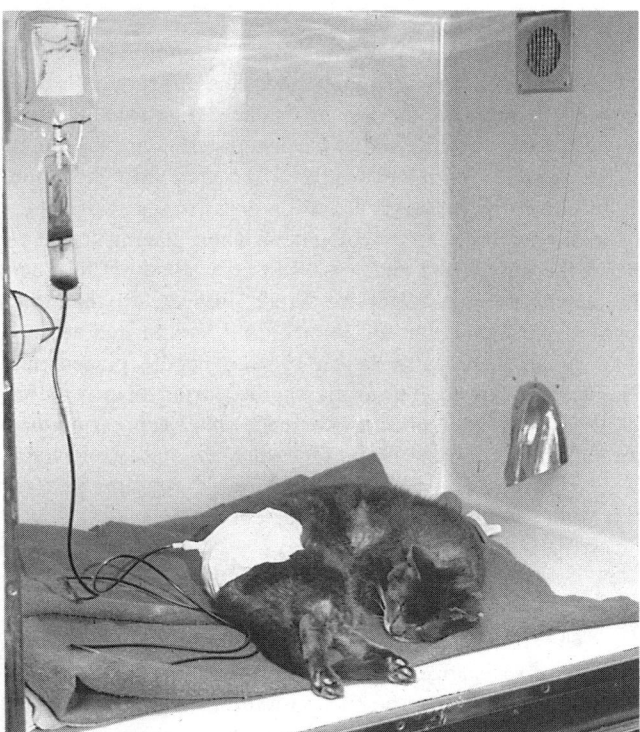

Figure 4—Intraosseous blood transfusion in a cat with poor peripheral blood pressure and peripheral vascular thrombosis secondary to repeated intravenous catheterization.

ever rapid access to the circulatory system is required and peripheral or central access is impossible or too time-consuming. It is an excellent route of administration of drugs for patients in cardiac arrest. It can be used as an interim therapy to expand the circulatory volume of patients with hemodynamic failure (e.g., arrest or shock) until circulatory function is recovered and a peripheral catheter can be placed. It is particularly beneficial for neonates or exotic animals (except birds) if small size makes routine catheter placement and maintenance difficult. Techniques for intraosseous infusion in birds are currently under investigation. Other indications for use of the intraosseous route include severe burns, edematous states, morbid obesity, and peripheral vascular thrombosis.[4,8,12,20,21]

CONTRAINDICATIONS

Contraindications for intraosseous fluids include skeletal abnormalities, skin and wound infections, abscesses over the bone, and recent fractures of the bone that is to be used for catheter placement.[4,12] Intraosseous infusion should not be used in pneumatic bones. Sepsis is the only systemic disease that is a contraindication for intraosseous administration of fluids.[4,12,21] In cases of septic shock, the risk of initiating osteomyelitis must be weighed against the increased risk of mortality from resuscitation with inadequate volumes of fluid.

METHODS

Successful intraosseous infusion requires the following equipment:

- Topical antiseptic
- Lidocaine 1%
- A No. 10 or No. 11 scalpel blade for making a stab incision
- An 18- to 25-gauge hypodermic needle, an 18- to 22-gauge spinal needle or bone marrow needle, or a Cooke® intraosseous catheter
- 10-ml syringe for aspiration of bone marrow
- Heparinized saline solution (2 IU/ml)
- Fluid with administration set or catheter cap
- Tape butterfly and suture material
- Triple antibiotic ointment or other appropriate antiseptic ointment or cream
- Bandaging material.

Cooke designed a needle (Cooke® Intraosseous Catheter—Cooke Catheters) with a stylet for this purpose; but a 20-gauge spinal needle (for cats, many exotics, or young dogs), a bone marrow needle (for mature dogs), or an 18- to 25-gauge hypodermic needle (for neonates of many species) can be used to pierce the bony cortex and establish quick access to the marrow sinusoids and vascular system. If a bony core obstructs the lumen of the needle, the needle can be withdrawn and a new needle (preferably one size larger) placed in the channel through the cortex.

The access site must be prepared aseptically. The most common sites are the flat medial surface of the proximal tibia approximately 1 to 2 cm distal to the tibial tuberosity, the tibial tuberosity itself, or the trochanteric fossa of the femur. The wing of the ilium, the ischium, and the greater tubercle of the humerus can be used. In humans, the sternum has been used.

In neonates that are in hypovolemic shock, a single intraosseous line may be sufficient to supply shock doses of fluids[15]; for larger animals, establishment of two lines in separate bones or pressurized flow should be considered.

Catheter Placement

For a stable animal, the skin and periosteum over the site are anesthetized with 1% lidocaine. The appendage is stabilized. To increase the life of the needle, a stab incision may be made over the site to be penetrated. For placement in the medial tibia, the needle is directed into the bone slightly distally and away from the proximal growth plate. To avoid sciatic nerve involvement when placing the needle in the femur, the needle should be walked off the medial aspect of the greater trochanter into the trochanteric fossa of the femur; the hip joint should remain in a neutral position and internally rotated during needle placement. Pressure is then applied to the needle during firm rotation in 30° turns. This maneuver creates a small depression that seats the needle in the bone. Once the seat has been established, increasing pressure on the same rotation pattern drives the needle through the near cortex.

As the needle passes through the cortex, a sudden loss of resistance is often felt. To test placement of the needle, the needle can be flicked with a finger on release. An appropriately placed needle is stable enough in the bone not to wobble when flicked. The limb should then be moved and the hub of the needle observed. The hub of the needle should move with the limb without being dislodged.

If the needle stands upright, a 10-ml syringe should be attached to the hub and gentle suction applied. Bone marrow (fat, bone spicules, and blood) should be aspirated into the needle. The apparatus is flushed with heparinized saline and should flow freely. The subcutaneous tissue must be observed for fluid extravasation. If the fluid fails to flow freely, the needle should be rotated 90° to 180° to move the beveled edge away from the inner cortex.

If more than one hole is placed through the cortex, extravasation of fluid into subcutaneous tissue may occur. If extravasation is attributable to leakage through a poorly created access channel, the needle is removed and another bone is chosen as the site. A bone should not be reused for 12 to 24 hours after perforation of a cortex.[21]

Once the needle is securely placed, the substance to be infused can be connected to the needle by a standard intravenous administration set or an intravenous catheter plug can be added and heparinized saline used to flush the needle, thus allowing continuous vascular access. The needle can be sewn into place by placing a tape butterfly near the hub and securing it to the skin or suturing the butterfly to the periosteum near the needle exit site. Cooke® intraosseous catheters have permanent butterflies for suturing. The area should be covered with triple antibiotic ointment or antiseptic ointment or cream on gauze; the needle should be protected from breaking or bending with a bulky wrap attached to the patient's body (Figure 4).

Using the greater trochanter of the femur of an active animal allows increased mobility without the risk of dislodging the needle. We have found that the tibia is more readily accessible in large or obese animals.

Rate of Administration

The rate of delivery of fluids by the intraosseous route is limited to 11 ml/min with gravity flow and 24 ml/min with 300 mm Hg pressure.[9,15,23] Pressure can be provided by a commercially available pressure-infusion cuff. The following recommendations are for delivering shock doses (90 ml/kg/hr):

- Gravity flow through a single catheter is used for animals that weigh up to 7.3 kg (16 lb)
- Pressurized flow through a single catheter or gravity flow through multiple catheters is used for animals that weigh between 7.3 and 16.4 kg (16 to 36 lb)
- Pressurized flow through multiple catheters is used for animals that weigh more than 16.4 kg (36 lb)
- A separate bone must be used for each catheter.

Restoration of peripheral pressure by rapid intraosseous fluid replacement enables routine intravenous catheter placement and continued volume fluid therapy.

Catheter Maintenance

Maintenance of an intraosseous catheter is identical to that of an intravenous catheter; routine flushing every six hours with 0.5 to 1.0 ml of heparinized saline is required to ensure patency. Although there are no published reports of recommended intraosseous catheter duration, extrapolations from intravenous catheter recommendations suggest that an intraosseous catheter can remain in place for as long as 72 hours without complications if aseptic technique, adequate bandaging, and routine catheter maintenance are used.[24]

COMPLICATIONS

The complication rate of intraosseous infusions in humans is approximately equal to that of routine vascular access. The most commonly reported complication of intraosseous infusion is infection.[4,9,21] Among 4000 reviewed cases in humans of all ages, there was a 0.6% incidence of osteomyelitis.[8,14] The most common risk factors for osteomyelitis are sepsis and catheter use that persists for several days.

There are no reported cases of fat embolism with gravitational or pressurized flow.[4,9,21] Other less frequently reported complications include epiphyseal damage from improperly directed catheters and extravasation of fluids from punctures of both cortices.[14] The risk of extravasation can be eliminated; when it is known that an intraosseous needle has pierced both cortices, that particular bone is rejected as an access site for 12 to 24 hours.[20] For large or adult dogs, a bone marrow needle may be necessary to prevent bending of the needle as it is driven through the bone.

Establishment of an intraosseous catheter can be painful for conscious animals; therefore, the periosteum is anesthetized with 1% lidocaine. Aspiration of marrow

Intraosseous Infusion of Fluids 151

TABLE I
Patients That Received Intraosseous Infusion

Species or Breed	Age	Sex	Average Weight	Rationale for Intraosseous Catheter Placement	Substances Given	Short-Term Outcome	Approximate Duration of Catheterization	Complications	Diagnosis	Long-Term Outcome
Domestic Shorthair cat	8 weeks	Male	500 g	Size, peripheral vascular collapse, dehydration (approximately 10%), hypoglycemia	50% dextrose	Increased perfusion, increased blood glucose	6 hours	Patient died of underlying disease process	Panleukopenia	Died
Samoyed	12 years	Female, spayed	25 kg	Peripheral vascular collapse, vascular thrombosis secondary to catheterization, dehydration (7%–8%), fever	Balanced electrolyte solution, antibiotics	Increased perfusion, rehydration, increased temperature	72 hours	Patient died of underlying disease process	Renal lymphosarcoma	Died
Domestic Shorthair cat	14 years	Male, castrated	5 kg	Poor peripheral perfusion, vascular thrombosis, anemia	Whole blood (30 ml)	No change	2 hours	None	Unknown	Died
Chihuahua	8 weeks	Female	300 g	Size, peripheral vascular collapse, dehydration, hypoproteinemia	Balanced electrolyte solution, plasma, antibiotics	Increased perfusion, increased plasma protein, increased maintenance hydration	24 hours	Catheter became dislodged, was replaced	Parvovirus infection	Died
Old English Sheepdog	10 years	Female, spayed	35 kg	Edema, vascular thrombosis	Balanced electrolyte solution	No change	4 hours	Pain[a]	Lymphosarcoma	Receiving chemotherapy
Domestic Shorthair cat	10 weeks	Male	500 g	Peripheral vascular collapse, hypothermia, 12% dehydration, anemia	T-61[b]	Euthanasia	5 minutes	Not applicable	Unknown	Died
Domestic Shorthair cat	6 years	Female, spayed	3 kg	Inability to catheterize vein, azotemia, dehydration	Balanced electrolyte solution	Rehydration	12 hours	Catheter obstruction by clots	Feline infectious peritonitis	Died
Doberman pinscher	3 months	Male	10 kg	Seizures	Diazepam	Control of seizures	8 hours	None	Unknown	Lost to follow-up
Domestic Shorthair cat	4 weeks	Male	100 g	Hypothermia, hypoglycemia, 12% dehydration, agonal respiration	Balanced electrolyte solution, 50% dextrose	Death	5 minutes	Patient died of underlying disease process	Unknown	Died
Guinea pig	2 years	Female	200 g	Hypothermia, dehydration, respiratory distress	Balanced electrolyte solution, dexamethasone, T-61[b]	Euthanasia	2 hours	Not applicable	Unknown	Died

TABLE I (continued)

Species or Breed	Age	Sex	Average Weight	Rationale for Intraosseous Catheter Placement	Substances Given	Short-Term Outcome	Approximate Duration of Catheterization	Complications	Diagnosis	Long-Term Outcome
Domestic Shorthair cat	2 months	Female	1 kg	Hemorrhage, shock, size	Balanced electrolyte solution, 20 ml blood	Increased perfusion, increased packed cell volume	1–2 hours	None	Trauma (dog attack)	Recovered
Old English sheepdog	18 days	Male	Unknown	Dehydration, unconsciousness, anemia, size	Balanced electrolyte solution, 30 ml blood	Rehydration	24	None	Hookworms, fleas	Recovered
Domestic Shorthair cat	5 months	Male	2 kg	Possible hemorrhage after orchidectomy, shock	Balanced electrolyte solution	Clinical improvement	3 hours	None	Postsurgical shock	Recovered
Domestic Shorthair cat	2.5 months	Female	800 g	Emaciation, dehydration, hypothermia	Balanced electrolyte solution, ketamine hydrochloride (after stabilization)	Rehydration, amputation of tail	18 hours	None	Gangrene of tail	Recovered
Mixed breed dog	6 weeks	Unknown	2.5 kg	Dehydration, weakness, anemia	Blood	Increased packed cell volume, rehydration	1–2 hours	None	Hookworms	Lost to follow-up
Domestic Shorthair cat	Unknown	Female	3 kg	Depression, dehydration	Balanced electrolyte solution	Ovariohysterectomy (after stabilization)	4 hours	Bent needle	Septic metritis	Recovered
Siamese cat	1.5 years	Female	Unknown	Shock, decreased perfusion, unconsciousness	Balanced electrolyte solution	Increased perfusion, stable condition, surgery to repair stomach and hernia, recovery	24–48 hours	None	Trauma	Lost to follow-up
Toy poodle	12.5 years	Female	1.5 kg	Uremia, dehydration, small size	Balanced electrolyte solution	Increased perfusion, rehydration, stable condition, ovariohysterectomy	24 hours	Patient refused to tolerate catheter after surgery	Pyometra	Recovered
Chihuahua	3 months	Unknown	500 g	Small size	Thiopental	Surgery	5 hours	None	Femoral fracture	Recovered

[a]Future recommendation for such large dogs would be to place the intraosseous catheter in the medial aspect of the tibia to decrease risk of sciatic nerve involvement and to facilitate catheter placement.
[b]T-61® Euthanasia Solution–Hoechst-Roussel.

contents creates an uncomfortable sensation in human patients, but transient constant infusion into human marrow is reportedly not painful.[8] We have found that such infusion is well tolerated by animals.

Radiographic follow-up in humans has shown no significant lesions in the bone following intraosseous catheter use.[12,13,22] Microscopic bone marrow examination demonstrated that patients that had received isotonic, normal pH substances had a slight decrease in cellularity. The use of alkaline or hypertonic solutions results in edema, pyknotic marrow nuclei, and decreased cellularity. These changes spontaneously resolve within four to six weeks.[19,22]

CLINICAL CASES

Nineteen patients receiving blood therapy or requiring vascular access and fluid or drugs were studied. In most of the cases, multiple attempts at intravenous catheterization had failed; but an intraosseous catheter was placed without difficulty in all cases. The technique effectively provided rapid access to the veins (Table I).

About the Authors

When this article was written, Dr. Otto and Dr. Kaufman were affiliated with the Veterinary Hospital of the School of Veterinary Medicine of the University of Pennsylvania, Philadelphia, Pennsylvania. Dr. Otto is currently affiliated with the Department of Small Animal Medicine of the College of Veterinary Medicine, University of Georgia. Dr. Kaufman is a Diplomate of the American College of Veterinary Internal Medicine and is currently in internal medicine practice in Bridgeton, New Jersey. Dr. Crowe is affiliated with the Small Animal Teaching Hospital of the College of Veterinary Medicine, University of Georgia, Athens, Georgia. He is a Diplomate of the American College of Veterinary Surgeons.

REFERENCES

1. Rosetti V, Thompson BM, Aprahamian C: Difficulty and delay in intravascular access in pediatric arrests. *Ann Emerg Med* 13:406, 1984.
2. Crowe DT: Cardiopulmonary resuscitation and advanced life support, in Zaslow IM (ed): *Veterinary Trauma and Critical Care*. Philadelphia, Lea & Febiger, 1984, p 527.
3. Orlowski JP: My kingdom for an intravenous line. *Am J Dis Child* 138:803, 1984.
4. Hodge D: Intraosseous infusions: A review. *Pediatr Emerg Care* 1:215-218, 1985.
5. Prete MR, Liannan CS, Burke FM: Plasma atropine concentrations via intravenous, endotracheal and intraosseous administration. *Am J Emerg Med* 5:101-104, 1987.
6. Spivey WH, Lathers CM, Malone D, et al: Comparison of intraosseous, central and peripheral routes of administration of sodium bicarbonate during CPR in pigs. *Ann Emerg Med* 14:1135-1140, 1985.
7. Tocantins LM, O'Neill JP, Price AH: Infusions of blood and other fluids via the bone marrow in traumatic shock and other forms of peripheral circulatory failure. *Ann Surg* 114:1085-1092, 1941.
8. Tarrow AB, Turkel H, Thompson MS: Infusions via the bone marrow and biopsy of the bone and bone marrow. *Anesthesiology* 13:501-509, 1952.
9. Shoor PM, Berryhill RE, Beaumof JL: Intraosseous infusion: Pressure-flow relationship and pharmacokinetics. *J Trauma* 19:772-774, 1979.
10. Tocantins LM: Rapid absorption of substances injected into the bone marrow. *Proc Soc Exp Biol Med* 45:292-296, 1940.
11. Berg RA: Emergency infusion of catecholamines into bone marrow. *Am J Dis Child* 138:810-811, 1984.
12. Papper EM: The bone marrow route for injecting fluids and drugs into the general circulation. *Anesthesiology* 3:307-313, 1942.
13. Tocantins LM, O'Neill JP, Jones HW: Infusion of blood and other fluids via the bone marrow. *JAMA* 117:1229-1234, 1941.
14. Rosetti VA, Thompson BM, Miller J, et al: Intraosseous infusion: An alternative route of pediatric intravascular access. *Ann Emerg Med* 14:885-888, 1985.
15. Hodge D, Delgado-Paredes C, Fleisher G: Intraosseous infusion flow rates in hypovolemic "pediatric" dogs. *Ann Emerg Med* 16:305-307, 1987.
16. Turkel H: *Trephine Technique of Bone Marrow Infusions and Tissue Biopsies*, ed 8. Detroit, Karl, Schallenbrand & Fine, 1957.
17. Drinker CK, Drinker KR, Lund CC: The circulation in the mammalian bone marrow. *Am J Physiol* 62:1-92, 1922.
18. Spivey WH, Unger HD, Lathers CM, McNamara RM: Intraosseous diazepam suppression of pentylenetetrazol-induced epileptogenic activity in pigs. *Ann Emerg Med* 16:156-159, 1987.
19. Macht DI: Studies on intraosseous injection of epinephrine. *Am J Physiol* 138:269-272, 1943.
20. Vlades MM: Intraosseous fluid administration in emergencies. *Lancet* 1:1235-1236, 1977.
21. Quilligan JJ, Turkel H: Bone and marrow infusion and its complications. *Am J Dis Child* 71:457-465, 1946.
22. Spivey WH, Unger HD, McNamara RM, et al: The effect of intraosseous sodium bicarbonate on bone in swine. *Ann Emerg Med* 16:773-776, 1987.
23. Hodge D, Delgado-Paredes C, Fleisher G: Central and peripheral catheter flow rates in "pediatric" dogs. *Ann Emerg Med* 15:1151-1154, 1986.
24. Maki DG, Boticelli JT, LeRoy ML, Thullke TS: Prospective study of replacing administration sets for intravenous therapy at 48 vs 72 hour intervals: 72 hours is safe and cost-effective. *JAMA* 258(13):1777-1781, 1987.

Pyrethrin and Pyrethroid Insecticide Intoxication in Cats

University of Illinois at Urbana/Champaign
Ted Whittem, BVSc, PhD

KEY FACTS

❑ Pyrethrins and pyrethroids are popular agents because of rapid insecticidal action and a relatively low toxicity for cats.

❑ The primary site of action of pyrethrins and pyrethroids is at the gated sodium channels in the cell membrane of excitable cells.

❑ Rapid mammalian metabolism of pyrethrins and pyrethroids is the primary mechanism by which mammals resist intoxication.

❑ No specific treatment for pyrethrin or pyrethroid intoxication in cats is known, and the general principles of treating toxicoses must be applied.

❑ Because pyrethrins and pyrethroids are not water soluble, copious application of mild detergent is necessary to ensure removal of the residual insecticide.

Pyrethrins—naturally occurring esters of chrysanthemic acid and pyrethric acid—are usually extracted for commercial purposes from the flowers of *Chrysanthemum cinerariaefolium*. Pyrethrins and their synthetic analogues, pyrethroids, are now the most commonly used insecticides for the treatment of ectoparasitic infestation of cats. These agents are popular because of rapid insecticidal action and a relatively low toxicity for cats, especially in contrast with other classes of insecticides (e.g., the organochlorines and organophosphates). Pyrethroids were developed to improve the stability of the pyrethrins, and the success of this chemical modification has led to widespread use of these agents as agricultural and industrial insecticides. As a result, pyrethroids are now used frequently in the domestic setting.

In cats, a common sequela to the use of pyrethrins and pyrethroids is intoxication. Despite the relatively low toxicity of pyrethrins and pyrethroids compared with other insecticides, toxicity does occur in individual cats. Veterinarians who use products that contain these agents should be aware of the signs of toxicity. In addition, an understanding of the pathophysiology of toxicity will help veterinarians to prescribe appropriate therapy and give an accurate prognosis.

MECHANISMS OF ACTION AND TOXICITY

Pyrethrins and pyrethroids are divided into two classes: class I and class II. This division is based on chemical structure and electrophysiologic differences at their sites of action.[1] Some authorities, however, attribute electrophysiologic differences to a dose-effect phenomenon for both classes.[2] The primary site of action of both classes is at the gated sodium channels in the cell membrane of excitable cells.[3-5] After the passage of an action potential in the excitable cells of nervous tissue and muscle, pyrethrins and pyrethroids block open a small percentage of the cell membrane sodium channels. These agents are therefore termed *open channel blockers*.[6] Normally, after the passage of an action potential, the initial cellular influx of sodium ions is rapidly curtailed. In the presence of pyrethrins and pyrethroids, however, some sodium influx continues.[7] With class I[1] and low doses of class II[2] pyrethrins and pyrethroids, the continued sodium ion influx results in a long tail current subsequent to the primary action potential. The tail current results in repetitive discharging of the excitable cell.[7] In addition, class II agents may further enhance the continued sodium ion influx, leading to the depolarization of the cell membrane. Persistent cell membrane depolarization inhibits the propagation of further action potentials.[3-5]

The mechanisms of action of pyrethrins and pyrethroids are common to insects and mammals; however, the activity of pyrethrins and pyrethroids at the cell membrane sodium channel is negatively correlated to temperature. Therefore, some selectivity in toxicity for insects versus mammals may be attributed to lower body temperatures of insects.[5,8]

In some mammals, class II pyrethroids have also been shown to act at γ-aminobutyric acid (GABA)$_A$ receptors in the central nervous system. Class II pyrethroids inhibit specific binding of GABA to GABA$_A$ receptors.[9,10] Therefore, class II pyrethroids inhibit GABA-induced chloride ion influx.[10,11] The physiologic function of GABA$_A$ receptor–mediated chloride ion influx is the induction of presynaptic inhibition. Therefore, this antiinhibitory action of pyrethroids could lead to hyperexcitability of nervous tissue and hence may contribute to or exacerbate some clinical signs of toxicity. Furthermore, this may also be the mechanism by which pyrethroids potentiate convulsive disorders.[12]

ABSORPTION, DISTRIBUTION, METABOLISM, AND ELIMINATION

Although information on the absorption and distribution of pyrethrins and pyrethroids in cats is limited, dermal exposure is the most frequent route that leads to intoxication. This may be simply because it is the most common route of application in cats. In a retrospective study of 116 cases of pyrethrin and pyrethroid exposure in cats, 94% of intoxicated cats were exposed by application to the skin and haircoat.[13] In these cases, toxicity may have resulted from percutaneous absorption rather than ingestion from grooming behavior. Although toxicity after oral exposure is believed to be less likely because of rapid hepatic metabolism (and hence a relatively high first-pass clearance from portal blood), oral exposure may be important in cats because of the peculiar metabolism of the species.

In mammals, pyrethrins and pyrethroids are rapidly biotransformed and detoxified by ester hydrolysis or oxidation. The particular reaction depends on the characteristics of each compound. Readers are referred elsewhere for a detailed review of the literature.[14] Phase I metabolic reactions occur in the plasma and the liver. Nonspecific plasma esterases are important for detoxification of most pyrethrins and pyrethroids, except allethrin and pyrethrum.[15] Because organophosphate insecticides inhibit plasma esterase activity, simultaneous exposure to organophosphate insecticides may render pyrethrin or pyrethroid toxicity more likely or more severe.[14,16] The hepatic reactions are carried out through the mixed-function oxidase system by various cytochrome P$_{450}$ enzymes. These reactions are inhibited by the α-cyano side chain of class II pyrethroids and are slower for *cis* stereoisomers.[2] In addition, some formulations include "synergist" agents, such as piperonyl-butoxide, that function to inhibit cytochrome P$_{450}$ and hence impede rapid phase I metabolism of pyrethrins and pyrethroids. Rapid mammalian metabolism of pyrethrins and pyrethroids is the primary mechanism by which mammals resist intoxication; therefore, conditions that slow phase I metabolism decrease the dose necessary for intoxication.[16] However, it should be noted that these strategies slow metabolism of pyrethrins and pyrethroids in insects also, thereby resulting in increased insecticidal efficacy.

Phase I metabolic transformations are followed by hydroxylation and conjugation to either glucuronides or sulfates, which in turn are eliminated primarily in the urine.[2] The feline liver is inefficient at glucuronide conjugations relative to other mammalian species. Slow conjugation may lead to relatively slow urinary excretion, thereby causing an accumulation of hydroxylated phase I metabolites of pyrethrins and pyrethroids. Through substrate inhibition of phase I pathways, this accumulation may slow the overall rate of pyrethrin and pyrethroid detoxification. This may be the reason that clinical intoxication by pyrethrin and pyrethroid insecticides is reported to be more common in cats than in other domesticated species.[17]

Pyrethrins and pyrethroids are almost insoluble in water. Probably as a consequence, these agents partition into tissues with a high lipid content, such as nervous tissue.[18] This property may well account for the rapid onset of clinical signs[13] and the apparent diphasic elimination of these insecticides.[18] The slow elimination phase ensures that, were these insecticides to be repeatedly administered, they could accumulate in fatty tissues.

CLINICAL SIGNS AND DIAGNOSIS

In a retrospective study of 87 cases of pyrethrin and pyrethroid intoxication in cats, central neuropathies were reported to be the most common clinical signs. Central neuropathies manifested primarily as hyperexcitability, tremors, or convulsions and occurred in 69% of intoxicated cats. Skeletal muscular weakness and fasciculations, which are signs of peripheral neuropathies, occurred in 28% of affected cats. Respiratory distress, which was reported in 18% of the cases, was not correlated to inhalation exposure and was believed to be secondary to weakness of the respiratory musculature. Other less frequently observed signs were vomiting, diarrhea, anorexia, and cardiovascular distress.[13] Clinical signs were evident only in cats younger than four years of age, with more than half the intoxicated cats younger than 12 months.[19] Although young cats seemed more likely to be intoxicated, there was no obvious explanation for such an age predilection. In addition, because no data have been published to describe the population distribution of the age of cats treated with insecticides, this predilection may reflect trends in insecticide use rather than a toxicologic phenomenon. Nevertheless, evidence for an age predilection exists and (although the evidence is inconclusive) should be considered when insecticides are prescribed for young cats.

Cats exposed to toxic doses of pyrethrins or pyrethroids were reported to have a rapid onset of clinical signs; 42% had an onset of signs in less than one hour.[13] In the same study, all remaining cats were affected within three hours of exposure.[19]

The particular compound used (and its formulation) may affect the pattern of clinical signs shown in intoxication. Formulations that included hydrocarbons, such as petroleum distillates, have been associated with the occurrence of cardiovascular distress. Formulations with alcohols, such as isopropyl alcohol, have been correlated to the occurrence of peripheral neuropathies[13]; however, prospective studies in which the effect of the formulation solvent on pyrethrin and pyrethroid intoxication have not been published. The presence of cytochrome P_{450} inhibitors did not effect the toxicity of the pyrethrins or pyrethroids for cats. It is possible that phase I metabolism is not the rate-limiting step in detoxification of these insecticides in cats, even subsequent to inhibition by synergists. Although the division of pyrethrins and pyrethroids into class I and II has been based on the pattern of clinical signs caused in experimental animals, no correlation was shown between the class of pyrethrin or pyrethroid and the nature of the observed clinical signs.[13]

The potential for alteration of expected clinical signs by formulations with other compounds has been demonstrated. In particular, a commercial formulation of the pyrethroid fenvalerate with diethyltoluamide (DEET) has been incriminated as a cause of intoxication in a large number of feline cases[20]; however, the clinical signs described are not consistent with pyrethroid intoxication and have been experimentally reproduced in cats and dogs by oral exposure to diethyltoluamide alone.[18]

Commercial products containing pyrethrins and pyrethroids intended for dermal application on cats vary greatly in formulation details. Varying characteristics include the type and concentration of pyrethrin or pyrethroid, the carrier solvents, the type and concentration of synergists, and the packaging and method of delivery (e.g., hand sprays, pressure sprays, shampoos, and dips). These differences, together with the expected variation in the administered dose by an owner, combine to make the calculation or estimation of dose-effect relationships difficult. Veterinarians should advise clients to follow the instructions on a particular product with care.

The diagnosis of pyrethrin or pyrethroid intoxication is difficult because veterinarians must rely solely on a history of exposure, clinical signs, and elimination of diagnostic differentials. At present, there are no practical diagnostic tests available to confirm a tentative diagnosis. Autopsy is unrewarding, with gross and histopathologic findings consistent only with agonal death. Tissue analysis for the presence of some pyrethrins and pyrethroids is available through some laboratories but serves only to confirm exposure, because tissue concentrations consistent with intoxication have not been defined for companion animal species.[1]

TREATMENT

No specific treatment for intoxication by pyrethrins or pyrethroids is known, and the general principles of treating toxicoses must be applied. First, the patient should be removed from access to further exposure; this includes provision for return of the patient to its normal habitat after remission of clinical signs. Therefore, residues on horizontal surfaces (e.g., carpets and floors) of domestic residences should be removed by appropriate cleaning while the cat is elsewhere (being treated). Further absorption of toxin by the cat should be prevented. If exposure was oral and recent, it is appropriate to induce emesis; this is followed by dosing with activated charcoal (2 g/kg). If the ingested formulation contained petroleum products, emesis is contraindicated.[1] Fatty meals should be avoided as they may aid in gastrointestinal absorption. Cats exposed topically should be washed with lukewarm water and a mild detergent. The use of very warm water is contraindicated because its use would increase dermal perfusion and thereby may increase the rate of transdermal absorption of insecticide. Because pyrethrins and pyrethroids are not water soluble, copious application of mild detergent is necessary to ensure removal of the residual insecticide.

Clinical signs may be controlled as necessary. The use of subcutaneous atropine (0.2–2.0 mg/kg) for excessive salivation and respiratory secretion, intravenous diazepam (0.5–1.0 mg/kg) administered incrementally to desired effect, and/or intravenous methocarbamol (44 mg/kg) administered incrementally to desired effect for seizures and muscle fasciculations have been advocated.[21] Attention should be paid to the body temperature of the cat. Elevation of core body temperature as a result of excessive muscular activity may lead to cerebral edema and continued convulsions.[22] Lowering of body temperatures as the patient becomes depressed (or subsequent to bathing) may exacerbate depression.[22] In addition, reduction in body temperature may lead to an increase in the toxicity of the pyrethrin or pyrethroid insecticide. Experimental use of local anesthetics, such as lidocaine in vitro, recently has shown selective depression of pyrethroid-induced tail currents.[23] Local anesthetics have not yet been used routinely in cases of clinical pyrethroid toxicity but may find use in the future. Basic supportive care should also include consideration of fluid and electrolyte requirements. Induction of diuresis through aggressive fluid therapy may aid in the elimination of metabolites of the toxin but should be undertaken with care to avoid iatrogenic pulmonary edema.

CONCLUSION

Recovery from moderate intoxication by pyrethrins and pyrethroids is usually expected for animals that are given appropriate treatment. In addition, because no residual tissue lesions are induced, successful recovery from intoxication is expected to be absolute. However, death does occur,[13] and because cats are more frequently intoxicated than other domesticated species, appropriate treatment is likely to be important to ensure recovery.

It is generally accepted that no satisfactory alternative insecticide to pyrethrins and pyrethroids is available for use on cats. Therefore, pyrethrins and pyrethroids will continue to be used for control of ectoparasites in this species. Recommendations for use of pyrethrins or pyrethroids must be made after careful consideration of the formulation of the particular product, the age and health of the patient, and the likelihood that appropriate dosing regimens are followed by the owner.

ACKNOWLEDGMENT

The author is indebted to Jodie Katz, DVM, for her assistance in preparing this manuscript.

About the Author

Dr. Whittem, who is a Diplomate of the American College of Veterinary Clinical Pharmacology, is an Assistant Professor of Veterinary Clinical Pharmacology at the College of Veterinary Medicine, University of Illinois at Urbana/Champaign.

REFERENCES

1. Valentine WM: Pyrethrin and pyrethroid insecticides. *Vet Clin North Am Small Anim Pract* 20(2):375–382, 1990.
2. Ray DE: Pesticides derived from plants and other organisms, in Hayes WJ, Laws ER (eds): *Handbook of Pesticide Toxicology*. New York, Academic Press, 1991, pp 585–636.
3. Vijverberg HPM, de Weille JR: The interaction of pyrethroids with voltage-dependent Na channels. *Neurotoxicology* 6:23–34, 1985.
4. Lombet A, Mourre C, Lazdunski M: Interaction of insecticides of the pyrethroid family with specific binding sites on the voltage-dependent sodium channel from mammalian brain. *Brain Res* 459:45–53, 1988.
5. Chinn K, Narashi T: Temperature-dependent subconducting states and kinetics of deltamethrin-modified sodium channels of neuroblastoma cells. *Pflugers Arch* 43:571–579, 1989.
6. Jacques Y, Romey G, Cavey MT, et al: Interaction of pyrethroids with the Na⁺ channel in mammalian neuronal cells in culture. *Biochim Biophys Acta* 600:882–897, 1980.
7. Narahashi T: Nerve membrane ionic channels as the primary target of pyrethroids. *Neurotoxicology* 6:3–12, 1985.
8. van den Bercken J, Akkermann LMA, Van der Zalm JJ: DDT-like action of allethrin in the sensory nervous system of *Xenopus laevis*. *Europ J Pharmacol* 21:95–106, 1973.
9. Lawrence LJ, Gee KW, Yamamura HI: Interactions of pyrethroid insecticides with chloride ionophore-associated binding sites. *Neurotoxicology* 6:87–98, 1985.
10. Crofton KM, Reiter LW, Mailman RB: Pyrethroid insecticides and radioligand displacement from GABA receptor chloride ionophore complex. *Toxicol Let* 35:183–190, 1987.
11. Bloomquist JR, Adams PM, Soderlund DM: Inhibition of γ-aminobutyric acid-stimulated chloride flux in mouse brain vesicles by polycycloalkane and pyrethroid insecticides. *Neurotoxicology* 7:11–20, 1986.
12. Devaud LL, Szot P, Murray TF: PK11195 antagonism of pyrethroid-induced proconvulsant activity. *Eur J Pharmacol* 121:269–273, 1986.
13. Whittem T, Katz JM: Pyrethrin and pyrethroid insecticide toxicity in cats: A retrospective case study (abstr). *Proc 9th Ann Vet Med Forum Am Coll Vet Intern Med*:890, 1991.
14. Leahey JP (ed): *The Pyrethroid Insecticides*. London, Taylor & Francis, 1985.
15. Cassida JE, Kimmel EC, Elliott M, Janes NF: Oxidative metabolism of pyrethrins in mammals. *Nature* 230:326–327, 1971.
16. Lawerence LJ, Casida JE: Pyrethroid toxicology: Mouse intracerebral structure-toxicity relationships. *Pestic Biochem Physiol* 18:9–14, 1982.
17. Beasley VR, Dorman DC, Fikes JD: Pyrethrum (pyrethrins) and pyrethroids, in Beasley VR (ed): *A Systems Affected Approach to Veterinary Toxicology*. Champaign, IL, Illinois Animal Poison Information Center, 1990, pp 111–116.
18. Marei AEM, Ruzo LO, Casida JE: Analysis and persistence of permethrin, cypermethrin, deltamethrin and fenvalerate in the fat and brain of treated rats. *J Agri Food Chem* 30:558–562, 1982.
19. Whittem T: Unpublished data, Department of Veterinary Clinical Sciences, Massey University, Palmerston North, New Zealand.
20. Dorman DC, Buck WB, Trammel HL, et al: Fenvalerate/N,N-diethyl-m-toluamide (Deet) toxicosis in two cats. *JAVMA* 196(1):100–102, 1990.
21. Dorman DC, Beasley VR: Neurotoxicology of pyrethrin and the pyrethroid insecticides. *Vet Hum Toxicol* 33(3):238–243, 1991.

22. Greene CE, Braund KG: Diseases of the brain, in Ettinger SJ (ed): *Textbook of Veterinary Internal Medicine*, ed 3. Philadelphia, WB Saunders Co, 1989, pp 578–623.
23. Oortigiesen M, van Kleef RG, Vijverberg HP: Block of deltamethrin-modified sodium current in cultured mouse neuroblastoma cells: Local anesthetics as potential antidotes. *Brain Res* 518(1-2):11–18, 1990.

4-Methylpyrazole: An Antidote for Ethylene Glycol Intoxication in Dogs

KEY FACTS

- Metabolism of ethylene glycol by the liver results in the formation of metabolic intermediates, particularly glycolic acid.
- Glycolic acid is responsible for severe metabolic acidosis, hyperosmolality, and elevated anion gap values.
- Therapy with ethanol has several disadvantages.
- More effective and safer treatment includes the administration of 4-methylpyrazole as an alcohol dehydrogenase inhibitor.

Ecole Nationale de Médecine Vétérinaire
Sidi Thabet, Tunisia
Lotfi El Bahri, DVM, MSc, PhD

ETHYLENE GLYCOL is a common cause of intoxication in small animals. Commercial automobile antifreeze preparations typically contain 95% ethylene glycol. The intoxication occurs most often during the autumn, when radiator fluid is changed and new antifreeze is placed into automobiles. The sweet taste of ethylene glycol encourages consumption by dogs and cats. Ethylene glycol poisoning is significant in clinical toxicology because the associated mortality is high. Of the animals with diagnosed ethylene glycol toxicosis at the Kansas State University Veterinary Teaching Hospital from 1975 to 1980, 74% died.[1] Ethylene glycol toxicosis is a medical emergency.

Ethylene glycol and its metabolites are extremely toxic to animals. The substance is a central nervous system depressant that may enter the cerebrospinal fluid and cause ataxia and signs of drunkenness.[2] Ethylene glycol induces osmotic diuresis and thus promotes dehydration. Other toxic effects result from metabolic conversion in the liver.

Metabolism in the liver begins with oxidation by alcohol dehydrogenase (a soluble cytoplasmic enzyme confined mainly to liver cells) to produce glycolaldehyde (Figure 1). Glycolaldehyde is readily metabolized to glycolic acid. Glycolic acid may accumulate in high concentrations in the blood (at least 30 mg/100 ml).[3] Glycolic acid is responsible for the severe metabolic acidosis (pH of 2% aqueous solution is 2.16)[4] associated with an extreme elevation of the anion gap (which may exceed 25 mEq/L) and the increased osmolal gap (more than 60 mOsm/L) observed in poisoned animals.[2]

The next step is the slow conversion of glycolic acid to glyoxylic acid. Glyoxylic acid is more toxic, but its half-life is short. The minor pathway from glyoxylic acid is decarboxylation to yield formic acid. Glyoxylic acid may also be metabolized to glycine. Some of the glycine conjugates with benzoic acid to form hippuric acid.

Another metabolic pathway of glyoxylic acid is oxidation to form oxalic acid. Most oxalic acid is excreted in the urine; some combines with calcium to form calcium oxalate crystals, a portion of which are precipitated in the vasculature and in renal tubules and (to a lesser degree) in cerebral blood vessels. Only 2% to 3% of the ethylene glycol ingested by a dog is metabolized to form oxalic acid.[5] Oxalate crystal production is greater in cats than in other species.[6]

Some ethylene glycol is excreted unchanged in the urine. In one investigation, 5.7% to 23.4% of administered ethyl-

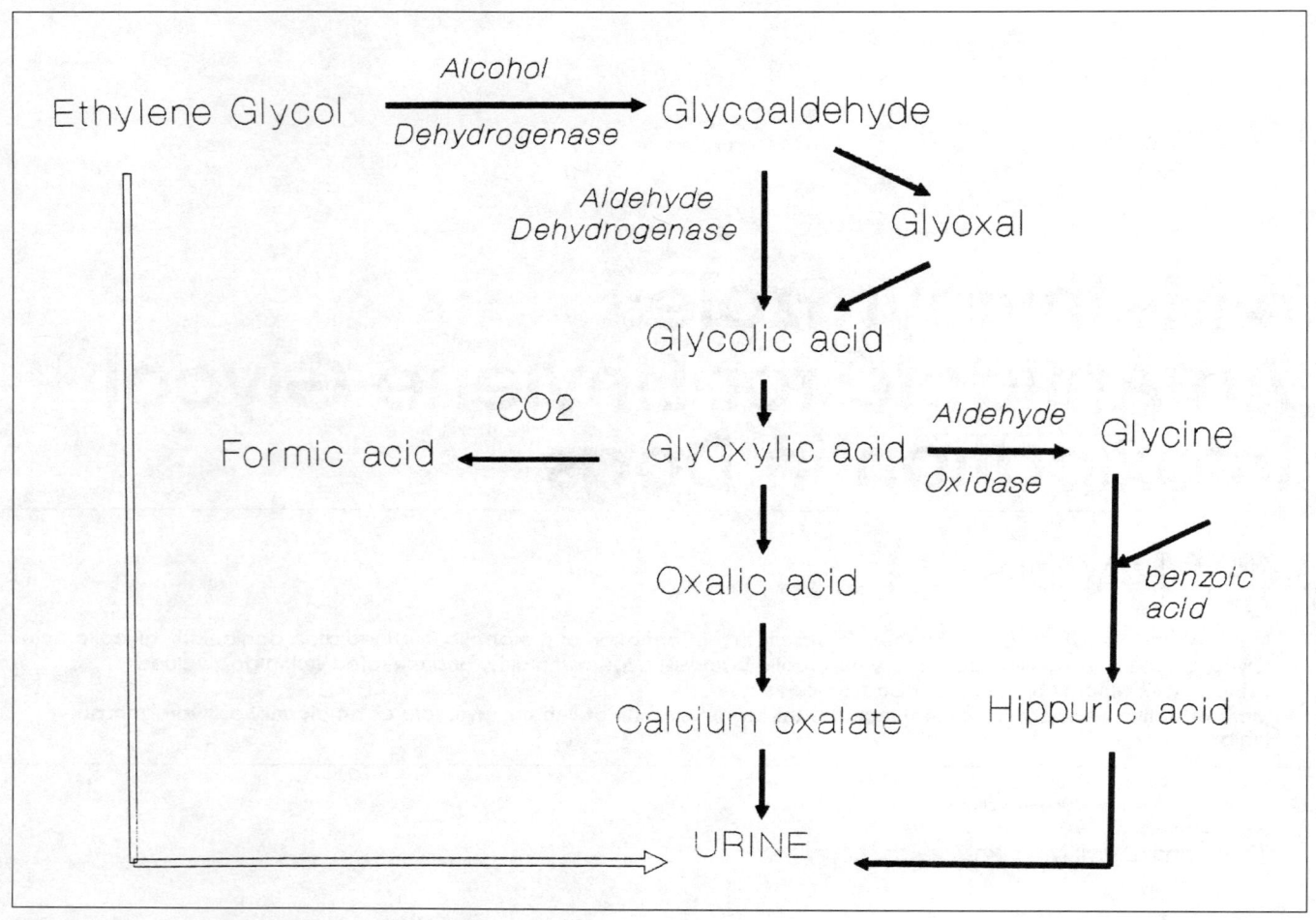

Figure 1—The metabolic pathway of ethylene glycol.

ene glycol was found in the urine during the first 24 hours.[7] The plasma half-life of ethylene glycol ranges from 2.5 to 6 hours in dogs.[7a] Certain metabolites of ethylene glycol have toxic effects on mitochondrial function.[8] The reported toxic dose of ethylene glycol in dogs is 4.2 to 6.6 ml/kg; the toxic dose in cats is 1.5 ml/kg.[9]

Ethanol interferes with ethylene glycol metabolism because alcohol dehydrogenase has a higher affinity for ethanol than for ethylene glycol.[10] Competitive inhibition of alcohol dehydrogenase results in the excretion of unmetabolized ethylene glycol by the kidneys. Ethanol is thus used in the treatment of ethylene glycol intoxication. The common treatment in dogs is 5.5 ml/kg of intravenous 20% ethanol every four hours for five treatments and then every six hours for four treatments.[11] Sodium bicarbonate (5% solution) is used to correct metabolic acidosis. Aggressive fluid therapy is required to compensate for the osmotic diuresis induced by ethanol.

EARLY TREATMENT of ethylene glycol toxicosis is important. Nephrotoxic metabolites of ethylene glycol can be detected in the serum of intoxicated dogs as early as three hours after ethylene glycol ingestion.[3] Changes in serum biochemistry that imply renal damage are apparent from 18 to 24 hours after ingestion,[3,12] and those demonstrating diminished renal excretory function are established at 46 hours.[13]

The prognosis depends on the amount of ethylene glycol absorbed and the time from ingestion to initiation of treatment. Treatment is most successful if administered within four hours after ingestion.[14,15]

Ethanol therapy has several disadvantages and side effects. Substantial technical difficulties arise if ethanol infusion is used to treat ethylene glycol poisoning. Considerable individual variation in the rate of ethanol metabolism demands careful and frequent patient monitoring to maintain an adequate blood ethanol level (100 mg/dl) for 46 to 72 hours.[15] The relationship between dose and steady-state plasma concentration is unpredictable.[16]

In addition, because a metabolic shunt pathway can operate if alcohol dehydrogenase is inhibited, ethylene glycol can be transformed to glyoxal and then to oxalic acid.[17] Furthermore, ethanol enhances many of the metabolic ef-

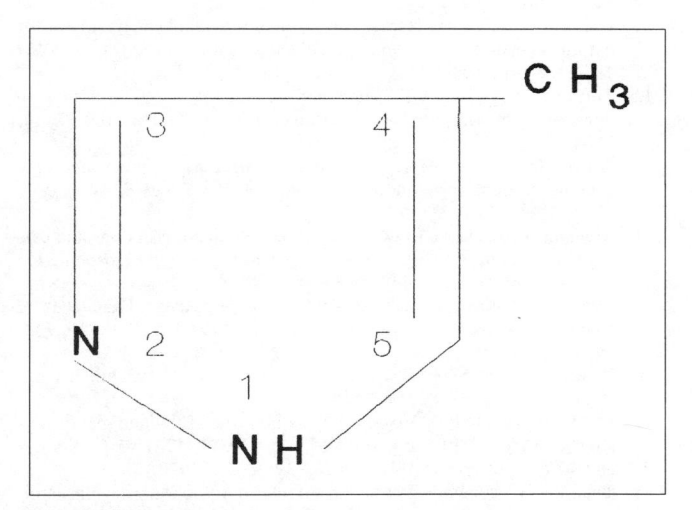

Figure 2—The structure of 4-methylpyrazole.

fects of ethylene glycol, such as central nervous system depression (to allow for ethylene glycol excretion, it is necessary to maintain an animal in a near-comatose state for as long as 72 hours). Ethanol increases plasma osmolality, prolongs diuresis (inhibiting secretion of antidiuretic hormone),[11] and creates hypoglycemia. Ethanol therapy is thus not ideal.

More effective treatment would inhibit alcohol dehydrogenase activity without producing the adverse effects of ethanol. Pyrazole, 4-methylpyrazole, and several alkyldiols (e.g., propylene glycol and 1,3-butanediol) are potent inhibitors of alcohol dehydrogenase.[18-23] The results of recent studies demonstrate that 4-methylpyrazole is the most efficient and least toxic inhibitor of alcohol dehydrogenase in dogs.[11]

CHEMISTRY

The inhibitor 4-methylpyrazole is a hygroscopic, white crystalline compound that is soluble in water and alcohol (Figure 2). The molecular weight is 82.11 daltons. The molecule is stable in light. The shelf-life at 4 °C is less than three years.[24]

PHARMACOKINETICS

There have been few studies of the pharmacokinetics of 4-methylpyrazole in animals. In dogs, after intravenous administration of 10mg/kg, peak concentrations in plasma reach 2 to 3 mg (17 to 25 µmol/L).[7a] In mice, 4-methylpyrazole is metabolized to 4-hydroxymethylpyrazole and 4-carboxypyrazole.[21] After the administration of a single dose of 4-methylpyrazole to healthy human volunteers, the elimination of the agent from plasma was of zero order (plasma levels decrease linearly with time).[25] The plasma half-life of 4-methylpyrazole in dogs is two hours.[7a]

MECHANISM OF ACTION

The inhibition of enzymatic activity is noncompetitive. The activity of alcohol dehydrogenase is markedly inhibited by 4-methylpyrazole.[26] By comparison, 4-methylpyrazole induces a competition with ethanol at a 3000:1 ratio of ethanol to 4-methylpyrazole, thus yielding a 50% inhibition of alcohol dehydrogenase activity.[24] Alcohol dehydrogenase has a relatively low affinity for ethanol.[16]

A relationship between the dose of 4-methylpyrazole and the degree of inhibition of alcohol dehydrogenase has been demonstrated in monkeys.[27] A blood concentration of 4-methylpyrazole above 10 µmol/L provides constant inhibition of alcohol dehydrogenase activity. The inhibitory effect of 4-methylpyrazole has rapid onset[27] and is prolonged.[28]

REPEATED DOSES of 4-methylpyrazole inhibit the metabolism of ethylene glycol and prevent the appearance of plasma and urinary metabolites of ethylene glycol.[29] The result is a great increase in the plasma half-life of ethylene glycol (from 3 to 15 hours).[24] The anion gap returns to the normal range within four hours after the start of 4-methylpyrazole therapy.[25] In addition, the agent is an effective reagent for stabilizing the redox state of cytosolic and mitochondrial spaces.[24,30]

TOXICITY

The acute toxicity is low. The LD_{50} of intravenous 4-methylpyrazole in rats and mice is 312 mg/kg.[24,31] Short- and long-term regimens of 4-methylpyrazole are well tolerated by these animals.[26,27] Pyrazole (1400 mg/kg orally in one dose) causes necrosis of follicular epithelial cells of rat thyroid[32] and has well-documented toxic effects.[33] No side effects have been reported in humans with the use of single doses as high as 20 mg/kg.[34]

INDICATIONS

Jubb and coworkers demonstrated that many dogs with experimentally induced ethylene glycol toxicosis survive if treated with 4-methylpyrazole within eight hours.[35] The agent is administered intravenously at a dose of 20 mg/kg initially, then 15 mg/kg at 12 and 24 hours, and finally 5 mg/kg at 36 hours.[35]

In another study, eight dogs with clinical signs suggesting ethylene glycol ingestion were treated with 4-methylpyrazole.[11] A 50 mg/ml solution of 4-methylpyrazole in propylene glycol was administered in intravenous boluses as follows: at initiation of therapy (20 mg/kg), at 17 hours after initiation (15 mg/kg), and at 25 hours after initiation (5 mg/kg). In two of the eight patients, an additional dose of 5 mg/kg was given at 36 hours after initiation of therapy.[11] All patients demonstrated clinical and metabolic improvement within 24 hours after admission. Of the eight dogs, seven were released within three days of admission.[11]

An increased use of 4-methylpyrazole in cases of possible ethylene glycol toxicosis may have contributed to the decrease in associated fatality (from 70% to 43%) at the Colorado State University Veterinary Teaching Hospital.[14] When a sufficient amount of ethylene glycol has been metabolized, use of 4-methylpyrazole does not prevent damage to renal tubules. Dogs diagnosed after the onset of azotemia should be given supportive treatment for acute renal failure.[11] In cats, 4-methylpyrazole is not recommended because ethanol is more effective in preventing ethylene glycol biotransformation.[36]

In humans, 4-methylpyrazole is used as an antidote to ethylene glycol intoxication.[25,29] The proposed dose regimen is 20 mg/kg/day orally or 7 mg/kg/day in an intravenous infusion of isotonic sodium chloride solution.[24]

Therapy with 4-methylpyrazole has the following potential advantages compared with ethanol therapy:

- 4-methylpyrazole can be administered within eight hours after the ingestion of ethylene glycol.[15,35]
- Inhibition of alcohol dehydrogenase by 4-methylpyrazole is more effective than with the use of ethanol as a competitive substrate.
- Complications of ethanol administration, such as central nervous system depression and prolonged osmotic diuresis, are not associated with 4-methylpyrazole administration.
- No adverse effects are associated with 4-methylpyrazole.

As a more effective antidote to ethylene glycol intoxication, 4-methylpyrazole represents a significant therapeutic advance.

About the Author
Dr. Bahri is affiliated with the Service de Pharmacie-Toxicologie, Ecole Nationale de Médecine Vétérinaire, Sidi Thabet, Tunisia.

REFERENCES

1. Barton J, Oehme FW: The incidence and characteristics of animal poisonings seen at Kansas State University from 1975 to 1980. *Vet Hum Toxicol* 23:101–102, 1981.
2. Beasley VR: Diagnosis and management of ethylene glycol (antifreeze) poisoning. *Feline Pract* 15(1):41–46, 1985.
3. Hewlett TP, Ray AC, Reagor TC: Diagnosis of ethylene glycol (antifreeze) intoxication in dogs by determination of glycolic acid in serum and urine with high pressure liquid chromatography and gas chromatography–mass spectrometry. *J Assoc Off Anal Chem* 66(2):276–283, 1983.
4. *The Merck Index: An Encyclopedia of Chemicals and Drugs*, ed 9. Rahway, NJ, Merck & Co, 1976.
5. Penumarthy L, Oehme FW: Treatment of ethylene glycol toxicosis in cats. *Am J Vet Res* 36:209, 1975.
6. Black RP: Ethylene glycol intoxication. *Feline Pract* 15(4):43–45, 1985.
7a. Pinault L, Joseph E: L'intoxication par l'éthylène glycol chez le chien. Diagnostic et traitement. *Rec Med Vet* 171(2/3):159–163, 1995.
8. Bachmann E, Goldberg L: Reappraisal of the toxicology of ethylene glycol. III. Mitochondrial effects. *Food Cosmet Toxicol* 9:31–55, 1971.
9. Oehme FW: Antifreeze (ethylene glycol) poisoning, in *Veterinary Internal Medicine: Diseases of the Dog and Cat*. Philadelphia, WB Saunders Co, 1983, pp 203–204.
10. Bostrom WF, Li T: Alcohol dehydrogenase enzyme, in Jakoby WB (ed): *Enzyme Basis of Detoxication*, vol 1. New York, Academic Press, 1980, pp 231–248.
11. Dial SM, Thrall MA, Hamar DW: 4-methylpyrazole as treatment for naturally acquired ethylene glycol intoxication in dogs. *JAVMA* 195(1):73–76, 1989.
12. Thrall MA, Grauer GF, Mero KN: Clinicopathologic findings in dogs and cats with ethylene glycol intoxication. *JAVMA* 184:37–41, 1984.
13. Grauer GF, Thrall MA, Henri BA, et al: Early clinicopathologic findings in dogs ingesting ethylene glycol. *Am J Vet Res* 45:2299–2303, 1984.
14. Rowland J: Incidence of ethylene glycol intoxication in dogs and cats seen at Colorado State University Veterinary Teaching Hospital. *Vet Hum Toxicol* 29(1):41–44, 1987.
15. Fuhrer L, George C: L'intoxication par l'ethylene glycol chez le chien. A propos d'un cas clinique. *Rec Med Vet* 165(8–9):715–720, 1989.
16. Rang HP, Dale MM: *Pharmacology*. New York, Churchill Livingstone, 1987, pp 87–88, 683–689.
17. Seeff LB, Hendler E, Hosten A, Shalhoub RI: Ethylene glycol poisoning: Survival after ingestion of 400 ml with 42 days of oliguria and 17 days of coma. *Med Ann DC* 39:31–35, 1970.
18. Theorell H, Yonetani T: On the effects of some heterocyclic compounds on the enzymatic activity of liver alcohol dehydrogenase. *Acta Chem Scand* 23:255–260, 1969.
19. Li TK, Theorell H: Human liver alcohol dehydrogenase inhibition by pyrazole and pyrazole analogs. *Acta Chem Scand* 23:892–902, 1969.
20. Pietruszko R: Human liver alcohol dehydrogenase. Inhibition activity by pyrazole, 4-methylpyrazole, 4-hydroxymethylpyrazole and 4-carboxypyrazole. *Biochem Pharmacol* 24:1603–1607, 1975.
21. Van Stee EW, Harris AM, Horton ML, Back KC: The treatment of ethylene glycol toxicosis with pyrazole. *J Pharmacol Exp Ther* 192:251–259, 1975.
22. Holman NW Jr, Mundy RL, Teague RS: Alkyldiol antidotes to ethylene glycol toxicity in mice. *Toxicol Appl Pharmacol* 49:385–392, 1979.
23. Murphy MJ, Ray AC, Jones LP, et al: 1,3-butanediol treatment of ethylene toxicosis in dogs. *Am J Vet Res* 45:2293–2295, 1984.
24. Likforman J, Brouard A, Philippe C, et al: 4-methylpyrazole. *J Toxicol Clin Exp* 7:373–382, 1987.
25. Baud FJ, Galliot M, Astier A, et al: Treatment of ethylene glycol poisoning with intravenous 4-methylpyrazole. *N Engl J Med* 319(2):97–100, 1988.
26. Blomstrand R, Ostling-Wintzell H, Lof A, et al: Pyrazoles as inhibitors of alcohol oxidation and as important tools in alcohol research: An approach to therapy against methanol poisoning. *Proc Natl Acad Sci* 76:3499–3503, 1979.
27. McMartin KE, Hedstrom KG, Tolf BR, et al: Studies on the metabolic interactions between 4-methylpyrazole and methanol using the monkey as an animal model. *Arch Biochem Biophys* 199:606–614, 1980.
28. Blomstrand R, Theorell H: Inhibitory effect on ethanol oxidation in man after administration of 4-methylpyrazole. *Life Sci* 9(2):631–640, 1970.
29. Baud FJ, Bismuth C, Garnier R, et al: 4-methylpyrazole may be an alternative to ethanol therapy for ethylene glycol intoxication in man. *J Toxicol Clin Toxicol* 24:463–483, 1986.
30. Theorell H, Chance B: The combustion of alcohol and its inhibition by 4-methylpyrazole in perfused rat livers. *Arch Biochem Biophys* 151:434–444, 1972.
31. Magnusson G, Nyberg JA, Bodin NO, Hansson E: Toxicity of pyrazole and 4-methylpyrazole in mice and rats. *Experentia* 28:1198–1200, 1972.
32. Szabo S, Horvath E, Kovacs K, et al: Pyrazole induced thyroid necrosis: A distinct organ lesion. *Science* 199:1209–1210, 1978.
33. Wilson WL, Bottiglieri NG: Phase I. Studies with pyrazole. *Cancer Chemother Rep* 21:137–141, 1962.
34. McMartin KE, Jacobsen D, Sebastian S, et al: Safety and metabolism of 4-methylpyrazole in human subjects. *Vet Hum Toxicol* 29:471, 1987.
35. Jubb KVF, Kennedy PC, Palmer N: *Pathology of Domestic Animals*, ed 3. New York, Academic Press, 1985, p 375.
36. *The Merck Veterinary Manual: A Handbook of Diagnosis, Therapy, and Disease Prevention and Control for the Veterinarian*, ed. 7. Rahway, NJ, Merck & Co, 1991, p 1650.

Management of Cholecalciferol Rodenticide Toxicity

Akron Veterinary Internal Medical Practice
Sharon Center, Ohio
Marcia Carothers, DVM

The Ohio State University
Columbus, Ohio
Dennis Chew, DVM

The use of cholecalciferol rodenticides (Quintox®, Bell Laboratories; Rampage®, CEVA Laboratories; and Ortho Rat and Mouse-Be-Gon®, Chevron) has recently increased[1] due to the lack of cholecalciferol resistance by the rodent population and no secondary toxicity to species who eat the poisoned rodents.[2] Although the LD_{50} in dogs was reported to be 88 mg/kg by one manufacturer, toxicity at much lower dosages (<10 mg/kg) has been reported.[3-9] No breed predilection has been noted; however, high-risk groups included dogs less than 12 kg and less than 9 months of age.[4,9] Feline toxicosis has been reported.[10-12]

PATHOGENESIS

Hypercalcemia is the major consequence of cholecalciferol toxicity due to the action of vitamin D on calcium homeostasis. Cholecalciferol is absorbed from the jejunum, bound to a carrier protein, and hydroxylated to 25 hydroxycholecalciferol (25 OH-CC) in the liver. This metabolite is further hydroxylated in the kidney to 1,25 dihydroxycholecalciferol (1,25 diOH-CC), the active metabolite of Vitamin D. The metabolite, 1,25 diOH-CC, increases calcium and phosphorus absorption in the intestines, mobilizes calcium from bone, and enhances the reabsorption of calcium and phosphorus by the kidneys. Although cholecalciferol and 25 OH-CC have little biologic activity, their plasma half-lives may last for days (1 to 30) and duration of effect may last for weeks.[6] When plasma 25 OH-CC concentrations are increased, this metabolite competes with 1,25 diOH-CC for sites of action in bone, jejunum, and kidneys.[6] In one report of canine cholecalciferol toxicosis, serum 25 OH-CC remained increased for 30 days, and the calculated half-life was 10.67 days.[7]

CLINICAL SIGNS

The clinical signs of hypercalcemia secondary to cholecalciferol toxicity are usually vague and include anorexia, depression, vomiting, constipation, polyuria, and polydipsia. Neurologic signs (seizures, muscle twitching, and stupor) may develop in cases with severe hypercalcemia. Hypercalcemia usually develops within 12 to 24 hours of intoxication and is the most consistent laboratory abnormality. Hyperphosphotemia (usually 7 to 8 mg/dl) often may oc-

TABLE I
Treatment for Cholecalciferol Toxicity

Treatment	Dose Regimen[a]	Rationale
Emetics		
Apomorphine	0.04 mg/kg IV or 0.08 mg/kg SQ or IM	Elimination of gastric contents with ingested pesticide
Ipecac syrup	1 to 2 ml/kg PO	
Activated charcoal	1 to 5 g/kg PO	Adsorption of pesticide in the stomach and intestines
Fluid therapy		
Intravenous saline (0.9%)	120 to 180 ml/kg/day initially, then 60 to 120 ml/kg/day	Correction of dehydration; enhancement of calciuresis
Furosemide	2.5 to 4.5 mg/kg IV, SQ, or PO twice to three times daily	Enhancement of calciuresis
Prednisone	1 to 2 mg/kg IV, SQ, or PO twice daily	Reduction of intestinal calcium absorption; inhibition of bone resorption; enhancement of calciuresis
Calcitonin	4 to 6 IU/kg SQ twice to three times daily	Inhibition of bone resorption
Phosphage binders (aluminum hydroxide)	10 to 30 mg/kg PO twice to three times daily	Reduction of phosphorus absorption in the intestinal tract
Low-calcium diet	As fed per label or veterinarian directions	Reduction of calcium absorption in the intestines

[a]IV = intravenously; SQ = subcutaneously, IM = intramuscularly; PO = orally.

cur simultaneously. Azotemia may develop secondary to the hypercalcemia and dehydration.[13] Pathologic changes occur in the gastrointestinal tract, kidneys, and cardiovascular system. Mucosal hemorrhage may be present in the stomach and small intestines. Renal changes include calcification of the glomeruli and tubular basement membrane. Myocardial necrosis and mineralization of the myocytes have been reported.[3] The exact pathogenesis of hypervitaminosis D is not known. The development of hypercalcemia and hyperphosphatemia are thought to be associated with metastatic calcification of previously normal soft tissues. However, a direct effect of hypervitaminosis D that results in widespread cellular degeneration and subsequent dystrophic mineralization may be operative; in these instances, organ failure and death may occur despite minimal or absent hypercalcemia.[5]

DIAGNOSIS

The diagnosis of cholecalciferol intoxication is usually based on a history of exposure, clinical signs of hypercalcemia, laboratory findings of hypercalcemia and hyperphosphatemia, and pathologic findings in terminal cases. Serum 25 OH-CC can be measured and provides conclusive evidence of cholecalciferol toxicity.

THERAPY

The goals of treatment are directed at decreasing the absorption of cholecalciferol in the gastrointestinal tract, correcting the fluid and electrolyte imbalance, reducing the hypercalcemia, and treating miscellaneous complications such as seizures and arrhythmias.[4–6,13] In recent intoxications (i.e., < 2 to 4 hours), emetics and activated charcoal may be the only treatment necessary.[4] If dehydration, vomiting, and hypercalcemia are present, aggressive treatment should be pursued.[4,5,15] Severe complications of hypercalcemia such as seizures and cardiac arrhythmias should be treated symptomatically (see Table I).

Detoxification of the gastrointestinal tract includes

the use of an emetic (apormorphine, ipecac syrup, etc.) if the patient is alert and responsive. Adsorbents (activated charcoal) and a saline cathartic (sodium sulfate, magnesium sulfate, etc.) are given following emesis; however, ipecac syrup negates some of the absorption properties of the activated charcoal if used in combination.[4] If a large quantity of the rodenticide is identified in the vomitus, further treatment is not necessary. Evaluation of the serum calcium, phosphorus, and creatinine is recommended 24, 48, and 72 hours post-treatment to ensure that absorption of the toxin has not occurred.

If the animal is showing signs of anorexia, vomiting, and dehydration, and/or is hypercalcemic, fluid therapy should be started immediately.[4,5,13] Correction of dehydration restores extracellular fluid volume, which increases glomerular filtration rate and enhances renal excretion of calcium. Saline (0.9%) is the fluid of choice as sodium decreases calcium reabsorption in the renal tubules.[4,13] Although the intravenous route is preferred, subcutaneous fluids may be adequate if the hypercalcemia is minimal (< 15 mg/dl). The initial fluid volume given should be two to three times maintenance needs to correct for dehydration, provide maintenance, and produce volume expansion. The duration of fluid therapy will depend on the magnitude of the hypercalcemia, the degree of azotemia, and severity of clinical signs. Evaluation of serum electrolytes (i.e., potassium, phosphorus) is important during therapy as fluid diuresis and anorexia may result in depletion of these electrolytes. Supplementation of potassium as dictated by serum concentrations is often necessary in many cases. In severe intoxications, intravenous fluids may be necessary for 7 to 10 days.

Furosemide (Lasix®) is beneficial in promoting calciuresis and helpful in cases with moderate to severe hypercalcemia.[4,13] The use of furosemide prior to rehydration and fluid volume expansion is contraindicated as diuretics may potentiate the dehydration and hypercalcemia.[13] Although furosemide therapy in cholecalciferol toxicity has not been studied, parenteral and oral furosemide BID to QID appear to be helpful. Furosemide therapy for two to four weeks may be necessary in most cases due to the prolonged effects of cholecalciferol and its metabolites.[4,13] The thiazide diuretics should not be used as this group of diuretics decreases the excretion of calcium in the renal tubules and may increase the serum calcium.[4,13]

Glucocorticoids will decrease the serum calcium by reducing bone resorption, decreasing intestinal calcium absorption, and enhancing calciuresis.[4,13] Oral prednisone and parenteral methylprednisolone have been reported to be beneficial in the treatment of cholecalciferol toxicity.[4,5,13] As with furosemide, the duration of treatment with glucocorticoids recommended is two to four weeks.

Calcitonin is recommended by the manufacturer as a treatment for subsequent hypercalcemia in cholecalciferol toxicosis.[2] Although calcitonin is not a specific antidote, this drug will reduce the serum calcium by inhibiting osteoclastic activity. The use of calcitonin in veterinary medicine has been infrequent, and dosages have been extrapolated from the use in humans.[4,13] Treatment with calcitonin has been reported in two cases of cholecalciferol toxicity.[7-9,11,15-17] In one dog, calcitonin (8 units/kg SQ q 24 hr) resulted in anorexia and was discontinued due to this proposed side effect.[15] In another dog, calcitonin (4–7 units/kg SQ q 6 to 8 hr) was continued for 27 days and was associated only with mild, intermittent vomiting.[7] Calcium concentrations returned to normal within two hours of administration when IV fluids, furosemide, and prednisone failed to significantly improve the hypercalcemia.[7] Calcitonin treatment is expensive, and the response time may be short. However, in animals with severe hypercalcemia (>18 mg/dl), calcitonin may be beneficial when used in conjunction with IV fluids, furosemide, and prednisone.

The use of sodium bicarbonate may be beneficial in cases of severe hypercalcemia (calcium >18 mg/dl). Improving the acidosis or creating a mild alkalosis favors the shifting of the ionized calcium (active form) to the protein-bound portion (non-active form). Infusions of 1 to 4 mEq/kg have been recommended.[13] The magnitude of serum calcium reduction is mild. Consequently, this therapy is most useful in combination with other treatments. Because the measurement of ionized calcium concentrations is not widely available, monitoring the acid-base status via blood gas analysis is the best method to evaluate the effectiveness of this treatment.

Intestinal phosphate binders that do not contain calcium may be useful in decreasing the effects of hyperphosphatemia (i.e., decreasing the calcium × phosphorus product and subsequent soft tissue mineralization). Aluminum hydroxide is recommended during the first two weeks, and the dosage may be adjusted depending on serial serum phosphorus concentrations.[9]

A low calcium diet is important to decrease the amount of intestinal absorption. Hill's k/d®, u/d®, and s/d® (Hill's Pet Products) or a homemade calcium restricted diet should be maintained for one month due to the prolonged half-life of 25 OH-CC. Milk products and growth diets should be avoided.[4,5,13]

Although decreased exposure to sunlight was thought to be beneficial by reducing the conversion of 7-dehydroxycholesterol to vitamin D in the skin, this pathway is not important in the dog. Other unproven methods for the treatment of cholecalciferol toxicity include anticonvulsants, intestinal calcium resin binders, and calcium channel blockers.[5]

In summary, the recommendations for treatment of cholecalciferol toxicity are:

1. Decrease gastrointestinal absorption with emetics and activated charcoal, if toxicity is detected early.
2. Correct fluid and electrolyte imbalances with IV 0.9% saline, potassium supplementation prn.
3. Prevent or reduce the hypercalcemia with the use of furosemide, prednisone, and/or calcitonin.
4. Decrease the intestinal absorption of phosphorus and calcium with the use of phosphate binders and a low calcium diet.

Prognosis depends on the degree and duration of toxicity. If aggressive therapy is maintained for several weeks, complete recovery usually is achieved.

References

1. Beasley VR, Trammel HL: Incidence of poisonings in small animals, in Kirk RW (ed): *Current Veterinary Therapy. X.* Philadelphia, WB Saunders Co, 1989, pp 97–113.
2. Bell Laboratories, Inc: Technical Release: Quintox® Rat and Mouse Bait, Madison, Wisconsin, 1987.
3. Gunther R, Felice LJ, Nelson RK, Franson AM: Toxicity of a vitamin D_3 rodenticide to dogs. *JAVMA* 193:211–214, 1988.
4. Dorman DC: Anticoagulant, cholecalciferol, and bromethalin-based rodenticides. *Vet Clin North Am [Small Anim Pract]* 20:339–352, 1990.
5. Carothers MA, Chew DJ, Nagode LA: 25 (OH) Vitamin D_3 intoxication: 14 episodes in 12 dogs, in preparation.
6. Dzanis DA, Kallfelz FA: Recent knowledge of vitamin D toxicity in dogs. *Proceedings of the 6th Annual Veterinary Medical Forum, ACVIM,* 1988, pp 289–292.
7. Dougherty SA, Center SA, Dzanis DA: Salmon calcitonin as adjunct treatment for vitamin D toxicosis in a dog. *JAVMA* 196: 1269–1272, 1990.
8. Scheftel J, Setzer S, Walser M, Pertile T, Hegstad RL, Felice L, Murphy MJ: Elevated 25-hydroxy and normal 1,25–dihydroxy cholecalciferol serum concentrations in a successfully-treated case of vitamin D_3 toxicosis in a dog. *Vet Hum Toxicol* 33(4): 345–348, 1991.
9. Talcott PA, Mather GG, Kowitz EH: Accidental ingestion of a cholecalciferol-containing rodent bait in a dog. *Vet Hum Toxicol* 33(3):252–256, 1991.
10. Moore FM, Kudisch M, Richter K, Faggella A: Hypercalcemia associated with rodenticide poisoning in three cats. *JAVMA* 193:1099–1100, 1988.
11. Peterson EN, Kirby R, Sommer M, Bovee KC: Cholecalciferol rodenticide intoxication in a cat. *JAVMA* 199:904–906, 1991.
12. Thomas JB, Hood JC, Gasck F: Cholecalciferol rodenticide toxicity in a domestic cat. *Aust Vet J* 67(7):274–275, 1990.
13. Chew DJ, Carothers MA: Hypercalcemia. *Vet Clin North Am [Small Anim Pract]* 19:265–288, 1989.
14. MacKenzie CP, Burnie AG, Head KW: Poisoning in four dogs by a compound containing warfarin and calciferol. *J Small Anim Pract* 28:433–445, 1987.
15. Fooshee SK, Forrester SD: Hypercalcemia secondary to cholecalciferol rodenticide toxicosis in two dogs. *JAVMA* 196:1265–1268, 1990.
16. Garlock SM, Matz ME, Shell LG: Vitamin D_3 rodenticide toxicity in a dog. *JAAHA* 27:356–360, 1991.
17. Livezey KL, Dorman DC, Hooser SB, Buck WB: Hypercalcemia induced by vitamin D_3 toxicosis in two dogs. *Canine Pract* 16(5):26–32, 1991.

Pathophysiology of Snake Envenomization and Evaluation of Treatments—Part I

Tucson Wildlife Rehabilitation Center
Tucson, Arizona
Stormy Hudelson, DVM
Paul Hudelson, MA

KEY FACTS

❏ Venom can be composed of different toxins, depending on the season, geographic location, species, and age of the snake.

❏ Many venoms contain phospholipase A_2, which may cause the patient's body to release large volumes of prostaglandins.

❏ The most common hemodynamic effects of envenomization include an immediate fall in systemic arterial blood pressure followed by an increase in total systemic resistance, decreased cardiac output, hypoproteinemia, and increased packed cell volume.

❏ No in vivo direct test of the histamine-releasing activity of rattlesnake venom has been reported.

The treatment of snakebite remains controversial. Although human medical literature contains a great many reports concerning the efficacy and advisability of particular treatment regimens, there is a relative paucity of refereed literature on the subject from the veterinary medical community. The articles in standard texts offer only a superficial overview of treatment protocols for envenomization.[1-4] The danger of relying on such articles is that the practitioner might assume that one treatment protocol is definitive and thus would be unprepared for the potentially dangerous sequelae that can develop in cases of severe envenomization. This three-part presentation of articles is intended to provide an understanding of the complex actions of the venoms in relation to the clinical context of treatment of the envenomized patient.

There is a distinction between venomous and poisonous animals. Poisonous animals, such as the Colorado River toad *(Bufo alvarius)*, have tissues in their bodies that are toxic when ingested. Venomous animals have specialized glands that produce venom that acts to immobilize and kill prey and begin the digestive process. There are five groups of venomous snakes (Table I): Colubridae (rigid rear-fanged snakes [opisthoglyphs], such as the boomslang and the bird snake), Elapidae (rigid front-fanged snakes [proteroglyphs], such as cobras, kraits, mambas, and coral snakes), Viperidae (true vipers, hinged, front-fanged [solenoglyphs], such as adders, asps, and vipers), crotalines[a] (pit vipers [named for the heat-sensitive pits on either side of the face] and solenoglyphs, such as rattlesnakes, copperheads, cottonmouths, and Asian lanceheads), and Hydrophiidae (rigid front-fanged sea snakes [proteroglyphs]).[5] The elapids, colubrids, and hydrophiids (rigid front or rear fangs) hold their prey after striking. For example, the coral

[a]Some taxonomies place crotalines in a separate family (Crotalidae) while others leave them as a subfamily of Viperidae.

Updated from original publication in Volume 17, Number 7, July 1995

TABLE I
Genera and Species and Common Names of Selected Venomous Snakes

Genera and Species	Common Names
VIPERIDAE	
Vipera russelli	Russell's viper
Echis carinatus	saw-scaled viper
CROTALINES	
Agkistrodon piscivorus piscivorus	eastern cottonmouth
Agkistrodon piscivorus conanti	Florida cottonmouth
Agkistrodon contortix contortix	southern copperhead
Agkistrodon contortix mokeson	northern copperhead
Agkistrodon rhodostoma	Malayan pit viper
Crotalus adamanteus	eastern diamondback rattlesnake
Crotalus atrox	western diamondback rattlesnake
Crotalus durissus terrificus	South American rattlesnake
Crotalus horridus horridus	timber rattlesnake
Crotalus molossus molossus	northern black tail rattlesnake
Crotalus scutulatus scutulatus	Mohave rattlesnake
Crotalus viridis viridis	prairie rattlesnake
Trimeresurus mucrosquamatus	Chinese habu
Bothrops jararaca	jararaca
Bothrops asper	fer-de-lance
Bothrops atrox	fer-de-lance
Sistrurus catenatus	massasauga rattlesnake
ELAPIDAE	
Bungarus multicinctus	Formosan krait
Haemachatus haemachatus	ringhals
Micrurus fulvius	eastern coral snake
Micruroides euryxanthus	western or Sonoran coral snake
Naja nigricollis	spitting cobra
Naja naja atra	Chinese cobra
Naja naja naja	Indian cobra
Notechis scutatus	tiger snake
COLUBRIDAE	
Dispholidus typhus	boomslang
Thelotornis kirtlandi	bird snake
HYDROPHIIDAE	
Hydrophis cyanocinctus	annulated sea snake
Hydrophis ornatus	reef sea snake
Pelamis platurus	pelagic sea snake

ing; their toxins are primarily proteolytic and hemotoxic.[6]

VENOM CONSTITUENTS

Snake venom is an extremely complex mixture of enzymes, proteins, and peptides. To date, at least 26 enzymes have been characterized. Ten of these enzymes appear to be common to all the venoms studied. Different families of snakes generally contain higher concentrations of some fractions of enzymes than other fractions of enzymes; for example, the venoms of Elapidae are rich in acetylcholinesterase, whereas those of Crotalinae have not demonstrated any acetylcholinesterase but are rich in endopeptidase.[5] Proteolytic enzymes are found in higher concentrations in the venom of crotalines than in viperids, while elapid and hydrophiid (sea snakes) venoms contain small amounts of proteolytic enzymes or none at all.

All venoms are not equal. There is variation in toxicity among species; geographic and seasonal variation of venom toxicity within species; and seasonal and age-related differences among individuals within a species. Also, the amount of venom injected can vary with each biting incident.[7] We will discuss the more prominent components of venoms and how these components react in the body so clinicians can make more informed decisions about the treatment of envenomized patients.

EFFECTS ON THE CARDIOVASCULAR SYSTEM

The most common clinical presentation of an envenomized patient is an immediate fall in arterial resistance (decrease in systemic arterial blood pressure) followed by an increase in total systemic resistance, decreased cardiac output, hypoproteinemia, and increased packed cell volume. Increased vascular permeability can occur, often with petechiae. By this time, metabolic acidosis may be apparent, accompanied by a drop in blood pressure and ensuing shock.[8]

After intramuscular injection of *Crotalus* venom, cats demonstrate initial hemoconcentration, lactic acidemia, and hypoproteinemia.[5] This is followed by a drop in the packed cell volume, hemolysis (dependent on venom dose), shock, and labored respiration. In some cases, oliguria, respiratory rales, and death ensue. The researcher believes that the hypovolemia is secondary to leakage of red blood cells and protein from the capillaries. Approximately one third of the total circulating fluid volume can be lost into an affected extremity within hours of envenomization.[5] Both cobra (*Naja* species) and Russell's viper (*Vipera russelli*) venoms cause pooling of blood in shock organs (i.e., the lungs of cats and the hepatosplanchnic

snake (elapid) hunts other snakes and its powerful neurotoxic venom is used to immobilize its prey.[6] Rattlesnakes and other viperids (hinged, moveable, front fangs) strike and release the prey and then search for the dying animal after it has ceased mov-

bed of dogs).[9] It has been suggested that the vasodilatation seen in humans is also a contributory factor in hypotensive shock.[10]

Prostaglandin and Bradykinin Activity of Venoms

All the rattlesnake venoms that have been analyzed contained kininogenases and small amounts of factors that destroy both bradykinins and bradykinin potentiating factors. Kininogenases act on plasma globulins to form bradykinins (potent vasodilators), via activation of factor XII of the intrinsic blood coagulation pathway (Figures 1 and 2). The bradykinin-potentiating factor acts on the lung kinases so that they are unable to inactivate the bradykinins. Despite this action, the bradykinins rapidly disappear from circulation,[8] presumably through normal metabolic pathways and because of the bradykinin-destroying factors found in the venom. Bradykinins may increase prostaglandin (PG) synthesis by stimulation of endogenous phospholipase A_2, which liberates arachidonic acid from membrane phospholipids. Through a series of reactions, arachidonic acid is converted to PGI_2, PGE_2, $PGF_{2\alpha}$, and thromboxane A_2 (Figure 2).

Prostaglandin I_2 is primarily produced in endothelial cells, PGE_2 and $PGF_{2\alpha}$ are primarily produced in the kidney and spleen, and all three are produced to some degree in the heart. Thromboxane A_2 is formed primarily in the platelets.[11] Venoms, especially those of *Crotalus* species, have their own phospholipase A_2 (PLA_2) enzyme. When exogenous PLA_2 from cobra venom was perfused over guinea pig lung tissue, prostaglandins (but no histamines) were released.[12] Prostaglandin E_2 and PGI_2 decrease systemic arterial pressure via vasodilatation and therefore exacerbate hypotension.[13] When Mohave rattlesnake venom was administered intravenously to anesthetized rabbits, the observed hypotension was decreased by the administration of indomethacin. Indomethacin blocks the action of cyclooxygenase, preventing the production of PGE_2, $PGF_{2\alpha}$, and PGI_2. A rapid recovery of diastolic and systolic pressures to prevenom injection levels was also observed in the presence of indomethacin.[8]

Phospholipase A_2 and Histamine Activity of Venoms

The PLA_2 activity of mojave toxin and crotoxin causes the release of prostaglandins. Prostaglandin levels may rise high enough to produce severe congestion in localized areas of the lungs and increase vascular permeability and hemorrhage; all of these pathologies are seen at autopsy in humans who have died from envenomization.[13] This may be seen in other animals, such as cats and horses, whose primary shock organs are the lungs.

Miller and Tu[14] found that both Taiwan cobra and Mohave rattlesnake venoms cause capillary permeability increasing (CPI) activity. Because the CPI activity could be blocked by pretreatment with histamine receptor (H_1) blockers, histamine release is implicated as a causal factor of CPI activity in these two venoms.[14] The reason this assumption differs from that of Damerau et al,[12] who found no histamine release on perfused guinea pig lung tissue, may be because Miller and Tu used a purified CPI factor at three times the concentration of the LD_{50} of the crude venom. They found that hydrocortisone partially inhibited the CPI activity of the mojave CPI fraction. This could imply that the CPI fraction contains at least some PLA_2 activity and that the hydrocortisone is interacting with this pathway.[14]

When purified PLA_2 enzymes from Formosan habu and cobra venoms were applied to rat peritoneal mast cells, histamine was released. As in the Miller and Tu study, however, the concentration of the purified PLA_2 far exceeded the LD_{50} of the crude venoms.[15,16] When the PLA_2 from the Formosan habu was injected into the hind paw of rats, maximum edema occurred in one to two hours, whereas the complete venom demonstrated maximum swelling in 15 to 30 minutes. When the rats were pretreated with dexamethasone (4 mg/kg), indomethacin (10 mg/kg), or diphenhydramine (at the exceedingly high dose of 100 mg/kg), there was a reduction in the extent of edema. Dexamethasone showed a more pronounced effect on PLA_2-induced swelling and diphenhydramine was more effective for venom-induced edema. It was suggested that the antihistamine inhibits the histamine-mediated edema, but no histamines were measured.[17] When venom from the South American rattlesnake, timber rattlesnake, and massasauga rattlesnake was applied to washed rabbit platelets, greater than 50% of the histamine and serotonin stored in the platelets was released. Ten times the concentration of the prairie, western, and eastern diamondback rattlesnake venoms demonstrated no stored histamine and serotonin release by the rabbit platelets.[18] No in vivo direct test of the histamine-releasing activity of a variety of fractions of *Crotalus* species venom has been reported.[5]

Effects of Venoms on Vascular Permeability

Western diamondback rattlesnake venom disrupts the basal lamina and collagen of the capillaries. The endothelial membrane becomes thin and develops gaps, allowing leakage of red blood cells through the membrane.[19] This per rhexis hemorrhage manifests as petechiae, whereas red blood cells moving through the intercellular junctions (diapedesis) appear as ecchymoses.[20] Both types of hemorrhage could be

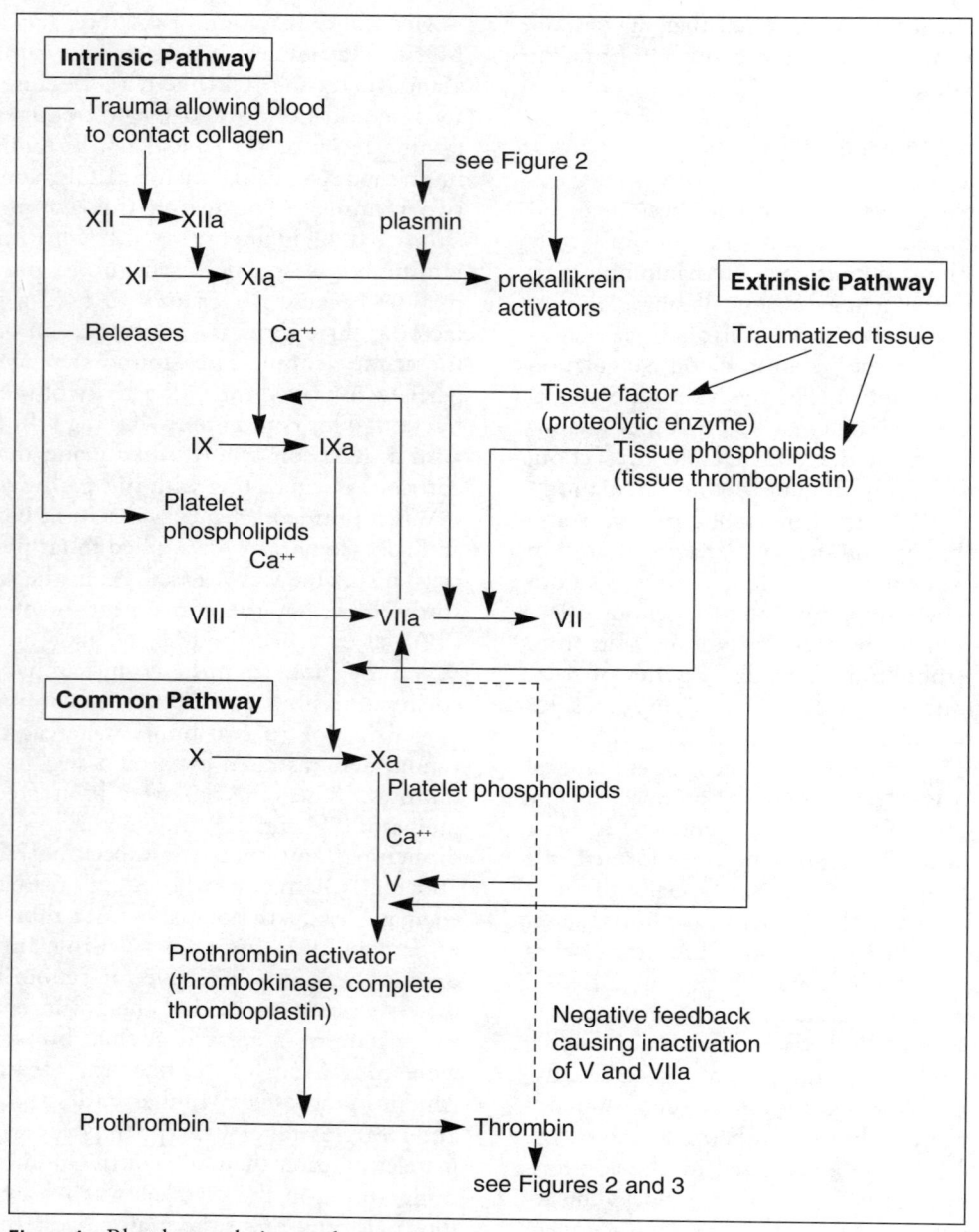

Figure 1—Blood coagulation pathways.

found in cases of western diamondback rattlesnake envenomization.[19] Systemic hemorrhage is seen in most organs when venom is injected intravenously.[8]

A lethal factor in *Crotalus* species venom transiently damages the endothelial cells of vascular walls causing a blebbing of the endothelium, dilatation of perinuclear spaces, and lysis of plasma membranes.[8,21] This microangiopathic vascular permeability allows plasma, plasma proteins, and red blood cells to leak into surrounding tissues. Affected capillaries in the skin may be seen clinically as bullae with clear serum transudate or hemorrhage, depending on the severity of the envenomization.[20] These synergistic actions of venom components ultimately cause hemoconcentration, lactic acidosis, and hypovolemic shock.[21] These could eventually lead to pulmonary edema and hemorrhage, which is most pronounced in cats, less so in rabbits, often delayed in dogs, and minor in monkeys.[5]

Cardiac, Hemolytic, and Thrombocytopenic Activity of Venoms

A cardiotoxin isolated from Taiwan cobra venom is most likely a group of substances. Among the wide variety of activities are those claimed to cause hemolysis and cardiac arrest. There is no evidence for direct action on the heart by either cobra or rattlesnake ven-

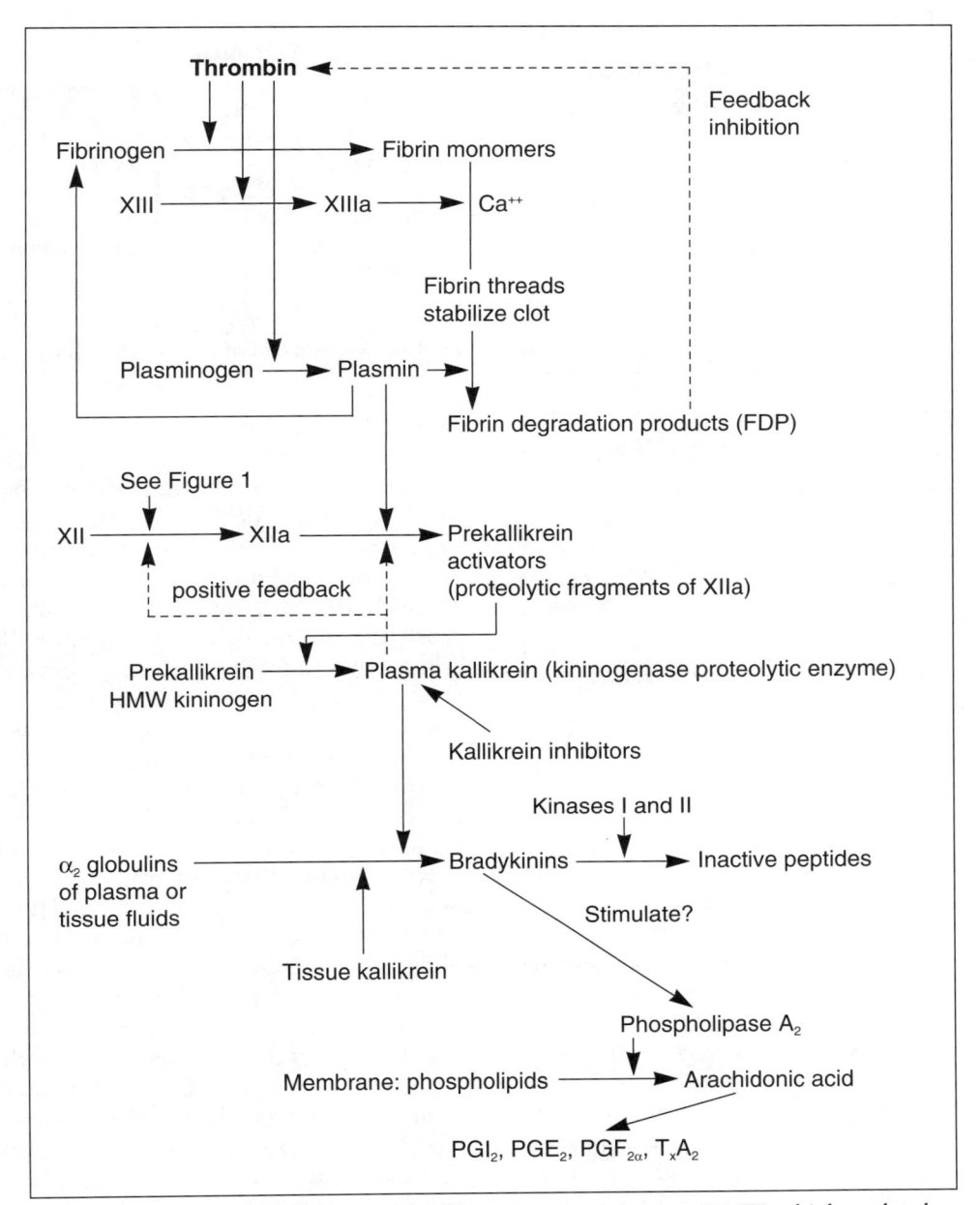

Figure 2—Simplified fibrinolytic and kinin-producing pathways. *HMW* = high-molecular-weight.

om; however, cardiac collapse could be secondary to decreased coronary perfusion.[8] In cats given intravenous eastern diamondback rattlesnake venom, myocardial ischemia, extensive subendocardial and myocardial hemorrhage, and edematous lungs with interstitial and alveolar hemorrhage have been reported.[22] The hyperkalemia associated with rhabdomyolysis could also affect cardiac performance.

Hemolysis occurs more frequently in cases of envenomization by the Elapids. South American rattlesnake venom can cause hemolysis, but envenomization by other rattlesnakes rarely, if ever, causes the condition.[8] The PLA$_2$ in venom is an esterolytic enzyme that catalyses the hydrolysis of the ester bond of lecithin, yielding fatty acids and lysolecithin, which is itself cytotoxic.[23] The PLA$_2$ reacts with the lecithin in the red blood cell membrane, thereby causing increased permeability of cell membranes and hemolysis. The precipitation of hemoglobin and red blood cell ghosts in the renal tubules is potentially toxic to the kidneys.

Thrombocytopenia can be seen in some envenomization patients. The venoms of the black tail rattlesnake, timber rattlesnake, western diamondback rattlesnake, and (to a minor degree) the Mohave rattlesnake have platelet-aggregating properties.[8,24–26]

Procoagulative Properties of Snake Venoms

Factor V activation
Factor IX activation
Factor X activation
Indirect prothrombin activation (requires phospholipids, Ca++, and factor V)
Direct prothrombin activation
Thrombinlike activity

Anticoagulative Properties of Snake Venoms

Inhibits or prevents activation of clotting proteins
Fibrinogenolytic activity
Fibrinolytic activity
Activates plasma proactivator of plasminogen
Directly activates plasminogen
Directly acts on phospholipids

$$(A\alpha)_2(B\beta)_2(\gamma)_2 \xrightarrow[H_2O]{Thrombin} \begin{cases} 2 \text{ A Fibrinopeptides} \\ + \\ 2 \text{ B Fibrinopeptides} \\ + \\ 2(\alpha\beta\gamma) \text{ Fibrin monomers} \end{cases}$$

Fibrinogen which consists of 2 tripeptides

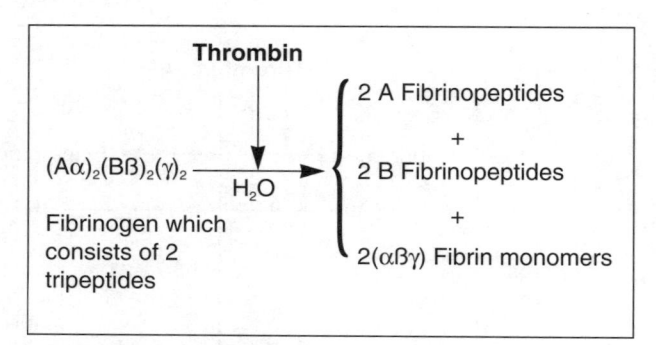

Figure 3—Conversion of fibrinogen to fibrin.

The venom of the black tail rattlesnake acts on the platelet membrane to form aggregations. Even at venom dilutions of 1:45,000, the platelets demonstrated 45% aggregation.[24] A platelet activating protein in timber rattlesnake venom has been characterized and called crotalocytin platelet aggregating protein (a serine protease).[26] Thrombocytopenia may be caused by some or all of the following: factors in the venom that cause platelet aggregation, the normal physiologic effect of platelets adhering to endothelial damaged vessels, and the production of PGE$_2$ and thromboxane A$_2$ from PLA$_2$. Prostaglandin E$_2$ and thromboxane A$_2$ cause platelet aggregation, whereas PGI$_2$ inhibits platelet aggregation.

PROCOAGULATIVE AND ANTICOAGULATIVE PROPERTIES OF VENOMS

Many studies have demonstrated procoagulative and anticoagulative properties of a variety of venoms[27] (see the boxes). The clotting proteins occur in blood as unactivated (zymogen) precursors, which are activated by surface contact with the collagen of blood vessels (e.g., factor XII) or by proteolysis. The proteolyzed and activated clotting proteins activate other zymogens in a cascadelike process within the intrinsic and extrinsic clotting pathways (Figure 1). The end result is the generation of thrombin, which converts fibrinogen to a fibrin clot, and also activates factor XIII, which stabilizes the clot (Figure 2). Thrombin also activates factors V, VII, and VIII (Figure 1). Factor X is activated in the presence of calcium by Russell's viper, northern pacific rattlesnake, and some South American and Asian pit viper venoms.[5] Factors V and X are also activated by some of the viper venoms. Elapids, viperids, and colubrids (but not crotalines) have direct prothrombin activation capabilities.[5] This prothrombin to thrombin conversion does not require calcium (Ca++), phospholipids, or factor V, although some venoms do require these cofactors for maximal activity. In vitamin K–deficient patients, elapid, viperid, and colubrid venoms convert prothrombin to thrombin. Some venoms form an intermediate product that is less easily converted to thrombin, in essence becoming anticoagulative in nature. Thrombin hydrolyzes the bonds between the fibrinopeptides and the α and ß portions of the A$_\alpha$ and B$_\beta$ chains of fibrinogen. The release of the fibrinopeptides by thrombin generates fibrin monomer (Figure 3). This exposes binding sites that allow the molecules of fibrin monomers to aggregate spontaneously and form an initially soluble clot, which traps platelets, red blood cells, and other components. Thrombin then activates factor XIII, which stabilizes the fibrin clot and renders it insoluble.[11] Thrombin also activates factor VII and factor VIII, which in turn activate factor X in the presence of Ca++ and phospholipids. The activated factor X, in turn, converts prothrombin to thrombin. Therefore, thrombin consumes platelets, fibrinogen, and Ca++ and activates factors V, VII, and VIII[28] (Figures 1 and 2).

Many snakes of the Viperidae family and Crotalinae subfamily have significant concentrations of a thrombinlike enzyme in the venom, whereas the venom of the Elapidae and Hydrophiidae families has little or none.[5] Most of the crotalid venoms studied (except that of the Mohave rattlesnake, which appears to have no hemorrhagic properties[8]) cleave only fibrinopeptide A from fibrinogen, thereby resulting in an imperfect fibrin clot. Factor XIII is not activated, so the clot is not plasmin resistant. This results in a high concentration of fibrin degradation products as well as pure defibrination. This can occur within hours[28] or as quickly as 30 minutes, as was observed in an envenomization by a Malayan pit viper.[29]

What differentiates pure defibrination from disseminated intravascular coagulation is that in defibrination, platelets and factor VIII are not consumed. In addition, this thrombinlike activity is not inhibited by heparin. Defibrination alone may be benign and self-limiting; however, it could aggravate hemorrhage due to trauma or cytolytic toxins (hemorrhagins) found in many of the venoms.

Cottonmouth venom cleaves fibrinopeptide B. Southern copperhead venom cleaves both fibrinopeptides A and B but cleaves fibrinopeptide B at a much faster rate. Therefore, these two snakes do not cause defibrination because fibrin is never formed but they do cause hypofibrinogenemia by fibrinogenolysis (dissolution of fibrinogen).[30] At high concentrations of black tail rattlesnake venom, clots are formed faster (three to four minutes) than the unstable clot can dissolve.[24] At lower venom concentrations, the reaction has enough time to cause fibrinolysis at a faster rate than fibrinogenolysis.[24] Venoms also have demonstrated fibrinolytic activity by direct action on plasminogen and/or the plasma proactivators of plasminogen. Venoms can also inhibit or prevent the activation of clotting proteins.[24] The venom PLA_2 enzymes form complexes with phospholipids, thereby rendering the phospholipids unavailable for use in the clotting cascade.[24] Proteolytic enzymes may also play a direct role in clot dissolution.[5] From this discussion it can be seen that although many venoms have coagulative properties, the combination of defibrinogenation, the continuous presence of fibrin degradation products (which themselves act as anticoagulants), and the anticoagulative nature of prothrombin intermediate products leads to an overall anticoagulative state.

SUMMARY

A familiarity with the venomous snakes in the geographic area and the most common pathologies associated with these snakes will guide the clinician toward rapid and efficient therapy for the envenomized patient. The most common clinical presentation of an envenomized patient is an immediate fall in arterial resistance (decrease in systemic arterial blood pressure) followed by an increase in total systemic resistance, a decrease in cardiac output, hypoproteinemia, and an increase in packed cell volume. Most of these effects appear to be associated with the activity of the PLA_2 enzyme present in those venoms studied.

ACKNOWLEDGMENT

The authors thank Lisa Marshall, graphic artist, for producing the figures used in this article.

About the Authors

Dr. Stormy Hudelson is a Diplomate of the American Board of Veterinary Practitioners, Avian Speciality. Mr. Paul Hudelson has been a veterinary technician and has an MA in English literature. Dr. Hudelson and Mr. Hudelson are currently affiliated with The Tucson Wildlife Rehabilitation Center in Tucson, Arizona.

REFERENCES

1. Peterson, ME, Meerdink GL: Bites and stings of venomous animals, in Kirk RW (ed): *Current Veterinary Therapy. X.* Philadelphia, WB Saunders Co, 1989, pp 177–186.
2. Blood DC, Radostits OH, Henderson JA: *Veterinary Medicine: A Textbook of the Diseases of Cattle, Sheep, Pigs, Goats and Horses*, ed 6. London, Bailliere Tindall, 1983, pp 1023–1025.
3. Ettinger SJ: *Textbook of Veterinary Internal Medicine.* Philadelphia, WB Saunders Co, 1975, pp 109–110.
4. Kirk RW, Bistner SI (eds): *Handbook of Veterinary Procedures and Emergency Treatment*, ed 4. Philadelphia, WB Saunders Co, 1985, pp 109–201.
5. Russell FE: *Snake Venom Poisoning.* Great Neck, New York, Scholium International Inc, 1983, pp 139–344.
6. Lowe CH, Schwalbe CR, Johnson TB: *Venomous Reptiles of Arizona.* Phoenix, Arizona Game and Fish Commission, 1986, pp 3–5.
7. Chippaux JP, Williams V, White J: Snake venom variability: Methods of study, results and interpretation. *Toxicon* 29(11): 1279–1303, 1991.
8. Tu AT (ed): *Rattlesnake Venoms: Their Actions and Treatment.* New York, Marcel Dekker Inc, 1982, pp 3–314.
9. Vick JA: Etiology of early endotoxin-induced bradycardia and hypotension. *Milit Med* 129:659, 1964.
10. Burch JM, Agarwal R, Hattox KL, et al: The treatment of crotalid envenomation without antivenin. *J Trauma* 28(1): 35–43, 1988.
11. Murray RK, Granner DK, Mayes PA, et al: *Harper's Biochemistry*, ed 22. Norwalk, CT, Appleton & Lange, 1990.
12. Damerau B, Lege L, Oldigs HD, et al: Histamine release, formation of prostaglandin-like activity (SRS-C) and mast cell degranulation by the direct lytic factor (DLF) and phospholipase A of cobra venom. *Naunyn Schiedebergs Arch Pharmac* 287:141–156, 1975.
13. Gopalakrishnakone P: Morphologic studies on the effects of a phospholipase A_2 complex (crotoxin) from *Crotalus durissus terrificus* venom on muscle, nerve and neuromuscular junction in the mouse. Unpublished data, PhD Thesis, University of London, 1979, pp 12–37.
14. Miller RA, Tu AT: Factors in snake venoms that increase capillary permeability. *J Pharm* 41:792–794, 1989.
15. Nagai H, Sakamoto T, Kondo M, et al: Extracellular phospholipase A_2 and histamine release from rat peritoneal mast cells. *Int Arch Allergy Appl Immunol* 96:311–316, 1991.
16. Wang JP, Teng CM: Rat paw oedema and mast cell degranulation caused by two phospholipase A_2 enzymes isolated

from *Trimeresurus mucrosquamatus* venom. *J Pharm Pharmacol* 42:846–850, 1990.
17. Chiu HF, Chen IJ, Teng CM: Edema formation and degranulation of mast cells by a basic phospholipase A_2 purified from *Trimeresurus mucrosquamatus* snake venom. *Toxicon* 27(1):115–125, 1989.
18. Markwardt F, Barthel W, Glusa E, et al: Über die freisetzung biogener amine aus blutplattchen dürch tierische fifte. *Naunyn Schmiedebergs Arch Exp Pathol Pharmak* 252:297–304, 1966.
19. Ownby CL, Bjarnason J, Tu AT: Hemorrhagic toxins from rattlesnake (*Crotalus atrox*) venom. *Am J Pathol* 93:201–210, 1978.
20. Snyder CC, Knowles RP: Snakebites: Guidelines for practical management. *Postgrad Med* 83(6):52–60, 65–68, 71–73, 75, 1988.
21. Wingert WA, Chan L: Rattlesnake bites in southern California and rationale for recommended treatment. *West J Med* 148(1):37–44, 1988.
22. Abel JH Jr., Nelson AW, Bonilla, CA: *Crotalus adamanteus* basic protein toxin: Electron microscopic evaluation of myocardial damage. *Toxicon* 11:59–63, 1973.
23. Smith TA II, Figge HL: Treatment of snakebite poisoning. *Am J Hosp Pharm* 48(10):2190–2196, 1991.
24. Hardy DL, Jeter M, Corrigan JJ Jr: Envenomation by the northern blacktail rattlesnake (*Crotalus molossus molossus*): Report of two cases and the in vitro effects of the venom on fibrinolysis and platelet aggregation. *Toxicon* 20(2):487–493, 1982.
25. Corrigan JJ Jr, Jeter MA: Mohave rattlesnake (*Crotalus scutulatus scutulatus*) venom: In vitro effect on platelets, fibrinolysis, and fibrinogen clotting. *Vet Hum Toxicol* 32(5):439–441, 1990.
26. Schmaier AH, Colman RW: Crotalocytin: Characterization of the timber rattlesnake platelet activating protein. *Blood* 56:1020–1028, 1980.
27. Denson KWE: Coagulant and anticoagulant action of snake venoms. *Toxicon* 7(1):5–11, 1969.
28. Van Mierop LHS, Kitchens CS: Defibrination syndrome following bites by the eastern diamondback rattlesnake. *J Fla Med Assoc* 67(1):21–27, 1980.
29. Reid HA, Chan HE, Thean PC: Prolonged coagulation defect (defibrination syndrome) in Malayan viper bite. *Lancet* 2:621–626, 1963.
30. Herzig RH, Ratnoff OD, Shainoff JR: Studies on a procoagulant fraction of southern copperhead venom: The preferential release of fibrin peptide B. *J Lab Clin Med* 76:451–465, 1970.

UPDATE

MYOCARDITIS

Myocarditis may be a concern for the first few days or week after envenomization, according to a report of two horses that developed myocarditis after being bitten by a Palestine viper (*Vipera palaestinae*). Electrocardiographs (ECGs) and cardiac auscultation can help monitor an animal following a bite. ECG diagnosed tachyrhythmia and ventricular premature depolarizations in one of the horses. A second horse was found dead 60 days after envenomization. Extensive diffuse necrosis of cardiac ventricular tissue was evident in both horses, consistent with exposure to toxins rather than the focal necrosis that is associated with hypoxic damage.[1]

REFERENCES
1. Hoffman A, Orgad U, Nyska A: Myocarditis following envenoming with *Vipera palaestinae* in two horses. *Toxicon* 31(12):1623–1628, 1993.

Pathophysiology of Snake Envenomization and Evaluation of Treatments—Part II

Tucson Wildlife Rehabilitation Center
Tucson, Arizona
Stormy Hudelson, DVM
Paul Hudelson, MA

KEY FACTS

❏ Neurotoxicity is primarily seen in envenomization by the elapids, by the Mohave rattlesnake and by the South American rattlesnake.

❏ The major neurotoxic effects of the venoms of the elapids and the Mohave and South American rattlesnakes are respiratory paralysis and general flaccid paralysis.

❏ It is believed that mojave toxin exerts its effect primarily on the motor nerve terminals of the diaphragm, which leads to respiratory paralysis.

❏ The extent of tissue necrosis from most rattlesnake envenomizations can be accurately evaluated 72 hours after envenomization.

❏ The primary causes of renal failure associated with snake envenomization are myoglobinuria, hemoglobinuria, defibrination syndrome, disseminated intravascular coagulation, toxic nephropathy, and hypovolemic shock.

Part I of this three-part series on snake envenomization presented an overview of the types of venomous snakes and venom constituents. The article also reviewed the effects of envenomization on the patient's cardiovascular system. The second article in this series will continue to review the pathophysiology of snake envenomization on the nervous, muscular, and urinary systems.

EFFECTS ON THE NERVOUS SYSTEM

Neurotoxicity is primarily seen in envenomization by elapids, by the Mohave rattlesnake *(Crotalus scutulatus scutulatus)*, and by the South American rattlesnake *(Crotalus durissus terrificus)*. Major peripheral nervous system effects of these venoms include respiratory paralysis and general flaccid paralysis. Convulxin, a protein isolated from South American rattlesnake venom,[1] can induce loss of equilibrium, nystagmus, and convulsions in cats. Gastrointestinal and respiratory disturbances also occurred, but subsided within 40 minutes. Because convulxin has been shown to aggregate platelets and release biogenic amines, the convulsions may result from cerebral ischemia secondary to the formation of microemboli or from massive release of autopharmacologic substances.[1] These conclusions seem to be substantiated by the results of Lomba.[2] Low amounts of ^{131}I-labelled crotoxin (a neurotoxic protein also present in Mohave rattlesnake venom) were found in the brains, spinal cords, and cerebral spinal fluid of experimentally envenomized dogs.[2]

Involvement of the autonomic nervous system is apparent from the signs of vomiting, salivation, urination, and defecation, which occur before paralysis in dogs after intravenous administration of venom from the timber rattlesnake *(Crotalus horridus horridus)* or the South American rattlesnake.[3]

Bradykinins, prostaglandins, or serotonin released in response to envenomizations by these snakes may, in part, cause these signs. The autonomic nervous system effects of notexin (a neurotoxin found in some elapids) and crotoxin (a neurotoxin from the South American rattlesnake) are not mediated by cholinergic or histaminergic mechanisms; however, the effects of crotoxin can be blocked with verapamil, a calcium channel blocker.[4,5]

Mojave toxin (venom A) interferes with neuromuscular transmission by a presynaptic nerve-blocking action. Because spontaneous release of only very small amounts of transmitter could be measured at severely intoxicated nerve end-plates, it is apparent that nerve impulses were unable to invade the motor axon terminal, thus interfering with neurotransmitter release. It seems that this effect is greatest on motor axon terminals of the diaphragm, which can lead to respiratory paralysis.[6]

Crotoxin is a neurotoxic protein that makes up 60% to 70% of the volume of crude venom from the South American rattlesnake[7] and is primarily responsible for the lethality.[8] Crotoxin consists of two components, an acidic crotapotin (crotoxin A) and a basic phospholipase A_2 (PLA_2)-like component (crotoxin B).[9] Crotoxin B from the eastern diamondback rattlesnake (*Crotalus adamanteus*) is less toxic than pure PLA_2. Crotoxin A alone has no toxic activity; however, when it is combined with crotoxin B, as it is in the crude venom, the neurotoxic effects are potentiated.[10] Crotoxin B blocks synaptic transmission by the PLA_2 moiety causing leakage of presynaptic acetylcholine vesicles within the presynaptic axon terminal.[11] The lethal toxin of the South American rattlesnake causes flaccid paralysis by interfering with depolarization-secretion coupling at the motor axon terminal, resulting in inhibition of the release of neurotransmitter.[12] Both PLA_2 and crotoxin act on the phospholipid structure of the presynaptic membrane. This action may result in the release of lysolecithin; may lead to alterations of the active zone of the axon terminal, including interference with conformation changes induced in the calcium channel by the arrival of a nerve impulse; and may increase susceptibility to transient changes in permeability in the less structured portion of the terminal membrane. Crotoxin and PLA_2 also induce alterations in the structure of the presynaptic membrane resulting, in formation of transient instabilities with an increased calcium ion (Ca^{++}) flux and a prolonged disturbance of the calcium channel and/or synchronized release of synaptic vesicles.[13]

The elapids, excluding the cobras, produce at least three neurotoxins, including taipoxin, ß-bungarotoxin, and notexin (a subunit of ß-bungarotoxin and crotoxin). These neurotoxins are homologous to either pancreatic PLA_2 or its proenzyme.[14] These toxins induce morphologic changes in the ultrastructure of the motor axon terminal, including an increase of omega-shaped profiles in the axolemma (coated pits), a depletion of synaptic vesicles, and progressive swelling and vacuolization of the mitochondria in the motor axon terminals.[15] It seems that much of the neurotoxic effect of venom PLA_2 of most of the elapids, the South American rattlesnake, and possibly the Mohave rattlesnake is due to the relative specificity for presynaptic membranes. The postsynaptic effect is considered to be of minor importance except when it contributes to total blockade.[16] Cobra venom acts by binding to receptors on the motor end-plate. This neurotoxicity can be reversed by the use of acetylcholinesterase inhibitors.[17]

EFFECTS ON THE MUSCULAR SYSTEM

Phospholipase A_2 damages the muscle cell plasma membrane, disrupts intracellular organelles, and allows an increased influx of Ca^{++} as well as an efflux of creatine and creatine kinase. The increase in Ca^{++} concentration may cause necrosis by triggering protease activity or by promoting the release of lysosomal enzymes.[18] Mojave toxins reduce the calcium sequestering activity of isolated vesicles of the sarcoplasmic reticulum.[19] This effect may cause an increase in the cellular calcium concentration and subsequently lead to cell death.[16]

When crotoxin or homologous PLA_2 was injected into the hindlimb of mice, dissolution of the muscle fibers was observed within 6 to 24 hours. By 72 hours, muscle regeneration was well established and complete in seven days.[15] The mojave toxin demonstrated a similar pattern of muscle necrosis.[6] The venom from the western diamondback rattlesnake (*Crotalus atrox*) seems to affect the fast-twitch muscle fibers preferentially.[20] Notexin occasionally causes myonecrosis if there are lesions in the plasma membrane. Myonecrosis does not occur when notexin is applied to in vitro growing, immature muscle cells or to in vivo regenerating muscles. This implies that muscle tissue in these states lacks either toxin-binding sites or an important substrate.[21] Taipoxin and venom from the spitting cobra (*Naja nigricollis*) also produce myonecrosis; however, ß-bungarotoxin does not.

The histologic appearance of muscle tissue in mice that received intramuscular injections of a variety of rattlesnake venoms demonstrated coagulative necrosis, myolytic necrosis, or a combination of the two. All the elapid venoms studied caused myolytic myonecrosis.[22] Myotoxin-α (isolated from prairie rattlesnake [*Crotalus viridis viridis*] venom)[23] given intramuscularly to mice caused complete vacuolation and loss of striation in muscle tissue at 48 and 72 hours.[1]

When the crude venom was administered, hemorrhage, hemolysis, severe mitochondrial changes, and destruction of external lamina and sarcolemma were seen. Crotoxin caused similar pathologic changes.[24] Some venoms, most notably those of the western diamondback rattlesnake and prairie rattlesnake, caused myonecrosis and hemorrhage. These effects may be caused, at least in part, by ischemia from hypotension and by capillary permeability–increasing activity, which cause a decrease in blood supply and oxygen and result in cellular death.[25] When rhabdomyolysis occurs, various intracellular muscle constituents are released into the circulation, thereby resulting in myoglobinemia, hyperphosphatemia, hyperkalemia, hyperuricemia, metabolic acidosis, and intravascular volume depletion.[26] These conditions can affect other organs and body systems, most notably the kidneys and the cardiovascular system.

In addition to factors that cause myonecrosis, many venoms also contain collagenase (which digests collagen) and hyaluronidase (which catalyzes the hydrolysis of hyaluronic acid). With the breakdown of the hyaluronic barrier, venom can more easily penetrate tissues.[27]

EFFECTS ON THE URINARY SYSTEM

Renal failure has been associated with snake envenomization. The primary causes include the nephrotoxic effects of myoglobinuria and hemoglobinuria, defibrination syndrome, disseminated intravascular coagulation, toxic nephropathy, and hypovolemic shock.

Any snake envenomization that causes muscular necrosis could cause the release of myoglobin. In the case of Mohave rattlesnake envenomization, there may be no local signs of tissue necrosis and only mild swelling.[28] In these cases, finding dark or red urine in conjunction with increasing serum creatinine levels should alert the clinician to myoglobinuric renal failure. Supportive laboratory findings may include myoglobinemia, myoglobinuria, hyperphosphatemia, hyperkalemia, hyperuricemia, metabolic acidosis, and hypocalcemia.

Low serum calcium levels are often associated with acute and chronic renal failure but may be the consequence of increased serum phosphate levels from the rhabdomyolysis, which induces a reciprocal depression of serum calcium levels.[29] Hypercalcemia may become apparent during the diuretic phase of recovery from tubular necrosis or, more rarely, before diuresis.[30] Metabolic acidosis may result from hypoxemia, hypovolemia, release of lactate from muscle, or the nephrotoxic effects of rhabdomyolysis.[31]

Hyperkalemia is associated with the release of potassium from damaged muscle tissue, decreased glomerular filtration rate, and myoglobinuric renal failure. Hyperkalemia is most pronounced in those animals developing oliguric renal failure.[26] Hyperuricemia may be caused (1) by the release of purines from muscle tissue, which are converted to uric acid in the liver or (2) from the decreased renal elimination of urates in animals that convert purines to uric acid.[26] A rapid increase in uric acid alone may cause acute renal failure.[32]

When myoglobin is released from damaged muscle tissue into the circulation, approximately 50% is bound to an α_2-globulin. The free myoglobin is filtered by the glomeruli of the kidneys. Myoglobinuria occurs when the renal threshold of myoglobin is exceeded.[33] At a urine pH less than 5.6, myoglobin dissociates to ferrihemate and globin. The ferrihemate fraction is nephrotoxic and can cause deterioration of renal function regardless of urine pH.[34] These effects are magnified by low urine flow states.

The histologic findings in myoglobinuric renal failure consist of epithelial degeneration and necrosis, basement membrane disruption (tubulorrhexis), heme casts (indicating acute tubular disease), interstitial edema, and leukocytic infiltration.[35]

Urinalysis often reveals red blood cells and protein. If myoglobin concentrations are high enough, the urine will be discolored. In alkaline urine, myoglobin appears red or pink; in acidic urine, the myoglobin dissociates and the ferriheme turns the urine a dark reddish-brown. If there is a low glomerular filtration rate with dilute urine being excreted, massive muscle necrosis can be present without visible myoglobinuria; with a normal glomerular filtration rate and concentrated urine being excreted, visible myoglobinuria may be present with minimal myonecrosis.[33]

Differentiating myoglobin from hemoglobin in the urine may be difficult with readily available methods. Hemoglobin is bound to haptoglobin in the plasma until concentrations exceed the renal threshold. Therefore, when the concentration of hemoglobin approaches the renal threshold, plasma can appear pink from the hemoglobin while the urine remains clear. The renal threshold for myoglobin is less than the protein-binding capacity. Therefore, at plasma concentrations above the protein-binding capacity of myoglobin, all myoglobin is filtered through the kidneys, which prevents pink discoloration of the plasma. Urine that is positive for occult blood in the absence of large numbers of red blood cells in the sediment and in conjunction with clear plasma would be indicative of myoglobinuria. Pink plasma indicates some degree of hemoglobinuria.[33]

Intravascular hemolysis can occur with some types of snake envenomization, releasing hemoglobin into circulation. Hemoglobin dissociates to ferrihemate and haptoglobin at a urine pH less than 5.6, and ferrihemate is directly nephrotoxic.[34,36] Because free hemoglobin is cleared from the circulation within hours, the absence of hemoglobinemia or hemoglobinuria does not necessarily indicate the absence of hemoglobinuric acute renal failure.[37] The hemoglobin molecule is too large to penetrate cells unless they are damaged, as they might be by anoxia or ischemia resulting from the hypotension of envenomization.[36] Fibrin strands occasionally develop in the glomerulus, adhering to and thickening the glomerular filtration membrane. This thickening, which may occur in cases of intravascular hemolysis, disseminated intravascular coagulation, and defibrination, decreases the glomerular filtration rate.[37] Histologic changes due to intravascular hemolysis are similar to those seen in myoglobinuric renal failure with the added changes that fibrin deposits can be seen within Bowman's space and epithelial cell proliferation may be present.[38] Fibrin degradation products and fibrinopeptide α, which results from the cleavage of fibrinogen to form fibrin monomers, are filtered and excreted in the urine. Serial measurements of fibrin degradation products and fibrinopeptide α can be helpful in following the course of the pathologic process.[38]

The microthrombi that occur with some envenomizations following disseminated intravascular coagulation[39–41] can lead to acute tubular necrosis or cortical necrosis.[37] Cortical necrosis is more likely when disseminated intravascular coagulation is accompanied by hypovolemic shock.[37] Anuria is a common feature of cortical necrosis. If urine is produced, it usually demonstrates moderate proteinuria, a low specific gravity, numerous red blood cells, red blood cell casts, white blood cells, and granular casts. Histologically, necrosis can range from focal to complete tubular or cortical involvement.[37]

Direct nephrotoxicity of snake venom has been difficult to prove because the resultant systemic disturbances of envenomizations can themselves induce acute renal failure.[42] ^{125}I-labelled venom from the saw-scaled viper (*Echis carinatus*) was shown to be excreted in the urine.[43] Isolated rat kidney perfused with venom of Russell's viper (*Vipera Russelli*) at concentrations most likely to occur in envenomization (less than 80 ng/g) demonstrated definite nephrotoxicity. The likely site of nephrotoxicity is the proximal tubules.[44]

CONCLUSION

As illustrated by this and the first article of this series, a thorough understanding of the pathophysiology of snake envenomization is crucial to adequately evaluate and treat the envenomized patient. Because some of the more serious effects of envenomization, such as respiratory paralysis and acute renal failure, may not develop for several hours after envenomization, it is imperative that the patient be monitored for a minimum of 24 hours in a hospital setting. The third article in this series will review the signs and diagnosis of envenomization and evaluate various treatment regimens.

About the Authors

Dr. Stormy Hudelson is a Diplomate of the American Board of Veterinary Practitioners, Avian Speciality. Mr. Paul Hudelson has been a veterinary technician and has an MA in English literature. Dr. Hudelson and Mr. Hudelson are currently affiliated with The Tucson Wildlife Rehabilitation Center in Tucson, Arizona.

REFERENCES

1. Brazil OV: Neurotoxins from the South American rattlesnake. *J Formo Med Assoc* 71:394–400, 1972.
2. Lomba MG: Estudios sobre a distriduicao e excrecao da crotoxinal-^{131}I em caes. Unpublished data. PhD thesis, State University of Campinas, Sao Paulo, Brazil, 1969, pp 7–74.
3. Brazil OV, Prado-Franceschi J, Waisbich E: Pharmacology of crystaline crototoxin: I. Toxicity. *Mem Inst Butantan Simp Internac* 33:973–980, 1966.
4. Harris JB, Zar HA: The effects of a toxin isolated from Australian tiger snake (*Notechis scutatus scutatus*) venom on autonomic neuromuscular transmission. *Br J Pharmacol* 62:349–358, 1978.
5. Muniz ZM, Diniz CR: The effect of crotoxin on the longitudinal muscle-myenteric plexus preparation of the guinea pig ileum. *Neuropharmacology* 28(7):741–747, 1989.
6. Gopalakrishnakone P, Hawgood BJ, Holbrooke SE, et al: Sites of action of Mojave toxin isolated from the venom of the Mojave rattlesnake. *Br J Pharmacol* 69:421–431, 1980.
7. Breithaupt H: Neurotoxin and myotoxic effects of Crotalus phospholipase A and its complex with crotapotin. *Naunvn Schiedebergs Arch Pharmac* 292:271–278, 1976.
8. Fortes-Dias CL, Fonesca BCB, Kochva E, et al: Purification and properties of an antivenom factor from the plasma of the South American rattlesnake (*Crotalus durissus terrificus*). *Toxicon* 29(8):997–1008, 1991.
9. Delot E, Bon C: Differential effects of presynaptic phospholipase A_2 neurotoxins on *Torpedo* synaptosomes. *J Neurochem* 58(1):311–319, 1992.
10. Hendon PA, Fraenkel-Conrat H: The role of complex formation in the neurotoxicity of crotoxin A and B. *Toxicon* 14:283–289, 1976.
11. Hanley MR: Crotoxin effects of *Torpedo californica* cholinergic excitable vesicles and the role of its phospholipase A activity. *Biochem Biophys Res Commun* 82:392–401, 1978.
12. Hawgood BJ, Smith JW: The mode of action at the mouse neuromuscular junction of the phospholipase A-crotapotin complex isolated from the venom of the South American rattlesnake. *Br J Pharmacol* 61:597–606, 1977.
13. Hawgood BJ, Santana de Sa S: Changes in spontaneous and evoked release of transmitter induced by the crotoxin complex and its component phospholipase A_2 at the frog neuromuscular junction. *Neuroscience* 4:293–303, 1979.
14. Chang CC, Lee JD, Eaker D, et al: The pre-synaptic neuromuscular blocking action of taipoxin: A comparison with β-

bungarotoxin and crotoxin. *Toxicon* 15:571–576, 1977.
15. Gopalakrishnakone P, Hawgood BJ: Morphological changes in murine nerve, neuromuscular junction, and skeletal muscle induced by the crotoxin complex. *J Physiol* (Lond) 291:5–6P, 1979.
16. Tu AT (ed): *Rattlesnake Venoms: Their Actions and Treatment*. New York, Marcel Dekker, 1982, pp 121–246.
17. Tu AT: *Venoms: Chemistry and Molecular Biology*. New York, John Wiley & Sons, 1977, pp 97–103.
18. Gutierrez JM: Myonecrosis induced by Bothrops asper venom-pathogenesis and treatment. *Proc 2nd Am Symp on Animal, Plant and Microbial Toxins*: 27–39, 1986.
19. Cate RL, Bieber AL: Effects of mojave toxin on rat skeletal sarcoplasmic reticulum. *Biochem Biophys Res Commun* 72:295–301, 1976.
20. Stewart RM, Page CP, Schwesinger WH, et al: Antivenin and fasciotomy/debridement in the treatment of the severe rattlesnake bite. *Am J Surg* 158(12):543–547, 1989.
21. Harris JB, Johnson HA, MacDonell CA: Muscle necrosis induced by some presynaptically active neurotoxins, in Eaker D, Wadstrom T (eds): *Natural Toxins: Toxicon Suppl No. 2*. Oxford, Pergamon Press, 1980, pp 569–578.
22. Homma M, Tu AT: Morphology of local tissue damage in experimental snake envenomation. *Br J Exp Pathol* 52:538–542, 1971.
23. Ownby CL, Cameron D, Tu AT: Isolation of myotoxic component from rattlesnake (*Crotalus viridis viridis*) venom. *Am J Pathol* 85:149–158, 1976.
24. Cameron DL, Tu AT: Chemical and functional homology of myotoxin-α from prairie rattlesnake venom and crotamine from South American rattlesnake venom. *Biochim Biophys Acta* 532:147–154, 1978.
25. Snyder CC, Knowles RP: Snakebites: Guidelines for practical management. *Postgrad Med* 83(6):52–60, 65–68, 71–73, 75, 1988.
26. Curry SC, Chang D, Connor D: Drug and toxin-induced rhabdomyolysis. *Ann Emerg Med* 18(Oct):1068–1084, 1989.
27. Russell FE: *Snake Venom Poisoning*. Great Neck, NY, Scholium International Inc, 1983, pp 168–172.
28. Jansen PW, Perkin PM, Van Stralen D: Mojave rattlesnake envenomation: Prolonged neurotoxicity and rhabdomyolysis. *Ann Emerg Med* 21(3):322–325, 1992.
29. Hood VL, Johnson JR: Acute renal failure with myoglobinuria after tiger snake bite. *Med J Aust* 2(Oct 18):638–641, 1975.
30. Gabow PA, Kaehny WD, Kelleher SP: The spectrum of rhabdomyolysis. *Medicine* 61:141–152, 1982.
31. McCarron DA, Elliot WC, Rose JS: Severe mixed metabolic acidosis secondary to rhabdomyolysis. *Am J Med* 67:905–908, 1979.
32. Smith WE, Steele TN: The hyperuricemic nephropathies, in Suki WN, Massry SG (eds): *Therapy of Renal Diseases and Related Disorders*. Boston, Martinus Nijhoff Publishers, 1984, pp 327–333.
33. Knochel JP: Rhabdomyolysis and myoglobinuria. *Semin Nephrol* 1:75–86, 1981.
34. Anderson WAD, Morrison DB, Williams EF Jr.: Pathologic changes following injections of ferriheme (hematin) in dogs. *Arch Pathol* 33:589–602, 1942.
35. Azevedo-Marques MN, Cupo P, Coimbra TN, et al: Myonecrosis, myoglobinuria and acute renal failure induced by South American rattlesnake (*Crotalus durissus terrificus*) envenomization in Brazil. *Toxicon* 23(4):631–636, 1985.
36. Braun AR, Weiss FR, Keller AI, et al: Evaluation of the renal toxicity of heme proteins and their derivatives: A role in the genesis of acute tubule necrosis. *J Exp Med* 131(3):443–460, 1970.
37. Dubrow A, Flamenbaum W: Acute renal failure associated with myoglobinuria and hemoglobinuria, in Brenner BM, Lazarus JM (eds): *Acute Renal Failure*, ed 2. New York, Churchill Livingstone, 1988, pp 264–293.
38. Vaziri ND, Kaupke CJ: Biochemical investigations of urine, in Massry SG, Glassock RJ (eds): *Textbook of Nephrology, Vol 2*, ed 2. Baltimore, Williams & Wilkins, 1989, 1613–1614.
39. Hatano M (ed): *Nephrology Volume I: Proceedings of the XIth International Congress of Nephrology*. Tokyo, Springer-Verlag, 1991, pp 794–803.
40. Harris ARC, Hurst PE, Saker BM: Renal failure after snake bite. *Med J Aust* 2(Sep 11):409–411, 1976.
41. White J, Fasset R: Acute renal failure and coagulopathy after snakebite. *Med J Aust* 2(Aug 6) 142–143, 1983.
42. Burdmann EA, Woronik V, Prado EBA, et al: Snakebite-induced acute renal failure: An experimental model. *Am J Trop Med Hyg* 48(1):82–88, 1993.
43. Greenwood BM, Warrel PA, Davidson NMcD, et al:Immunodiagnosis of snake bite. *Br Med J* 4:743–745, 1974.
44. Ratcliffe PJ, Pukrittayakamee S, Ledingham JGG, et al: Acute renal failure in the isolated perfused kidney, induced by Russell's viper venom. *Clin Sci Suppl II* 68(SII):39–40, 1985.

UPDATE

CENTRAL NERVOUS SYSTEM

Results from 96% of electroencephalograms (EEGs) of human patients bitten by either a Russell's viper (*Vipera russelli*), a common cobra of Sri Lanka (*Naja naja*), a hump-nosed viper (*Hypnale hypnale*), or a dogfaced freshwater snake suggest onset of an encephalopathy within hours of the bite. Abnormalities persisted for several days without clinical neurological effects. These changes, primarily of the temporal lobe, occurred with or without the use of antivenin.[1]

REFERENCES

1. Ramachandran S, Ganaikabahu B, Pushparajan K, Wijesekera J: Electroencephalographic abnormalities in patients with snake bites. *Am J Trop Med Hyg* 52(1):25–28, 1995.

Pathophysiology of Snake Envenomization and Evaluation of Treatments—Part III

Tucson Wildlife Rehabilitation Center
Tucson, Arizona
Stormy Hudelson, DVM
Paul Hudelson, MA

KEY FACTS

❏ If rhabdomyolysis occurs, lactic acidosis and hyperkalemia are special problems that should be considered when selecting fluids for intravenous administration.

❏ The number of vials of the appropriate antivenin used is directly related to the clinical signs, body fluid volume of the patient, and the location of the bite.

❏ Antivenin administration may still be beneficial 60 hours after envenomization.

❏ Antihistamines are of little value in the treatment of snake envenomization.

❏ Corticosteroid therapy is beneficial for the treatment of anaphylaxis, inflammation, and capillary permeability; it also blocks the action of phospholipase A_2.

The first two articles in this series focused on the pathophysiology of snake envenomization by examining the effects of venom and venom constituents on the cardiovascular, nervous, muscular, and urinary systems. This last article reviews the diagnosis, signs, and treatment of the envenomized patient. We cannot sufficiently emphasize the fact that each case of envenomization is unique. No one treatment protocol is recommended; instead, treatment is directed toward the clinical signs with the understanding that vigilant patient monitoring is a crucial component of successful treatment.

DIAGNOSIS AND CLINICAL SIGNS

The in vivo effects of venoms of snakes vary from species to species. The composition of venom can vary dramatically among individuals of a single species and even between serial samples from a venom specimen.[1] Therefore, no single set of characteristic signs diagnoses snake envenomization successfully. Some laboratories can perform blood analysis to determine the concentration and type of venom injected. This can help to determine whether antivenin is appropriate and what type and how much antivenin to use; however, levels of venom do not necessarily correlate with levels of the individual toxic compounds except in bothropic envenomizations.[2] Signs of envenomization can vary from mild discomfort at the site of envenomization to profound hemorrhagic and neurologic alterations. Copperhead bites are typically minimally painful and symptomatic. Conversely, in some areas, envenomization by Mohave rattlesnakes *(Crotalus scutulatus scutulatus)* can cause rapid death from respiratory paralysis.

In general, pit viper envenomization demonstrates local effects, such as fang marks (one to several with repeated striking); pain, which normally develops immediately; and rapid swelling primarily from edema. Most bites can be considered dry or nonpoisonous if no pain or swelling occurs within one hour of envenomization[3]; however, some envenomizations by the Mohave rattlesnake can be life-threatening even if there is no pain and only slight swelling.[4] Additional local signs may include erythemia, petechia, ecchymosis, bullae, cyanosis, myonecrosis, and tissue slough.[3,5] Systemic signs may include all to none of the following: nausea, vomiting, mental confusion, hypotension, respiratory distress, bleeding disorders, weakness, tachycardia, increased thirst, perioral numbness, fever, arrhythmia, and nystagmus.[5–7]

Large animals are usually bitten on the muzzle and develop extensive facial, muzzle, and submandibular swelling and edema, which may cause inspiratory dyspnea. Epistaxis may also be seen.[8] Tiger snake (*Notechis scutatus*) envenomization in horses often demonstrates pronounced pupillary dilatation, negative pupillary light reflex, positive menace response, and drooping eyelids (ptosis). Trembling is evident in standing equine patients and may even progress to paralysis in recumbent horses. Sweating may be pronounced.[9] Mohave rattlesnake envenomization in some areas (such as southern California) may manifest primarily as respiratory paralysis and myoglobinuric renal failure with minimal swelling. A dark or red change in urine color and rising serum creatinine levels can help in diagnosing rhabdomyolysis and myoglobinuric renal failure when there is little or no local reaction.[10,11] In other areas, a Mohave rattlesnake bite may be more benign, causing only hypotension and ptosis.[12]

The elapids, most notably the coral snakes (*Micrurus* and *Micruroides* species), leave tiny fang or tooth marks with little or no local swelling. No signs may appear for 1 to 7½ hours, but once evident, they can progress very rapidly. Signs may start with salivation, vomiting, and apprehension and progress into convulsions, bulbar paralysis involving cranial motor nerves, and death from respiratory paralysis. In human patients, respiratory paralysis usually resolves after three days of mechanically assisted respiration.[3,13]

Special note should be made for those patients with repeated exposure to venom (e.g., hunting dogs). IgE antibodies have been found in the blood of some human patients who have had previous exposure to snake venom from working in a laboratory with lyophilized venom, who have received multiple snake bites, or who were handling venomous snakes. One snake handler, who was bitten in the hand by a rattlesnake, collapsed and developed cyanosis and wheezing but no urticaria. Another handler developed acute dyspnea, rhinorrhea, conjunctivitis, and thickening of the tongue and palate after a nonbite exposure to rinkals (*Hemachatus haemachatus*) venom. This patient had specific IgE antibodies to numerous snake venoms.[14,15] Repeated exposure to venom does not necessarily cause hypersensitivity—certain Ecuadorian Indians were found to have protective antibodies against the venoms of snakes in that area.[16]

EVALUATION OF TREATMENTS

With the numerous in vivo reactions that can occur with various snake venoms, there is no single treatment regimen appropriate for the care of the envenomized patient. Blood and urine should be collected for baseline data at the time of patient presentation. Routine urinalysis can help to identify rhabdomyolysis and/or urinary tract bleeding. Complete blood cell count and platelet count as well as evaluation of serum chemistries, electrolytes, and bleeding profile can help in monitoring the progress of the patient. Early blood crossmatching for transfusion is important because if defibrination occurs, the red blood cell clumping makes crossmatching impossible.[17] A culture of the wound is also helpful if bacterial infection develops. With the predominance of anaerobic bacteria found in the mouth of the snake, anaerobic cultures should be considered in addition to aerobic cultures. Marking the levels of the swelling every 15 minutes can help the clinician determine the severity of envenomization.[18]

Intravenous Fluid Therapy

Intravenous fluid administration is generally accepted as appropriate first-line treatment, because hypovolemic shock and decreased cardiac output occur with most envenomizations. The appropriate type of fluids depends on the electrolyte imbalance, degree of hypovolemia, and whether coagulopathy is present. With rhabdomyolysis, increased lactic acid and K^+ are special problems. Lactated Ringer's solution is contraindicated if lactic acidosis is present. Because some degree of lactic acidosis is present in most envenomizations, this fluid would be contraindicated in the treatment of snake bite. Normasol-R® and Plasmalyte® are good fluid choices because of the pH (5.5 to 8.0), absence of lactate and calcium, and mild systemic antiacidotic action. Solutions containing potassium should be used cautiously, if at all, in patients with hyperkalemia and/or renal failure.

In severe cases of hypovolemic shock, the use of colloids may be warranted. Six percent hetastarch (a plasma volume expander) in 0.9% sodium chloride has a pH of 5.9 (3.5 to 7.0). The main disadvantage of hetastarch is that it is contraindicated, as are many of the colloids, if bleeding disorders are present because it transiently prolongs prothrombin, partial thromboplastin, and clotting times. In the presence of coagulopathies, platelet-rich plasma, fresh or frozen plasma, or whole blood may be the most appropriate fluids for rapid normalization of clotting factors.[7] Blood products may be ineffective in cases of pit viper envenomization if defibrination has occurred.[17]

Antivenin Therapy

Antivenin therapy is rarely contraindicated; however, it may be inappropriate for patients with a history of anaphylaxis to antivenin. Many large animals are treated solely with supportive therapy because of the expense of administering adequate volumes of antivenin.[8,9] Some cases of mild envenomization may be successfully treated with supportive therapy. Careful monitoring of the patient is important because an apparently mild case of envenomization may rapidly progress to a moderate or severe case over a period of hours.[19]

There is no correlation between intradermal skin testing and predictability of early antivenin reactions (anaphylaxis).[20] This may be due to the anticomplementary activity of the commercial antivenins seen in vitro; however, no evidence of complement activation or the appearance of immune complexes after antivenin treatment could be found in 11 human patients with generalized anaphylaxis. All 11 patients had a negative skin test reaction.[20]

Antivenin Administration

The administration of antivenin begins by reconstituting the antivenin with the accompanying diluent or sterile water. If the diluent is warmed before reconstitution, the antivenin dissolves faster.[6] If intravenous envenomization has not occurred, the antivenin can be delivered in the intravenous fluids and administered over a period of one or more hours, depending on the severity of signs and the number of vials to be used. The number of vials used is directly related to the clinical signs, body fluid volume of the patient, and the location of bite. In humans bitten by rattlesnakes, a minimum of 20 vials of antivenin is routinely used. Snake bites on digits or in small animals may require 50% more antivenin than bites in larger animals or bites excluding digits.[6] More antivenin is needed in these cases because of the relatively small volume of body fluid in smaller animals, which results in higher absolute venom concentrations and the difficulty of attaining high antivenin concentrations in digits.[6,21,22] There is no maximum dose of antivenin. The total dose is based on the monitoring of clinical signs and treatment effects.[18] The end point is usually interpreted as the point when the pain associated with the bite is relieved.[5]

In veterinary medicine, this end point may be difficult to recognize and, as mentioned, some Mohave rattlesnake bites are accompanied by very little pain. It may be more appropriate to perform serial neurologic, physical, and coagulopathy examinations and discontinue the antivenin when there seems to be no further progression of the envenomization. More antivenin may be needed if signs return. This situation can occur if one fang has penetrated a vessel or muscle and the other fang has deposited venom in adipose tissue, which results in different venom absorption rates.[7,11,17,21] The analysis of six lots of a commercial antivenin found one to two grams of equine protein per vial. An average of 18% of this was protective IgG.[19] In addition, significant amounts of specific neutralizing IgG are lost during the ammonium sulfate processing. It is no wonder that large volumes of antivenin may be required.

In most cases, if signs of envenomization are evident, antivenin should be given as soon as possible. Patients that have been intravenously inoculated with venom require an immediate intravenous push of antivenin. Humans treated for intravenous rattlesnake envenomization required an average of 20 vials of antivenin intravenously administered as rapidly as the antivenin was reconstituted. At this time methylprednisolone was also given, and no adverse reactions to the antivenin were seen.[23]

In less severe cases, antivenin can be diluted in fluids and given at a slower rate. Initial antivenin doses should be given within two hours of envenomization. A study of eastern diamondback rattlesnake (*Crotalus adamanteus*) envenomization in dogs found that if antivenin, without other supportive treatment, was given 30 minutes after the venom was injected subcutaneously, eight out of eight dogs survived. If the antivenin was given four hours after envenomization, five out of eight survived; if given at eight hours, only one dog survived. The degree of tissue necrosis followed a similar pattern.[24] Mice and rabbits administered ^{131}I-labeled venom still had detectable levels of venom 72 hours after venom injection. Consequently, antivenin may still have therapeutic benefits for at least 60 hours after envenomization.[18]

Treatment delays may be more hazardous in digit bites and in envenomizations of smaller animals because of the lack of venom dilution. Patients envenomized by coral snakes or Mohave rattlesnakes may have delayed neurologic signs, but these signs can progress at an alarming rate. Human patients bitten by coral snakes had a much lower recovery rate if they were treated after signs of envenomization occurred.[6,13] Antivenin should be administered immediately, and the patient should be hospitalized for at least 24 hours for observation.[6] It is also important to remember that the antivenin for eastern coral snakes is not effective against the Arizona or Sonoran coral snakes (Micruroides euryxanthus).

Anaphylaxis

Anaphylaxis may occur with the administration of antivenin or in cases where there has been repeated exposure to venom. We could find no case reports in the veterinary field concerning this phenomenon. This may be due to the fact that, until recently, most animal envenomization cases were treated with rapid-acting steroids with or without concurrent antivenin therapy. In the rare case where an animal presented in anaphylaxis due to circulating IgE levels from previous exposure to venom, epinephrine is considered the preferred initial therapy.[14,25,26] Epinephrine can be given intravenously in life-threatening situations. Because the half-life of epinephrine is only two minutes, an epinephrine infusion may be necessary, or a subcutaneous dose given at the same time as the initial intravenous dose may be appropriate. The subcutaneous route will result in bronchodilatation within 5 to 10 minutes with maximum effect in 20 minutes.

Epinephrine also can be administered endotracheally; however, this route achieves one tenth the plasma concentration and hemodynamic effects of the intravenous route.[27] The β and α adrenergic properties of epinephrine cause vasoconstriction, which directly antagonizes the generalized vasodilatation produced by histamine release; epinephrine also reverses the increased permeability to plasma of dilated vessels. These combined effects can rapidly restore circulating blood volume and blood pressure. Epinephrine also causes smooth muscle relaxation thus relieving bronchospasms, wheezing, and dyspnea due to anaphylaxis.[28] Corticosteroids should be given concurrently with epinephrine to reduce bronchospasms and inflammatory edema.[14,26]

Antihistamines are of little value in cases of antivenin anaphylaxis because histamine may already be present at receptor sites, and there are many mediators responsible for anaphylaxis that are not affected by antihistamines.[26] Antihistamines would be partially protective if they could be administered before the antigen (i.e., antivenin). Antihistamines that are H_1–receptor blockers (e.g., diphenhydramine) antagonize all the actions of histamine when given before the antigen, except the stimulation of hydrochloric acid secretion in the stomach and the part of vasodilatation mediated by H_2–receptors.

Antihistamines may have the added benefit of sedation, but in some individuals agitation or restlessness may occur,[29] as seen in cats. Antihistamines may also potentiate the effects of central nervous system depressant drugs.[29] If appropriate sedation is not obtained with the use of antihistamines, further sedation may be difficult to control. A leading manufacturer of Crotalidae polyvalent antivenin warns against the use of antihistamines, claiming that they may potentiate the effect of snake venom. In mild cases of anaphylaxis, slowing the rate of administration of the antivenin may be effective in stopping the anaphylactic signs.[23]

In experimental envenomizations using Chinese habu (Trimeresurus mucrosquamatus) venom and the purified PLA_2 from that venom, there was some evidence that suggested a mild, histamine-mediated edema. Pretreatment of rats with diphenhydramine at a dose of 100 mg/kg was beneficial in decreasing the edema, and dexamethasone given at 4 mg/kg was equally beneficial. The antihistamine had little or no effect on the PLA_2 portion of the venom.[30]

Serum Sickness

In humans, approximately 50% of snake bite victims who were treated with antivenin developed serum sickness, a type III hypersensitivity. Serum sickness can occur up to 30 days after antivenin administration. In humans, the typical signs of serum sickness include elevated body temperature, swollen lymph nodes, generalized urticarial rash, and painful joints.[46] Patients treated with steroids at the time of antivenin administration developed serum sickness only 13% of the time.[5] When antihistamines were administered for serum sickness, the disease progressed until steroid therapy was instituted.[18,46] Because type III hypersensitivity reactions are a result of antigen–antibody complexes formed in the presence of relative antigen excess rather than histamine reactions, it is not surprising that antihistamines are ineffectual.

A literature review revealed that 83% of human patients who did not receive steroid therapy developed serum sickness. Consequently, the reviewers recommended dispensing a two-week course of methylprednisolone at gradually tapering doses for patients treated with more than seven vials of antivenin.[21] In veterinary medicine, serum sickness may not be a significant problem because of the cost of antivenin in light of the number of vials needed for treatment.

Steroid Therapy

A review of the literature concerning steroid use in snake envenomization revealed little information regarding contraindications other than general statements claiming steroids may be contraindicated. The most notable concerns with steroid use were in early human literature. According to these sources, human patients were treated with one to three vials of antivenin, corticosteroids, and massive excision of the tissues surrounding the bite site with or without fasciotomy. The outcome of this regimen often resulted in superinfections. These infections were especially difficult to resolve because the newer generation antibiotics were not available at the time. Russell tested the efficacy of intramuscular injections of cortisone given in conjunction with monovalent *Crotalus* antivenin in a rabbit model[31,32]; Reid et al tested oral prednisone with no antivenin administration in humans bitten by Malayan pit vipers (*Agkistrodon rhodostoma*).[33] Neither Reid et al nor Russell believed that steroids were beneficial, and Russell was especially concerned that steroids might mask important clinical signs. Conversely, Glass advocated large intravenous doses of hydrocortisone every four to six hours in cases of severe rattlesnake envenomization.[34] The contraindications for conventional short-term corticosteroid use would also apply to their therapeutic use in snake envenomization.

Prolonged use of large doses of corticosteroids may lead to some of the following side effects: salt and water retention, producing hypertension and congestive heart failure; excessive K^+ loss in the urine; excessive bicarbonate retention, resulting in hypochloremic alkalosis; negative nitrogen balance and impaired glucose utilization; osteoporosis; impaired wound healing; masking of infections by suppression of basic inflammatory processes; increased hydrochloric acid and pepsin secretion, leading to perforated ulcers; and suppression of corticotropin secretion. Few of these effects are seen in short-term corticosteroid use, with the exception of the masking of infections. Concurrent use of appropriate antibiotics would minimize this risk.[35,36]

Glucocorticoid therapy is selected for its antiinflammatory and/or immunosuppressive actions. In anaphylactic shock, steroids suppress circulating antibody production that is caused by antigenic stimulation and inhibit antigen–antibody interaction, which can then lead to the release of mediators responsible for anaphylaxis.[37]

Corticosteroids reduce the binding of complement, IgE, and IgG antibodies to inflammatory cell receptor sites. Corticosteroids also have a bronchodilatory effect that has been attributed to their ability to increase the sensitivity of the bronchi and bronchioli to β-adrenergic agents[38]; reduce cellular infiltrates and exudates[38]; reduce target tissue responsiveness to inflammatory mediators (i.e., histamine, leukotrienes, platelet activating factor, and cyclooxygenase prostaglandin derivatives)[38]; inhibit mucus production[39]; decrease epithelial cell permeability[40]; decrease IgE receptor binding[41]; and alter Ca^{++} transmembrane movement, which decreases smooth muscle reactivity.[36]

Glucocorticoids exert their antiinflammatory effects by altering the immune response to stimuli. Steroids reduce the ability of granulocytes to leave the intravascular site for areas of inflammation, reduce granulocyte adherence to the endothelial wall, and reduce the granulocytic production of plasminogen activator. Plasminogen activator forms plasmin, and the plasmin hydrolyzes fibrin, which allows neutrophils to move more easily into inflammatory sites. Corticosteroids do not seem to affect the phagocytosis and chemotaxis of polymorphonuclear cells. Fever is suppressed via reduced leukocyte pyrogen production and/or the inhibition of interleukin-1 release from monocytes. Because the use of corticosteroids may also suppress the fever response, the clinician loses this parameter for monitoring the infectious process. Complete blood cell counts remain helpful in the monitoring of infection because they can reveal an increase in the number of bands as well as the appearance of toxic neutrophils.

Corticosteroids also are helpful in reducing increased capillary permeability by decreasing the adherence of granulocytes to the endothelium and increasing vasoconstriction by augmenting adrenergic activity. The augmentation of adrenergic activity helps stabilize the cardiovascular system and may increase cardiac contractility and cardiac output. In addition, steroids block the release of vasoactive kinins, thereby lessening the local immune response to stimuli.

Corticosteroids block the action of PLA_2. Phospholipase A_2 is the primary active component of most venoms and causes most of the pathophysiology. Phospholipase A_2 liberates arachidonic acid from membrane phospholipids. Arachidonic acid is the common precursor of prostaglandins, leukotrienes, and platelet-activating factor, all of which are part of the inflammatory process. Phospholipase A_2 also stimulates granulocytes to respond to stimuli.[42]

It is likely that the most important role of corticosteroids in snake envenomization therapy is blocking the action of PLA_2. This action diminishes the inflammatory response and hypotension while stabilizing membranes and promoting renal excretion of K^+ and Ca^{++} and retention of bicarbonate. Membrane stabilization greatly reduces red blood cell lysis, release of enzymes from lysosomes, capillary permeability, damage of muscle cell plasma membranes, and synaptic membrane damage. There is some evidence that low concentrations of cephaloridine may inhibit PLA_2 activity by interacting with phospholipids of lysosome membranes, but its use may be limited because it is nephrotoxic.[43]

A study of the effects of western diamondback rattlesnake (*Crotalus atrox*) envenomization in sheep found that administering the venom intravenously caused hemoconcentration, hypoventilation, and a decrease in cardiac output and systemic arterial pressure. When the sheep were premedicated with antivenin, they were unaffected by the venom. When the sheep were premedicated with hydrocortisone (3 to 5 mg/kg), betamethasone (0.15 to 0.20 mg/kg), or corticotropin (12.5 to 25.0 IU), a still-evident but attenuated protection against the effects of the venom remained. When steroids or corticotropin were given 30 minutes after venom administration, they produced stabilization of hemodynamic parameters within a few minutes and this effect peaked after 60 to 90 minutes. Sheep only receiving antivenin after venom administration failed to show improvement in any of the parameters. Three of the seven sheep in this group died of respiratory failure. Only one of the 24 sheep that received only steroids died. The one sheep that died received corticotropin. Sheep treated with steroids 50 to 75 minutes after venom infusion demonstrated no clinical improvement without concurrent fluid therapy.[44]

A review of 375 cases of venomous snake bite in domesticated animals, all of which were treated with steroids (with or without antivenin), revealed no problems with the use of steroids.[45] A treatment combination of dexamethasone (0.1 mg/kg subcutaneously), procaine penicillin G (25,000 IU/kg subcutaneously, once or twice a day for five to six days), and vaccination with clostridium and tetanus toxoid resolved eight cases of prairie rattlesnake *(C. viridis viridis)* envenomization in captive Rocky Mountain elk *(Cervus elaphus nelsoni)*.[8] Steroids and fluids without the use of antivenin were effective in 81 human patients envenomized by massasauga and pygmy rattlesnakes *(Sistrurus* species). Three patients had coagulopathies and received concurrent blood component therapy.[7]

Antibiotic Therapy

The choice of antibiotic is based on bacterial culture and sensitivity testing of the wound as well as the ability of the antibiotic to produce appropriate tissue level concentrations without toxic side effects. It would be prudent to start antibiotic therapy immediately, while culture results are pending. Some practitioners start patients on intravenous first- or second-generation cephalosporins pending culture results.[6]

Staphylococcus aureus, Staphylococcus epidermis, group A *Streptococcus, Acinetobacter* species, *Citrobacter* species, and *Pseudomonas* species were the predominant isolates from cultures from snake bite wounds of 36 human patients. It was not clear from the paper if anaerobic cultures were also performed.[47] According to Jarchow, the flora of major concern in the mouths of rattlesnakes in Arizona are *Clostridium* species including *C. tetani*.[a] Procaine penicillin G is the most effective antibiotic for the treatment of *C. tetani* infections.

Pseudomonas and other gram-negative bacteria as well as anaerobic bacteria are predominant in the mouths of captive snakes and in wounds caused by snakes. Third-generation cephalosporins may thus be an appropriate first choice for antibiotic therapy; however, caution should be observed if coagulopathy is present because some of the third-generation cephalosporins could exacerbate the problem. First- and second-generation cephalosporins are generally inactive against *Pseudomonas* and *Acinetobacter*, while certain second-generation cephalosporins are active against some anaerobes (e.g., *Clostridium*). Ciprofloxacin (the active metabolite of enrofloxacin) is active against most gram-negative organisms (including *Citrobacter, Acinetobacter*, and some *Pseudomonas* species) and most *Staphylococcus* species but is inactive against anaerobes and *Streptococcus* species. Aminoglycoside antibiotics and ciprofloxacin are contraindicated in patients that are myoglobinuric or have any other type of renal failure.

Tetanus toxoid should be considered in species that are especially sensitive to *Clostridium tetani* because of the predominance of this microbe as the normal oral flora of snakes and because fangs often cause deep puncture wounds. Elk envenomized by the prairie rattlesnake were treated with both clostridium and tetanus toxoids as well as procaine penicillin G, because clostridial infections are likely sequelae to snake bites in domesticated ruminants.[8]

Sedation and Analgesia Therapy

Patients requiring sedation present a special problem. Diazepam is reasonably safe except in cases of respiratory depression. Phenothiazines (e.g., acepromazine) can cause hypotension, which may aggravate the hypotension seen in most cases of snake envenomization. Barbiturates may be useful, but they also cause respiratory depression. If the pain of envenomization is tempered, the anxiety level of the patient may lessen. Human patients report that antivenin alone provides substantial analgesia.

The opiates provide some sedation and reasonably effective analgesia, but they can cause respiratory depression. Excitation may occur in some species, such as cats, horses, pigs, and cows. Most opiates also provoke histamine release, which causes peripheral arterial and venous dilatation. Morphine may be indicated in bite cases with pulmonary edema. Morphine causes a rapid decrease in pulmonary arterial flow and pressure, and left ventricular and diastolic pressure, which results in increased myocardial contractility. Morphine

[a]Jarchow J: Personal communication, Arizona-Sonora Desert Museum, 1993.

also has the cardiovascular effects of splanchnic pooling, decreased cardiac preload and afterload, and decreased respiratory effort.[25] In humans, the decrease in peripheral vascular resistance returns to normal in approximately 20 minutes, and a 60% increase in myocardial contractility is maintained for more than 30 minutes.[25] Aspirin and other nonsteroidal antiinflammatory agents may be beneficial but caution should be observed in patients with coagulopathies.[48]

Other Therapeutic Considerations

Wound excision has been advocated by some physicians.[3,5,7,34,47] Up to 79% of the radioactively labelled venom from eastern diamondback and cottonmouth moccasin (Agkistrodon piscivorus) was recovered from tissues excised from dogs 10 minutes after envenomization.[49]

Fasciotomies rarely seem to be indicated. The only time fasciotomy should be performed is in the presence of verified compartment syndrome. If rising compartment pressures are evident, a fasciotomy should be performed only after coagulopathies are under control.[19] In dogs given intramuscular injections of crotalid venom, intracompartmental muscle necrosis was not prevented by fasciotomy performed before the venom injection.[50] A study using New Zealand white rabbits found that, after intramuscular injection of western diamondback rattlesnake venom in a hindlimb, the combination of antivenin plus fasciotomy and debridement improved adjacent soft tissue edema but resulted in substantially poorer limb function when compared with antivenin therapy alone. Fasciotomy and debridement without antivenin did not improve survival, adjacent soft tissue edema, or limb function.[51]

There are other therapies that may prove useful in the treatment of envenomization. Antiprostaglandin therapy may be effective because of the increase in prostaglandin formation.[52] Indomethacin was demonstrated to rapidly restore diastolic and systolic pressures to preenvenomization levels.[53] Calcium channel blockers may also be indicated because of the increased calcium flux seen in presynaptic membranes that are altered by PLA_2 and crotoxin, and muscle cell membranes damaged by PLA_2. Electric shock therapy has received a great deal of coverage in the popular press, but scientific investigation into this therapy regimen indicates it is of no value and may be life-threatening.[55-58] Therapy with purified antivenins will be of great importance in the future.[19,54]

CONCLUSION

One can infer from the variety of possible sequelae to snake envenomization that there is no single therapy of choice. A clinician must take into consideration the effect of envenomization on each of the body systems and be prepared to respond accordingly. Familiarity with the venomous snakes in the area and the most common pathologies associated with these snakes will guide the clinician toward rapid, efficient therapy. As new drugs become available, especially purified antivenins, therapy may become more specific and have fewer complications.

About the Authors

Dr. Stormy Hudelson is a Diplomate of the American Board of Veterinary Practitioners, Avian Speciality. Mr. Paul Hudelson has been a veterinary technician and has an MA in English literature. Dr. Hudelson and Mr. Hudelson are currently affiliated with The Tucson Wildlife Rehabilitation Center in Tucson, Arizona.

REFERENCES

1. Chippaux JP, Williams V, White J: Snake venom variability: Methods of study, results and interpretation. *Toxicon* 29(11):1279–1303, 1991.
2. Barral-Netto M, Schriefer A, Barral A, et al: Serum levels of bothropic venom in patients without antivenom intervention. *Am J Trop Med Hyg* 45(6):751–754, 1991.
3. Snyder CC, Knowles RP: Snakebites: Guidelines for practical management. *Postgrad Med* 83(6):52–60, 65–68, 71–73, 75, 1988.
4. Jansen PW, Perkin RM, Van Stralen D: Mojave rattlesnake envenomation: Prolonged neurotoxicity and rhabdomyolysis. *Ann Emerg Med* 21(3):322–325, 1992.
5. Sabback MS, Cunningham ER, Fitts CT: A study of the treatment of pit viper envenomization in 45 patients. *J Trauma* 17(8):569–573, 1977.
6. Smith TA II, Figge HL: Treatment of snakebite poisoning. *Am J Hosp Pharm* 28(1):35–43, 1988.
7. Burch JM, Agarwal R, Mattox KL, et al: The treatment of crotalid envenomation without antivenin. *J Trauma* 28(1):35–43, 1988.
8. Miller MW, Wild MA, Baker BJ, et al: Snakebite in captive Rocky Mountain elk (Cervus elaphus nelsoni). *J Wildlife Dis* 25(3):392–396, 1989.
9. Fitzgerald WE: Snakebite in a horse. *Aust Vet J* 51(1):37–39, 1975.
10. Curry SC, Chang D, Connor D: Drug and toxin–induced rhabdomyolysis. *Ann Emerg Med* 18(10):1068–1084, 1989.
11. Jansen PW, Perkin RM, Van Stralen D: Mojave rattlesnake envenomation: Prolonged neurotoxicity and rhabdomyolysis. *Ann Emerg Med* 21(3):322–325, 1992.
12. Hardy DL: Envenomation by the mojave rattlesnake (Crotalus scutulatus scutulatus) in southern Arizona, USA. *Toxicon* 21(1):111–118, 1983.
13. Parrish HM, Khan MS: Bites by coral snakes: Report of 11 representative cases. *Am J Med Sci* 253(5):561–568, 1967.
14. Hogan DE, Dire DJ: Anaphylactic shock secondary to rattlesnake bite. *Ann Emerg Med* 19(7):814–816, 1990.
15. Wadee AA, Rabson AR: Development of specific IgE antibodies after repeated exposure to snake venom. *J Allerg Clin Immun* 80(11):695–698, 1987.
16. Theakston RDG, Reid HA, Larrick JW, et al: Snake venom antibodies in Ecuadorian indians. *J Trop Med Hyg* 84:199–

202, 1981.
17. Van Mierop LHS, Kitchens CS: Defibrination syndrome following bites by the eastern diamondback rattlesnake. *J Flor Med Assoc* 67(1):21–27, 1980.
18. Wingert WA, Chan L: Rattlesnake bites in southern California and rationale for recommended treatment. *West J Med* 148(1):37–44, 1988.
19. Sullivan JB Jr: Past, present, and future immunotherapy of snake venom poisoning. *Ann Emerg Med* 16(9):938–944, 1987.
20. Malasit P, Warrell DA, Chanthavanich P, et al: Prediction, prevention, and mechanism of early (anaphylactic) antivenom reactions in victims of snake bites. *Brit Med J* 292(Jan 4):17–20, 1986.
21. Jurkovich GJ, Luterman A, McCullar K, et al: Complications of crotalidae antivenin therapy. *J Trauma* 28(7):1032–1037, 1988.
22. Stolpe MR, Norris RL, Chisholm CD, et al: Preliminary observations on the effects of hyperbaric oxygen therapy on western diamondback rattlesnake *(Crotalus atrox)* venom poisoning in the rabbit model. *Ann Emerg Med* 18(8):871–874, 1989.
23. Davidson TM: Intravenous rattlesnake envenomation. *West J Med* 148(1):45–47, 1988.
24. Ya PM, Perry JF: Experimental evaluation of methods for the early treatment of snakebite. *Surgery* 47:975–981, 1960.
25. Zaritsky AL, Chernow B: Catecholamines and other inotropes, in Chernow B (ed): *The Pharmacologic Approach to the Critically Ill Patient*, ed 2. Baltimore, Williams & Wilkins, 1988, pp 584–602.
26. Mahon WA: Drugs and the respiratory system, in Kalant H, Roschlau WHE, Sellers EM (eds): *Principles of Medical Pharmacology*, ed 4. Toronto, Dept of Pharmacology, University of Toronto, 1985, pp 451–462.
27. Chernow B, Holbrook P, D'Angona DS Jr, et al: Epinephrine absorption after intratracheal administration. *Anesth Anlg* 63:829, 1984.
28. *Physicans Desk Reference*, ed 47. Medical Economics Data: Montvale, NJ, 1993, p 2550.
29. Kadar D: Histamine and antihistamines, in Kalant H, Roschlau WHE, Sellers EM (eds): *Principles of Medical Pharmacology*, ed 4. Toronto, Dept of Pharmacology, University of Toronto, 1985, pp 375–382.
30. Chiu HF, Chen IJ, Teng CM: Edema formation and degranulation of mast cells by a basic phospholipase A_2 purified from *Trimeresurus mucrosquamatus* snake venom. *Toxicon* 27(1):115–125, 1989.
31. Russell FE: Effects of cortisone during immunization with Crotalus venom. *Toxicon* 3:65–67, 1963.
32. Russell FE: Use of Crotalus monovalent antivenin from rabbit serum. *Curr Therap Res* 3:438, 1961.
33. Reid HA, Thean PC, Martin WJ: Specific antivenin and prednisone in viper-bite poisoning: Controlled trial. *Br Med J* 2(Nov 30):1378–1380, 1963.
34. Glass TG: Cortisone and immediate fasciotomy in the treatment of severe rattlesnake bite. *Tex Med* 65:41–46, 1969.
35. Schimmer BP, Sellers EA: Adrenocorticotropic hormone and adrenal steroids, in Kalant H, Roschlau WHE, Sellers EM (eds): *Principles of Medical Pharmacology*, ed 4. Toronto, Dept of Pharmacology, University of Toronto, 1985, pp 553–562.
36. Chin R Jr: Corticosteroids, in Chernow B (ed): *The Pharmacological Approach to the Critically Ill Patient*, ed 2. Baltimore, Williams & Wilkins, 1988, pp 559–562.
37. Rosenthale ME: Evaluation for immunosuppressive and antiallergic activity in, Scherrer RA, Whitehouse MW (eds): *Antiinflammatory Agents: Chemistry and Pharmacology*, vol 2. Medicinal Chemistry vol 13. New York, Academic Press, 1974, pp 123–142.
38. Morris HG: Mechanisms of glucocorticoid action in pulmonary disease. *Chest* 88(suppl):133S, 1985.
39. Maron Z, Shelhamer, Alling D, et al: The effects of corticosteroids on mucous glycoprotein secretion from human airways in vitro. *Am Rev Respir Dis* 129:62, 1984.
40. Schleimer RP: The mechanisms of antiinflammatory steroid action in allergic diseases. *Ann Rev Pharmacol Toxicol* 25:381, 1985.
41. Ziment I: Steroids. *Clin Chest Med* 7:341, 1986.
42. Flower RJ: The mediators of steroid action. *Nature* 320:20, 1986.
43. Fry M, Plummer DT: The stabilization of renal lysosomes by cephaloridine: The role of a membrane-bound phospholipase A_2, in Fillastre J-P (ed): *Nephrotoxicity*, New York, Masson Publishing, 1977, pp 193–211.
44. Halmagyi DFJ, Starzecki B, Horner GJ: Mechanism and pharmacology of shock due to rattlesnake venom in sheep. *J Appl Physiol* 20(4):709–718, 1965.
45. Gonzalez D: Snake bites in domestic animals. *Toxicon* 28(2):149, 1990.
46. Wetzel WW, Christy NP: A king cobra kite in New York City. *Toxicon* 27(3):393–395, 1989.
47. Downey DJ, Omer GE, Moneim MS: New Mexico rattlesnake bites: Demographic review and guidelines for treatment. *J Trauma* 31(10):1380–1386, 1991.
48. Russell FE: *Snake Venom Poisoning*. Great Neck, New York, Scholium International, 1983, p 315.
49. Snyder CC, Knowles RP, Pickens JE, et al: Pathenogenesis and treatment of poisonous snake bites. *JAVMA* 151(12):1635–1637, 1967.
50. Garfin SR, Castilonia RR, Mubarak SJ, et al: Rattlesnake bites and surgical decompression: Results using a laboratory model. *Toxicon* 22(2):177–182, 1984.
51. Stewart RM, Page CP, Schwesinger WH, et al: Antivenin and fasciotomy/debridement in the treatment of the severe rattlesnake bite. *Am J Surg* 158(12):543–547, 1989.
52. Damerau B, Lege L, Oldigs HD, et al: Histamine release, formation of prostaglandin-like activity (SRS-C) and mast cell degranulation by the direct lytic factor (DLF) and phospholipase A_2 of cobra venom. *Naunyn Schiedebergs, Arch Pharm* 287:141–156, 1975.
53. Tu AT ed: *Rattlesnake Venoms: Their actions and treatment*. New York, Marcel Dekker, 1982, p 128.
54. Russel FE, Sullivan JB, Egen NB, et al: Preparation of a new antivenin by affinity chromatography. *Am J Trop Med Hyg* 34(1):141–150, 1985.
55. Johnson EK, Kardong KV, MacKessy SP: Electric shocks are ineffective in treatment of lethal effects of rattlesnake envenomation in mice. *Toxicon* 25:1347–1349, 1987.
56. Howe NR, Meisenheimer JL: Electric shock does not save snakebitten rats. *Ann Emerg Med* 17:254–256, 1988.
57. Dart RC, Lindsey D, Schulman A: Snakebites and shocks. *Ann Emerg Med* 17:1262, 1988.
58. Russell FE: A letter on electroshock for snakebite. *Vet Hum Toxicol* 29:320, 1987.

UPDATE

CLINICAL SIGNS

Occasionally, a bite from a nonvenomous snake may present with local effects similar to those of a poisonous bite. Garter snakes (*Thamnophis elegans vagrans*) may cause localized swelling, ecchymosis, and hemorrhagic vesicles at the site of the bite without systemic signs. This appearance easily could be misinterpreted as a crotaline bite.[1]

Experimental subcutaneous exposure of dogs to the venom of a common tiger snake (*Notechis scutatus*, an elapid) revealed preparalytic signs of envenomization, including vomiting, defecation, salivation, and/or sudden collapse. Occurring shortly after envenomization, these signs generally subside before paralysis set in, even in seriously envenomized dogs. Such clinical signs indicate a lethal or near lethal dose of venom. Hemolysis occurred quite rapidly at all the doses tested. It did not progress significantly, however, and is not of clinical concern when fluid therapy is part of the treatment protocol.[2]

DIAGNOSTICS

An ELISA kit (Snake Venom Detection Kit, CSL Ltd, 45 Poplar Rd., Parkville, Victoria, Australia 3052) adapted for field use is being used in Australia. The ELISA detects venom in a sample from a swab of the bite, urine, or blood (preference in this order) and can identify the type of snake.[3]

Blood films made from 28 dogs bitten by rattlesnakes in Colorado (genus species not given) demonstrated that echinocytosis in dogs supports a diagnosis of rattlesnake envenomation (Brown et al, 1994).[4]

A simple whole blood clotting test (WBCT20) is useful in assessing the effectiveness of antivenin therapy in relation to restoration of blood coagulability. Two milliliters of venous blood are placed in a new glass test tube and left upright at room temperature for twenty minutes. The tube is then tipped gently to see whether the blood has clotted. WBCT20 seems simpler, faster, more reliable and less expensive than laboratory estimation of plasma fibrinogen concentrations. Fibrinogen levels inversely correlate to these testing times.[5]

Findings from a study of human patients bitten by a Papuan taipan (*Oxyuranus scutellatus canni*, an elapid)[6] provide a simple and objective means of assessing interventions in the management of neurotoxicity following this type of snakebite. Evoked compound muscle action potentials decreased and increased in direct correlation to clinical deterioration and recovery.

TREATMENTS

Dogs experimentally injected with tiger snake venom exhibited reduced muscle damage when maintained under general anesthesia in order to reduce muscular activity. Myoglobinuria was delayed for 24 hours, suggesting that maintaining fluid therapy for at least 48 hours would be prudent.[7]

In 93% of rats experimentally envenomized with Russell's viper venom, antivenin supplemented with antithrombin III (AT-III) prevented abnormal clotting.[8] The venom is associated with activation of coagulation and consumption of AT-III. AT-III, the most important plasma inhibitor of the coagulation cascade activation, counters most activated clotting factors and has no effect unless used in combination with antivenin. This study's findings emphasize the necessity of antivenin in combating the coagulopathies associated with bothropic and crotaline envenomization. Heparin therapy, aimed at disseminated intravascular coagulation, would have no effect once AT-III is consumed.

A pilot study of humans with coagulopathies following envenomization (types of snakes not mentioned) found that adding intravenous immunoglobulin to antivenin therapy diminished the volume of antivenin needed to control the coagulopathies.[9]

Polyclonal ovine Fab antivenin appears superior to other monospecific antivenins. Experiments show that Fab monospecific antivenin for the treatment of carpet viper (*Echis ocellatus*) envenomization has the advantage of wide distribution and theoretically low immunoreactivity.[10]

Antivenin Polyvalent Crotalid (ovine) Tab (Crotab®, Therapeutic Antibodies, Inc., Nashville, TN) appears to be 3.1 times to 9.6 times more potent than equine origin polyvalent crotalidae antivenin (ACP) (Wyeth Laboratories, Philadelphia, PA) for the prevention of the lethal effects of the nine crotaline venoms tested. Fab antivenin was efficacious against envenomization by Southern Pacific rattlesnake (*Crotalus viridis helleri*) while ACP was not.[11]

This new product causes less serum sickness, less hypersensitivity, but may require dosage every six hours for 24 to 48 hours to insure that signs of envenomization do not return. Local effects of venom are attenuated and coagulopathies respond within a few hours.

Peoples in areas where venomous snakes are endemic have used remedies prepared from local plants in the treatment of snakebites. While commercial application of such remedies is not likely in the near future, ethnopharmacologists are beginning to investigate the efficacy of these folk remedies by systematically testing plant extracts in the treatment of envenomization.[12–14]

References

1. Gomez HF, Davis M, Phillips S, et al: Human envenomation from a wandering garter snake. *Ann Emerg Med* 23(5):1119–1122, 1994.
2. Lewis PF: Some toxicity thresholds for the clinical effects of common tiger snake (*Notechis scutatus*) envenomation in the dog. *Aust Vet J* 71:133–135, 1994.
3. McColl M: Snake envenomation in Australia. *Aust Vet J* 71(5):1385, 1994.
4. Brown DE, Meyer DJ, Wingfield WE, Walton RM: Echinocytosis associated with rattlesnake envenomation in dogs. *Vet Pathol* 31:654–657, 1994.
5. Sano-Martins IS, Fan HW, Castro CB, et al: Reliability of the simple 20-minute whole blood clotting test (WBCT20) as an indicator of low

plasma fibrinogen concentration in patients envenomed by *Bothrops* snakes. *Toxicon* 32(9):1045–1050, 1994.
6. Trevett AJ, Lalloo DG, Nwokolo NC, et al: Electrophysiological findings in patients envenomed following the bite of a Papuan taipan (*Oxyuranus scutellatus canni*). *Trans Roy Soc Trop Med Hyg* 89:415–417, 1995.
7. Lewis PF: Myotoxicity and nephrotoxicity of common tiger snake (*Notechjs scutatus*) venom in the dog. *Aust Vet J* 71(5):136–139, 1994.
8. Clemens R, Pukritayakamee S, Vanijanonta S, et al: Therapeutic effects of antivenom supplemented by antithrombin III in rats experimentally envenomated with Russell's viper (*Daboia russelli siamensis*) venom. *Toxicon* 33(1):77–82, 1995.
9. Sellahewa KH, Kumararatne MP, Dassanayake PB: Intravenous immunoglobulin in the treatment of snake bite envenoming: A pilot study. *Ceylon Medical J* 39(4):173–175, 1994.
10. Laing GD, Lee L, Smith DC, et al: Experimental assessment of a new low-cost antivenom for treatment of carpet viper (*Echis ocellatus*) envenoming. *Toxicon* 33(3):307–313, 1995.
11. Consroe P, Egen NB, Russell FE, et al: Comparison of a new ovine antigen binding fragment (Fab) antivenin for United States Crotalidae with the Commercial antivenin for protection against venom-induced lethality in mice. *Am J Trop Med Hyg* 53(5):507–510, 1995.
12. Reyes-Chilpa R, Gomez-Girabay F, Quijano L, et al: Preliminary results on the protective effect of (—)-edunol, a pterocarpan from *Brongniartia Podalyrioides* (Leguminosae), against *Bothrops atrox* venom in mice. *J Ethnopharm* 42:199–203, 1994.
13. Mors WB, de Nascimiento MC, Parente JP, et al: Neutralization of lethal and myotoxic activities of South American rattlesnake venom by extracts and constituents of the plant *Eclipta prostrata* (Asteraceae). *Toxicon* 27:1003–1009, 1989.
14. Houghton PJ, Skari KP: The effect on blood clotting of some West African plants used against snakebite. *J Ethnopharm* 44:99–108, 1994.

KEY FACTS

- Cases of mycetismus (mushroom poisoning) are encountered infrequently in small animal practice.
- The toxins of major importance in North American mushrooms can be divided into four categories based on their physical effects and time of onset of clinical signs.
- Treatment of mushroom poisoning is largely supportive regardless of the type ingested.
- Accurate identification by an experienced mycologist of the type of mushroom involved is desirable if possible.

Mushroom Poisoning

Ronald B. Wilson, DVM
Diplomate, ACVP
C. E. Kord Animal Disease Laboratory
Tennessee Department of Agriculture
Nashville, Tennessee

John A. Holladay, DVM
Brentwood Veterinary Clinic
Brentwood, Tennessee

Cases of mycetismus (mushroom poisoning) are encountered infrequently in small animal practice.[1,2] Given the ubiquitous nature of mushrooms during warm seasons and the indiscriminate eating habits of many dogs, it is somewhat surprising that clinical toxicity relating to the ingestion of wild mushrooms is not seen more frequently in small animals. In this article, reports of mushroom poisoning in the veterinary literature are reviewed and a case of suspected mycetismus in a litter of puppies that was presented with acute diarrhea is reported.

Review of the Literature

Approximately 350 cases of mushroom poisoning are reported in the United States each year, most of which occur in children under five years of age.[3] The incidence of mycetismus in Europe is higher, presumably reflecting the increased practice of mycophagy and perhaps better reporting of cases of intoxication. Reports in the veterinary literature detailing mycetismus are limited. Cases of fatal poisoning in cattle have been reported.[4,5] A fatal hemolytic episode in a 10-week-old dog was associated with the ingestion of *Gyromitra esculenta*.[6] Suspected mushroom poisoning was reported in two cats,[2] in which vomiting and excess salivation were followed by a near comatose state four hours after ingestion. The second cat died 30 hours after the onset of clinical signs.

The toxins of major importance in North American mushrooms can be divided into four categories based on physical effects and time of onset of clinical signs; they may be further divided into seven groups (Table I) on the basis of the toxins they contain.[7] Toxins from mushrooms that cause cellular destruction (Category A), most often of liver and kidney, include the cyclopeptides (Group I) and monomethylhydrazine (Group II). The cyclopeptide group includes the genera *Amanita* and *Galerina*, while *Gyromitra* is the genus associated with monomethylhydrazine toxicity.[7]

Mushrooms that manifest their toxicity by affecting the autonomic nervous system (Category B) include the genus *Coprinus* (coprine poisoning, Group III) and the genera *Clitocybe* and *Inocybe*, which produce muscarinic effects (Group IV). A third classification (Category C) of toxins that affect the central nervous system includes Groups V (ibotenic acid-muscimol) and VI (psilocybin-psilocin). Group V includes differing species of the genus *Amanita*, ingestion of which results in delirium. The Group VI toxins (genera

TABLE I
Classification of Toxins in North American Mushrooms

A. Cellular Destruction
    I. Cyclopeptides (*Amanita*, *Galerina*)
    II. Monomethylhydrazine (*Gyromitra*)

B. Autonomic Nervous System Effects
    III. Coprine poisoning (*Coprinus*)
    IV. Muscarinic effects (*Clitocybe*, *Inocybe*)

C. Central Nervous System Effects
    V. Ibotenic acid-muscimol (delirium) (*Amanita*)
    VI. Psilocybin-psilocin (hallucinogenic) (*Psilocybe*, *Panaeolus*)

D. Gastrointestinal Irritants
    VII. Numerous genera, including *Agaricus*, *Amanita*, *Lepiota*

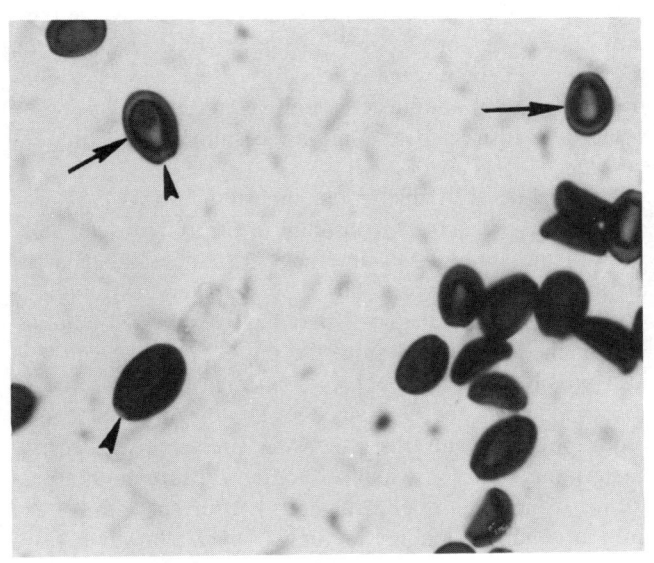

Figure 1—These brownish-red spores have a thick wall (*arrow*) and operculum (*arrowhead*). (×2100)

Psilocybe and *Panaeolus*) cause hallucinogenic effects upon their ingestion. The final classification, Category D, includes the Group VII toxins. Gastrointestinal irritation occurs 30 minutes to 3 hours following their consumption.[7] Among the many genera that produce these signs are *Agaricus* species, *Amanita* species, and *Lepiota* species.[7] An eighth group is sometimes added to encompass miscellaneous components that produce exotic effects.[3]

Treatment of mushroom poisoning is largely supportive regardless of the type ingested. Reduction of absorption by induced vomition may be beneficial if accomplished within one hour of exposure. Orally administered activated charcoal (1 g/kg body weight) may also reduce absorption and can be repeated every six to eight hours if necessary. Increased excretion of toxins may be obtained by forced diuresis and catharsis. Cardiovascular and respiratory function must be monitored closely with appropriate therapy being instituted if problems occur. Renal and hepatic parameters must be evaluated for at least 48 hours following ingestion as the onset of clinical signs resulting from Group I toxins may be delayed.[7,8]

The use of atropine is generally limited to muscarinic (Group IV) poisoning, and then only when cholinergic signs are life threatening.[1,8]

Differentiation between toxic and nontoxic mushrooms presents a challenge for even the well-trained mycologist.[3,7] Some mushrooms are poisonous only when consumed in large quantity while others may be toxic only when old, decayed, or altered by frost.[7] Other mushrooms are edible in some geographic areas and toxic in other locations.[7] While a history of mushroom ingestion and the accompanying clinical signs may be helpful in determining the type of mushrooms involved, accurate identification by an experienced mycologist is desirable if possible.

Report of a Case

A litter of five, seven-week-old boxer puppies was presented to the Brentwood Veterinary Clinic with recent onset of a black, tarry diarrhea. The puppies had been successfully treated for coccidia at three weeks of age; no other parasites had been detected at that time. The pups had been weaned at six weeks of age. Their diet consisted of a commercially available, dry ration formulated for puppies; the food had been available to the pups since they were three weeks old. Each pup reportedly had been eating and drinking normally before the illness. All pups had access to the outdoors. The owner indicated that there was no known exposure to toxicants.

Physical examination revealed all the puppies to be alert and responsive; pupillary reflexes were normal and excessive lacrimation and salivation were not present. The abdomen of all pups was easily palpated and there were no detectable abnormalities. Each pup's rectal temperature was within the normal range. The owner reported that none of the pups had vomited and there was little straining during attempted defecation. Fecal material collected for examination was black and pastelike in consistency. Ingested grass was mixed with the feces. Fecal flotation and direct smears performed on feces from three of the puppies revealed numerous (several hundred per high-powered field), brownish-red spores measuring approximately 5×7 μm (Figure 1). Parasite eggs were not present. Many spores were elliptical although several were centrally indented, resulting in a reniform appearance. A single spore was present at the apex. The spores had thick walls, yet their surface was smooth. Based on morphology, the spores were subsequently identified as being derived from ingested mushrooms; a more precise identification was not possible.[a] A consulted mycologist, however, indicated that they were not members of the genus *Amanita*, which contains many of the toxic species of mushrooms.[b]

[a]Sauve R: Personal communication, Division of Plant Industries, Tennessee Department of Agriculture, Nashville, Tennessee, 1984.
[b]Wolfe F: Personal communication, Department of Biology, Vanderbilt University, Nashville, Tennessee, 1984.

Based on the mild clinical disease exhibited by the puppies, the owner elected not to pursue further diagnostic tests. The puppies were successfully treated with kaolin-pectin (1 ml/kg) administered orally three times daily. The owner was instructed to confine the animals until they recovered.

The diagnosis of mushroom ingestion in this case was delayed as a result of consultation efforts to accurately identify the spores. Mushrooms were not found in areas accessible to the puppies; however, the interval from clinical presentation to diagnosis may have resulted in elimination of the mushrooms from the pups' environment. It is also possible that the puppies consumed all of the mushrooms to which they had access. The diagnosis of mushroom poisoning in this case was presumptive because bacteriology, virology, and serologic studies were not performed. The onset of clinical signs concurrent with the excretion of large numbers of fungal spores, however, suggests a causal relationship. The diagnosis of mycetismus in humans may be based on the presence of spores in vomitus, gastric contents, or feces.[8] As blood was not detected in the feces, the spores may have been responsible for the black discoloration.

REFERENCES

1. Ridgeway RL: Mushroom (*Amanita pantherina*) poisoning. *JAVMA* 172:681–682, 1978.
2. Atkins CE, Johnson RK: Clinical toxicities of cats. *Vet Clin North Am* 5:623–652, 1975.
3. Rippon JW: Allergic and toxic diseases associated with fungi, in Rippon JW (ed): *Medical Mycology: The Pathogenic Fungi and the Pathogenic Actinomycetes*. Philadelphia, WB Saunders Co, 1982, pp 701–720.
4. Burton HA: Mushroom poisoning in cattle. *Vet Med* 39:290, 1944.
5. Piercy PL, Hargis G, Brown CA: Mushroom poisoning in cattle. *JAVMA* 105:206–208, 1944.
6. Bernard MA: Mushroom poisoning in a dog. *Can Vet J* 20:82–83, 1979.
7. Lincoff G, Mitchell DH (eds): Introduction, in *Toxic and Hallucinogenic Mushroom Poisoning*. New York, Van Nostrand Reinhold Co, 1977, pp 1–24.
8. Lincoff G, Mitchell DH (eds): Diagnosis and treatment of mushroom poisoning, in *Toxic and Hallucinogenic Mushroom Poisoning*. New York, Van Nostrand Reinhold Co, 1977, pp 174–200.

Managing Epileptic Dogs

University of Tennessee
William B. Thomas, DVM, MS

KEY FACTS

❏ Poor seizure control may result from inaccurate diagnosis of underlying disease, insufficient client education, selection of an inappropriate antiepileptic medication or inadequate dose, and seizures that are refractory to standard therapy.

❏ A thorough physical and neurologic examination as well as a laboratory profile consisting of a complete blood count, serum chemistry profile, and urinalysis is indicated in any dog presented for evaluation of seizures.

❏ Phenobarbital is the drug of choice for the initial management of idiopathic epilepsy in dogs.

❏ Periodic reevaluation and therapeutic drug monitoring often are necessary to determine the dose of antiepileptic medication that controls the seizures and avoids side effects.

❏ Administration of bromide improves control of seizures in many epileptic dogs that are refractory to phenobarbital.

Epilepsy generally refers to recurrent seizures of any cause, although many authors restrict the meaning to recurrent seizures unrelated to an underlying progressive disease.[1–4] Successful management of epilepsy is often difficult, as is evident by estimates that approximately 20% to 50% of canine epileptics treated at referral centers are not satisfactorily controlled.[5–7] Factors that contribute to therapeutic failure include the presence of underlying disorders that cause the seizures or complicate management, insufficient client education, improper selection of medication and dose, intolerable side effects of medication, and seizures that are refractory to medication.[8–11] This article discusses how to identify and avoid common causes of unsuccessful management of epileptic dogs.

IDENTIFYING UNDERLYING DISEASE

Epilepsy can be classified as idiopathic or symptomatic.[12] Idiopathic epilepsy, also called primary or true epilepsy, is the most common type of epilepsy in dogs.[1,2,4,13] The pathophysiology of idiopathic epilepsy is incompletely understood, but a genetic defect in the neuronal membrane or neurotransmitter function is suspected.[4,14–17] Symptomatic epilepsy, also referred to as acquired or secondary epilepsy, is caused by previous or current intracranial or extracranial disease.[1,2] Causes of intracranial disease may be congenital, neoplastic, inflammatory, traumatic, or vascular in origin. The principal extracranial disorders are caused by metabolic and toxic diseases[2,3,18] (Table I).

Identification of an underlying intracranial or extracranial disease is extremely important. Therapy of seizures due to progressive disease requires not only medical control of seizures but management of the underlying disease.[3] Because a definitive diagnosis of idiopathic epilepsy is seldom possible, the diagnostic approach is designed to identify any underlying disease.

The initial evaluation of any dog presented for evaluation of seizures should include a complete history; physical and neurologic examination; and laboratory profile consisting of a complete blood count, serum chemistry profile, and urinalysis.[3,19] Selection of other diagnostic tests should be based on the results of this initial evaluation.

History

Because many dogs presented for evaluation of seizures are normal on examination and laboratory evaluation, the history often is the most impor-

TABLE I
Common Causes of Seizures in Dogs

Cause	<1 Year	1–5 Years	>5 Years
IDIOPATHIC EPILEPSY		X	
SYMPTOMATIC EPILEPSY			
Extracranial			
Metabolic			
Hypoglycemia	X		X
Hypocalcemia		X	X
Hepatic encephalopathy	X		X
Hyperlipoproteinemia		X	X
Toxic	X	X	X
Intracranial			
Developmental			
Hydrocephalus	X		
Lissencephaly	X		
Metabolic storage diseases	X		
Neoplastic			X
Inflammatory			
Rabies	X	X	X
Distemper	X	X	X
Rickettsial diseases	X	X	X
Protozoal diseases	X	X	X
Fungal diseases	X	X	X
Granulomatous meningoencephalitis		X	
Trauma	X	X	X
Vascular			X

tant component of the assessment. The age of onset is useful in narrowing the list of diagnostic differentials. In dogs with idiopathic epilepsy, the first seizure usually occurs between one and five years of age.[4,19,20] When the onset of seizures occurs at younger than one year or older than five years of age, an underlying disease usually is responsible for the seizures.[19,20]

Seizures can usually be classified as generalized or focal on the basis of the owner's description of the seizure. Generalized seizures, which are the most frequently recognized type, are usually characterized by unconsciousness, symmetric motor activity (e.g., opisthotonos or extension of the limbs followed by paddling and chewing movements) and autonomic signs (e.g., salivation, urination, and defecation). Milder generalized seizures sometimes are recognized. With such seizures, the dog may remain conscious and have limited involuntary movement.

Focal seizures, also called partial seizures, are manifested by asymmetric motor activity (e.g., twitching of one side of the body) or bizarre, complex behavior (e.g., tail chasing, "fly biting," or aggression).[1,21,22] Consciousness may or may not be impaired during a focal seizure. A focal seizure may progress to a generalized seizure. Classification of seizures is important because focal seizures usually indicate the presence of an underlying disease.[1,3]

The history may provide evidence of a previous or current disorder that is responsible for the seizures. The owner should be questioned about illnesses or trauma, the possibility of intoxication, and vaccination history.

Physical Examination

Many underlying metabolic, infectious, and neoplastic diseases may be detected by careful physical examination, which includes examination of the ocular fundi. The neurologic examination should include assessment of behavior and gait, proprioception in all limbs, and cranial nerves (including the menace response in each eye and conscious facial sensation). Asymmetric deficits, such as circling, hemiparesis, blindness in one eye, or decreased sensation on one side of the face strongly suggest a focal intracranial lesion, such as neoplastic, inflammatory, or vascular disorders.[19]

Generalized deficits suggest an extracranial or diffuse intracranial disorder. Because transient generalized deficits, such as blindness, depression, and ataxia, may result from any seizure (even in dogs with idiopathic epilepsy), the examination should be repeated if generalized abnormalities are detected soon after a seizure.[3,19] Dogs with idiopathic epilepsy do not have interictal neurologic deficits.

Laboratory Examination

A complete blood count, serum chemistry profile, and urinalysis are indicated primarily to detect metabolic disorders. Liver function tests, such as serum bile acids or blood ammonia concentrations, should be performed if hepatic encephalopathy is suspected. Blood lead evaluation is indicated in young dogs and dogs from areas with a high incidence of lead poisoning.[3]

Additional Diagnostic Tests

Other diagnostic procedures, such as radiography and serum titers for infectious diseases, may be indicated based on the initial evaluation.[3,13,19] Computed tomography or magnetic resonance imaging is indicated in dogs older than five years of age and in dogs with persistent neurologic deficits; these procedures are able to detect intracranial lesions, such as tumors. Cerebrospinal fluid analysis should be considered to detect inflammatory disorders in dogs younger than one year of age and in dogs with persistent neurologic deficits. Computed tomography or magnetic resonance imaging should precede cerebrospinal fluid collection in dogs with suspected intracranial masses because removal of cerebrospinal fluid from dogs with increased intracranial pressure can cause dangerous shifts in brain tissue.[23]

A diagnosis of idiopathic epilepsy is appropriate in dogs that have (1) generalized seizures, (2) an onset of seizures between one and five years of age, (3) no abnormalities on physical and neurologic examination, and (4) normal laboratory evaluations.[1,2,18] Idiopathic epilepsy is always a tentative diagnosis; if other abnormalities develop or if seizures become unresponsive to therapy, the diagnosis should be reconsidered.

PRECIPITATING FACTORS

Concurrent disease, stress, or drug administration may complicate the management of epileptic dogs. Infections or metabolic disturbances may increase seizure activity in an otherwise well-controlled epileptic.[9,24,25] Because estrogen increases susceptibility to seizures, estrus may provoke seizures in some epileptic dogs.[4,25,26] Some medications, including phenothiazine tranquilizers, ketamine, and ivermectin, may increase seizure activity.[25,27,28] Changes in the dog's normal routine, such as travel, may cause sleep deprivation, which has been shown to precipitate seizures in humans.[29] A previously well-controlled epileptic should be evaluated for precipitating factors if seizures suddenly increase.

INSUFFICIENT CLIENT EDUCATION

Insufficient client education may result in client anxiety, unrealistic expectations, or noncompliance. The decision to begin drug therapy should be based on the frequency and severity of seizures and the owner's concerns.[3] Because epilepsy refers to recurrent seizures, the term is correctly applied only after more than one seizure has occurred. In dogs with idiopathic epilepsy, treatment after the second seizure should be considered because early treatment may improve the prognosis for successful control of epilepsy.[1,15] Some authors recommend antiepileptic drug therapy for dogs with seizures that occur more frequently than every four to eight weeks, episodes of status epilepticus, or clusters of several seizures daily.[3,30,31]

Before drug therapy is started, the owner should understand the goals of therapy, potential side effects, and the cost and effort involved in managing an epileptic dog.[3,11,14] Although completely eliminating seizures is ideal, a more realistic goal of therapy is to decrease the frequency and severity of seizures without causing unacceptable side effects.[3,8] Many antiepileptic drugs cause mild sedation, polydipsia, polyuria, and polyphagia. The sedative effect usually diminishes after several weeks of therapy.[7] Unless informed of the nature of these side effects, owners may become alarmed and stop therapy or reduce the dose.

Owners should also understand that several weeks of therapy are usually required to achieve a therapeutic serum concentration and that it is unrealistic to expect immediate reduction in seizure activity. Periodic evaluations and dose adjustments usually are required to achieve optimum effects. Long-term therapy with most antiepileptic drugs, especially at high doses, can produce hepatotoxicity that may limit therapy.[32,33] Owners must understand that their dogs may require daily medication for the remainder of their lives. Maintenance antiepileptic drug therapy is inappropriate if the owner is unable or unwilling to commit the necessary time, effort, and expense.

INEFFECTIVE DRUGS

The choice of antiepileptic drugs ideally should be based on results of well-controlled clinical studies. The sporadic natural history of seizures, subjective criteria usually used to evaluate efficacy, and the reluctance to withhold therapy in lieu of a placebo have precluded well-designed clinical trials.[34] Nevertheless, based on clinical experience and pharmacokinetic data, phenobarbital is currently considered the drug of choice for the initial management of epilepsy in

TABLE II
Antiepileptic Drugs for Dogs

Drug[a]	Dose Regimen	Time to Reach Steady State	Target Serum Concentration	Reference
Phenobarbital	2–5 mg/kg two times daily	10–18 days	20–45 µg/ml	5,31
Primidone	5–10 mg/kg three times daily	10–18 days	20–45 µg/ml (phenobartibal[c])	7
Potassium bromide	20 mg/kg one time daily	4 months	0.7–1.9 mg/ml (bromide[c])	10,44
Chlorazepate	2 mg/kg two times daily	NA[b]	500–1900 ng/ml[d] (nordiazepam[c])	49
Valproate	60 mg/kg three times daily	NA[b]	50–150 µg/ml[d]	47
Mephenytoin	10 mg/kg three times daily	5–7 days	25–40 µg/ml[d] (5-phenyl hydantoin)	20

[a]Currently, primidone and phenytoin are the only drugs labeled for the treatment of canine epilepsy. Other antiepileptic drugs must be used in an extralabel fashion. Bromide must be custom formulated, and suppliers may require the veterinarian to contact the U.S. Food and Drug Administration.
[b]Not applicable; steady state is not reached at the indicated dosage frequency.
[c]Represents the active metabolite or compound that should be measured.
[d]Human values; canine values are not known.

dogs.[3,5,7,8] Primidone is also effective but may be more likely to cause hepatotoxicity.[6,7] The short half-lives of phenytoin, carbamazepine, diazepam, and valproic acid in dogs limit their use as single agents for the control of canine epilepsy.[35]

INADEQUATE DOSE

One of the most common causes of poor seizure control is a dose that is too low.[5,9,36] The oral dose of phenobarbital or primidone correlates poorly with serum concentrations because of variability in metabolism among dogs.[5,37] Ideal management therefore requires measuring serum concentrations in each patient to help determine the proper dose.

The serum concentration should be measured when a steady state has been reached (that is, when the amount of drug eliminated is replaced by drug being administered). After starting therapy or after any change in dose, five to six half-lives are required to achieve a steady state. Thus, for phenobarbital, serum concentration should be measured during the second week of therapy and two weeks after any change in dose. Therapeutic monitoring also should be done when there are signs of toxicity or poor seizure control; in addition, routine monitoring should be done every six months.[2,9]

An adjustment in dose can be made based on analysis of serum collected immediately before the next dose (i.e., trough concentration).[9] If the seizures are poorly controlled and the serum concentration is low, the owner should be questioned to make sure that the dog is consistently receiving the recommended dose. If compliance is good, the dose should be increased. For drugs that are cleared by first-order kinetics (e.g., phenobarbital), the new dose can be calculated by the following formula[9]:

$$\text{New dose} = \text{Current dose} \times \frac{\text{Target concentration}}{\text{Measured concentration}}$$

The target range for phenobarbital is 20 to 45 µg/ml (Table II). Although monitoring serum concentrations is a useful guide, target ranges are average values, and seizure control and side effects should be assessed carefully on an individual basis. Rigid adherence to the target range should be avoided. Some dogs may be managed well with serum concentrations below the expected target range; others may suffer unacceptable side effects at serum concentrations within the target range.[2,3]

HEPATOTOXICITY

Occasionally, the development of hepatotoxicity complicates management of epileptic dogs. Most dogs receiving long-term antiepileptic drug therapy have moderate increases in serum alkaline phosphatase (SAP) and alanine transaminase (ALT) without serious liver dysfunction.[26,38–40] Less commonly, severe and even fatal hepatotoxicity occurs.[26,40,41] With the use of phenobarbital, prolonged serum concentrations of greater than 35 µg/ml may increase the risk of serious liver disease.[40]

A physical examination, complete blood count, serum chemistry profile, serum phenobarbital concentrations, and bile acids should be assessed every 6 to 12 months in dogs receiving phenobarbital or primidone. Evidence of hepatotoxicity includes lethargy, ataxia, icterus, ascites, decreased albumin, proportionately larger increases of alanine transaminase than serum alkaline phosphatase, increased bile acids, and rising serum concentrations of phenobarbital despite a constant oral dose.[8,32,38,40] If hepatotoxicity is suspected, potassium bromide should be used instead of phenobarbital.[8] If phenobarbital is discontinued early enough, liver changes are potentially reversible.[40,41]

REFRACTORY EPILEPSY

Epileptic dogs should not be considered refractory to medication until (1) secondary causes of seizures and precipitating factors have been excluded and (2) either serum concentrations are within the target range or the dog is suffering from unacceptable side effects. A common mistake is to add a second drug before adequate serum concentrations of the first drug are achieved.[9] Several alternative medications are available for the management of epileptic dogs that are truly refractory to phenobarbital.

The addition of potassium bromide improves seizure control in approximately 80% of dogs with epilepsy that is refractory to phenobarbital or primidone; 21% to 26% of dogs will become seizure-free.[9,10,42–44] Because of its minimal effects on liver function, bromide is also indicated in epileptic dogs with liver disease.[8,45] The long half-life of bromide (16.5 to 25 days) means that two to three weeks are required before bromide levels enter the target range and three to four months are required before a steady state is attained.[44,45] Bromide concentrations should be measured at one and four months after initiating therapy.[45]

Side effects of combined therapy with phenobarbital and bromide include polyuria, polydipsia, polyphagia, transient sedation, and rarely, pancreatitis.[9,20,42] Ataxia may occur at serum concentrations of bromide greater than 1.5 mg/ml.[42] If seizures become well controlled, the phenobarbital dose can be gradually tapered to the lowest dose that controls seizures. Some dogs can be managed with bromide alone.[44] In fact, there is ample evidence that treatment of human epileptics with multiple drugs is usually no more effective than therapy with a single agent.[46]

Several other drugs have been used to improve seizure control in dogs refractory to standard therapy. Specific recommendations are not feasible because the clinical usefulness, and in some cases the pharmacokinetics, of these drugs have not been fully studied. Because of drug interactions, serum concentrations of each medication should be carefully monitored when administering multiple drugs. Chlorazepate, valproate, or mephenytoin may improve seizure control when administered in addition to phenobarbital.[11,20,47]

In some epileptic dogs (especially large breeds) that are appropriately managed, seizures cannot be adequately controlled without unacceptable side effects.[11,25] Some owners may accept partial control if they understand that seizures of short duration are rarely life-threatening. Frequent or severe seizures, especially episodes of status epilepticus, may severely compromise the dog's quality of life and necessitate euthanasia.

As research increases our understanding of the cellular pathogenesis of seizures and mechanisms of antiepileptic drug actions, newer antiepileptic drugs are becoming available.[34] Although not yet routinely used in veterinary medicine, surgical therapy is indicated in human patients with certain types of medically intractable epilepsy.[48] Improvements in imaging and electrophysiologic techniques in veterinary medicine may allow surgery to be considered for epileptic dogs refractory to medical management.

CONCLUSION

Appropriate management of epileptic dogs entails obtaining an accurate diagnosis, ensuring proper client education, selecting an appropriate antiepileptic medication, and periodic evaluation and therapeutic drug monitoring to determine a dose that controls the seizures and avoids side effects. If seizures are still poorly controlled, the use of bromide is often beneficial. By following these principles, seizures can be controlled in most dogs with idiopathic epilepsy.

ACKNOWLEDGMENT

The author thanks Robert Selcer, DVM, MS, and Elizabeth Shull, DVM, of the Department of Clinical Sciences, University of Tennessee, for their assistance in the preparation of this manuscript.

About the Author

Dr. Thomas is affiliated with the Department of Small Animal Clinical Sciences, College of Veterinary Medicine, University of Tennessee, Knoxville, Tennessee. Dr. Thomas is a Diplomate of the American College of Veterinary Internal Medicine (Neurology).

REFERENCES

1. Shell LG: Understanding the fundamentals of seizures. *Vet Med* 88:622–628, 1993.
2. Forrester SD, Boothe DM, Troy GC: Current concepts in the management of canine epilepsy. *Compend Contin Educ Pract Vet* 11(7):811–820, 1989.
3. LeCouteur RA, Child G: Clinical management of epilepsy in dogs and cats. *Probl Vet Med* 1:578–595, 1989.

4. Oliver JE: Seizure disorders and narcolepsy, in Oliver JE, Hoerlein BF, Mayhew IG (eds): *Veterinary Neurology.* Philadelphia, WB Saunders Co, 1987, pp 285–302.
5. Farnbach GC: Serum concentrations and efficacy of phenytoin, phenobarbital, and primidone in canine epilepsy. *JAVMA* 184:1117–1120, 1984.
6. Farnbach GC: Efficacy of primidone in dogs with seizures unresponsive to phenobarbital. *JAVMA* 185:867–868, 1984.
7. Schwartz-Porsche D, Loscher W, Frey H-H: Therapeutic efficacy of phenobarbital and primidone in canine epilepsy: A comparison. *J Vet Pharmacol Ther* 8:113–119, 1985.
8. Dyer KR, Shell LG: Anticonvulsant therapy: A practical guide to medical management of epilepsy in pets. *Vet Med* 88:647–653, 1993.
9. Schwartz-Porsche D: Management of refractory seizures, in Kirk RW, Bonagura JD (eds): *Current Veterinary Therapy. XI.* Philadelphia, WB Saunders Co, 1992, pp 986–991.
10. Schwartz-Porsche D: Seizures, in Braund KG: *Clinical Syndromes in Veterinary Neurology,* ed 2. St. Louis, CV Mosby Co, 1994, pp 234–251.
11. Hass JA, Fenner WR: Epilepsy resistant to anticonvulsant therapy. *Probl Vet Med* 1:596–605, 1989.
12. Wyllie E, Luders H: Classification of the epilepsies, in Wyllie E (ed): *The Treatment of Epilepsy: Principles and Practice.* Philadelphia, Lea & Febiger, 1994, pp 492–493.
13. Knecht CD, Sorjonen DC, Simpson ST: Ancillary tests in the diagnosis of seizures. *JAAHA* 20:455–458, 1984.
14. Lane SB, Bunch SE: Medical management of recurrent seizures in dogs and cats. *J Vet Intern Med* 4:26–39, 1990.
15. Russo ME: The pathophysiology of epilepsy. *Cornell Vet* 71:221–247, 1981.
16. Meldrum BS: Anatomy, physiology, and pathology of epilepsy. *Lancet* 336:231–234, 1990.
17. Cunningham JG, Farnbach GC: Inheritance and idiopathic canine epilepsy. *JAAHA* 24:421–424, 1988.
18. Shell LG: The differential diagnosis of seizures. *Vet Med* 88:629–640, 1993.
19. Shell LG: The diagnostic approach to seizures. *Vet Med* 88:641–646, 1993.
20. Sisson A: Diagnosis and treatment of seizure disorders of dogs and cats. *Proc 8th ACVIM Forum* 8:349–356, 1990.
21. Dodman NH, Miczek KA, Knowles K, et al: Phenobarbital-responsive episodic dyscontrol (rage) in dogs. *JAVMA* 201:1580–1583, 1992.
22. Breitschwerdt EB, Breazile JE, Broadhurst JJ: Clinical and electroencephalographic findings associated with ten cases of suspected limbic epilepsy in the dog. *JAAHA* 15:37–50, 1979.
23. Oliver JE, Lorenz MD: *Handbook of Veterinary Neurology,* ed 2. Philadelphia, WB Saunders Co, 1993, p 93.
24. Indrieri RJ: Status epilepticus. *Probl Vet Med* 1:606–618, 1989.
25. Chrisman CL: *Problems in Small Animal Neurology,* ed 2. Philadelphia, Lea & Febiger, 1991, pp 177–205.
26. Newmark ME, Penry JK: Catamenial epilepsy: A review. *Epilepsia* 21:281–300, 1980.
27. Modica PA, Tempelhoff R, White PF: Pro- and anticonvulsant effects of anesthetics (Part II). *Anesth Analg* 70:433–444, 1990.
28. Lipka LJ, Lathers CM: Psychoactive agents, seizure production, and sudden death in epilepsy. *J Clin Pharmacol* 27:169–183, 1987.
29. Gunderson CH, Dunne PB, Feyer TL: Sleep deprivation seizures. *Neurology* 23:678–686, 1973.
30. Bunch SE: Anticonvulsant drug therapy in companion animals, in Kirk RW (ed): *Current Veterinary Therapy. VIII.* Philadelphia, WB Saunders Co, 1983, pp 836–844.
31. Selcer RR, Shull Selcer E: A practical approach to seizure management in dogs and cats. *Prog Vet Neurol* 1:147–156, 1990.
32. Bunch SE, Baldwin BH, Hornbuckle WE, Tennant BC: Compromised hepatic function in dogs treated with anticonvulsant drugs. *JAVMA* 184:444–448, 1984.
33. Bunch SE, Conway MB, Center SA, et al: Toxic hepatopathy and intrahepatic cholestasis associated with phenytoin administration in combination with other anticonvulsant drugs in three dogs. *JAVMA* 190:194–198, 1987.
34. Porter RJ: New antiepileptic agents: Strategies for drug development. *Lancet* 336:423–424, 1990.
35. Frey H-H: Anticonvulsant drugs used in the treatment of epilepsy. *Probl Vet Med* 1:558–577, 1989.
36. Morton DJ, Honhold N: Effectiveness of a therapeutic drug monitoring service as an aid to the control of canine seizures. *Vet Rec* 122:346–349, 1988.
37. Ravis WR, Pedersoli WM, Wike JS: Pharmacokinetics of phenobarbital in dogs given multiple doses. *Am J Vet Res* 50:1343–1347, 1989.
38. Bunch SE, Castleman WL, Baldwin BH, et al: Effects of long-term primidone and phenytoin administration on canine hepatic function and morphology. *Am J Vet Res* 46:105–115, 1985.
39. Meyer DJ, Noonan NE: Liver tests in dogs receiving anticonvulsant drugs (diphenylhydantoin and primidone). *JAAHA* 17:261–264, 1981.
40. Dayrell-Hart B, Steinberg SA, VanWinkle TJ, Farnbach GC: Hepatoxicity of phenobarbital in dogs: 18 cases (1985–1989). *JAVMA* 199:1060–1066, 1991.
41. Poffenbarger EM, Hardy RM: Hepatic cirrhosis associated with long-term primidone therapy in a dog. *JAVMA* 186:978–980, 1985.
42. Podell M, Fenner WR: Bromide therapy in refractory canine idiopathic epilepsy. *J Vet Intern Med* 7:318–327, 1993.
43. Pearce LK: Potassium bromide as an adjunct to phenobarbital for the management of uncontrolled seizures in dogs. *Prog Vet Neurol* 1:95–101, 1990.
44. Trepainier LA: Pharmokinetics and clinical use of bromide. *Proc 11th ACVIM Forum* 11:878–880, 1993.
45. Podell M, Fenner WR: Use of bromide as an antiepileptic drug in dogs. *Compend Contin Educ Pract Vet* 16(6):767–774, 1994.
46. Troupin AS: Antiepileptic drug therapy: A clinical overview, in Wyllie E (ed): *The Treatment of Epilepsy: Principles and Practice.* Philadelphia, Lea & Febiger, 1994, pp 785–790.
47. Nafe LA, Parker A, Kay WJ: Sodium valproate: A preliminary clinical trial in epileptic dogs. *JAAHA* 17:131–133, 1981.
48. Ojemann GA: Surgical therapy for medically intractable epilepsy. *J Neurosurg* 66:489–499, 1987.
49. Forrester SD, Brown SA, Lees GE, Hartsfield SM: Disposition of chlorazepate in dogs after single- and multiple-dose oral administration. *Am J Vet Res* 51:2001–2005, 1990.

UPDATE

Several other drugs may be useful in dogs with refractory epilepsy. In a small clinical study, the addition of felbamate improved seizure control in 75% of dogs with epilepsy that was refractory to standard medication.[1] A recommended dose is 15 mg/kg orally three times daily. If necessary, the dose can be titrated upward every two weeks by 7.5 mg/kg increments to a maximum of 45 mg/kg. Optimal dose and serum concentration have not been determined for the dog. Serum concentrations of phenobarbital should be monitored, as they may increase during concomitant administration with felbamate. An advantage of felbamate is that it is relatively nonsedating, compared to many other antiseizure drugs. Disadvantages include a high risk of liver disease (approximately 25%) and possible risk of bone marrow suppression. Because of the limited clinical experience and potential risks associated with felbamate, this drug should be considered only in dogs with severe, refractory seizures.

Many dogs with refractory epilepsy suffer clusters of seizures during a short time. Owner administration of diazepam per rectum is often effective in preventing multiple seizures.[2] After rectal administration of diazepam, there is rapid absorption with relatively high bioavailability of active metabolites.[3] The parenteral solution can be administered rectally using a syringe with an attached teat cannula or soft rubber catheter. Alternatively, some pharmacies will formulate diazepam suppositories. Owners are instructed to administer 0.5 to 10 mg/kg when the first seizure occurs.

REFERENCES

1. Daryell-Hart B, Tiches D, Vite C, Steinberg SA: Efficacy of felbamate as an anticonvulsant in dogs with refractory seizures. *Proc 14th ACVIM Forum*, 14:756, 1996.
2. Podell M: The use of diazepam per rectum at home for the acute management of cluster seizures in dogs. *J Vet Intern Med* 1995, 8:68–74.
3. Papich MG, Alcorn J: Absorption of diazepam after its rectal administration in dogs. *Am J Vet Res* 1995, 56:1629–1636.

Seizure Disorders in Companion Animals

J. E. Oliver, Jr, DVM
Professor and Head
Department of Small Animal Medicine
College of Veterinary Medicine
University of Georgia
Athens, Georgia

Seizure disorders are among the most frequently seen neurologic problems in small animal practice. Seizures often present a diagnostic dilemma because they are episodic, frequently not observed by the veterinarian and often present with no other clinical abnormality. A protocol for diagnosis and management is presented which can be adapted to the capabilities of the practice and the interest of the client.

Definitions

Seizures, epilepsy, fits or convulsions are terms used to describe a disorder of brain function characterized by paroxysmal, stereotyped alterations in behavior. The term epilepsy indicates that the seizures are recurring but does not imply the cause of the seizures.

Several components of the seizure may be described. The actual seizure is called the *ictus*. Prior to the seizure (preictal), there may be a period of altered behavior called the *aura*. People with seizures report varying sensations, apprehension and other symptoms during the aura. Animals may hide, appear nervous or seek out the owner at this time. The ictus usually only lasts 1 to 2 minutes but this is variable. Following the seizure, the postictal phase, the animal may return to normal in seconds to minutes or may be restless, lethargic, confused, disoriented or blind for minutes to hours.[1] The aura and postictal phase do not seem to have any relationship to the severity or cause of the seizures.[1]

Two components are recognized as the basis for seizure disorders, the *seizure focus* and *spread* of the activity to other areas of the brain. The paroxysmal alterations in behavior are associated with synchronous excessive discharge in large aggregates of neurons, the *seizure focus*.[2] If the activity of the seizure focus *spreads* to other parts of the brain, a generalized cerebral dysrhythmia results which produces the behavioral change recognized as a seizure.

Seizure foci are apparently present in many individuals who do not have seizures. Some populations of neurons in the brain (e.g., hippocampus) are much more likely to develop seizure activity than others. The seizure focus has been studied extensively in a variety of experimental models and in naturally occurring epilepsy. Neurons in seizure foci are characterized by having large-amplitude, prolonged membrane depolarizations with associated high frequency bursts of spikes. These changes cause paroxysmal discharges in the electroencephalogram (EEG).[2]

Seizures can be generated in any individual by pharmacologic, metabolic or electrical changes. However, the threshold of stimulation required varies widely. Normal individuals may require potent convulsant drugs (e.g., pentylenetetrazol) or electric shock to exceed the threshold. A lower seizure

TABLE I
CLASSIFICATION OF SEIZURES—CLINICAL SIGNS*

Clinical Manifestation	EEG	Etiology	Anatomical Location
Generalized Seizures, Bilateral Symmetrical Seizures, or Seizures without Local Onset			
Tonic-Clonic (Grand Mal, Major Motor)	Generalized dysrhythmia from onset. Symmetrical. Often normal interictal unless activated or has organic or toxic origin.	1) Genetic predisposition 2) Diffuse or multiple organic lesions 3) Toxic or metabolic	1) Unlocalized 2) Diencephalic (centrencephalic)
Absences with or without motor phenomena (Petit Mal) Rare or rarely recognized in animals	Generalized 3 per second spike and wave dysrhythmia. Symmetrical (human).	Usually genetic (human)	1) Unlocalized 2) Diencephalic (centrencephalic)
Partial Seizures or Seizures Beginning Locally			
Partial Motor (may generalize to tonic-clonic seizure). Signs depend on site of discharge	Focal dysrhythmia (spikes, slow waves). May generalize secondarily.	Acquired organic lesion. See Table II.	Focal cortical or subcortical
Psychomotor (may generalize or appear as complex behavioral change—running, fear, aggression)	Dysrhythmia related to temporal lobe (unproved in animals).	Acquired organic lesion. See Table II.	Limbic system (hippocampus, temporal or pyriform lobe)

*Modified from JE Oliver.[9]

threshold may allow production of seizures by conditions such as fever, photic stimulation or minor alterations in body chemistry (e.g., hypoglycemia, hypocalcemia, hyperventilation). Finally, there are individuals who have seizures with no apparent stimulus required. The range from normal individuals to those with spontaneous seizures is a continuum without sharply defined boundaries.

The behavioral changes of seizures are composed of one or more of the following involuntary phenomena: (1) loss or derangement of consciousness or memory (amnesia); (2) alteration of muscle tone or movement; (3) alteration of sensation, including hallucinations of special senses (e.g., visual, auditory, olfactory); (4) disturbances of the autonomic nervous system (e.g., salivation, urination, defecation); and (5) other psychic manifestations, abnormal thought processes or moods (recognized as behavioral changes, e.g., fear, rage).[3]

One or more of the above are present in a seizure. For example, loss of consciousness is usually associated with a generalized motor seizure but may not be a part of a seizure with behavioral manifestations. Behavioral or psychic changes are not necessarily seizure disorders. However, if the changes are paroxysmal, seizures should be strongly considered.

Classification of Seizures

Numerous classifications of seizures have been proposed based on clinical signs, etiology, location of the abnormality, age or circumstance of occurrence, and electrophysiology.[4-11] Two schemes are of primary benefit for clinical purposes, one based on clinical signs and one on the cause of the seizures.

Clinical Signs

Classification of seizures, based on clinical signs, is useful from both a descriptive and diagnostic standpoint (Table I).

Gastaut has proposed that generalized seizures be called *primary generalized epilepsy*, if no cause can be ascertained, and *secondary generalized epilepsy*, if any organic cause can be found.[5] Primary generalized epilepsy corresponds to essential epilepsy, true epilepsy, idiopathic epilepsy, genetic epilepsy and centrencephalic epilepsy.

Partial or focal seizures are usually acquired, thus ruling out primary generalized epilepsy.

Generalized Seizures

Tonic-Clonic Seizures (grand mal, major motor)—These are the most frequently recognized seizures in animals. The seizure is frequently preceded by an aura. The animal falls and becomes unconscious, the limbs are extended rigidly, opisthotonos is usually seen and respiration stops (apnea). The tonic phase is usually brief (10 to 30 seconds) and is rapidly followed by clonic limb movements in the form of running or paddling activity. Chewing movements of the mouth are common. Visceral activity may start in the tonic or clonic phase of the ictus and may include pupillary dilatation, salivation, urination, defecation and piloerection. The clonic phase may alternate with tonic activity. The ictus usually lasts 1 to 2 minutes. The postictal phase may be

TABLE II
Classification of Seizures—Causes of Seizure Disorders

Classification	Most Frequent Causes	Diagnostic Tests*
Genetic	Genetic	Breed, age, history
Developmental	Hydrocephalus	PE, EEG, Ventriculography
	Lissencephaly	Breed, PE, EEG
	Porencephaly	Ventriculography
Infectious	Viral: Canine Distemper	History, EEG, CSF
	Feline Infectious Peritonitis	CSF
	Bacterial: Any Type	CSF
	Mycotic: Cryptococcosis	CSF
	Protozoan: Toxoplasmosis	CSF, Titer
Metabolic	Electrolyte: Hypocalcemia	Serum Calcium
	Carbohydrate: Hypoglycemia,	Fasting Blood Glucose
	Functional Insulinoma	Fasting Blood Glucose
	Glycoprotein Storage Disease (Lafora)	Biopsy, Necropsy
	Fat: Lipid Storage Diseases	Breed, Biopsy
	Cardiovascular: Arrhythmia	EKG
	Vascular	Arteriography
	Renal	PE, BUN, UA
	Hepatic: Cirrhosis	PE, BSP, SGPT, Serum NH_3
	Portacaval Shunt	Same + Angiography
	Nutritional: Thiamine	History, Treatment
	Parasitism (Multiple factors)	PE, Treatment
Neoplastic	Primary: Gliomas, Meningioma	NE, EEG, Radiography
	Secondary: Metastatic	Same
Toxic	Heavy Metal: Lead	History, Blood Lead
	Organophosphates	History, NE
	Chlorinated Hydrocarbon	History, NE
	Strychnine	History, NE
Traumatic	Acute: Immediately after head injury	History, PE
	Chronic: Weeks to years after injury	History, EEG

*Definitions: PE = physical examination, EEG = electroencephalography, CSF = cerebrospinal fluid, BUN = serum urea nitrogen, UA = urine analysis, BSP = Bromsulphalein test, SGPT = serum glutamic pyruvic transaminase, NE = neurologic examination, EKG = electrocardiography.

a few minutes of rest followed by normal activity or may include confusion, disorientation, restlessness and pacing, or blindness lasting for minutes to hours.

Careful questioning of the owner is required to determine if the seizure starts as generalized, symmetrical activity or has a focal component. The aura should not be confused with focal seizure activity. Any indication of focal motor activity, such as chewing, forced turning of the head or clonic jerks of muscle groups, implies a focal component, even if it generalizes secondarily.

Absences (petit mal seizures)—These are either very uncommon in animals or, more likely, they are uncommonly recognized. They are characterized by brief (seconds) loss of contact with the environment, but without motor activity. Variations seen in humans include minor motor components such as facial twitching, loss of postural tone or autonomic activity. Redding has reported one dog with absence attacks and characteristic EEG changes (4 Hz spike-wave complexes).[6] Unless these attacks are frequent or the owner is very observant, they would probably be unnoticed.

Partial Seizures

Partial Motor Seizures (focal motor, Jacksonian)—These reflect the activity of a local seizure focus in an area producing motor activity. Movements are restricted to one part of the body, such as the face or one limb. Partial seizures frequently spread, resulting in a generalized seizure. The focal component of the onset is the key differential feature. Since partial seizures are invariably acquired, primary generalized epilepsy can be ruled out from consideration.

The true Jacksonian seizure, which includes a focal onset followed by a progression of motor activity to adjacent structures ultimately terminating in a generalized motor seizure, is rare in animals. The motor area of the cerebral cortex of domestic animals is so small that such a progression occurs very rapidly. Patients with partial motor seizures are more likely to have focal EEG abnormalities in interictal periods than those with generalized seizures. Partial sensory and autonomic seizures are not commonly recognized. Psychomotor seizures may have a predominance of autonomic signs.[5,12] Animals that have repetitive episodes of *fly-biting* may be having focal sensory seizures in the visual cortex. Psychomotor seizures with a sensory component is the explanation generally accepted.

Psychomotor Seizures (partial seizures with complex symptomatology, behavioral seizures, emotional disorders)—These are paroxysmal episodes of abnormal behavior. Examples include hysteria, rage, autonomic reactions such as salivation, or hallucinations such as *fly-biting*.

Differentiating psychomotor seizures from pure behavioral changes can be difficult. Psychomotor seizures will usually be preceded by an aura and followed by a postictal phase. The ictus should be stereotyped and repetitive. Autonomic components of the ictus are common.

Causes of Seizures

Seizures may be caused by any process which alters the normal function of neurons in the brain. As with all neurologic diseases, the etiology should be considered in broad categories with the most common diseases within that category as a secondary consideration. Table II outlines the major categories of diseases that are likely to produce seizures.

Genetic

Primary, generalized epilepsy (idiopathic, cryptogenic) is inherited and has no demonstrable pathologic cause. Although it is thought to occur in a number of species,[13] the most comprehensive studies have been in man (Robb[14]) and dogs.[15-19]

Primary generalized epilepsy usually occurs in the form of generalized tonic-clonic seizures in animals. Absence attacks are a common form in man but are apparently rare in dogs.[10] Breeds of dogs which have been shown to have a genetic basis for epilepsy are listed in Table III. Also listed are those breeds reported to have a high incidence of seizure disorders but not having reported genetic studies. Whether these breeds have genetic epilepsy is yet to be proven.

The first seizure in a dog with primary, generalized epilepsy will usually occur between the ages of 6 months and 5 years.[20] In a large Beagle colony, 29 dogs had their first seizure at a mean age of 30 months (range, 11 to 70 months).[15] However, many of the dogs with abnormal EEG's had not been observed to have seizures by the age of 6 years and therefore could be at risk for future seizures. Males had a significantly higher incidence rate than females in this colony.[15] The incidence of seizures in each of three different reports relating to other breeds was approximately 1%.[1,20,21]

The diagnosis of primary, generalized seizures can only be made by excluding other causes. There are no positive diagnostic findings that will substantiate the diagnosis. The breed, age and history may be highly suggestive, especially if there is a familial history of seizures. Abnormality in the EEG is not consistent.[11,18,22] Activation techniques may prove useful in detecting latent abnormalities.[18,22]

Developmental

Disorders in this group may or may not be inherited but are distinguished from primary, generalized epilepsy (genetic) by having demonstrable pathologic changes in the brain. Hydrocephalus is probably the most common developmental disorder causing seizures. Other developmental defects that may produce seizures are lissencephaly[23] and porencephaly (Tables IV and V).

Hydrocephalus is characterized by an excess of cerebrospinal fluid (CSF) in the cranium, usually associated with enlargement of the ventricular system (internal hydrocephalus). It may be congenital or acquired. Decreased absorption or obstruction to the flow of CSF are the usual causes.[6,24]

Lissencephaly is a congenital absence of the convolutions of the cerebral cortex.[6,23] It has only been reported in the Lhasa Apso dog and in one cat. Affected animals can have behavioral, visual and slight proprioceptive deficits in addition to seizures.

Porencephaly is a cystic malformation of the cerebrum which usually communicates with the ventricle or subarachnoid space. It may be congenital or acquired (degenerative).

Infectious

Almost any infectious disease has the potential for causing seizures if it invades the central nervous system (CNS). The most common diseases are listed in Table II. Canine

TABLE III
Genetic Epilepsy—Primary Generalized Epilepsy

Genetic factor proven or highly suspicious
- Alsatian (German Shepherd)[17]
- Beagle[15,34]
- Keeshond[35]
- Tervuren (Belgian) Shepherd[13]

Breeds reported to have a high incidence of seizure disorders[1,6,16,21]
- Poodle
- Wirehaired Terrier
- Cocker Spaniel
- St. Bernard
- Irish Setter
- Collie
- Boxer
- Dachshund

TABLE IV
Common Causes of Seizures at Different Ages

Less Than 1 Year

Developmental	—Hydrocephalus, Lissencephaly
Toxic	—Heavy metals—lead, Organophosphates, Chlorinated hydrocarbons
Infectious	—Canine distemper, encephalitis
Metabolic	—Hypoglycemia, Portacaval shunt, hepatic encephalopathy, Storage diseases—lipodystrophy, gangliosidosis, glycogen, Leukodystrophy, Nutritional—thiamine, parasitism
Traumatic	—Acute

1-3 Years
Genetic—primary generalized epilepsy
Others as above

Over 4 Years

Metabolic	—Hypoglycemia secondary to insulinoma, Cardiovascular—arrhythmia, thromboembolism
Neoplastic	—Primary or metastatic brain tumor

TABLE V
CAUSES OF SEIZURES—BREED PREDISPOSITION

Breed	Cause
Alsatian (German Shepherd)	Genetic
Beagle	Genetic
Belgian (Tervuren) Shepherd	Genetic
Boston Terrier	Hydrocephalus, Neoplasia
Boxer	Neoplasia
Cairn Terrier	Globoid cell leukodystrophy
Chihuahua	Hydrocephalus
English Setter	Lipodystrophy
German Shepherd (Alsatian)	Genetic
German Shorthaired Pointer	Lipodystrophy
Irish Setter	Genetic
Keeshond	Genetic
Lhasa Apso	Lissencephaly
Miniature Pinscher	Hydrocephalus
Miniature Schnauzer	Hyperlipoproteinemia, Portacaval shunts
Pekingese	Hydrocephalus
Poodle, Miniature & Standard	Genetic (suspected)
Poodle, Toy	Hydrocephalus
St. Bernard	Genetic (suspected)
West Highland White Terrier	Globoid cell leukodystrophy
Yorkshire Terrier	Hydrocephalus

distemper is probably the most common cause of seizures in dogs. The CNS manifestations may appear without any noticeable clinical illness. Diagnosis may require an EEG.[6,24]

Metabolic

Failure of one of the major organs may result in alterations in electrolytes and glucose, or accumulation of toxic products resulting in seizures. Some animals have a lower seizure threshold so that relatively minor alterations may cause seizures. Abnormal cellular metabolism from deficiencies in specific enzymes causes accumulation of metabolic products, the storage diseases. Storage diseases often affect neurons which may produce seizures as one part of the clinical picture. Nutritional deficiencies may also alter the metabolic state. Table II lists the most common metabolic abnormalities.

Neoplastic

Intracranial neoplasia, either primary or metastatic, may cause seizures. The seizure activity is caused by abnormality in neurons adjacent to the neoplasm which are compressed, distorted or have an insufficient blood supply. The tumor is not electrically active, but often induces modification of surrounding electrical activity.

Seizures may be the first sign of brain tumor. Neurologic deficit may not be apparent until weeks to months after the onset of seizures, especially if the mass is in the cerebral cortex. Arteriography, ventriculography or brain scan may be required for diagnosis.

Toxic

Many toxins affect the CNS and most can cause seizures. Diagnosis usually depends on history, identification of the toxic substance from body tissues or intestinal contents, and response to treatment.

Heavy Metals—Lead poisoning is a frequent intoxication in animals. Other clinical signs include depression, tremor and ataxia, sometimes associated with gastrointestinal signs. Seizures are often psychomotor. Peripheral blood changes may include nucleated erythrocytes (RBC) and basophilic stippling of RBC without anemia. The changes in the RBC are transient and cannot be used to rule out lead poisoning. Blood lead determination is diagnostic. Treatment is with calcium ethylenediamine-tetraacetic acid.[6,25]

Strychnine—Malicious or accidental poisoning with strychnine causes a tonic seizure which is exacerbated by stimulation. The animal remains conscious unless respiration stops. Strychnine blocks inhibitory interneurons in the spinal cord causing a release of motor neuron activity.

Traumatic

Seizures may be seen immediately after acute head injury as a direct effect on neurons. Post-traumatic seizures may occur many weeks to several years after a head injury. Post-traumatic epilepsy may be focal or generalized depending on the location of the brain lesion. The focus develops secondary to a scar in the brain at the site of initial injury. The focal abnormality may be recognized on EEG.

Data Base for Seizure Disorders[9]

The recommended data base is formulated at three levels (Table VI). The minimum data base (MDB) can be obtained at a veterinary clinic with available clinical pathology service. The specific chemistries might be modified to fit those available in an automated service. The only cost other than the initial examination is the cost of laboratory studies. Risk to the patient is minimal.

The MDB is designed to screen for primary neurologic disease (neurologic examination) and metabolic or systemic disorders (physical examination, laboratory examination).

The more complete data base includes CSF analysis, skull radiography and EEG (Table VI). CSF analysis and radiography can be performed at most clinics but EEG is not usually available except at referral centers. These tests are indicated if the MDB indicates the presence of neurologic disease or if the seizures have not been controlled with medication. These procedures are not recommended as a part of the MDB because of the low yield in animals with

TABLE VI
Data Base for Seizure Disorders*

Minimum Data Base
  Patient Profile
    Breed, age, sex
  History
    Immunizations: kind, dates, by whom
    Age of onset
    Frequency, course
    Description of seizure
      General; partial; duration; aura; postictal; time of day; relation to exercise, food, sleep and stimuli
    Previous or present illness or injury
    Behavioral changes
  Physical Examination
    Complete systems examination including specifically:
      Musculoskeletal—size, shape of skull, evidence of trauma, atrophy of any muscles
      Cardiovascular—color of mucous membranes, arrhythmias, murmurs
  Neurologic Examination
    Complete with emphasis on cerebral signs including:
      Vision, pupils
      Tactile and visual placing
      Hopping
      All cranial nerves
      Spinal reflexes
  Clinical Pathology
    CBC   Urinalysis
    BUN   Alkaline Phosphatase
    Calcium   SGPT
    Fasting Blood Glucose
    Others if indicated

More Complete Data Base (in addition to Minimum Data Base)
  CSF: Cell count, total and differential, protein, pressure
  Skull Radiographs: Ventrodorsal, lateral, frontal
  EEG

Focal Brain Disease Suspected
  Contrast Radiography
  Brain Scans

*Modified from JE Oliver.[9]

normal findings on the MDB, the increased risk because anesthesia is required and the increased cost to the client.

Procedures to evaluate structural alterations in the brain, including contrast radiography and radioisotopic brain imaging, are reserved for animals with a high probability of focal brain disease. The only exception is ventriculography which may be used to make a definitive diagnosis of hydrocephalus. These procedures are more dangerous, more expensive and generally should be done at referral centers.

Plan for Diagnosis and Management

A MDB should be completed on every patient having more than one seizure. Patients having only one isolated seizure should be given a thorough physical and neurologic examination. If no abnormalities are found, the owners should be advised to watch for further seizures.

Information from the MDB should lead to one of three alternatives: (1) a diagnosis of the cause of the seizure, (2) a possible cause of the seizure requiring confirmation with further tests or (3) no suggestion of the cause of the seizure (Table VII).

The history should provide information relating to the onset and progression of the disease (Table VIII). Seizures, by definition, are acute in onset. However, the owner may be able to recognize a chronic progression of signs with seizures being only one component. Diagnostic tests that are most likely to be useful in each disease are listed in Table II. The MDB will rule out most metabolic diseases. Other diseases may or may not be suggested by the data accumulated.

If there are no positive or suggestive findings on the MDB, the animal should be treated with anticonvulsant medications, as described below.

If the seizures are not controlled with anticonvulsants, a more complete data base should be obtained. Chronic encephalitis and occult hydrocephalus can usually be detected with EEG. Chronic subclinical encephalitis and occult hydrocephalus are the most common causes of seizures that are refractory to medication.

Some dog breeds have primary, generalized epilepsy which is difficult to control. The most common examples are German Shepherds, St. Bernards and Irish Setters.[1,11]

Negative findings on the complete data base in an animal that has been poorly controlled with anticonvulsant medication suggests a poor prognosis. Treatment may be altered by changing dosage or drugs, combining drugs and changing the schedule of administration. Reevaluation periodically may reveal progressive disease which was missed originally.

Contrast radiography and radioisotope brain scans are indicated if there is evidence of focal brain disease or hydrocephalus. Mass lesions or alterations in the ventricular system are necessary for these tests to be positive.

Therapy

The probability of successful treatment depends more on successful client education than on any other single factor. Treatment failures are usually the result of (1) progressive disease, (2) refractory epilepsy, (3) inadequate client education, and (4) inadequate blood levels of anticonvulsant. Progressive disease will be identified by repeated examinations. Refractory epilepsy may be expected in those breeds previously listed. Client education is a variable that can be controlled by the veterinarian.

The client should understand what successful treatment is. Successful treatment is defined by the author to be (1) reduced frequency of seizures, (2) shorter duration of seizures and/or (3) reduced severity of seizures. Note that elimination of seizures is not listed. Complete elimination of seizures is certainly a goal but its successful achievement is frequently not possible.

The client should be given some basic rules for treating epileptics.

1. Efficacy of medication should not be judged for at least 2 weeks, thus allowing the medication a chance.
2. Medication should not be changed or discontinued suddenly. Status epilepticus may follow.
3. Phenothiazine tranquilizers are *contraindicated* in epileptics.
4. Changes in the animal's environment must be taken into consideration—more medication when increased excitement is expected, etc.
5. Medication may be required for life; it should not be discontinued prematurely.
6. No single drug or combination works in all cases. Each case must be treated individually. Adjustments of dosage, schedule or drugs will probably be required.

TABLE VII
Plan for Diagnosis and Management of Patient with Seizures*

Minimum Data Base†

Positive Findings	Suggestive Findings		Negative Findings
R/o Metabolic	Metabolic	Developmental	Developmental
R/i Infectious	Toxic	Genetic	Genetic
Distemper	R/o with specific	Infectious	Infectious
Toxoplasmosis	tests	Neoplastic	Neoplastic
Other		Traumatic	Traumatic
R/i Developmental			
Hydrocephalus			Treat with anticonvulsants
R/i Toxic			
R/i Traumatic		Complete Data Base ← If poorly controlled	

Complete Data Base

Positive Findings	Negative Findings
R/o Developmental	Assume *Genetic*
R/o Infectious	Repeat Evaluations
R/o Neoplastic	at intervals or
R/o Traumatic	if change in status

Treat primary problem
Supplement with anticonvulsants
if necessary

Treat with anticonvulsants

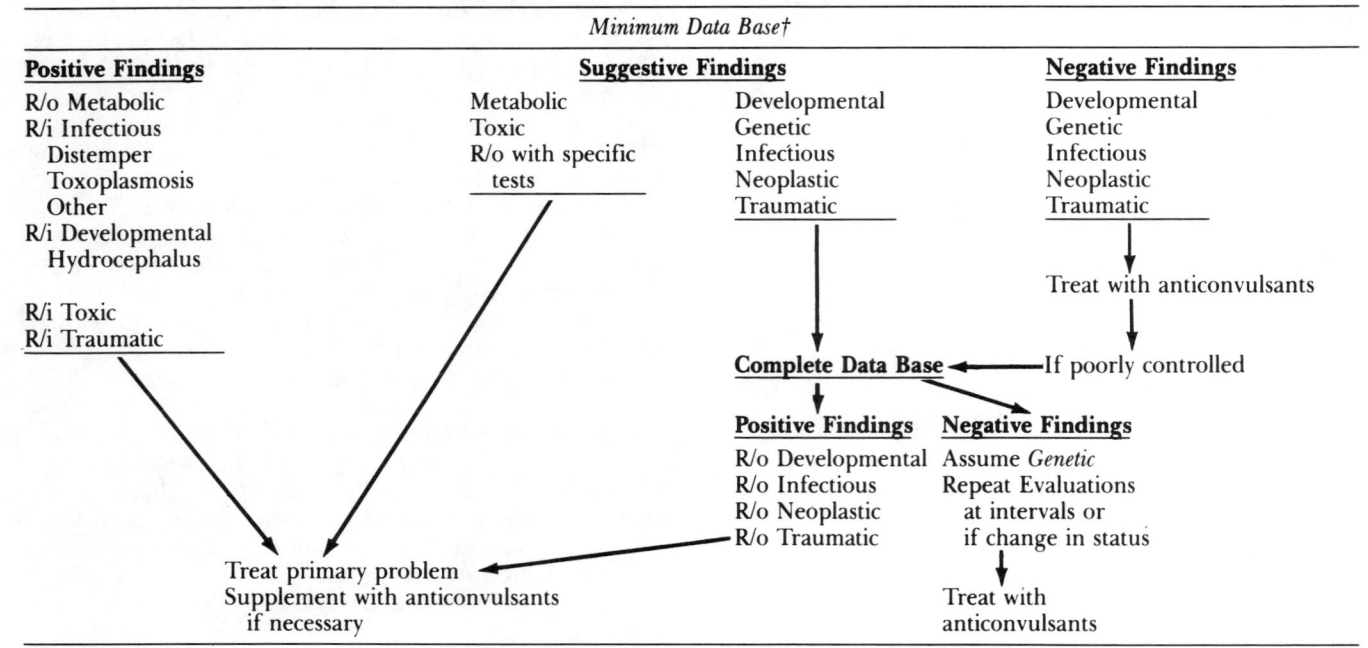

*Modified from JE Oliver[9]
†*Definitions:* R/o—Rule out. Positive findings confirm the diagnosis, negative findings eliminate the diagnosis. R/i—Rule in. Positive findings confirm the diagnosis, negative findings *not* adequate diagnosis.

Finding the right combination can almost be a research project.

Treatment of animals that have had only one seizure is not usually recommended. Also, treatment is not initiated while establishing a diagnosis, unless the seizures are frequent and severe (more than one per day).

Treating frequent or severe seizures is recommended, especially if they tend to cluster (several in one day). Owners should be advised that each time a seizure discharge spreads, it increases the probability that it will spread again.

The final decision on treatment must be made by the client. In essence, *if the client feels that the seizures are more of a problem than giving the medication, then treatment is in order.* Clients with small dogs in large yards will tolerate more seizures than those with giant breeds in small apartments.

The ideal anticonvulsant would completely suppress seizures without side effects or toxicity. Unfortunately, such a drug is not known. There are three primary drugs used in the chronic treatment of seizures: phenobarbital, primidone and phenytoin (diphenylhydantoin). Additionally, diazepam and short-acting barbiturates may be used in the treatment of status epilepticus.

Phenobarbital is generally the first drug used. Phenobarbital raises the threshold for seizure discharge and inhibits the spread of discharge from the epileptic focus.[26] It is safe, inexpensive and has few side effects other than sedation. An initial period of sedation is usually followed by a return to normal activity in a few days. Polyphagia, polydipsia and polyuria may be seen in some patients. The usual dose is 1 to 2 mg/kg/day given in divided doses twice daily.[1]

If phenobarbital is not effective, **primidone** is used. A portion of the primidone molecule is metabolized to phenobarbital, while the remainder is phenylethylmalonamide (PEMA). The phenobarbital component has been reported to be as little as one-fourth and as much as three-fourths of the total.[1,26,27] Published studies of primidone metabolism, blood levels and half-life in the dog have not been found. Primidone's probable major function is to suppress the epileptic focus. Efficacy of primidone in patients with seizures has been demonstrated clinically for years. It is probably the most effective drug available for seizures resulting from encephalitis. Side effects include depression, polydipsia, polyphagia and hepatic necrosis (the latter in a small number of patients). The side effects may be dramatic but they are usually transient, despite continuing medication. Hepatic necrosis, however, is an indication for immediate termination of therapy. The usual dose is 10 mg/kg/day divided in two doses. One-half to twice this dose may be used depending on the individual.

Phenytoin is probably the most widely used anticonvulsant in man. Proper use of the drug in animals is being questioned because of studies showing marked differences in metabolism of the drug between species. Pharmacokinetics vary depending on route of administration, pretreatment, treatment with other drugs, and on the individual case (even within the same breed).[28] Approximate plasma half-life of phenytoin is: man—22 to 28 hours, dogs—3 to 4 hours, cats—24 to 108 hours. Therefore, humans are on a once or twice a day schedule, and cats should be medicated once weekly. Treatment of cats is not recommended until chronic toxicity studies have been performed. Phenytoin has not been approved for use in cats. Combination of phenytoin with phenobarbital may further reduce the half-life of phenytoin.

TABLE VIII
The Differential Diagnosis Based on Course of Disease

	Seizures		
	Acute Nonprogressive	*Acute Progressive*	*Chronic* Progressive*
Developmental	Genetic epilepsy Lissencephaly Porencephaly	Hydrocephalus	
Degenerative			Storage diseases Demyelinating diseases
Infectious		Viral: Canine Distemper FIP Bacterial: Any Mycotic: Any Protozoan: Toxoplasmosis	
Metabolic		Hypocalcemia Hypoglycemia Cardiac arrhythmia Hepatic encephalopathy Renal failure	Hepatic encephalopathy
Neoplastic		Metastatic	Primary
Nutritional		Thiamine deficiency	Parasitism—Puppies
Toxic		Organophosphates Chlorinated hydrocarbons Strychnine Tetanus	Heavy metals
Traumatic		Head Injury: Immediately after injury	Head Injury: Weeks to years after injury

*Seizures may have acute onset but syndrome as a whole is chronic.

In addition, blood levels in the dog do not reach therapeutic levels (10 µg/ml based on human clinical and canine research data) at the same dosage levels prescribed in man.[28] One study indicates that at least 30 mg/kg/TID is needed to reach therapeutic levels.[28,29] Another study reports that therapeutic levels were achieved with 1.5-2.5 mg/lb/TID, but the reported therapeutic levels were only 1.5-3.0 µg/ml.[30] Clinical studies of therapeutic blood levels are needed to resolve the problem. Until they are available, it is recommended that phenytoin be used only after phenobarbital and primidone have proven unacceptable. Side effects of phenytoin have been rare, possibly due to the dose which has been too low to be therapeutic. Ataxia, elevated liver enzymes and gingival hyperplasia have been reported. The recommended dosage varies from 5 to 50 mg/kg/TID.

Mephobarbital is longer acting than phenobarbital and therefore may be given once daily. Its efficacy is essentially the same as that of phenobarbital since it is metabolized into two molecules of phenobarbital. It offers once a day medication at a greater expense.

Diazepam is used in treatment of status epilepticus and may be used in conjunction with other drugs in treatment of epilepsy. The duration of action is short, requiring TID or QID administration. Phenobarbital and diazepam are the only anticonvulsants recommended for cats.

Other drugs that may be beneficial, although not currently approved for use in animals, include parametha-dione,[31] carbamazepine[32] and sodium valproate. Progestational agents have been beneficial in some cases, especially those with psychomotor-type seizures.

A protocol for treatment of seizures is outlined in Table IX.

Status epilepticus is the condition of rapidly recurring convulsions without recovery of consciousness in the inter-

TABLE IX
Protocol for Anticonvulsant Medication

Seizures less than 1 per week
1. Phenobarbital 1 mg/kg/BID. Reduce dose after 1 week if sedation is a problem. Increase to point of sedation if seizures not controlled.
2. Primidone 5 mg/kg/BID. Increase or decrease dose as above. If seizures are not controlled with primidone:
3. Phenytoin 10 mg/kg/TID. Increase dose if seizures are not controlled. Check blood levels if possible, adjusting dose to provide 10 µg/ml. If seizures are not controlled:
4. Try combinations of above or consider use of drugs not approved (with owner's consent), i.e., carbamazepine or paramethadione.

Seizures more than 1 per week
1. Phenobarbital 2 mg/kg/BID or primidone 10 mg/kg/BID. Proceed as above.

vals between convulsions.[33] It must be treated as a serious emergency because death can result. Causes of status epilepticus include (1) toxicities or metabolic abnormalities, (2) withdrawal of anticonvulsant medication, (3) ineffective anticonvulsant medication and (4) progressive brain disease. A protocol for treatment of status epilepticus is presented in Table X.

TABLE X
PROTOCOL FOR TREATMENT OF STATUS EPILEPTICUS

1. Stop the seizure. Diazepam, 10-35 mg in 10 mg boluses, IV. Diazepam will usually give at least temporary remission allowing time for succeeding steps. If not, phenobarbital sodium is given (1-2 mg/kg IV). If neither is effective, sodium pentobarbital is given to effect (estimated dose 10-15 mg/kg). Administration of pentobarbital must be done cautiously as diazepam and phenobarbital may potentiate its effect. Ultrashort barbiturates should not be used as they may potentiate seizure activity.
2. With the seizures stopped, assure ventilation of the patient. An endotracheal tube should be placed if the patient is unconscious.
3. Place an IV catheter, draw blood for hematology and chemistries and start a drip with lactated Ringer's solution. Do blood glucose as soon as possible.
4. Give 50% dextrose IV (2-3 ml for toy breeds, 50 ml for giant breeds). If seizures are not violent or there are interictal quiet periods, steps 3 and 4 may be done first. Hypoglycemia is the one cause of status that can be treated directly.
5. If hypocalcemia is suspected, give an intravenous calcium preparation. Monitor the heart rate.
6. Once seizures are under control, evaluate the animal to try to determine the cause. Treat specifically if a cause can be found (e.g., toxicity).
7. Monitor body temperature. If it reaches 106°F, cool the animal with ice to a temperature of 103°F. Maintain temperature in a normal range.
8. Continue control of seizures. Intravenous or intramuscular phenobarbital is preferred until oral medication can be used.

REFERENCES

1. Kay WJ, Fenner WR: Epilepsy, in Kirk RW (ed): *Current Veterinary Therapy VI*. Philadelphia, WB Saunders Co, 1977, pp 853-867.
2. Prince DA: Neurophysiology of epilepsy. *Annu Rev Neurosci* 1:395-415, 1978.
3. Lennox WG: *Epilepsy and Related Disorders*. Boston, Little Brown and Co, 1960.
4. de Lahunta A: *Veterinary Neuroanatomy and Clinical Neurology*. Philadelphia, WB Saunders Co, 1977.
5. Gastaut H: Clinical and electroencephalographical classification of epileptic seizures. *Epilepsia* (Suppl) 10:S12-S13, 1969.
6. Hoerlein BF: *Canine Neurology*. 3rd ed. Philadelphia, WB Saunders Co, 1978.
7. Masland RL: Comments on the classification of epilepsy. *Epilepsia* (Suppl) 10:S22-S28, 1969.
8. Oliver JE Jr, Hoerlein BF: Convulsive disorders of dogs. *J Am Vet Med Assoc* 146:1126-1133, 1965.
9. Oliver JE Jr: Protocol for the diagnosis of seizure disorders in companion animals. *J Am Vet Med Assoc* 172:822-824, 1978.
10. Parker AJ: Epilepsy in the dog, causes, classification and diagnosis. *Ill Vet* 16:5-10, 1973.
11. Redding RW: The diagnosis and therapy of seizures. *J Am Anim Hosp Assoc* 5:79-92, 1969.
12. Breitschwerdt EB, Breazile JE, Broadhurst JJ: Clinical and electroencephalographic findings associated with ten cases of suspected limbic epilepsy in the dog. *J Am Anim Hosp Assoc* 15:37-50, 1979.
13. Van der Velden NA: Fits in Tervueren Shepherd dogs: A presumed hereditary trait. *J Small Anim Pract* 9:63-70, 1968.
14. Robb P: Epilepsy, a review of basic and clinical research. NINDB Monograph No 1, DHEW Publ No (NIH) 73-415, Washington, DC, 1965.
15. Biefelt SW, Redman HC, McClellan RO: Sire and sex-related differences in rates of epileptiform seizures in a purebred beagle dog colony. *Am J Vet Res* 32:2039-2048, 1971.
16. Croft PG: Fits in dogs: A survey of 260 cases. *Vet Rec* 77:438-445, 1965.
17. Falco MJ, Barker J, Wallace ME: The genetics of epilepsy in the British Alsatian. *J Small Anim Pract* 15:685-692, 1974.
18. Redman HC, Weir JE: Detection of naturally occurring neurologic disorders of beagle dogs by electroencephalography. *Am J Vet Res* 30:2075-2082, 1969.
19. Wiederholt WC: Electrophysiologic analysis of epileptic beagles. *Neurology* 24:149-155, 1974..
20. Cunningham, JG: Canine seizure disorders. *J Am Vet Med Assoc* 158:589-597, 1971.
21. Eberhart GW: Epilepsy in the dog. Gaines Symposium, pp 18-20, 1959.
22. Holliday TA, Cunningham JG, Gutnick MJ: Comparative clinical and electroencephalographic studies of canine epilepsy. *Epilepsia* 11:281-292, 1970.
23. Greene CE, Vandevelde M, Braund K: Lissencephaly in two Lhasa Apso dogs. *J Am Vet Med Assoc* 169:405-410, 1976.
24. Oliver JE Jr, Knecht CD: Diseases of the brain, in Ettinger SJ (ed): *Textbook of Veterinary Internal Medicine*. Philadelphia, WB Saunders Co, 1975, pp 357-400.
25. Kirk RW: *Current Veterinary Therapy VI*, Philadelphia, WB Saunders Co, 1977.
26. Berman PH: Management of seizure disorders with anticonvulsant drugs: Current concepts. *Pediatr Clin North Am* 23:443-459, 1976.
27. Kutt H: Interactions of antiepileptic drugs. *Epilepsia* 16:393-402, 1975.
28. Sanders JE, Yeary RA: Serum concentrations of orally administered diphenylhydantoin in dogs. *J Am Vet Med Assoc* 172:153-156, 1978.
29. Sanders JE, Yeary RA, Powers JD, deWet P: Relationship between serum and brain concentrations of phenytoin in the dog. *Am J Vet Res* 40:473-476, 1979.
30. Pasten TJ: Diphenylhydantoin in the canine: Clinical aspects and determinations of therapeutic blood levels. *J Am Anim Hosp Assoc* 13:247-254, 1977.
31. Parker AJ: A preliminary report on a new anti-epileptic medication for dogs. *J Am Anim Hosp Assoc* 11:437-438, 1975.
32. Troupin A, Ojemann LM, Halpern L, Dodrill C, Wilkus R, Friel P, Feigl P: Carbamazepine—a double-blind comparison with phenytoin. *Neurology* 27:511-519, 1977.
33. Duffy FH, Lombroso CT: Treatment of status epilepticus, in Klawans HL (ed): *Clinical Neuropharmacology*. Vol. 3. New York, Raven Press, 1978.
34. Koestner A, Rehfeld CE: Idiopathic epilepsy in a beagle colony. Argonne National Laboratory (Lemont, IL), Biol. and Med. Res. Div. Annual Report, pp 178-179, 1968.
35. Wallace ME: Keeshonds: A genetic study of epilepsy and EEG readings. *J Small Anim Pract* 16:1-10, 1975.

UPDATE

Since the original publication of this article in January 1980, the terminology for seizure disorders, the classification of seizure types, and the known causes of seizures have changed little; however, significant advances have been made in the diagnosis and therapy of seizures. The purpose of this update is to provide the reader with the latest information regarding these advances.

DIAGNOSIS: COLLECTING A DATABASE FOR SEIZURE DISORDERS

The minimum database for seizure patients remains largely unchanged since the original publication of this article. A thorough history, physical examination, and neurologic examination, as well as a complete blood count, serum chemistry profile, urinalysis, and possibly liver function testing are still the starting point for the investigation into the cause of seizures in dogs and cats. Today, however, a more complete database includes CT or MRI imaging of the brain (rather than skull radiographs), as well as an electroencephalogram and cerebrospinal fluid analysis. In addition, the patient population, for whom a more complete database is recommended, has expanded. Following the previous recommendations of this article, a young adult canine patient with normal bloodwork, physical, and neurologic examinations would have been considered a likely idiopathic epileptic (with no "positive or suggestive findings" on the minimum database) and anticonvulsant therapy without further diagnostics recommended. Although it remains true that the most likely diagnosis in such a circumstance is idiopathic epilepsy, a recent study documented a significant number (7/24; 26%) of otherwise normal young adult dogs with seizures to have structural cerebral abnormalities underlying their seizure disorders.[1] A more complete database that includes advanced imaging (CT scan or MRI) of the brain, therefore, should be offered to the owner of any pet with recurrent seizures, along with a frank discussion of the cost-effectiveness of such an approach.

THERAPY

Although phenobarbital remains the drug of first choice for the management of seizures in dogs, potassium bromide (KBr) has replaced primidone and phenytoin as drug of second choice. Potassium bromide was first used as an anticonvulsant in humans in the 1850s, but was largely abandoned in the early part of this century as more effective anticonvulsants with less sedative side effects were developed.[2] In a recent retrospective study, 83% (19/23) of refractory canine idiopathic epileptics were found to have a reduction in the number of seizures after KBr was added to the anticonvulsant regimen.[3] The severity of seizures was subjectively observed by the owners of 15 of the 23 dogs (65%) to be reduced in this same study, and 18 of 23 owners (78%) reported that they were satisfied with KBr therapy for their pet, as regarded improved quality of life or decreased seizure frequency or severity.

Recommended initial dosages of KBr range from 20 mg/kg/day[3] to 40 mg/kg/day.[4] Since the elimination half-life is extremely long (24 days), the medication can be administered as a single daily dose. KBr appears to be a safe anticonvulsant that does not undergo hepatic metabolism or induce hepatic enzymes. The most common side effect is sedation, to which the patient usually accommodates within three weeks.[4] Uncommon side effects may be more serious and include dermatitis, mental and neurologic disturbances, and gastrointestinal symptoms.[2] Like other anticonvulsants, the maintenance dosage of KBr should be determined by monitoring serum levels of the drug. Although not yet definitively established, the therapeutic serum level of KBr for dogs appears to be approximately the same as that for humans (500 to 1900 µg/ml). Young, otherwise healthy dogs have been observed to safely tolerate serum levels as high as 2500 µg/ml when necessary to control their seizures.[4] It has been recommended that trough serum levels be measured 30 and 120 days (approximately one and five half-lives, respectively) after initiating therapy, and dosage adjusted accordingly to maintain a therapeutic serum level.[3] KBr most often is used in combination with phenobarbital, although it is occasionally used with success as a sole anticonvulsant in patients with hepatic dysfunction.

The use of diazepam per rectum at home for the management of cluster seizures in dogs represents a second advance in seizure management. In a recent prospective study of 11 idiopathic epileptic dogs with cluster seizures, eight (73%) had no further seizures in the subsequent 24-hour period after a single 0.5 mg/kg dose of diazepam, given per rectum at home by the owner.[5] No adverse effects were reported and overall client compliance rate was 88%.

The currently recommended protocol for anticonvulsant therapy in dogs therefore begins with phenobarbital (2.5 mg/kg PO q12h initial dosage, with maintenance dosage adjusted to achieve steady-state trough serum levels of 20 to 40 µg/ml) as the drug of first choice. If seizure control is inadequate, phenobarbital maintenance dosage is adjusted to achieve steady-state serum trough levels at a slightly higher level of 30 to 40 µg/ml. KBr is added to the regimen (20 to 40 mg/kg PO q24h initial dosage, with maintenance dosage adjusted to achieve steady-state trough serum concentrations of 1000 to 1500 µg/ml, possibly up to 2500 µg/ml for refractory cases) if seizure control remains inadequate. Phenobarbital and diazepam remain the only anticonvulsants recommended for use in cats.

—*Stacey A. Sullivan, DVM*
University of Georgia

REFERENCES

1. Podell M, Fenner WR, Powers JD: Seizure classification from a nonreferral-based population. *J Am Vet Med Assoc* 206(11):1721–1728, 1995.
2. Lane SB, Bunch SE: Medical management of recurrent seizures in dogs and cats. *J of Vet Int Med* 4(1):26–39, 1990.
3. Podell M, Fenner WR: Bromide therapy in refractory canine idiopathic epilepsy. *J of Vet Int Med* 7(5):318–327, 1993.
4. Schwartz-Porsche D: Management of refractory seizures, in Kirk RW, Bonagura JD (eds): *Current Veterinary Therapy XI*. Philadelphia, WB Saunders, 1992, 986–991.
5. Podell M: The use of diazepam per rectum at home for the acute management of cluster seizures in dogs. *J of Vet Int Med*, 9(2): 68–74, 1995.

Assessment and Management of the Ophthalmic Emergency in Cats and Dogs

Colorado State University
Steven M. Roberts, DVM

Emergency veterinary medicine has progressed to the point that specialized acute-care treatment facilities can be found throughout the United States. Although true ophthalmic emergencies (i.e., situations in which delay of diagnosis and therapy for a few hours can permanently jeopardize the ocular function) are infrequent, urgent cases often are presented. These cases require diagnosis and therapy as soon as possible, but a delay of several hours may not alter the outcome significantly. This article reviews procedures for assessing and managing the acute-care ophthalmic patient. Other articles in the literature discuss ophthalmic examination equipment as well as the pathophysiology, diagnosis, and management of ophthalmic problems.[1–11,86]

An algorithm approach separating emergency and urgent cases into adnexal injuries and injuries to the globe is followed in this article (see Supplements A and B).[a] General therapeutic management schemes that reinforce general principles of therapy are presented to encourage rational use of the various treatments. Clinicians should avoid always following rigid therapeutic protocols. Additional information on ocular emergencies can be found in the literature.[5,6,12,13]

INITIAL CONSIDERATIONS

Severe ocular problems require timely, appropriate management. Delaying treatment for a few hours to allow accurate assessment of the problem and to formulate a treatment plan is better than initiating inappropriate therapy.

---

[a]Because of the nature of ophthalmic injuries and the physiology of the eye, an adnexal injury frequently is linked to a problem, disease, or condition involving the globe and vice versa. Practitioners are urged to recognize these ocular interrelationships and follow Supplements A and B (pages 220 to 223) accordingly.

Because many ophthalmic emergencies are caused by trauma that could be life-threatening, overall patient evaluation cannot be overlooked, especially if chemical restraint or general anesthesia is to be used to facilitate the ocular examination or treatment. Often the outcome of the ocular problem (i.e., either preservation or loss of vision) is determined at the time of injury and inappropriate emphasis on ocular treatment at the expense of overall patient health is inexcusable.

Medical and/or surgical intervention can enhance (or delay) the healing process, but improvement of visual function may not be possible. Surgical intervention requires experience, proper use of instruments, and availability of suitable equipment and materials; otherwise, the case should be referred to a specialist. Temporary protection (bandages, tarsorrhaphy, or restraint devices) can augment appropriate topical and/or systemic therapy.

Classification, or staging, of ophthalmic emergencies depends on the information obtained from the patient history and physical examination. Historical information on the type of trauma, time of injury, previous attempts at therapy, visual function present following the insult, and previous problems with either eye must be considered when selecting the examination procedure and therapeutic regimen and when presenting a prognostic evaluation. The clinician sometimes is presented with an ophthalmic emergency that is an acute exacerbation of a subacute or chronic problem. Accurate assessment and therapy are mandatory but can be made only after evaluating the visual system thoroughly and determining whether the condition is a recurrence of a previous problem (i.e., a subacute or chronic problem that has become acute).

A systemic examination of the ocular tissue should be conducted[7-11] (i.e., from anterior to posterior and extraocular to intraocular). Ophthalmic emergencies then can be classified into one of four categories according to the potential for vision loss:

1. Non-vision threatening—Minimal loss of function
2. Latently vision threatening—Loss of vision if the disease progresses
3. Imminently vision threatening—Loss of vision probable; hospitalization and therapy recommended
4. Directly vision threatening—Loss of vision on presentation; emergency therapy necessary.

Staging the problem is a valuable method of facilitating application of general principles of diagnosis and therapy. The practitioner should avoid relying totally on a cookbook of diagnostic and therapeutic recipes.

ADNEXAL INJURIES

Adnexal injuries (Supplement A) are less likely to cause functional alteration of the eye than injuries occurring directly to the globe (Supplement B). Although blunt or sharp trauma to the eyelids and conjunctiva may not be considered directly vision threatening, proptosis should be. Thus, an adnexal injury can be a true ocular emergency or an urgent case.

Eyelids

Injuries to this adnexal tissue can be the result of blunt trauma, allergy, or sharp trauma (Supplement A). Blunt trauma is the most common but is infrequently presented as an acute emergency; instead, the owner concerned about blunt injury to soft tissue may contact the veterinarian by telephone for information on first-aid management. If an animal is presented, the practitioner must realize that ecchymotic hemorrhage, subcutaneous bruising, edema, and ocular discharge are not serious by themselves. These findings serve as indicators of potential orbital involvement (i.e., fractures) and/or intraocular involvement. After more serious injuries have been ruled out, I recommend conservative treatment (i.e., cool compresses the first 24 hours, followed by warm compresses) with or without systemic and/or topical antibiotics and corticosteroids.

Injuries related to allergy are often associated with insect bites or general urticaria. The tissue reaction can be quite dramatic. Treatment of the clinical signs with systemic and topical antiinflammatory products (corticosteroids, antiprostaglandins, antihistamines, or dimethyl sulfoxide) usually provides relief. Moist compresses may be equally as effective as systemic and topical therapy. Improvement should be noted within 24 hours.

Sharp injuries include puncture wounds and lacerations. Puncture wounds are the most common in companion animal practice. Wound cleansing coupled with topical and/or systemic antibiotics are usually adequate for treating punctures. Lid lacerations, whether partial or full thickness, are closed after minimal debridement using meticulous wound-closure procedures. Wound healing is promoted by the tremendous vascular supply of the facial region (Figure 1). If the animal presents with a nasal canthal laceration, careful evaluation of the nasolacrimal system patency by passage of fluorescein dye, irrigation, and/or catheterization is in order. For canalicular lacerations, placement of retention catheters (for mechanical support and maintenance of duct patency) as well as suture apposition of severed ductule ends are recommended. Functional patency of the lower canaliculus and punctum may be more important than that of the upper to allow tear excretion and to prevent epiphora.

Primary wound repair of sharp injuries can be done several hours to days after the injury was sustained if the tissue is protected and kept moist and free of contamination. Closure of tissue in two layers (tarsoconjunctiva and skin/muscle) is optimal. Conjunctival closure can be best achieved using continuous patterns with absorbable suture materials (5-0 or 6-0) by burying the knots in the subconjunctival tissue. The free lid margin should be apposed carefully using 4-0 to 6-0 sutures in a simple interrupted or cruciate pattern that incorporates the tarsal plate for maximum strength. If apposition is precise, minimal notching and scarring occur. If loss of eyelid tissue has occurred, blepharoplastic procedures may be useful.[14–23] Unless more than 30% of the eyelid has been lost, simple procedures, such as direct closure, should be tried.

If the nictitans is lacerated, direct surgical repair is feasible using small absorbable suture material. If only 1 to 2 mm of the free margin is involved, the tissue can be amputated. The entire third eyelid should be removed only when neoplasia is present.[24] If necessary, autogenous tissue can be used to replace the nictitans.[25–27]

Conjunctiva

Injuries to the conjunctiva (Supplement A) frequently can be associated with injuries to the lid and globe (refer to Supplement B). Although generally considered latently vision threatening, the presence of conjunctival lacerations, subconjunctival hemorrhage, and conjunctival vascular hyperemia would suggest evaluating the globe for injury.

Small lacerations may not require suturing because healing usually occurs rapidly (similar to the other mucosal surfaces). Second-intention healing results in little scarring. Large lacerations should be sutured with 5-0 or 6-0 absorbable material and the knots buried to avoid corneal irritation. The extra time required to suture this type of injury can minimize symblepharon formation. As with any conjunctival injury, folds of conjunctiva as well as the laceration itself should be inspected to rule out the possibility of a trapped foreign body.

Topical antibiotics are adequate for treatment. The question of whether treatment with ointments or solutions is preferred is subject to considerable debate. Although ointments ideally should not be used on open wounds, studies of wound healing indicate minimal delays in healing. The advantages of ointments include prolonged tissue contact, lubrication, formation of a barrier against microorganisms, and decreased drug loss through the nasolacrimal system. On the other hand, solutions offer simpler instillation, less interference with vision, fewer skin reactions, and minimal inhibition of corneal epithelial mitotic activity.[28–32] Both forms of therapy are beneficial, and selection of products should be based on clinician familiarity with each product and anticipated owner compliance.

Vascular change frequently is associated with conjunctival injuries. One such change is subconjunctival hemorrhage, which by itself is not an emergency and generally requires no specific therapy (Figure 2). This finding, however, may indicate a more serious ocular or systemic problem (e.g., bleeding or clotting disorders, vasculitis, septicemia, or cellulitis).[33] Resorption is usually complete in one to three weeks with or without topical corticosteroid therapy. A more important vascular-related change is hyperemia. This finding suggests conjunctivitis, episcleritis, anterior uveitis, or glaucoma. Obviously, the treatment of each condition differs considerably, and rapid assessment is required to handle the latter two conditions appropriately.

If the hyperemic vessels have a branching pattern, are mobile, and appear bright red, only conjunctival involvement is likely. If the vessels appear to be more numerous near the corneal limbus, show minimal branching, are immobile in relation to the conjunctiva, and look dark red, episcleral hyperemia is present.[33] Topical epinephrine or phenylephrine can be useful in differentiating superficial conjunctival vessels from deeper episcleral vessels by observing the vasoconstriction of the former, which is induced within 15 to 30 seconds after topical instillation. Episcleral hyperemia indicates episcleral or intraocular involvement (anterior uveitis or glaucoma). Evaluation of the pupillary light reflex as well as intraocular pressure should be considered. An abnormal pupillary light reflex with an increase or decrease in intraocular pressure would indicate intraocular disease. Abnormal pupillary light reflexes without ocular disease could be associated with an extraocular problem (i.e., orbit or central nervous system).

Orbit

The orbit, which is a cavity surrounded by bone, protects the globe and separates it from the cranial cavity (Supplement A). Domestic animals do not have a complete bony floor of the orbit as primates and humans do. In contrast to horses and oxen, dogs and cats have an incomplete lateral orbital wall. Because of the variety of tissues contained within the orbit, there are many causes of orbital disease. Such disease may be classified by its effect on the globe position (i.e., enophthalmos or exophthalmos). Many instances of enophthalmos and/or exophthalmos do not represent emergency cases, but a globe prolapse (proptosis) is a true emergency.

Proptosis (Figure 3) is an exaggerated exophthalmic condition resulting when the globe is forced anteriorly beyond the bony orbital rim and eyelids. This problem is directly vision threatening and occurs most often secondary to crushing head trauma. The potential for functional vision is determined by the severity of initial injury. Response of the periocular tissues includes chemosis, subconjunctival hemorrhage, retrobulbar hemorrhage, and blepharospasm. These changes, especially blepharospasm, prevent the globe from returning to a normal position. Prompt replacement of the globe to prevent corneal and conjunctival desiccation gives the animal the best chance of retaining ocular function.

Before reducing the proptosis, the degree of ocular injury must be evaluated, including assessment of damage to muscular, nervous, and vascular tissue. The following generalizations can guide the practitioner in this evaluation[3–6, 12,13,34]:

- If more than two extraocular muscles are ruptured, replacement may be difficult. The medial rectus and inferior oblique muscles usually rupture first, followed by the dorsal rectus and superior oblique muscles.
- If only conjunctival attachments remain and the optic nerve is severed, enucleation is indicated.
- Hyphema represents an unfavorable finding because severe damage to the ciliary body may have resulted and because phthisis bulbi is common.
- Pupillary light reflexes are useful but not completely reliable until 7 to 10 days after the injury. A direct reflex is rarely noted in the injured eye, but the presence of a contralateral indirect reflex is a favorable sign.
- The pupil size in the injured eye can be used to determine underlying nerve damage. If the oculomotor nerve or optic nerve is disrupted, mydriasis results (a guarded prognosis). A pupil that is near normal in size indicates loss of both the sympathetic and oculomotor nerves (a poor prognosis). A miotic pupil may represent the typical response of an injured eye or loss of sympathetic innervation (a favorable response).
- Most globes will be blind as a result of optic nerve damage.

In most situations, reduction of the proptosis should be attempted. If necessary, enucleation can be performed later. Reduction is based on drawing the infolded eyelids over the displaced globe and securing the eyelids with a temporary tarsorrhaphy. A lateral canthotomy may be used to facilitate globe replacement. Following reduction, topical antibiotic and atropine ointments, systemic corticosteroids, and warm followed by cool compresses are indicated. Systemic antibiotics may be used but are not warranted in most cases. Retrobulbar injection of corticosteroids has been recommended but tends to increase tissue swelling. Because of the bruising, hemorrhage, and vascular stasis within the orbital space, the use of systemic corticosteroids is a more appropriate therapy. The tarsorrhaphy should be maintained until retrobulbar swelling subsides (10 to 21 days) and appreciable exophthalmos is no longer noticed beneath the lids. Sequelae to proptosis include blindness, exposure keratitis secondary to lagophthalmos, phthisis bulbi, permanent strabismus, and keratoconjunctivitis sicca.

On occasion, other forms of orbital disease may present as an acute ocular problem. Such problems as exophthalmos associated with orbital cellulitis or abscess and enophthalmos following blunt trauma represent urgent cases that need complete evaluation. Although unlikely to present as emergencies, eosinophilic myositis of the extraocular muscles or muscles of mastication and retrobulbar neoplasia should be considered causes of exophthalmos to avoid a mistaken diagnosis.

INJURIES TO THE GLOBE

Of all ophthalmic problems, those involving the globe are the most confusing to diagnose and assess (Supplement B). Any traumatic injury should at least be considered an urgent case. True emergencies consist of corneal laceration, deep corneal ulcer, endophthalmitis, glaucoma, lens luxation, optic neuritis, and retinal detachment. A systematic approach to the ophthalmic examination and assessment allows problem management to be directed toward the specific pathophysiologic mechanisms (although not always successfully).

Anterior Segment

The most anterior aspect of the globe (corneal aspect) is often involved either with diseases affecting primarily the cornea (e.g., ulcerative keratitis) or with conditions occurring secondary to intraocular problems (e.g., iridocyclitis, glaucoma, or anterior lens luxation). The unique physical properties of relative dehydration and precise lamellar stromal arrangement impart transparency to corneal tissue. Alteration of the epithelial and/or endothelial surface results in a loss of transparency (edema).[35–37] Edema should be classified according to whether it is epithelial or endothelial in origin. If edema of epithelial origin is suspected, fluorescein stain can determine the integrity of the corneal surface.

Corneal Ulceration or Laceration

Fluorescein retention by the cornea indicates loss of epithelial integrity (Supplement B). Once a break in

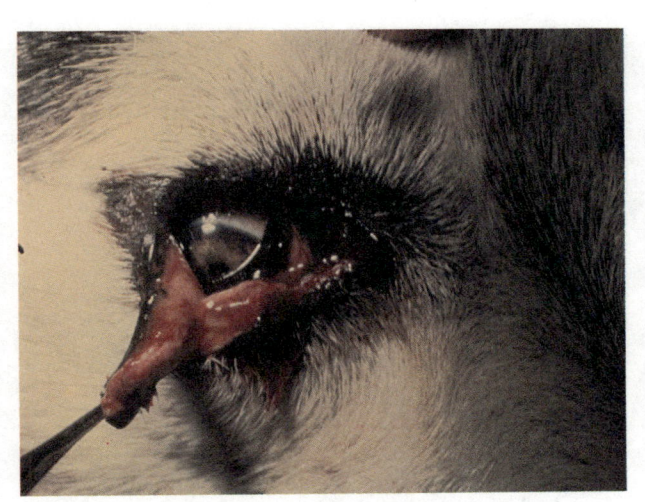

Figure 1—Management of eyelid lacerations includes minimal debridement to preserve as much tissue as possible and meticulous wound closure to restore anatomic configuration and function. Remarkable healing capabilities are possible because of the vascular nature of this tissue.

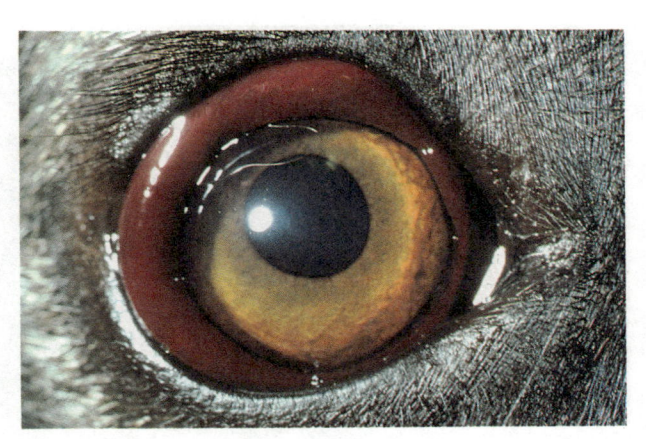

Figure 2—Subconjunctival hemorrhage can occur after blunt trauma to the eye or from choking injuries. Despite marked adnexal injury, the practitioner may encounter little evidence of intraocular damage.

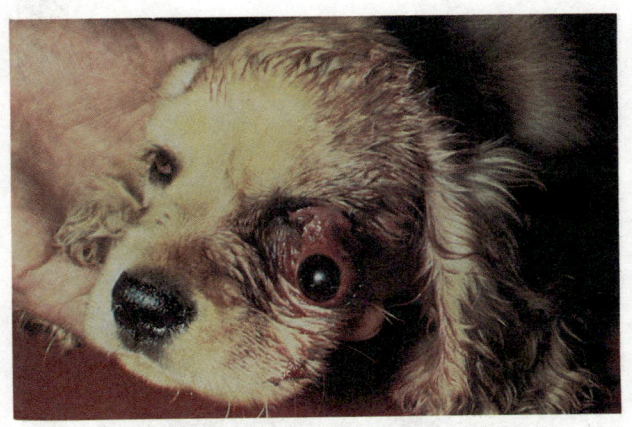

Figure 3—Proptosis with complete avulsion of the extraocular muscles and optic nerve offers few options. Enucleation is indicated because ischemic necrosis of the globe likely will result.

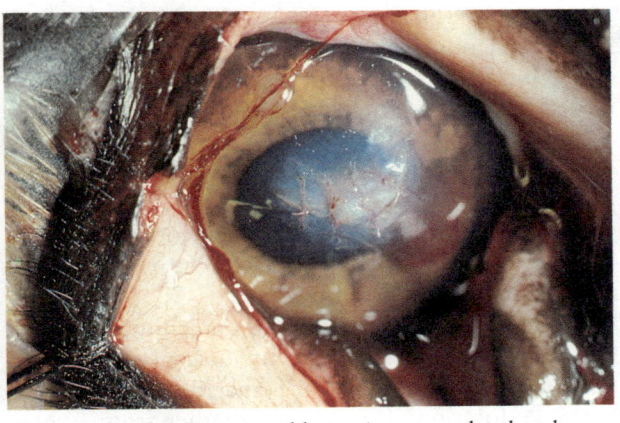

Figure 4—Perforating corneal lacerations must be closed accurately using 7-0 to 9-0 absorbable or nonabsorbable suture material. The prognosis for retained vision depends on the amount of damage that occurred to the uvea and/or lens.

the corneal epithelium is realized, the depth and extent should be determined. Assessment and management depend on the nature of the injury (i.e., superficial versus deeply penetrating or perforating versus nonperforating). Perforations cause the most severe corneal damage because of disruption of the stromal and endothelial layers. Any situation involving these lesions requires rapid, aggressive management if the animal's vision is to be maintained. Determination of the cause of corneal ulcers is essential. Specimens collected from wound margins and submitted for cytologic and bacteriologic evaluation may be helpful in determining specific therapeutic agents to use.[38,39] The causative agent may not be found in some cases, and the host tissue response (e.g., neutrophil infiltration) can be more important in propagating the tissue-destructive processes.

The most important aspects of management are mechanical support of damaged tissue, control and prevention of sepsis, protection of the globe, and promotion of healing.[2–6,12,13,16,40–48,87] Mechanical support can be achieved by using conjunctival grafts/flaps, keratoplasty, tissue adhesives, soft hydrophilic contact lenses, and nictitans flaps. Sepsis can be controlled or prevented with antimicrobials used at frequent intervals (i.e., as often as every 15 to 60 minutes). Frequency of use can be decreased and finally discontinued when the sepsis is controlled. Globe protection

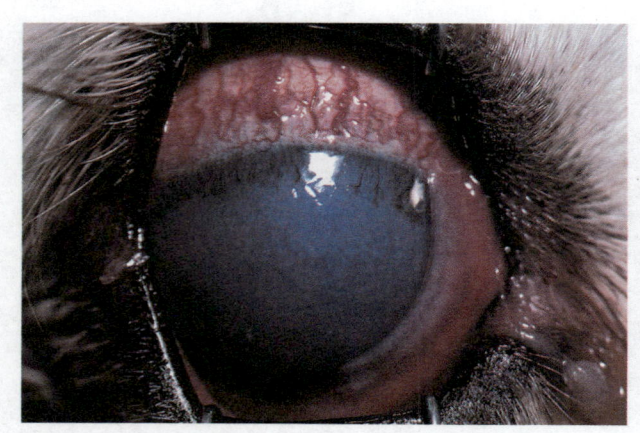

Figure 5—Subacute to chronic glaucoma is evidenced by diffuse corneal edema of endothelial origin, perilimbal vascular keratitis, episcleral vascular injection, and an intraocular pressure of 65 mm Hg.

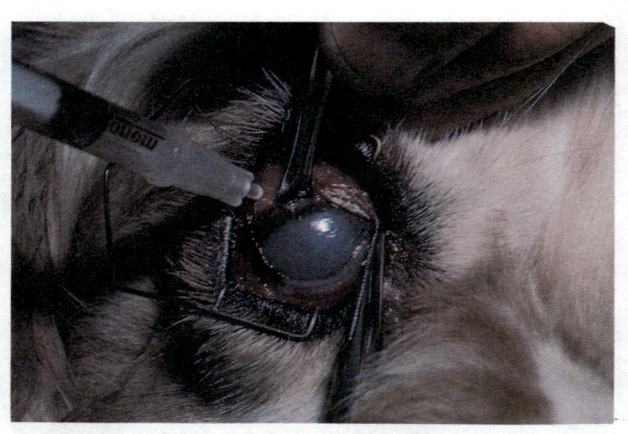

Figure 6—Intravitreal injection of gentamicin can sometimes be useful to destroy the secretory epithelium of the ciliary bodies. Any potential for vision will be lost because gentamicin destroys the retina.

includes the use of protective collars, tarsorrhaphy, conjunctival grafts/flaps, nictitans flaps, and pharmacologic control of painful intraocular smooth muscle spasm (using topical atropine) and inflammation (using topical nonsteroidal antiinflammatory and systemic antiinflammatory agents). Healing can be promoted by use of proteolytic enzyme inhibitors (i.e., acetylcysteine or EDTA), endogenous or exogenous growth factors (i.e., topical plasma eye drops, fibronectin, epidermal growth factor, keratinocyte growth factor), and wound debridement (i.e., epithelial curettage, superficial punctate keratotomy, or superficial linear grid keratotomy).[88]

Corneal lacerations involving one third or less of the corneal thickness can be handled using conventional medical techniques for managing ulcerative keratitis. Perforations (Figure 4), whether from lacerations or ulcers, with or without iris prolapse require direct closure with 7-0 to 9-0 absorbable or nonabsorbable suture material. Any prolapse of uveal tissue should be reduced or amputated to facilitate wound closure and restoration of the anterior chamber. Medical management should be directed toward controlling the iridocyclitis and promoting corneal healing. Iridocyclitis therapy consists of cycloplegic agents (atropine) and antiinflammatory agents (systemic corticosteroids or nonsteroidal prostaglandin inhibitors, such as aspirin, phenylbutazone, or flunixin meglumine). Corneal wound healing is aided by broad-spectrum topical antibiotics (bacitracin-neomycin-polymyxin B combinations, gentamicin, or tobramycin), mucolytic and anticollagenase agents (acetylcysteine or EDTA), as well as emollients and demulcents (ointment and artificial tear preparations).

Corneal edema lacking significant fluorescein retention indicates endothelial damage; intraocular dis-

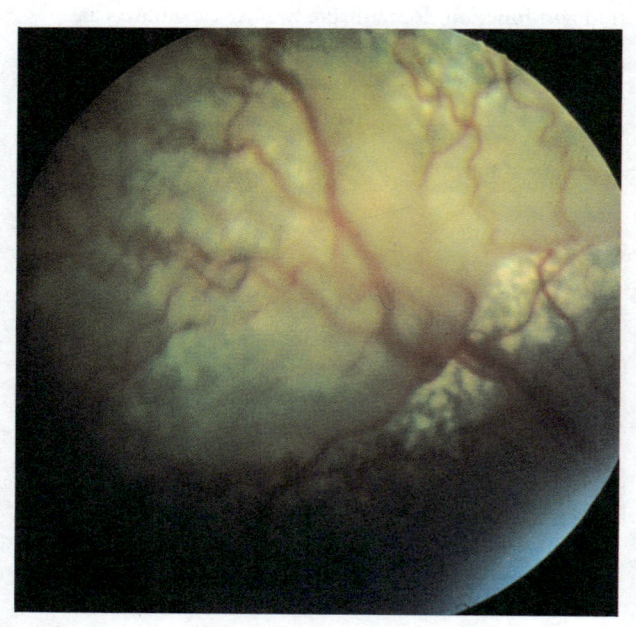

Figure 7—Serous retinal detachment of idiopathic inflammatory origin presents as a gray veil containing blood vessels suspended in the vitreous chamber. If a direct ophthalmoscope is focused on the optic nerve, the detachment will not be in focus. Eye movements will cause the detached tissue to drift and flutter within the vitreous.

ease therefore should be considered. Evaluation of conjunctival or episcleral hyperemia, pupillary light reflexes, intraocular pressure, contents of the anterior chamber, and position of the lens should follow. Acute to subacute glaucoma, acute endophthalmitis, and anterior lens luxation constitute true emergencies. Hyphema, hypopyon, iridocyclitis, lens subluxations, and posterior luxations should be considered urgent. Chronic glaucoma is neither an urgent nor an emergency case because the outcome cannot be altered by early treatment intervention.

Acute Glaucoma

Acute glaucoma is an emergency problem that requires quick assessment and appropriate therapy if globe function is to be restored (Supplements A and B). By definition, glaucoma exists if intraocular pressure is elevated beyond that compatible with vision (usually > 25 to 30 mm Hg). Increased intraocular pressure rapidly damages the retinal nerve fiber layer and optic nerve. Often blindness caused by permanent optic nerve damage is present at the time of initial examination. Thus, glaucoma should be considered an optic nerve disease in addition to a disease of increased intraocular pressure. This problem is more common in dogs than in cats; cats with glaucoma often present with chronic rather than acute glaucoma because they rarely demonstrate the cardinal signs, which are easily observed in dogs. Acute glaucoma in dogs presents as an acutely red, painful, blind eye with a cloudy cornea. Corneal clouding is diffuse (edema) but is not necessarily present until the intraocular pressure approaches 50 mm Hg or greater. Ocular redness results from episcleral as well as conjunctival vascular engorgement (Figure 5). Care is necessary to avoid confusion with conjunctival hyperemia. Conjunctival vessels are freely movable, are branched dichotomously, and blanch rapidly after instillation of topical epinephrine or phenylephrine; while episcleral vessels are poorly mobile, are branched minimally, and resist blanching. Most glaucomatous globes have an abnormal pupillary light reflex, with the pupil being dilated (midrange or widely).

Glaucoma can be confirmed by measuring the intraocular pressure using tonometry. Although some clinicians attempt digital tonometry by palpating the globe, this method is crude and can be misleading. Instead, mechanical indentation tonometry with the Schiötz tonometer is recommended. Although designed for the human eye, conversion tables are available for dogs and cats.[49,89] The instrument is accurate if an effort is made to keep the scale reading between 3 and 15 by using one of the several loading weights that accompany the device.

After making a diagnosis, either medical or surgical therapy must be selected.[50–52] Response to medical therapy can be frustrating because long-term control is difficult to maintain. Surgical procedures thus are frequently required (i.e., enucleation, evisceration, cyclocryosurgery, laser trans-scleral ciliary body coagulation, implantation of an anterior chamber shunt, or ciliary body chemical ablation).[90]

Emergency medical treatment should always be attempted in cases that are acute to subacute. The case should be reevaluated several times during the first 12 to 48 hours to assess not only response to medical therapy but whether surgery is indicated. If a surgical procedure to increase aqueous humor outflow is elected, it should be performed within a few days of the hypertensive crisis. In light of the optic nerve damage occurring with glaucoma and the evidence suggesting that ionized calcium promotes or is involved in the nerve damage process, treatment with calcium channel blockers may be beneficial.

Glaucoma is classified as *primary* (no discernible abnormalities to explain the elevation in intraocular pressure), *secondary* (a definite traumatic, lens-associated, inflammatory, or neoplastic cause is present), or *congenital* (anomalous iridocorneal angle structures). In cases of secondary glaucoma with associated lens problems or intraocular neoplasia, the specific cause must be dealt with as part of the therapy. Many cases of glaucoma in dogs have an inflammatory component. Medical treatment should be directed at decreasing ocular inflammation as well as reducing the elevated intraocular pressure. Initial medical treatment can be divided into four broad categories: (1) antiinflammatory agents, (2) osmotic diuretics, (3) carbonic anhydrase inhibitors, and (4) topical autonomic drugs.

Antiinflammatory therapy can be based on steroidal or nonsteroidal agents. Corticosteroids are effective but have been documented to elevate the intraocular pressure in primates, cats, and rabbits; however, this problem has not been observed in dogs. Nonsteroidal antiprostaglandin agents (such as aspirin, phenylbutazone, and flunixin meglumine) have been used successfully. Rapid reduction of intraocular pressure is best achieved with osmotic diuretics (parenteral mannitol or sodium ascorbate as well as oral glycerin at a dose of 1 g/kg). These agents create a hyperosmotic state within the extracellular fluid compartment, thus drawing water from the vitreous chamber (volume reduction) and decreasing the formation of aqueous humor. A single dose of mannitol can decrease the intraocular pressure for four to six hours. Water should be withheld for two to four hours after initiating osmotic therapy; otherwise, the hypotension is negated by fluid expansion within the extracellular compartment. Because these agents become less effective when administered repeatedly, they are not intended for use in chronic cases.

Long-term medical control relies on use of carbonic anhydrase inhibitors and topical autonomic drugs. Carbonic anhydrase inhibitors decrease active secretion of aqueous humor by the ciliary body epithelium as much as 50% to 60%. Although they are diuretics, other classes of diuretics (e.g., furosemide) do not decrease the intraocular pressure. Table I lists carbonic

TABLE I
Carbonic Anhydrase Inhibitors

Product	Dose (mg/kg)	Onset of Action (minutes)	Maximum Effect (hours)	Duration of Action (hours)
Acetazolamide	22	30	2–4	4–6
Dichlorphenamine	2.2	30	2–4	6–12
Methazolamide	5.5	60	7–8	10–14

anhydrase inhibitors and appropriate doses. Autonomic drug therapy to increase aqueous humor outflow and decrease humor production is often used with carbonic anhydrase inhibitors. Autonomic drugs include sympathomimetics, parasympathomimetics, and adrenergic beta blockers. A combined therapeutic plan using several agents is frequently required to control the intraocular pressure successfully. Table II lists available products and the frequencies of instillation. If medical therapy fails to maintain a hypotensive or normotensive eye, surgery is indicated. Historically, filtering procedures to increase aqueous humor outflow (posterior sclerotomy, cyclodialysis, and iridencleisis)[53,54] have been tried with limited short-term success. Traditionally, cyclocryosurgery,[55–58] evisceration,[1,16] or enucleation[1,16] has been most successful. Only the last two procedures require no special instruments.

Rapid chemical ablation of the ciliary body, on a nonselective basis, can be accomplished by intravitreal injection of gentamicin.[59] Intraocular injection of antibiotics has been used in humans to manage severe bacterial endophthalmitis that usually results in destruction of the globe.[60,61] Work with rabbits demonstrated that intravitreal injection of amounts equal to or greater than 0.4 mg damaged the retina.[62] Subsequent studies detected lysosomal inclusions in the retinal pigment epithelial cells as well as necrosis, hyperplasia, and disruption of the photoreceptor outer segments. Doses greater than 2 mg produced marked retinal necrosis.[63] Injection of 25 mg of gentamicin reportedly produced loss of nonpigmented ciliary body epithelium[59] in addition to retinal necrosis.

Following chemical ciliary body ablation, the intraocular pressure decreases either immediately or in three to four days, and buphthalmia regresses because of the persistent hypotonia. Chemical ablation of the ciliary body with gentamicin can be used if the practitioner elects to avoid enucleation or evisceration procedures. The method of injection is not difficult but does destroy the retina in addition to the ciliary body. If there were a chance to retain vision before the injection, there certainly would be no chance afterward. If the glaucomatous process is secondary to an intraocular tumor or septic endophthalmitis, the underlying cause will remain.

The procedure can often be done with mild sedation and topical anesthesia, although some patients require general anesthesia. Topical epinephrine or phenylephrine can be used to decrease conjunctival hemorrhage. The injection technique uses two tuberculin syringes with attached 25-gauge needles. One syringe and needle is used to initially tap the anterior chamber at the limbus and withdraw a volume of aqueous humor equal to the volume to be injected. The second syringe and needle is used to enter the vitreous compartment by penetrating the sclera 8 to 10 mm posterior to the corneoscleral junction (Figure 6). The needle should be directed toward the optic papilla to avoid puncturing the lens. Gentamicin (10 to 12.5 mg) then is injected. The needle can be withdrawn and compression applied to the site for several minutes. Slight vitreous leakage into the subconjunctival tissues may occur. An alternative to a single massive injection is to use several smaller injections (4 to 5 mg of gentamicin each) every two to four weeks until the intraocular pressure is at an acceptable level. The line between inadequate and excessive gentamicin administration is imprecise. If too much gentamicin is given, the globe becomes phthisical and may require enucleation for cosmetic reasons. In addition, the cornea can become edematous and opaque; and if a lens luxation or subluxation is present along with glaucoma, the likelihood of severe corneal edema is greatly increased.

Acute Iridocyclitis

Acute iridocyclitis (Supplements A and B) presents as a painful, red, possibly visually impaired eye that resembles glaucoma. Ocular signs of iridocyclitis include miosis, flare, conjunctival and episcleral hyperemia, perilimbal to generalized corneal edema, and inflammation of the iris (edema, neovascularization, and synechia).[64–66] Diagnosis is confirmed if the intraocular pressure is less than 14 mm Hg. An attempt should be made to determine the cause (viral, bacterial, fungal, parasitic, protozoan, neoplastic, immune mediated, or

TABLE II
Autonomic Drugs for Treating Glaucoma

Drug Class	Ocular Effects	Products	Duration of Hypotension	Frequency of Use
Sympathomimetic	Increase in outflow and small decrease in production of aqueous humor; mydriasis	Epinephrine	12–24 hours	Twice daily
		Dipivalyl epinephrine	14–18 hours	Twice daily
Parasympathomimetic	Increase in outflow and small decrease in production of aqueous humor; miosis	Pilocarpine	8–14 hours	Three or four times daily
		Carbachol	8 hours	Three or four times daily
		Demecarium	9 hours	Once a day
		Echothiophate	1–2 days	Once a day
Sympatholytic	Decrease in production of aqueous humor	Betaxolol	24 hours	Twice daily
		Carteolol	24 hours	Twice daily
		Levobutanol	24 hours	Twice daily
		Metipranolol	24 hours	Twice daily
		Timolol	24 hours	Twice daily

traumatic). Many cases are classified as idiopathic. Therapy should be directed toward resolving any underlying problems. Uncontrolled inflammation can rapidly destroy the globe function; thus, aggressive topical and/or systemic antiinflammatory therapy (steroidal or nonsteroidal) is necessary. Intraocular pain and formation of synechia can be reduced by using cycloplegics (atropine) to produce paralysis of the ciliary body musculature as well as mydriasis.[67]

Hyphema

Hyphema (Supplement B) refers to hemorrhage in the anterior chamber. Traumatic injuries frequently are the cause, with other causes including bleeding disorders, complications following intraocular surgery, chronic glaucoma, chronic iridocyclitis, intraocular neoplasia, and congenital ocular anomalies (e.g., collie eye anomaly or retinal dysplasia). If trauma is the suspected cause, the globe should be examined carefully to rule out ocular penetration or perforation. Inspection of the posterior segment may be difficult if the anterior chamber is filled with blood (eight-ball hemorrhage). Profuse hyphema does not clot completely because the iris produces fibrinolysin, which prevents hemorrhage from organizing into a true clot. It is generally believed that blood is removed through the iridocorneal angle with the exit of intact erythrocytes. Hyphema causes little inherent damage to the eye, and surgical removal is rarely indicated.[12,13,68]

Recommendations for medical treatment vary, and no controlled studies have been reported in the veterinary literature. Therapeutic recommendations include parasympathomimetics (pilocarpine) to increase outflow of red blood cells through the iridocorneal angle, sympathomimetics (epinephrine or phenylephrine) for mydriasis and vasoconstriction, and corticosteroids and cycloplegics (atropine) for any existing iridocyclitis. Experimentally induced hyphema in rabbits demonstrates no change in the clearance rate when the eyes are treated with 1% atropine, 1% pilocarpine, or 2% pilocarpine or when no treatment was initiated.[69] A study in humans demonstrated that 40 mg of prednisolone per day failed to resolve the traumatic hyphema.[70] Aminocaproic acid has been advocated in human medicine to minimize the incidence of secondary hemorrhage occurring after a traumatic injury. Secondary hemorrhage is believed to be related to blood clot lysis and retraction from the traumatized blood vessels several days after the trauma. Aminocaproic acid is an antifibrinolytic agent that presumably can prevent or delay clot dissolution and allow more time for the traumatized blood vessels to regain their integrity.[71] Secondary hemorrhage is not a major problem in veterinary medicine, however; and the use of antifibrinolytic agents may not be necessary. Recently the use of tissue plasminogen activator, either injected into the anterior chamber or administered topically, has been shown effective or potentially effective in clot dissolution.[91,92] The drug is administered by anterior chamber injection of 0.1 ml (25 µg) with an insulin syringe. The most important aspect of treating hyphema is the control of coexisting uveal inflammation.

Posterior Segment

Emergency or urgent cases involving the posterior segment (Supplement B) center around the retina (retinal detachment) and optic nerve (optic neuritis).

Ophthalmic Emergency Algorithm
Supplement A

EYELIDS

Blunt Trauma

SOFT TISSUE INJURY

SIGNS
  Bruising
  Discharge
  Edema
  Epiphora

TREATMENT OPTIONS
  None
  Warm/cold compresses
  Topical antibiotics
    & corticosteroids

IS CONJUNCTIVA INVOLVED?

ORBITAL FRACTURES

(zygomatic arch most frequent)

DIAGNOSE BY
  Palpation
  Radiography

TREATMENT OPTIONS
  None
  Fracture reduction

IS GLOBE INVOLVED?
(see Supplement B)

EVALUATE AMOUNT OF LAGOPHTHALMOS

Allergy

SIGNS
  Chemosis
  Conjunctival hyperemia
  Blepharoedema
  Epiphora

TREATMENT OPTIONS
  Moist compresses
  Systemic & topical
    antiinflammatory agents

Sharp Trauma

LACERATIONS & PUNCTURES

(upper, lower, nictitans)

MINOR—skin involvement
  & small wound
    Clean wound
    Topical antibiotics

SEVERE—skin defect &
  gaping wound
    Clean wound
    Minimal debridement
    Accurate wound closure

IS CONJUNCTIVA INVOLVED?

IS ANTERIOR SEGMENT INVOLVED?
(see Supplement B)

CONJUNCTIVA

Lacerations

MINOR WOUND
  No sutures
  Topical antibiotic solutions

SEVERE WOUND
  Suture with absorbable 5-0 to 7-0 material
  Prevent corneal irritation from suture knots

IS GLOBE INVOLVED?
(see Supplement B)

Vascular Changes

HEMORRHAGE

DIFFUSE SUBCONJUNCTIVA
  Phase I—rule out foreign bodies
  Phase II—treatment options
    None
    Topical antibiotics & steroids
    Cold/warm compresses

PETECHIAL
  Rule out bleeding disorder

HYPEREMIA

LOCALIZED
  Inflammatory granuloma
  Healing injury
  Episcleritis

Check whether intraocular pressure decreased

GENERALIZED

Conjunctival → Check pupillary light response

Normal
  Conjunctivitis
  Rule out
    Laceration
    Cellulitis
    Viral or bacterial infection
  Are lids involved?
  Is globe involved? (see Supplement B)

Abnormal
  Miotic pupil; low or normal
    intraocular pressure
  Anterior uveitis
    (see Supplement B)
  Episcleritis
  Mydriatic pupil; high
    intraocular pressure
  Glaucoma

Ciliary/Episcleral → Check intraocular pressure

Normal
  Excitement
  Concussion
  Shock
  Subclinical uveitis

RETROBULBAR (ORBITAL) TISSUE

Exophthalmos

Pain on opening mouth

NO

ORBITAL EDEMA
　Rule out tumor if unilateral
　Rule out trauma, allergy, or circulatory disturbance

Signs
　Chemosis, blepharoedema
　See Unilateral Pain, Retrobulbar Mass

YES

BILATERAL PAIN
　Signs—myositis; muscles swollen, firm, & warm; secondary eyelid edema
　Diagnosis based on biopsy & CBC changes
　Treatment—corticosteroids

UNILATERAL PAIN
　Retrobulbar mass
　　Signs—pain if necrosis is present, nictitans protrusion, possible strabismus
　　Diagnosis based on cytology, biopsy, radiographic changes

　Cellulitis and/or abscess
　　Rule out foreign body
　　Signs—Severe pain, protrusion of nictitans, pyrexia
　　Diagnosis based on CBC changes; may point posterior to third molar
　　Treatment options—warm compresses, drain & culture, topical & systemic antibiotics

Enophthalmos

CAUSES
　Microophthalmic or phthisis bulbi
　Globe rupture (see Supplement B)
　Ocular pain (see Conjunctiva and Supplement B)
　Dehydration
　Chronic wasting disease
　Horner's syndrome

Proptosis
(prognostic indicators)

STRABISMUS—if more than 2 extraocular muscles ruptured (poor prognosis)

HYPHEMA—indicates ciliary body damage (poor prognosis)

PUPIL SIZE
　Normal—sympathetic & parasympathetic innervation loss (poor prognosis)
　Mydriatic—parasympathetic innervation loss (guarded prognosis)

CONSENSUAL PUPILLARY LIGHT RESPONSE IN NORMAL EYE
　Present (good prognosis)
　If returns in 7-10 days (good prognosis)
　Absent (poor prognosis)

IS THE CORNEA NORMAL?
　(see Supplement B)

TREATMENT OPTIONS
　Topical antibiotics & atropine
　Replace globe
　Tarsorrhaphy
　Systemic corticosteroids

Ophthalmic Emergency Algorithm
Supplement B

ANTERIOR SEGMENT

Cornea

LEUKOMA (Focal or Diffuse)

No Fluorescein Retention

CORNEAL VASCULARIZATION

Superficial
- Keratoconjunctivitis sicca
- Healing ulcer
- Keratitis

Deep
- Interstitial keratitis
- Anterior uveitis (see Supplement A & Anterior Chamber)
- Glaucoma (see Supplement A, Vascular Changes)
- Episcleritis

NO CORNEAL VASCULARIZATION

No conjunctival hyperemia
- Dystrophy
- Scar tissue
- Degeneration

Conjunctival hyperemia (see Supplement A)
- Anterior uveitis (see Supplement A & Anterior Chamber)
- Glaucoma (see Supplement A, Vascular Changes)
- Episcleritis

Fluorescein Retention

SUPERFICIAL ULCER
- Adherent margins
  - Topical therapy
  - Protection
- Nonadherent margins
  - Debridement
  - Topical antibodies
  - Hyperosmotics
  - Protection

DEEP ULCER (see Laceration)
- Descemetocele
  - Surgical repair
  - Protection
  - Topical ulcer therapy
- No descemetocele
  - Mechanical support
  - Protection
  - Topical ulcer therapy

TRANSPARENT

Normal

LACERATION
- Perforation
  - Surgical repair
  - Ulcer & uveitis therapy
- No perforation
  - Surgical repair if greater than ½ thickness
  - Protection
  - Mechanical support
  - Ulcer therapy

POSTERIOR SEGMENT

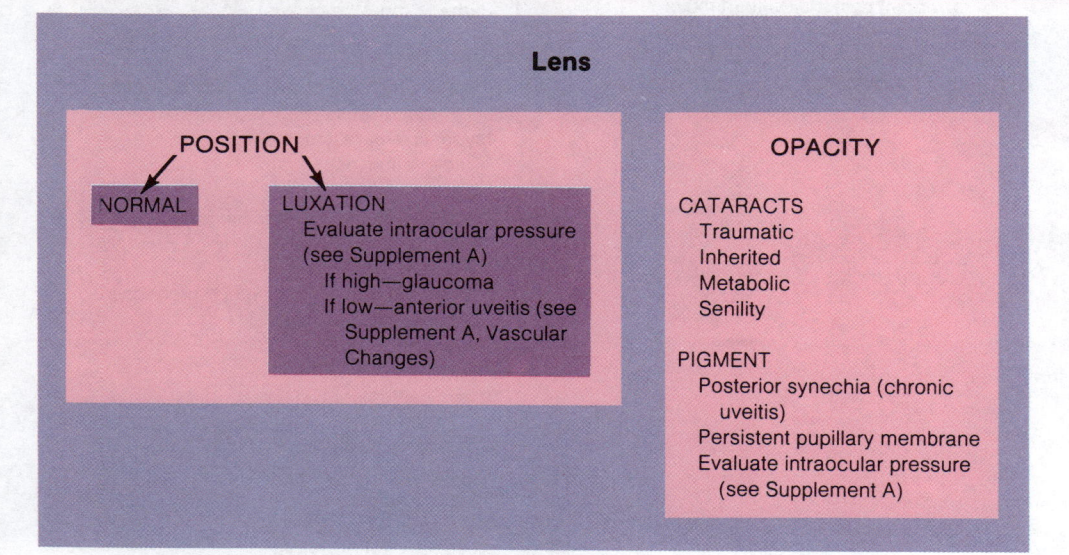

Lens

POSITION

NORMAL

LUXATION
- Evaluate intraocular pressure (see Supplement A)
- If high—glaucoma
- If low—anterior uveitis (see Supplement A, Vascular Changes)

OPACITY

CATARACTS
- Traumatic
- Inherited
- Metabolic
- Senility

PIGMENT
- Posterior synechia (chronic uveitis)
- Persistent pupillary membrane
- Evaluate intraocular pressure (see Supplement A)

Vitreous

FLOATERS
- Rule out uveitis

HEMORRHAGE OR EXUDATE
- Collie eye anomaly
- Endophthalmitis (see Anterior Chamber)
- Retinal hemorrhage
- Retinitis

Anterior Chamber
(abnormal contents)

AQUEOUS FLARE (hazy aqueous)
  Blood aqueous barrier breakdown with
    plasma protein leakage
  Evaluate intraocular pressure
    (see Supplement A)
  Evaluate iris and pupil
  Anterior uveitis
    (see Supplement A, Vascular Changes)

HYPOPYON (leukocytes within chamber)
  Sterile inflammatory response
    Diagnosis—anterior uveitis (see
      Supplement A, Vascular Changes)
    Treatment Options
      Systemic & topical antiinflammatory agents
        (i.e., corticosteroids, antiprostaglandins)
      Cycloplegics
      May or may not require topical
        or systemic antibiotics
  Septic inflammatory response
    Diagnosis—endophthalmitis (poor prognosis)
    Treatment options
      Aggressive therapy necessary
      Systemic antibiotics and corticosteroids
      Intraocular agents or antibiotics and corticosteroids
      Vitrectomy or intraocular lavage

HYPHEMA (RBCs within chamber)
  Rule out laceration

  Diffuse (acute or ongoing)
    Antiinflammatory therapy
    α-adrenergics (epinephrine or
      phenylephrine)
    May or may not require
      carbonic anhydrase inhibitors

  Stratified/clotted (chronic or resolving)
    Antiinflammatory therapy
    Cycloplegics

LENS
  Lens luxation
  Determine if glaucoma or uveitis present
    (see Supplement A, Vascular Changes)

Iris and Pupil

IRIS CONTOUR
  Swollen
    Anterior uveitis
      (see Supplement A,
      Vascular Changes)
    Neoplasia
    Granuloma
  Smooth
    Normal

PUPIL
  Miotic
    Synechia (chronic uveitis)
    Anterior uveitis
  Mydriatic
    Lens luxation
      (see Posterior Segment)
    Optic neuritis
    Detached retina

IRIS MOTION (iridodonesis)
  Lens subluxation or luxation
    (see Posterior Segment, Lens)

Retinal and Optic Nerves

RETINAL DETACHMENT

IDENTIFY ANY SYSTEMIC DISEASE

CAUSES
  Dysplasia or collie eye anomaly
  Chorioretinitis
  Neoplasia
  Idiopathic

TREATMENT OPTIONS
  Antiinflammatory diuretic
  May or may not require
    tranquilization
  May or may not require
    antihypertensive medication

OPTIC NEURITIS

RULE OUT INFECTIOUS OR
NEOPLASTIC CAUSE

TREATMENT OPTIONS
  Antimicrobial agents
  Antiinflammatory agents
  May or may not require
    detachment therapy

OTHER DIFFERENTIALS

RETINAL HEMORRHAGE
  Rule out systemic disease
    or local inflammation
  Treat underlying cause

CHORIORETINITIS
  Active
    Edema
    Exudate
    Hemorrhage
    Vascular congestion
  Inactive
    Hyperreflective retinal lesions
    No active signs

  Treatment options
    Antibiotics & antiinflammatory
      agents

A presenting sign of acute blindness occurring within hours or days is typical. If the disorder involves the retina or optic nerve, the pupillary light reflex will be abnormal. Blindness with a normal pupillary light reflex implies a lesion of the optic radiation or vision cortex. Difficulty often is encountered in determining whether the animal is acutely blind or has become acutely decompensated as a result of a chronic progressive loss of vision. This problem is common when dealing with dogs with advancing cataracts or progressive retinal atrophy. Owners may perceive a particular event that calls their attention to vision impairment as representing acute onset of blindness in their pets. Subacute to acute vision loss over the course of several weeks has been documented with increasing frequency in the past few years. Currently, such terms as *metabolic toxic retinopathy*,[72] *silent retinal syndrome*,[73] and *sudden acquired retinal degeneration syndrome*[74] have been used to describe this syndrome. The cause is currently unknown but may be connected with excitotoxin-induced neuronal damage. The syndrome involves rapid degeneration of photoreceptor cells. The ocular fundus appears normal during early ophthalmoscopic examination. The pupillary light reflex is reduced or absent, and electroretinogram signals are nonrecordable.

Retinal Detachment

Blindness is noted by the owner when the animal has complete bilateral detachments. Causes vary but include congenital (collie eye anomaly[75] and retinal dysplasia[76-78]), immune-mediated inflammatory,[79] infectious, neoplastic, systemic (renal hypertension),[80] or toxic (ethylene glycol) diseases.[81] Most cases are classified, however, as *idiopathic*.[82] Diagnosis is not difficult with indirect ophthalmoscopy. Complete detachments are often visible with a focal light source. A grayish veil containing blood vessels can be observed (Figure 7), and variable amounts of retinal hemorrhage may be present. Idiopathic cases associated with uveal inflammation frequently respond to treatment. In this situation, inflammation of the choroid has caused serous fluid to accumulate between the photoreceptors and the retinal pigment epithelium. Aggressive therapy with high levels of corticosteroids coupled with diuretics can produce a dramatic response. Before initiating this treatment, however, infectious causes must be ruled out. A guarded prognosis for complete restoration of vision must be given because degeneration and death of photoreceptors occur with retinal detachment. In cats, cell degeneration and death begin within 12 hours to 3 days after the onset of retinal detachment.[83]

Optic Neuritis

Inflammation involving any part of the optic nerve (bulbar, retrobulbar, or intracranial) is referred to as *optic neuritis*.[84,85] Ophthalmoscopic evidence is present only when the bulbar portion of the optic nerve is involved (optic disk). These cases demonstrate hyperemia of the optic nerve head as well as vascular congestion, edema, and hemorrhage of the retina immediately surrounding the optic nerve. If the condition is bilateral, acute blindness will be a presenting sign. Although the cause often cannot be determined, the clinician should rule out canine distemper, granulomatous meningoencephalitis (reticulosis), neoplasia, retrobulbar cellulitis, systemic mycosis, toxoplasmosis, and trauma. Infectious processes require specific therapy; but if the cause is inflammatory in origin, systemic antiinflammatory therapy is indicated. Depending on the inflammation severity, conventional antiinflammatory dosing or pulse-therapy (15 to 30 mg/kg of methylprednisolone sodium succinate) is implemented. Corticosteroid therapy should be continued for three to four weeks, decreasing the dose as the inflammation resolves. Rapid response to treatment within 2 to 10 days suggests a favorable prognosis. The intensity and duration of inflammation before treatment, however, determine the extent of optic nerve demyelination and atrophy that eventually result. Vision may deteriorate over weeks to months following therapy, as optic nerve degeneration and atrophy occur. In cases of granulomatous meningoencephalitis, rapid response to systemic corticosteroids may be noted initially, with relapses occurring later.

CONCLUSION

The assessment and management of emergency ophthalmic cases in cats and dogs need not be difficult or confusing if the problem is approached logically. Specific problems must be identified, a diagnosis made, and therapy instituted. The disastrous sequelae to uncontrolled inflammation always should be remembered and specific attempts must be made to arrest and suppress this process. When the clinician determines that vision cannot be salvaged, enucleation or intraocular prosthetic surgical procedures should be considered from the standpoint of alleviating unnecessary discomfort to the animal and treating the specific disease.

About the Author

Dr. Roberts is affiliated with the Department of Clinical Sciences, College of Veterinary Medicine and Biomedical Sciences, Colorado State University, Fort Collins, Colorado. He is a Diplomate of the American College of Veterinary Ophthalmologists.

REFERENCES

1. Gelatt KN (ed): *Textbook of Veterinary Ophthalmology.* Philadelphia, Lea & Febiger, 1981.
2. Magrane WC: *Canine Ophthalmology.* Philadelphia, Lea & Febiger, 1977.
3. Severin GA: *Veterinary Ophthalmology Notes,* ed 2. Fort Collins, CO, College of Veterinary Medicine and Biomedical Sciences, Colorado State University, 1982.
4. Slatter DH: *Fundamentals of Veterinary Ophthalmology.* Philadelphia, WB Saunders Co, 1981.
5. Kirk RW (ed): *Current Veterinary Therapy VII.* Philadelphia, WB Saunders Co, 1980.
6. Kirk RW (ed): *Current Veterinary Therapy VIII.* Philadelphia, WB Saunders Co, 1983.
7. Gelatt KN: Orbit and adnexa: Diagnostic methods in small animal ophthalmology (part I). *Compend Contin Educ Pract Vet* 2(5):413–419, 1980.
8. Gelatt KN: Anterior segment: Diagnostic methods in small animal ophthalmology (part II). *Compend Contin Educ Pract Vet* 2(6):489–496, 1980.
9. Gelatt KN: Posterior segment: Diagnostic methods in small animal ophthalmology (part III). *Compend Contin Educ Pract Vet* 2(7):556–562, 1980.
10. Bedford PGC: The diagnosis of ocular disease in the dog and cat. *Br Vet J* 138:93–119, 1982.
11. Hacker DV: Ophthalmology for the clinician. *Calif Vet* 10:12–19,24, 1984.
12. Winston SM: Ocular emergencies. *Vet Clin North Am* 11(1):59–76, 1981.
13. Morgan RV: Ocular emergencies. *Compend Contin Educ Pract Vet* 4(1):37–45, 1982.
14. Barrie KP, Gelatt KN: Disease of the eyelids (part I). *Compend Contin Educ Pract Vet* 1(5):405–410, 1979.
15. Martin CL: Feline ophthalmologic diseases. *Mod Vet Pract* 62:865–870, 1981.
16. Bojrab MJ, Crane SW, Arnoczky SP (eds): *Current Techniques in Small Animal Surgery.* Philadelphia, Lea & Febiger, 1983.
17. Gwin RM: Selected blepharoplastic procedures of the canine eyelid. *Compend Contin Educ Pract Vet* 2(4):267–272, 1980.
18. Gelatt KN, Blogg JR: Blepharoplastic procedures in small animals. *JAAHA* 5:67–78, 1969.
19. Doherty MJ: A bridge-flap blepharorrhaphy method for eyelid reconstruction in the cat. *JAAHA* 9:238–241, 1973.
20. Blanchard GL, Keller WF: The rhomboid graft-flap for the repair of extensive ocular adnexal defects. *JAAHA* 12:576–680, 1976.
21. Brightman AH II, Helper LC: Full thickness resection of the eyelid. *JAAHA* 14:483–485, 1978.
22. Munger RJ, Gourley IM: Cross lid flap repair of large upper eyelid defects. *JAVMA* 178:45–58, 1981.
23. Pavletic MM, Nafe LA, Confer AW: Mucocutaneous subdermal plexus flap from the lip for lower eyelid restoration in the dog. *JAVMA* 180:921–926, 1982.
24. Bromberg NM: The nictitating membrane. *Compend Contin Educ Pract Vet* 2(8):627–632, 1980.
25. Kuhns EL: Oral mucosal grafts for membrana nictitans replacement. *Mod Vet Pract* 58:768–771, 1977.
26. Kuhns EL: Reconstruction of canine membrana nictitans with an autograft. *Mod Vet Pract* 62:697–700, 1981.
27. Kuhns EL: Replacement of canine membrana nictitans with a lip graft. *Mod Vet Pract* 62:773–776, 1981.
28. Hanna C, Fraunfelder FT, Cable M, et al: The effect of ophthalmic ointment on corneal wound healing. *Am J Ophthalmol* 76:193–200, 1973.
29. Fraunfelder FT, Hanna C: Ophthalmic drug delivery systems. *Survey Ophthalmol* 18:292–298, 1974.
30. Robin JS, Ellis PP: Ophthalmic ointments. *Survey Ophthalmol* 22:335–340, 1978.
31. Campbell CB: Ophthalmic agents: Ointments or drops? *VM SAC* 74:971–974, 1979.
32. Shell JW: Pharmacokinetics of topically applied ophthalmic drugs. *Survey Ophthalmol* 26:207–218, 1982.
33. Helper LC: The canine nictitating membrane and conjunctiva, in Gelatt KN (ed): *Textbook of Veterinary Ophthalmology.* Philadelphia, WB Saunders Co, 1981, pp 320–342.
34. Carter JD: Diseases of the canine orbit, in Gelatt KN (ed): *Textbook of Veterinary Ophthalmology.* Philadelphia, WB Saunders Co, 1981, pp 265–276.
35. Maurice D: The structure and transparency of the cornea. *J Physiol* 136:263, 1957.
36. Maurice D, Giardini A: Swelling of the cornea in vivo after destruction of its limiting layers. *Br J Ophthalmol* 35:791, 1951.
37. Dice PF: The canine cornea, in Gelatt KN (ed): *Textbook of Veterinary Ophthalmology.* Philadelphia, WB Saunders Co, 1981, pp 343–374.
38. Bistner S: Clinical diagnosis and treatment of infectious keratitis. *Compend Contin Educ Pract Vet* 3(12):1056–1063, 1981.
39. Startup FG: Corneal ulceration in the dog. *J Small Anim Pract* 25:737–752, 1984.
40. Peiffer RL, Gelatt KN: Complete bulbar conjunctival flap in the dog. *Canine Pract* 2:15–18, 1975.
41. Peiffer RL, Gelatt KN, Gwin RM: Tarsoconjunctival pedicle grafts for deep corneal ulceration in the dog and cat. *JAAHA* 13:387–391, 1977.
42. Parshall CJ: Lamella corneal-scleral transposition. *JAAHA* 9:270–277, 1973.
43. Kublin KS, Refojo MF: Closure of ocular lacerations with an adhesive. *JAVMA* 156:313–318, 1970.
44. Fogle JA, Kenyon KR, Foster CS: Tissue adhesive arrests stromal melting in the human cornea. *Am J Ophthalmol* 89:795–802, 1980.
45. Peruccio C, Bosio P, Cornaglia E: Indications and limits of the cyanoacrylate tissue adhesives in corneal ulcers and perforations. *Fourteenth Annu Scientific Meet Am Coll Vet Ophthalmol* 14:135–153, 1983.
46. Schmidt GM, Blancahrd GL, Keller WF: The use of hydrophilic contact lenses in corneal disease of the dog and cat: A preliminary report. *J Small Anim Pract* 18:773–777, 1977.
47. Tammeus J, Krall CJ, Rengstorff RH: Therapeutic extended wear contact lens for corneal injury in a horse. *JAVMA* 182:286, 1983.
48. Morgan RV, Bachrach A, Ogilvie GK: An evaluation of soft contact lens usage in the dog and cat. *JAAHA* 20:885–888, 1984.
49. Peiffer RL, Gelatt KN, Jessen CR, et al: Calibration of the Schiotz tonometer for the normal canine eye. *Am J Vet Res* 38:1881–1889, 1977.
50. Gelatt KN: Canine glaucomas. *Compend Contin Educ Pract Vet* 1(2):150–155, 1979.
51. Brooks DE, Dzieyc J: The canine glaucomas: Pathogenesis, diagnosis, and treatment. *Compend Contin Educ Pract Vet* 5(4):292–300, 1983.
52. Brightman AH: Pharmacologic management of glaucoma in the dog. *JAVMA* 177:326–328, 1980.
53. Bedford PG: The surgical treatment of canine glaucoma. *J Small Anim Pract* 18:713–730, 1977.
54. Peiffer RL, Gwin RM, Gelatt KN, Schenk M: Combined posterior sclerectomy, cyclodialysis and trans-scleral iridencleisis in the management of primary glaucoma. *Canine*

Pract 4(3):54–61, 1977.
55. Brightman AH, Vestre WA, Helper LC, Tomes JE: Cryosurgery for the treatment of canine glaucoma. *JAAHA* 18:319–322, 1982.
56. Vestre WA: Use of cyclocryotherapy in management of glaucoma in dogs. *Mod Vet Pract* 65:93–97, 1984.
57. Roberts SM, Severin GA, Lavach JD: Cyclocryotherapy Part I: Evaluation of a liquid nitrogen system. *JAAHA* 20:823–827, 1984.
58. Roberts SM, Severin GA, Lavach JD: Cyclocryotherapy Part I: Clinical comparison of liquid nitrogen and nitrous oxide cryotherapy on glaucomatous eyes. *JAAHA* 20:828–833, 1984.
59. Vainisi SJ, Schmidt GM, West CS, Vernot J: Intraocular gentamicin for the control of endophthalmitis and glaucoma in animals. *Fourteenth Annu Scientific Meet Am Coll Vet Ophthalmol* 14:134, 1983.
60. May DR, Ericson ES, Peyman GA, Axelrod AJ: Intraocular injection of gentamicin. Single injection therapy of experimental bacterial endophthalmitis. *Arch Ophthalmol* 91:487–489, 1974.
61. Peyman GA, May DR, Ericson ES, Apple D: Intraocular injection of gentamicin. Toxic effects and clearance. *Arch Ophthalmol* 92:42–47, 1974.
62. Zachary IG, Forster RK: Experimental intravitreal gentamicin. *Am J Ophthalmol* 82:604–611, 1976.
63. D'Amico DJ, Libert J, Kenyon KR, et al: Retinal toxicity of intravitreal gentamicin. *Invest Ophthalmol Vis Sci* 25:564–572, 1984.
64. Keller WF: The canine anterior uvea, in Gelatt KN (ed): *Textbook of Veterinary Ophthalmology*. Philadelphia, WB Saunders Co, 1981, pp 375–389.
65. Fischer CA: Diseases of the uveal tract, uveitis and immunologically mediated ocular disease, in Kirk RW (ed): *Current Veterinary Therapy VI*. Philadelphia, WB Saunders Co, 1977, pp 638–646.
66. Bistner S, Shaw D, Riis RC: Diseases of the uveal tract—Inflammations (part II). *Compend Contin Educ Pract Vet* 1(12):899–906, 1979.
67. Bistner S, Shaw D, Riis RC: Diseases of the uveal tract (part III). *Compend Contin Educ Pract Vet* 2(1):46–53, 1980.
68. Bistner S, Shaw D, Riis RC: Diseases of the uveal tract (part I). *Compend Contin Educ Pract Vet* 1(11):868–875, 1979.
69. Rose SW, Coupal JJ, Simmons G, et al: Experimental hyphema clearance in rabbits. Drug trials with 1% atropine and 2% and 4% pilocarpine. *Arch Ophthalmol* 95:1442–1444, 1977.
70. Spoor TC, Hammer M. Belloso H: Traumatic hyphema: Failure of steroids to alter its course; a double-blind prospective study. *Arch Ophthalmol* 98:116–119, 1980.
71. McGetrick JJ, Jampol LM, Goldberg MF, et al: Aminocaproic acid decreases secondary hemorrhage after traumatic hyphema. *Arch Ophthalmol* 101:1031–1033, 1983.
72. Vainisi S, Schmidt G, West C, et al: Metabolic toxic retinopathy—A preliminary report. *Fourteenth Annu Scientific Meet Am Coll Vet Ophthalmol* 14:76–81, 1983.
73. Irby NL: Silent retina syndrome, in *Case Reports Forum*. Lake Tahoe, NV, American College of Veterinary Ophthalmology, 1982.
74. Acland GM, Irby NL, Aguirre GD, et al: Sudden acquired retinal degeneration in the dog: Clinical and morphologic characterization of the silent retina syndrome. *Fifteenth Annu Scientific Meet Am Coll Vet Ophthalmol* 15:86–104, 1984.
75. Freeman MH, Donovan RH, Schepens CL: Retinal detachment, chorioretinal changes, and staphyloma in the collie. *Arch Ophthalmol* 76:412–421, 1966.
76. Lavach JD, Murphy JM, Severin GA: Retinal dysplasia in the English springer spaniel. *JAAHA* 14:192–199, 1978.
77. Rubin LF: Heredity of retinal dysplasia in Bedlington terriers. *JAVMA* 152:260–262, 1968.
78. Nelson DL, MacMillan AD: Multifocal retinal dysplasia in field trial Labrador retrievers. *JAAHA* 19:388–392, 1983.
79. Bussanich MN, Rootman J, Dolman CL: Granulomatous panuveitis and dermal depigmentation in the dog. *JAAHA* 19:388–392, 1983.
80. Gwin RM, Gelatt KN, Terrell TG, Hood CI: Hypertensive retinopathy associated with hypothyroidism, hypercholesterolemia, and renal failure in a dog. *JAAHA* 14:200–209, 1978.
81. Barclay SM, Riis RC: Retinal detachment and reattachment associated with ethylene glycol intoxication in a cat. *JAAHA* 15:719–724, 1979.
82. Gwin RM, Wyman M, Ketring K, Winston S: Idiopathic uveitis and exudative retinal detachment in the dog. *JAAHA* 16:163–170, 1980.
83. Anderson DH, Stern WH, Fisher SK, et al: Retinal detachment in the cat: The pigment epithelial-photoreceptor interface. *Invest Ophthalmol Vis Sci* 24:906–926, 1983.
84. Barrie KP, Lavach JD, Gelatt KN: Diseases of the posterior segment, in Gelatt KN (ed): *Textbook of Veterinary Ophthalmology*. Philadelphia, WB Saunders Co, 1981, pp 474–517.
85. Nafe LA, Carter JD: Canine optic neuritis. *Compend Contin Educ Pract Vet* 3(11):978–981, 1981.
86. Severin GA: *Severin's Veterinary Ophthalmology Notes*, ed 3. Fort Collins, CO, College of Veterinary Medicine and Biomedical Sciences, Colorado State University, 1995.
87. Kern TJ: Ulcerative keratitis. *Vet Clin North Am [Small Anim Pract]* 20:643–666, 1990.
88. Kirschner SE: Persistent corneal ulcers. What to do when ulcers won't heal. *Vet Clin North Am [Small Anim Pract]* 20:627–642, 1990.
89. Pickett JP, Miller PE, Majors LT: Calibration of the Schiotz tonometer for the canine and feline eye. *Trans Am Coll Vet Ophthalmol* 19:47–51, 1988.
90. Roberts SM: Glaucoma in companion animals: Current management and new trends. *Calif Vet* 48(1):9–16, 1994.
91. Martin C, et al: Ocular use of tissue plasminogen activator in companion animals. *Vet Compar Ophthalmol* 3:29–36, 1993.
92. Gerding PA, Eurell T: Evaluation of intraocular penetration of topically administered tissue plasminogen activator in dogs. *Am J Vet Res* 54:836–839, 1993.

Respiratory Emergencies

KEY FACTS

- Treatment of respiratory emergencies depends on prompt recognition and positive therapeutic intervention.
- Management of bacterial bronchopneumonia, aspiration pneumonia, and pneumonia associated with smoke inhalation requires accurate diagnosis and aggressive life-saving medical treatment.
- Emergency techniques (e.g., tracheostomy, oxygen therapy, blood pressure monitoring, determinations of central venous pressure, insertion of a chest tube, and positive-pressure ventilation) can save lives.
- Respiratory arrest is a medical emergency that demands immediate correction and should take precedence over all other emergency care.
- Patients presented with pleural cavity disease (e.g., pneumothorax, pyothorax, chylothorax, or hemothorax) must be differentiated from patients presented with congenital or acquired diaphragmatic hernia.

Louisiana State University
Joseph Taboada, DVM
Johnny D. Hoskins, DVM, PhD

Rawley Memorial Animal Hospital
Springfield, Massachusetts
Rhea V. Morgan, DVM

HYPOXEMIA is the cardinal manifestation of all respiratory emergencies. Effective therapy often depends on prompt recognition and immediate positive therapeutic intervention. The clinical signs associated with hypoxemia are characterized by changes in respiratory rate, character, and effort. The respiratory rate may be increased or decreased, the depth may be impeded or exaggerated, and effort is often multiplied to the point that the animal is weak and exhausted from the increased work. Mucous membrane color is often abnormal, ranging from cyanotic to pale. Cyanosis, although most common, may be absent in patients with severe anemia, shock, or carbon monoxide poisoning and methemoglobinemia.

The astute clinician may listen for abnormal respiratory sounds or note abnormal posture during attempts to breathe. The phase of respiration in which these sounds are heard may be helpful in localizing the respiratory disease to the upper or lower airway. In an attempt to maximize air intake, the patient may assume an abnormal posture. Orthopnea, extension of the head and neck, abduction of the forelimbs, and sternal recumbency signal severe respiratory disease.

Cats in severe respiratory distress often do not show the same degree of obvious difficulty as dogs. Tachypnea and less-apparent increases in respiratory effort herald respiratory distress in cats. The clinician must take great care not to stress animals that have respiratory disease, especially cats. Many dyspneic cats have died after the stress of evaluation by a clinician who failed to recognize the severity of the respiratory condition immediately. Radiology is an especially prominent stressor for many dyspneic animals.

AIRWAY OBSTRUCTION
Causes

Airway obstruction is a common respiratory emergency. Trauma involving the upper airway may result in obstruction through facial and mandibular fracture, epistaxis, laryngeal and tracheal lacerations and fractures, and soft tissue swelling. Infections, including abscess formation, may compromise the nasal passage, pharynx, and larynx.[1] Occlusion with foreign material (e.g., bones, stones, wood, food, vomitus, or exudate) is also common. Rarely, such allergic phenomena as angioneurotic edema can cause airway narrowing at the level of the larynx. In addition, tumors of the airway and surrounding soft tissue and metastatic neoplasms have caused airway obstruction.[2-6]

Common causes of airway obstruction in brachycephalic canine breeds include stenotic nares, elongated soft palate, laryngeal malformation, everted laryngeal saccules, and hypoplastic trachea (Table I). These defects collectively have been referred to as the brachycephalic airway syndrome. Stenosis of the nares may be pivotal in creating many of the problems that develop in the brachycephalic dogs as they age.[7] Stenotic nares are resected while the dog

TABLE I
Anatomic Causes of Respiratory Distress

Anatomic Conformation	Breed
Stenotic nares	Brachycephalic breeds, shar pei
Elongation of soft palate	Brachycephalic breeds, beagle, shar pei, cocker spaniel
Eversion of the lateral ventricles of larynx	Brachycephalic breeds, especially English bulldog
Laryngeal paralysis	
Congenital	Bouvier des Flandres, bullterrier, Siberian husky
Acquired	Giant-breed dogs, especially Saint Bernard; golden retriever, Irish setter; Labrador retriever; German short-haired pointer; cats of any breed
Hypoplasia of trachea	English bulldog, shar pei
Tracheal collapse	Yorkshire terrier, Chihuahua, Pomeranian, toy and miniature poodle, other nonbrachycephalic toy breeds

is young to minimize problems as it matures.

Chronic excessive negative pressure within the upper airway may be responsible for elongation and thickening of the soft palate to the point that it overlies the epiglottis and partially or completely obstructs the glottis. Eversion of the lateral ventricles of the larynx and hypertrophy of pharyngeal tissue probably result from a similar negative pressure during inspiration in dogs with narrow airways.[7] In chronic cases, complete laryngeal collapse is possible. The brachycephalic airway syndrome is common in English bulldogs, boxers, Boston terriers, pugs, Shih Tzus, shar peis, and Himalayan cats.

Animals with the brachycephalic airway syndrome usually have a history of stridor and stertor that are often first noticed while the animal is excited or sleeping. Although the respiratory noise has often been present for a long time, severe clinical signs of distress may not be apparent until the animal is stressed or allowed to overheat. Acute distress associated with the brachycephalic airway syndrome may be seen in association with heat stress or excitement (as associated with trips to the veterinary facility) or as a complication following anesthesia.

Brachycephalic animals should always be monitored closely while they are recovering from an anesthetic procedure. The endotracheal tube should be left in place for as long as the animal will safely tolerate the tube's presence.

Laryngeal paralysis is another cause of upper airway stertor and obstruction. It may be congenital or acquired; clinical signs occur by the time the animal is 14 months of age in most congenital cases.[8,9] Congenital laryngeal paralysis has been identified in the Bouvier des Flandres, bullterrier, and Siberian husky breeds.[10] In the Bouvier des Flandres breed, the condition is transmitted by an autosomal dominant gene and is bilaterally symmetrical; clinical signs occur at four to six months of age.[11–13]

Acquired laryngeal paralysis can occur at any age and be unilateral or bilateral. Unilateral paralysis is often idiopathic but may result from trauma to the recurrent laryngeal nerve associated with bite wounds or placement of a pharyngostomy tube.[8] Nontraumatic causes include polyneuropathy, meningitis, and hypothyroidism.[8,14] Complete response to thyroid hormone supplementation has been noted in some dogs.

Lymphosarcoma has been reported to cause unilateral paralysis in cats.[15] Idiopathic bilateral laryngeal paralysis has also been reported to occur in cats.[16]

Although airway obstruction from the nares to the proximal trachea is usually associated with inspiratory stridor, obstructive disease of the intrathoracic trachea or large bronchi is typically associated with expiratory dyspnea or dyspnea noted throughout the respiratory cycle. Cough is also often a prominent feature of the history. Obstructive tracheal disease secondary to an inhaled foreign body in the airway is uncommon but should be considered if an animal with sudden onset of cough and respiratory distress is presented.[17]

Tracheal foreign bodies most commonly lodge at the tracheal bifurcation and include such things as pebbles, bones, plant material, nails, marbles, and safety pins.[18] Patients that have recently inhaled a foreign body should be suspended in a head-down position, and sharp pressure should be applied to the cranial abdomen in a manner that resembles the Heimlich maneuver. If this maneuver fails to dislodge the foreign object, endoscopic removal or thoracotomy is needed.

TRACHEAL OBSTRUCTION may occur secondary to tracheal stenosis. Obstruction may occur as a congenital lesion or may result from trauma or neoplastic disease. Scar tissue formation following blunt or penetrating trauma, aspiration of a foreign body, tracheostomy, tracheal surgery, or pressure from an endotracheal tube may result in stenosis and obstructive disease. Stenosis secondary to parasitic granulomas, abscesses, vascular anomalies, or tracheal tumors is rare.[18]

Hypoplasia of the trachea is a congenital defect in which the tracheal rings are inadequately developed.[19] This condition occurs in brachycephalic dogs, especially English bulldogs; along with the rest of the brachycephalic airway syndrome, it predisposes affected dogs to acute occlusion of the airway.

Tracheal collapse may present as either cough or acute

airway obstruction. It most often affects dogs of toy breeds and is noted less frequently in larger dogs and cats.[20] Although the disease is seen in animals of all ages, the average age at diagnosis is 7.5 years.[18] The causes of tracheal collapse are unknown, but proposed causes include hereditary predisposition, obesity, demineralization of tracheal cartilage, and weakness and stretching of the trachealis muscle; these factors allow the tracheal rings to flatten.[21] Chronic small airway disease may be important in the pathogenesis.

Small airway disease may result in increased transtracheal pressure and may eventually lead to tracheal collapse, especially in animals with preexisting weakness of the tracheal wall.[21] Collapse of the cervical trachea is more likely to occur during inspiration. Intrathoracic collapse usually occurs during expiration as a result of increased transtracheal pressure.[21] A cough that sounds like a goose honk is observed in approximately 50% of dogs with tracheal collapse and is often noted when the animal pulls on a leash or gets excited. The cough alone can become severe enough, or annoying enough, that the dog is presented as an emergency.

In advanced stages of the disease, true emergency presentations are likely because the dogs may become dyspneic and cyanotic at rest. Syncope may occur in a severely affected dog.

Clinical Signs

Airway obstruction is characterized by noisy stridulous or stertorous breathing. Slow, deep, forceful inspiratory effort is typical of upper-airway obstruction; whereas forceful expiratory effort is more representative of lower-airway obstruction. A history of decreased exercise tolerance, cyanosis, increased respiratory effort, and collapse may be given. Choking, retching that produces white froth, and vomiting may be noted. Severely distressed animals may paw or claw at their faces and throats. Animals with obstructive disease of the upper airway, especially the brachycephalic breeds, are predisposed to heat prostration.

Localization of the source of the noise may aid in determining the cause of the obstruction. Most upper airway obstructions produce stridulous sounds that are loudest at the larynx and pharynx. Tracheal obstruction and collapse produce a low-pitched honking sound that is accompanied by a cough.

Diagnosis

Most of the information required in the diagnosis of obstructive airway disease can be obtained from the case history and physical examination. Extreme care must be used in examining all animals with airway obstruction. Their hypoxic state predisposes them to collapse and respiratory arrest when they are stressed. A history of voice change may indicate pharyngeal or laryngeal disease. Upper airway obstruction should be suspected if a dyspneic animal has obvious facial injuries, epistaxis, or wounds to the neck. The animal should be thoroughly examined for stenotic nares, oral foreign bodies or masses, soft tissue swelling of the head and neck, and other systemic problems.

Radiography is helpful in defining facial fractures, laryngeal trauma, and injuries or tumors of the trachea. Dorsoventral flattening of the trachea may be evident in animals with tracheal collapse, but fluoroscopy and sometimes endoscopy are often necessary to delineate cervical and intrathoracic narrowing definitively. Great care must be taken during radiographic examination of the dyspneic animal. The positions necessary for diagnostic evaluation often impede respiration. Although the short time necessary for taking a diagnostic radiograph may not dramatically increase hypoxemia, stress and excitement will—especially in dyspneic cats, for which sedation is often necessary to relieve the stress and anxiety associated with the examination. The clinician must walk a fine line between the importance of gathering diagnostic information and the dangers of compromising the patient.

The nasopharynx and larynx should be examined directly if pharyngeal or laryngeal disease is suspected. Sedation is necessary if the animal is conscious. Elongation of the soft palate may be diagnosed by visualization of tissue overlying the epiglottis and extending beyond the tonsillar crypts. It is often thickened, redundant, and inflamed. Pharyngeal edema may accompany any of the obstructive diseases of the upper airway and may contribute significantly to the severity of the problem.

Everted laryngeal saccules are part of the brachycephalic airway syndrome and are seen as thin, pink membranous tissue that prolapses into the laryngeal inlet, especially during inspiration. In animals with laryngeal paralysis, vocal folds fail to abduct during inspiration, retain a midline position, and obviously narrow the laryngeal opening. Examination of the larynx should be performed with the patient lightly sedated so that laryngeal function can be more completely assessed. If laryngeal paralysis is diagnosed, hypothyroidism should be ruled out by use of the thyrotropin response test.

Diagnosis of tracheal collapse is usually based on the signalment, case history, and ruleout of other obvious causes of dyspnea and cough. Endoscopy may be necessary to confirm the presence of tracheal collapse, lower airway obstruction from tumors, or airway obstruction resulting from a foreign body.

Treatment

The major objectives in treating airway obstructions are to establish a patent airway, institute or assist ventilation, and maintain adequate oxygen tension to maximize oxygen delivery to the tissue. For animals with upper airway obstructions but normal pulmonary parenchymal function, maintaining adequate ventilation with room air may be all that is necessary. If ventilation cannot be completely normalized or pulmonary function is abnormal, however, oxygen therapy is critical to maintaining adequate tissue oxygenation. A protocol for the treatment of airway obstruction appears on this page. Table II lists drugs and doses for use in patients with airway obstruction.

The animal should be separated from its owner and taken to a central treatment area or intensive care unit. If the animal is unconscious, intratracheal intubation and oxygen therapy are instituted. All foreign material, saliva, and blood are suctioned or removed from the mouth and upper airway. If the obstruction appears to be partial, so that some air exchange is taking place, the animal may be sedated to relieve anxiety and oxygen is then administered. Handling and excitement should be kept to a minimum in order to minimize stress.

From the initial assessment, the clinician must determine as quickly as possible where the obstruction is. Obstructions of the upper airway that fail to respond to the described measures may be bypassed with a tracheostomy. If obstruction of the lower airway is suspected, radiographs are taken with the utmost care. Tracheal collapse is treated initially with strict cage confinement, oxygen, bronchodilators, and sedation (if necessary). Antitussives are usually needed to stop the cough. Coughing associated with the collapse results in tracheitis that perpetuates the cough and maintains a vicious circle of collapse–cough–tracheitis–cough–more-severe collapse and so forth.

Secondary bacterial infections are treated with antibiotics. The choice of antibiotic is based on bacterial culture and sensitivity testing. If endoscopic or transtracheal aspirate cannot be obtained, a broad-spectrum antibiotic (e.g., a trimethoprim-sulfonamide combination) is used initially.

If the clinician suspects tracheal collapse, the animal should be treated even if radiographic confirmation is lacking—survey thoracic radiographs (inspiratory and expiratory films) are diagnostic in less than 60% of cases.[22] Fluoroscopic evaluation facilitates diagnosis, but definitive diagnosis is best done by endoscopy.

Animals that do not respond to medical management may require surgery.[18,22] Surgery designed to open the glottis by widening the laryngeal opening is usually required for animals with laryngeal paralysis. The prognosis following surgery is generally fair to good if laryngeal function is good and the major bronchi are not involved.[18]

Technique for Tube Tracheostomy

If the animal is severely hypoxic or unconscious and the obstruction prohibits easy endotracheal intubation, tube tracheostomy should be performed immediately. The tracheostomy tube may be inserted using local anesthesia; but in most instances, the animal can be carefully anesthetized and intubated before insertion of the tracheostomy tube. General anesthesia ensures a patent airway, allows controlled ventilation, enables a more-aseptic procedure to be performed, and is usually less stressful for the animal in respiratory distress.

The animal is positioned in dorsal recumbency. The hair

Protocol for the Treatment of Airway Obstruction

1. Separate animal from owner; move animal to an intensive care area
2. Establish patent airway
   a. Intubate if the animal is in collapse or unconscious
   b. Remove oral foreign material and blood
   c. Perform tracheostomy if intubation is not easily accomplished
3. Begin oxygen therapy
   a. A mask can be used if obstruction is not severe
   b. A nasal catheter or oxygen cage is less likely to cause excitement
   c. With a transtracheal catheter, close to 100% inspired oxygen can be achieved with high oxygen flow rates
   d. Endotracheal intubation or tracheostomy may be necessary
4. Start supportive care (as appropriate)
   a. Intravenous fluid therapy
   b. Sedation
   c. Antibiotics
   d. Corticosteroids
   e. Bronchodilators
   f. Maintenance of normal body temperature
5. Perform further diagnostic procedures
   a. Radiography—survey films
   b. Laryngoscopic examination—limited to light sedation for proper assessment of laryngeal function
   c. Fluoroscopy for possible tracheal collapse
   d. Bronchoscopy
6. Assess and treat coexisting problems
7. Prepare patient for surgery
   a. Removal of foreign bodies or masses
   b. Repair of fractures and wounds
   c. Incision and drainage of abscesses
   d. Correction of anatomic defects
      i. Stenotic nares—resection of lateral alar cartilage
      ii. Elongated soft palate—surgical resection
      iii. Everted laryngeal ventricles—saccule resection
      iv. Laryngeal paralysis—partial laryngectomy or lateralization of arytenoid cartilage
      v. Tracheal collapse—prosthetic ring support
8. Continue postoperative care of tracheostomy tube
   a. Suction every two to four hours using aseptic technique
   b. Nebulize with saline solution or acetylcysteine diluted with saline solution
   c. Maintain normal hydration
   d. Consider antibiotics
   e. Monitor body temperature
   f. Periodically radiograph thorax

TABLE II
Drug Doses for Use in Patients with Airway Obstruction

Drug	Dose
Butorphanol tartrate	*Dogs*: 0.1–0.2 mg/kg intravenously or 0.4 mg/kg subcutaneously or intramuscularly every eight hours *Cats*: 0.1–0.4 mg/kg subcutaneously or intramuscularly every 12 hours
Morphine sulfate	*Dogs*: 0.1–0.4 mg/kg subcutaneously or intramuscularly every 8–12 hours *Cats*: 0.05–0.1 mg/kg subcutaneously or intramuscularly every 12 hours
Midazolam	*Dogs*: 0.1–0.2 mg/kg intramuscularly or subcutaneously
Meperidine hydrochloride	*Dogs*: 5–10 mg/kg intramuscularly *Cats*: 2–4 mg/kg intramuscularly
Fentanyl citrate–droperidol	*Dogs*: 0.1–0.3 ml per 20 kg intramuscularly
Oxymorphone hydrochloride	*Dogs*: 0.05–0.1 mg/kg intravenously or 0.1–0.2 mg/kg subcutaneously or intramuscularly (to maximum of 3 mg) *Cats*: 0.02 mg/kg intravenously
Dexamethasone	0.02–0.2 mg/kg intravenously or subcutaneously every 12 hours
Prednisolone	0.25–0.5 mg/kg intramuscularly or orally every 12 hours
Aminophylline	*Dogs*: 6–11 mg/kg intravenously or orally every six to eight hours *Cats*: 4 mg/kg orally or slowly intravenously every 12 hours
Theophylline	*Dogs*: 6–11 mg/kg intravenously or orally every six to eight hours *Cats*: 1–2 mg/kg slowly intravenously every eight hours

is shaved and the skin prepared from the point of the jaw to the thoracic inlet directly over the midline. An incision is made over the trachea immediately caudal to the larynx or below the obstruction (Figure 1A), and the proximal cervical trachea is exposed. An incision is made into the trachea between the cartilaginous rings through the membranous tissue (Figure 1B). Although which tracheal incision to use is controversial, it probably is of minimal importance in the formation of tracheal stenosis.[18] For high obstructions, the incision is made between the second and third, third and fourth, or fourth and fifth tracheal rings. The tracheal incision is widened using forceps or retracting sutures to facilitate tube placement.

The endotracheal tube is then withdrawn, and a tracheostomy tube [e.g., Portex®, Portex, Inc., Wilmington, MA] is inserted (Figure 1C). If the tracheostomy tube is supplied with an obturator, the obturator is then removed. The tracheostomy tube is sutured to the skin of the neck or is tied in place using umbilical tape. Sterile endotracheal tubes may be used in giant-breed and thick-necked dogs in which ordinary tracheostomy tubes cannot be adequately secured. After insertion of the tube, the airway is suctioned and patency of the tracheostomy tube is ensured.

Anesthesia may be maintained through the tracheostomy tube if further surgical procedures are to be performed at the same time. Continuous intensive-care monitoring is essential after placement of a tracheostomy tube. A patient with a tracheostomy tube may quickly asphyxiate if the tube becomes dislodged or occluded with mucus, blood, or exudate.

Mucoid secretions may adhere to the free end of the tube and compromise its patency. The tracheostomy tube is often irritating to the trachea, thus stimulating increased production of thick, viscid secretions. It also bypasses the normal humidifying and warming mechanisms of the nasal passages, thus further contributing to mucus formation.

The tracheostomy tube should be suctioned every two to four hours or as necessary using aseptic technique. To liquefy secretions, sterile saline solution or acetylcysteine [Mucomyst®—Mead Johnson] diluted in sterile saline solution may be administered by nebulization. If patency of the tube becomes poor, it should be replaced.

The tracheostomy tube is removed when the animal is able to breathe adequately around the manually occluded tube. Following removal of the tracheostomy tube, the site is left open to heal by second intention.

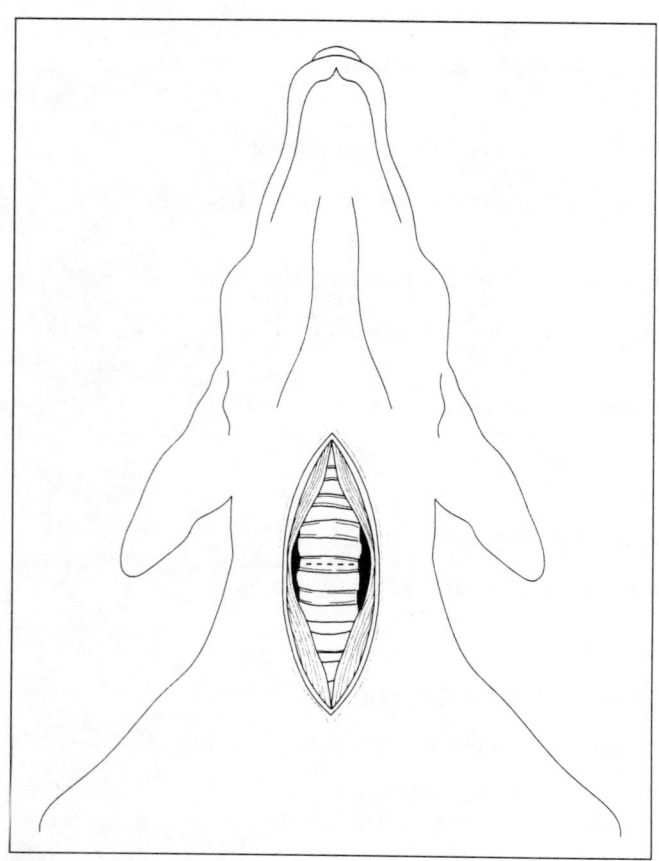

Figure 1A

Figure 1—Tracheostomy tube insertion. (**A**) Positioning of a dog in dorsal recumbency. The skin incision is made over the midline of the trachea and extending from the first through the fourth tracheal rings. (**B**) An incision is made between tracheal rings and enlarged with a hemostat or Trousseau dilator. (**C**) Insertion of the tracheostomy tube.

Once a patent airway and oxygen therapy have been established, other supportive care is instituted. Animals in shock are treated with intravenous fluids and corticosteroids.[23] Hyperthermic animals are rapidly cooled, and the protocol for heat exhaustion is followed.[24] Angioneurotic edema of the larynx usually responds to corticosteroids alone.

PARENCHYMAL EXCHANGE DISEASES

Oxygen and carbon dioxide pass through several layers of respiratory membrane as they are exchanged in the lungs. These layers are the alveolar surfactant and fluid layer, the alveolar epithelium with basement membrane, the thin interstitial space, and the capillary basement membrane and endothelium. Any process that alters the thickness or surface area of these layers and the pressure difference across these membranes or affects the regional perfusion alters the overall rate of gas exchange.[25] When ventilation–perfusion abnormalities result in severe impairment of oxygenation, a respiratory emergency exists.

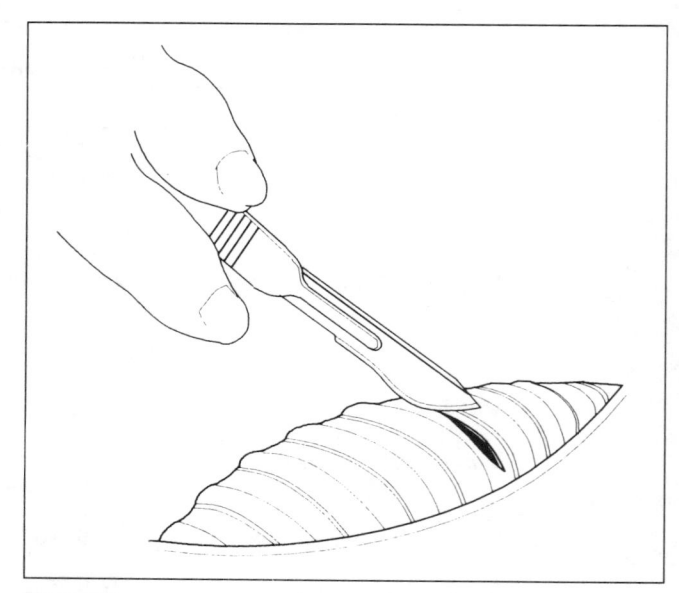

Figure 1B

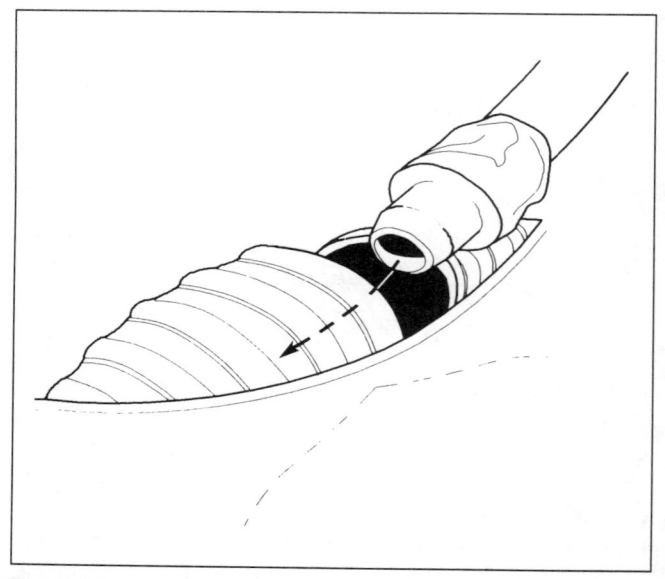

Figure 1C

Pneumonia

The most common life-threatening pneumonias are acute fulminating bacterial bronchopneumonia, aspiration pneumonia, and pneumonia associated with smoke inhalation.[19,26–28] Inflammatory exudate and/or aspirated foreign material occlude the alveoli, thus effectively decreasing the total surface area for exchange. Carbon monoxide poisoning associated with smoke inhalation dramatically changes gas pressures across the pulmonary membrane.[27,28]

Bacterial Pneumonia

Bacterial pneumonia may occur secondary to immunosuppression, defective airway defense mechanisms, chronic tracheobronchial disease, inhalation of toxic gases or smoke, or aspiration of foreign material or gastric contents.[26,27] Neuromuscular disorders, such as myasthenia gravis and idiopathic megaesophagus, may contribute to aspiration and subsequent bacterial infection. In a review of 42 dogs with bacterial bronchopneumonia, sporting dogs, working dogs, and hounds younger than one year old were most often affected.[29] Cats are affected less often than dogs.[26]

Clinical signs may include cough, fever, weakness, dyspnea, depression, and nasal discharge. Cough does not seem to be as common in cats as it is in dogs. Fever may be present because of the bacterial infection and the increased work associated with the exaggerated respiratory effort. Tachypnea and dyspnea are the most common clinical signs noted in cats and dogs.[26,29] Severely affected animals may be cyanotic, breathe with their mouths open, and appear apprehensive.

Diagnosis depends on demonstration of an alveolar or mixed interstitial pattern on thoracic radiography and the presence of suppurative inflammation and bacteria in a transtracheal aspirate or bronchoalveolar lavage specimen. Abnormal lung sounds characterized as increased breath sounds and crackles are often present, but normal thoracic auscultation does not rule out pneumonia. Even patients with severe cases of bacterial bronchopneumonia may sound normal on auscultation.[29] Leukograms typically are characterized by neutrophilia with left shift and monocytosis. Blood gases can be used as a sensitive indicator of severity of pulmonary dysfunction. The PaO_2 typically decreases initially, with $PaCO_2$ decreasing as ventilation–perfusion abnormalities worsen.

Samples should be obtained from all severely affected animals by transtracheal aspiration or bronchoalveolar lavage for cytologic examination and bacterial culture and sensitivity testing. Samples are ideally collected before antibiotic therapy is begun. Initial therapy should be based on Gram stains of lavage samples; more-definitive therapy is based on culture and sensitivity testing. Gram-negative organisms and staphylococci are the most common isolates from dogs with bacterial pneumonia.[29,30] The spectrum of inciting bacteria in cats is not well characterized. *Pasteurella* organisms and other gram-negative organisms are thought to be most common. Eugonic fermenter-4 bacteria may cause fulminant pneumonia and death in affected cats.[31]

The major treatment objectives are to (1) maintain adequate tissue oxygenation, (2) sustain airway patency, (3) maximize mucociliary clearance, (4) preserve hydration, and (5) treat infection. Oxygen should be administered to any animal that is cyanotic or has a PaO_2 below 60 mm Hg.[32] The choice of oxygen administration technique depends on the animal's needs and demeanor and the availability of equipment. An oxygen-delivery mask may be used initially and can achieve inspired oxygen concentrations of 30% to 60%.[32] Oxygen masks require high flow rates and are generally only tolerated for short periods. For longer periods, oxygen administration by nasal or transtracheal catheters or oxygen cages are used.

Oxygen cages that permit complete control of the patient's environment are expensive and may not be feasible for many practices. Care must be taken when inexpensive models are used—the closed environment often results in hyperthermia in large patients.

Nasal oxygen is easily administered and is well tolerated by most animals. A soft, flexible catheter is placed through the nares to the level of the oropharynx. A suture or cyanoacrylate glue can be used to anchor the tube to the skin adjacent to the nares and on the bridge of the nose. The tube is then secured to the animal's collar or an Elizabethan collar and connected to an oxygen source. Nasal administration can maintain inspired oxygen at a level equal to or greater than that provided by a mask or oxygen cage.[32] Flow rates of 6 to 8 L/min should be maintained. Transtracheal oxygen administration has the advantage of allowing lower flow rates (1 to 2 L/min) and maintaining extremely high inspired oxygen (approximating 100%) when high oxygen flow rates are used. The disadvantage is the increased rate of catheter-induced infection and posttherapy tracheitis, especially if humidification is insufficient and oxygen flow rates are high.[32]

AIRWAY PATENCY is preserved in animals with pneumonia through fastidious care of the upper airway and pharmacologic manipulation of the lower airways. Exudate should be suctioned and cleaned away from the nares and oral cavity frequently. Patency of the lower airways is maximized through the use of bronchodilators. Such ß$_2$-adrenergic agents as terbutaline sulfate or such methylxanthine phosphodiester hydrolase inhibitors as aminophylline are useful.

Improvement in mucociliary clearance is also important. This is best accomplished by encouraging expectoration and maintaining hydration. Intravenous fluids are an essential part of the initial management of pneumonia. Dehydration is corrected during the first three to six hours followed by 1.5 to 2 times maintenance fluid rates to maintain maximum airway hydration. Ultrasonic nebulization with sterile saline is also an ideal means of providing airway hydration.[32] Mild forced exercise or percussion (coupage) is indicated, especially if nebulization is used.

Antitussive therapy of any kind is contraindicated in animals with bacterial pneumonia. The cough is the primary means of evacuating the thick mucopurulent exudate from the lower airways of patients with pneumonia. Suppression of this important defense mechanism may result in prolonged recovery and potentially severe consolidation and abscess formation of one or more lung lobes.

Primary treatment of the infection with antibiotics begins immediately after a diagnosis of pneumonia has been made. Antibiotic therapy is ideally directed by results of Gram stains and the results of bacterial culture and sensitivity testing, but initial therapy should begin while the clinician is waiting for results. Trimethoprim-sulfonamide combinations, cephalosporin, chloramphenicol, and enrofloxacin are widely used antibiotics of first choice because of their high activity against gram-negative infections. Ampicillin, amoxicillin, or amoxicillin potentiated with clavulanic acid are additional choices if the initial Gram stain reveals gram-positive cocci. Tetracycline, chloramphenicol, and aminoglycosides are effective against *Bordetella bronchiseptica*.

Animals with severe bacterial pneumonia and marked respiratory insufficiency must be treated aggressively from the beginning. Ampicillin, amoxicillin, or a third-generation cephalosporin combined with an aminoglycoside are indicated. Fluorinated quinolones are used if a *Pseudomonas* species is suspected.

Aspiration Pneumonia

Aspiration pneumonia is the pulmonary sequela of aspiration of foreign material into the lower respiratory tract. It is most commonly seen in animals with altered states of consciousness, oropharyngeal or esophageal disease, or persistent vomiting. The veterinary facility is a common place for aspiration to occur, either in animals recovering from anesthesia or because of inadvertent pulmonary administration of material that was supposed to be placed in the gastrointestinal tract.

The severity of aspiration pneumonia depends on the pH, volume, and particle size of the inhaled material. Gastric acid is the most frequently encountered cause of aspiration pneumonia.[26,27] Acid pH, large volume, the presence of particulate matter, and septic exudate worsen the prognosis. Aspiration of such inert substances as saline, water, barium, and gastric fluid with a pH exceeding 3.0 causes severe pneumonia only if large volumes are aspirated or secondary bacterial infection occurs.

TREATMENT PRINCIPLES for aspiration pneumonia are the same as those discussed for bacterial pneumonia. Airway patency is initially maintained by suction of as much of the aspirated material as possible from the trachea and upper airway. Hypoxia is treated aggressively with oxygen therapy. Bronchodilators may be helpful in minimizing postaspiration bronchoconstriction.

The use of corticosteroids in animals with aspiration pneumonia is controversial.[27,28] Corticosteroids are indicated along with intravenous fluids in animals that require treatment for shock, but they may cause immunosuppression and decrease tracheobronchial clearance. Corticosteroids should therefore not be used after the shock has been reversed. Studies of aspiration pneumonia in animal models and humans have not shown benefit from the use of corticosteroids when shock is not present.[27] The choice of antibiotic is determined by the results of bacterial culture and sensitivity tests. Most cases of aspiration of an inert substance or chemical pneumonitis do not require antibiotic therapy.[27]

Prevention is the best approach to the problem of aspiration pneumonia. Ensuring that food and water have been withheld from an animal before an anesthetic procedure and using a cuffed endotracheal tube during anesthesia help prevent aspiration. If emergency anesthesia is required for an animal that has not fasted, metoclopramide hydrochloride (0.2 to 0.4 mg/kg intravenously to a maximum dose of 10 mg) can be used 30 to 45 minutes before induction. Metoclopramide hydrochloride promotes gastric emptying and increases tone at the gastroesophageal junction. Any animal that has oropharyngeal or esophageal dysfunction and is predisposed to regurgitation and aspiration of gastric contents is pretreated with a histamine$_2$ antagonist, such as cimetidine (5 mg/kg intravenously or intramuscularly) or ranitidine (2 mg/kg intramuscularly), 45 to 60 minutes before anesthesia. Raising the pH of gastric contents minimizes pulmonary damage should aspiration occur.

Smoke-Inhalation Injury

The injury resulting from smoke inhalation is less commonly encountered than either bacterial bronchopneumonia or aspiration pneumonia. Carbon monoxide poisoning and toxicity from noxious gases in the smoke result in most of the damage to the lower respiratory tract. Additionally, thermal injury to the nasal and oral cavities and pharynx often results in upper-airway obstruction secondary to edema and swelling.

Treatment principles are the same as those outlined above. Shock is aggressively treated, and it is important to administer 100% oxygen to an animal in severe respiratory distress. The half-life of carboxyhemoglobin is four hours when the animal is breathing room air but only 30 minutes when it is breathing 100% oxygen.[28] Carbon monoxide's affinity for hemoglobin is 240 times greater than that of oxygen; the resultant carboxyhemoglobin is unable to function as an oxygen carrier to tissue.

Adequate oxygen therapy can only be accomplished through endotracheal intubation, transtracheal catheterization with high oxygen flow rates, or positive end-expiratory pressure. Placement of a tracheostomy tube may be necessary if upper-airway edema is severe. Analgesics may be used for extreme pain or apprehension in selected patients. A protocol for treatment of pneumonia appears on the following page.

Pulmonary Contusion

Pulmonary contusion is bruising or hemorrhage into lung parenchyma and is most often caused by blunt tho-

Protocol for the Treatment of Pneumonia

1. Ensure patent airway
   a. Suction to remove foreign material and secretions
   b. Intubate if necessary
   c. Consider tracheostomy for patients with airway obstruction caused by secretions or laryngeal spasm
2. Begin oxygen therapy
3. Perform diagnostic evaluation
   a. Radiography of thorax
   b. Transtracheal aspiration
   c. Complete blood count
   d. Determination of arterial blood gases
   e. Bronchoscopy and bronchoalveolar lavage
4. Begin treatment of the pneumonia
   a. Nebulization with normal saline solution
   b. Physiotherapy
      i. Positive-pressure ventilation
      ii. Chest percussion (coupage)
      iii. Mild exercise to induce deep breathing
   c. Fluid therapy
   d. Bronchodilators
   e. Antibiotics
   f. Analgesics
   g. Possibly corticosteroids for patients with acute inhalation injury
5. Monitor the patient
   a. Mucous membrane color
   b. Capillary refill time
   c. Respiratory rate and effort
   d. Type of lung sounds
   e. Body temperature
   f. Arterial blood gases
   g. Periodic radiography of the thorax

Protocol for the Treatment of Pulmonary Contusion

1. Ensure patent airway
2. Treat for shock, control hemorrhage, and correct life-threatening injuries
3. Institute oxygen therapy
4. Start medical therapy
   a. Bronchodilators
   b. Corticosteroids
   c. Antibiotics
5. Consider further diagnostic evaluation
   a. Thoracic radiography
   b. Blood-gas determination
6. Monitor patient
   a. Respiratory rate and effort
   b. Mucous membrane color, capillary refill time
   c. Lung sounds
   d. Repeated radiographs after 24 to 48 hours

racic trauma.[33] Pulmonary contusions result from blunt impact on the thoracic wall when the glottis is closed. Blunt trauma to the abdomen when the glottis is open typically results in diaphragmatic hernia.[34] Pulmonary contusion was the most common thoracic injury noted in two studies of dogs and cats presented for limb fractures that resulted from motor-vehicle accidents; the condition was present in 44% of the dogs and 50% of the cats.[35,36] Other common thoracic injuries noted in these studies included rib fractures, pneumothorax, hemothorax, and pneumomediastinum.

Other causes of pulmonary contusions include blunt trauma associated with crush injuries, falls from extreme heights (i.e., the so-called high-rise syndrome), and abuse by humans.[34,37] Air exchange is reduced because of ventilation–perfusion mismatch as in patients with pneumonia.

Mild pulmonary contusions may cause only tachypnea and apprehension. Severe pulmonary contusions are accompanied by cyanosis, dyspnea, shock, and weakness. Hemoptysis is infrequent but when present warrants a grave prognosis.

Diagnosis of pulmonary contusion is based on the case history, physical findings, and thoracic radiography (Table III). At initial presentation after trauma, radiographic and clinical signs may be minimal. The clinician must remain vigilant, however, because animals may continue to deteriorate during the first 24 hours following the injury.

The therapeutic approach to the animal with pulmonary contusions (see the protocol above) is controversial. Shock and other life-threatening problems are treated immediately. Specific therapy for pulmonary contusion includes oxygen therapy and bronchodilators. The use of prophylactic antibiotics and steroids remains controversial and is probably not warranted.

Pulmonary Edema

Pulmonary edema is the accumulation of excessive amounts of fluid within the lung. The barrier to alveolar fluid accumulation consists of pulmonary capillary endothelium, alveolar–capillary interstitial space, and a delicate alveolar epithelium. Loose junctions between endothelial cells allow movement of fluid, electrolyte, and some protein. Tight junctions between alveolar epithelial cells normally prevent movement of fluid into the alveoli. These tight junctions are easily broken down when pressure in the interstitium exceeds the alveolar pressure. The result is flooding of the alveolar spaces and fulminant pulmonary edema.[38]

As alveolar fluid accumulates, lung compliance decreases and the animal has to work harder to breathe. Tachypnea and exercise intolerance result. As the edema worsens, ventilation–perfusion mismatching occurs and hypoxemia results.

TABLE III
Radiographic Changes in Animals with Parenchymal Disease[a]

Disease	Radiographic Signs
Pneumonia	
Bacterial	Alveolar or mixed alveolar–interstitial pattern; air bronchograms may be present; changes are present in multiple lobes and may be focal or multifocal
Aspiration	Most commonly affects ventral portions of middle lobes but depends on the animal's position at the time of aspiration; may be uni- or bilateral, focal or multifocal; mixed alveolar–interstitial pattern; air bronchograms may be present if a large amount of material is aspirated
Inhalation	Early changes confined to interstitial pattern with peribronchial infiltrates; late changes show mixed alveolar–interstitial pattern with air bronchograms present; early changes are widespread and diffuse; later changes may affect dependent portions of lungs, mimicking aspiration
Pulmonary contusion	Irregular, patchy areas of mixed alveolar–interstitial patterns or consolidation; interstitial disease is indicative of lung contusion, and alveolar pattern indicates alveolar bleeding; may be associated with rib fractures, pneumothorax, or atelectasis
Pulmonary edema	
Cardiogenic	*Dogs*: Hilar mixed alveolar–interstitial densities; pulmonary venous distension *Cats*: Diffuse, peripheral alveolar or mixed pattern
Electric shock, snakebite	Generalized, severe mixed pattern; often most pronounced in diaphragmatic lobes; bilateral, symmetrical; air bronchograms present
Feline asthma	Increased interstitial densities and peribronchial markings; pulmonary hyperlucency; straightening of diaphragm and increased thoracic size

[a]From Morgan RV: *Manual of Small Animal Emergencies.* New York, Churchill Livingstone, 1985. Modified with permission.

Under normal physiologic conditions, a small amount of fluid is continuously leaking from pulmonary capillaries into the interstitium, where it is rapidly drained by the lymphatic vessels and pulmonary capillaries back into the venous return. The amount of fluid that accumulates depends on the balance between (1) capillary hydrostatic and oncotic pressure, (2) interstitial hydrostatic and oncotic pressure, (3) the integrity of the normal capillary wall ultrastructure (permeability to blood solutes), and (4) normal lymphatic function. Changes in any of these factors can contribute to excessive interstitial (and eventually alveolar) fluid accumulation.

Primary causes of pulmonary edema include increased pulmonary venous pressure, increased capillary permeability, and combinations of the two.[38,39] Edema begins as increased water in the interstitium and progresses to fluid within the alveoli. An emergency arises when this fluid accumulation diminishes oxygenation of the blood to a level that is life-threatening. The causes of pulmonary edema (see the outline on the following page) are often classified according to their major pathophysiologic mechanism.

Increased pulmonary venous pressure is the most common cause of pulmonary edema in dogs and cats. Causes include failure of the left side of the heart as a result of cardiomyopathy; chronic volume overload, as in patients with mitral regurgitation, patent ductus arteriosus, or ventricular septal defects; chronic pressure overload, as in patients with aortic stenosis; and obstruction to ventricular filling, as seen in patients with hypertrophic cardiomyopathy or thyrotoxic heart disease. Neurogenic pulmonary edema (an uncommon finding associated with seizures and elevated intracranial pressure resulting from head trauma), overzealous intravenous fluid administration, and acute increase in pulmonary interstitial pressure (as seen when a large amount of pleural fluid or gas is aspirated quickly or in cases of acute extrathoracic airway obstruction) are other causes of increased pulmonary venous pressure.

Pulmonary edema attributable to increased capillary permeability is called permeability pulmonary edema. It is most often associated with aspiration and inhalation pneu-

> **Causes of Pulmonary Edema**
>
> 1. Increased pulmonary capillary pressure
>   a. Cardiac disease, especially left-sided heart failure
>   b. Excessive parenteral fluid administration
>   c. Head injury
>   d. Seizures
>   e. Electric shock
>   f. Laryngeal paralysis and other causes of severe upper airway obstruction
> 2. Decreased capillary oncotic pressure (hypoproteinemia) in combination with other factors
>   a. Liver disease
>   b. Protein-losing enteropathy
>   c. Protein-losing nephropathy
>   d. Chronic blood loss
>   e. Burns
> 3. Altered capillary permeability
>   a. Smoke inhalation
>   b. Near-drowning
>   c. Aspiration
>   d. Acute respiratory distress syndrome (shock lung)
>   e. Bacterial endotoxins
>   f. Toxins
>   i. Snake venom
>   ii. Alphanaphthyl thiourea (ANTU)
>   iii. Paraquat
>   g. Uremia
>   h. Hemorrhagic pancreatitis
>   i. Electric shock
> 4. Lymphatic insufficiency—infiltrative neoplasia
> 5. Unknown mechanisms
>   a. Electric shock
>   b. Head injuries
>   c. Seizures
>   d. Drug induced

monia and acute respiratory distress syndrome (ARDS).[39,40] Toxins (including alphanaphthyl thiourea, paraquat, bacterial endotoxins, and some snake venoms) may result in permeability pulmonary edema. Endogenous toxins present in severely uremic animals or animals with hemorrhagic pancreatitis can also result in pulmonary edema.

Electric shock may result in pulmonary edema because of increased pulmonary venous pressure as well as increased capillary permeability. The edema associated with electric shock most commonly occurs in young dogs and cats after they chew on an electric cord. The edema usually begins to develop within the first 12 hours after electric injury and is typically confined to the caudal lung fields radiographically. Direct electric injury to the capillary walls and massive sympathetic stimulation resulting in pulmonary venous vasoconstriction probably account for edema formation. In addition, myocardial failure may occur.

Regardless of the cause of pulmonary edema, clinical signs are typically the same: moist cough, dyspnea, cyanosis, moist end-inspiratory crackles and expiratory wheezes, orthopnea, signs of apprehension, and hemorrhagic froth from the nose and mouth. The clinical findings and a suspicious case history may allow a presumptive diagnosis to be made.

Once the animal has been stabilized, thoracic radiographs should be taken to confirm the diagnosis. Radiographically, pulmonary edema is initially characterized by venous engorgement, followed by lymphatic engorgement and perivascular and interstitial clouding. Coalescing fluffy airspace edema, eventually with formation of air bronchograms, is the end result. Cardiogenic edema tends to be located in the perihilar region, whereas permeability edema is characterized by symmetric involvement of all the lung lobes. The animal should also be examined for evidence of trauma, oral or facial burns, snakebites, and other systemic illnesses to help in establishing a cause.

Successful treatment of pulmonary edema (see the protocol on the following page as well as Table IV) requires removal or reversal of the cause and improved oxygenation of the blood. The animal must be treated immediately and rigorously. The consequences of overzealous treatment are minimal when compared with the results of inadequate therapy. The principal objectives of therapy include: (1) decreasing oxygen demands (cage rest); (2) improving alveolar oxygen delivery (oxygen therapy, bronchodilators); (3) decreasing excessive pulmonary fluid (diuretics); (4) supporting and maintaining pulmonary circulation (myocardial support); and (5) treating the underlying disorder.

Oxygen is administered via mask, cannula, cage, or endotracheal tube. If the animal is in collapse, it is intubated, the airway suctioned, and ventilation with positive pressure and 100% oxygen begun. Specific treatment of cardiogenic edema includes furosemide (2 to 4 mg/kg intravenously, intramuscularly, subcutaneously, or orally every six to eight hours) to reduce intravascular volume by diuresis and increase systemic venous capacitance.

Sedation may be necessary to improve the efficiency of gas exchange and reduce oxygen demand. Sedation is especially important for animals that are extremely restless and agitated. Morphine may be used in dogs (0.04 to 0.11 mg/kg [dose to effect] subcutaneously, intramuscularly, or intravenously) because it also increases systemic venous capacitance and reduces the massive sympathetic barrage that is present in patients with heart failure. Note that morphine will increase intracranial pressure and is thus contraindicated for the treatment of neurogenic pulmonary edema or edema resulting from electric shock. Acepromazine maleate is preferred in cats.

Acute preload reduction can be enhanced through the use of venodilators, such as nitroglycerin. In severe cases, phlebotomy of up to 25% of blood volume may save the patient's life. Specific therapy for myocardial disease is also instituted as soon as possible.

Protocol for the Treatment of Pulmonary Edema

1. Ensure patent airway and institute oxygen therapy
   a. Mask
   b. Oxygen cage
   c. Nasal cannula
   d. Transtracheal catheter
   e. Intubation, positive-pressure ventilation
2. Establish an intravenous catheter
3. Start medical therapy for the pulmonary edema
   a. Decrease cardiac workload
      i. Cage rest
      ii. Sedation
      iii. Inotropic support
   b. Improve ventilation
      i. Bronchodilators
      ii. Endotracheal suctioning
      iii. Nebulization with 40% ethanol
   c. Eliminate excessive fluid
      i. Diuretics
      ii. Vasodilators
      iii. Phlebotomy (dogs: remove 8 ml/kg, may be repeated in two hours; cats: remove 6 to 10 ml/kg)
4. Begin diagnostic evaluation when patient is stable
   a. Radiography
   b. Electrocardiography
   c. Echocardiography
   d. Complete blood count, biochemical profile, and urinalysis
   e. Blood gas determinations
5. Monitor patient
   a. Respiratory rate and effort
   b. Pulse and heart rate
   c. Blood pressure
   d. Central venous pressure
   e. Packed cell volume, total solids, blood urea nitrogen
   f. Urine output
   g. Body weight

TABLE IV
Common Drugs and Doses for Patients with Parenchymal Disease

Drug	Dose
Bronchodilators	
Aminophylline	*Dogs*: 6–11 mg/kg intravenously or orally every eight hours *Cats*: 4 mg/kg orally or slowly intravenously every 12 hours
Theophylline	*Dogs*: 6–11 mg/kg intravenously or orally every six to eight hours *Cats*: 1–2 mg/kg slowly intravenously every eight hours
Analgesics, sedatives	
Morphine	*Dogs*: 0.1–0.4 mg/kg subcutaneously or intramuscularly every 8–12 hours
Diazepam	*Dogs*: 5–15 mg intravenously *Cats*: 2.5–5.0 mg intravenously
Butorphanol tartrate	*Dogs*: 0.1–0.2 mg/kg intravenously or 0.4 mg/kg subcutaneously or intramuscularly every eight hours *Cats*: 0.1–0.4 mg/kg subcutaneously or intramuscularly every 12 hours
Hydrocodone bitartrate	*Dogs*: 0.2 mg/kg orally every eight hours
Diuretics	
Furosemide	2–5 mg/kg intravenously, intramuscularly, or orally every 4–12 hours
Spironolactone	2–4 mg/kg orally every 12 hours
Inotropic agents	
Digoxin	*Dogs*: 0.11 mg/M^2 orally every 12 hours
Dobutamine hydrochloride	*Dogs*: 2.5–10 µg/kg/min intravenously *Cats*: 0.5–3 µg/kg/min intravenously
Other agents	
Nitroglycerin ointment (2%)	1/8–1/2 inch topically every six hours
Hydralazine hydrochloride	*Dogs*: 0.5–3 mg/kg orally every 8–12 hours *Cats*: 2–5 mg orally every 12 hours
Captopril	*Dogs*: 0.5–1.5 mg/kg orally every 8–12 hours *Cats*: 6.25 mg orally every 8–12 hours
Enalapril maleate	*Dogs*: 0.5 mg/kg orally every 12–24 hours *Cats*: 0.25–0.5 mg orally every 48 hours
Sodium nitroprusside	*Dogs*: 1–10 µg/kg/min intravenously

The treatment of noncardiogenic edema is similar but generally less effective. Improved oxygen delivery is the most critical part of treatment in these cases. Mannitol may improve diuresis and decrease intracranial pressure in animals with neurogenic pulmonary edema. Mechanical ventilation with positive end-expiratory pressure (PEEP) is useful in improving oxygenation and increasing lung volume for distribution of the edema. Corticosteroids may be useful in cases of acute respiratory distress syndrome. Many cases of noncardiogenic edema are mild; cage rest, oxygen therapy, furosemide, and time often result in an uneventful recovery.

Feline Asthma

Feline allergic bronchitis or feline asthma is an obstructive lung disease of cats; the pathophysiology of the specific underlying disease process is not entirely understood. Cytologic evidence of a high incidence of eosinophils and clinical similarities to allergic asthma in humans have led to speculation concerning a possible allergic cause.[41,42] Anecdotal accounts of association of clinical signs with litter type, bedding material, and house dust also tend to support an allergic cause.

Clinical signs of feline asthma include wheezing, gagging, dyspnea, and coughing. Most cats are anxious and dyspneic at presentation but do not show evidence of cyanosis unless stressed during the clinical evaluation. A chronic history of coughing or respiratory difficulty may be present, but severe signs can occur acutely despite the absence of a previous history of respiratory disease. Wheezes and increased breath sounds are often heard during thoracic auscultation, but normal or muffled sounds are not unusual.

Diagnosis is based on clinical signs, radiographic evidence of peribronchial interstitial infiltrates, and cytologic examination of tracheobronchial aspirate. Other radiographic findings may include increased pulmonary radiolucency, increased thoracic size, flattening of the diaphragm, and aerophagia.[42] Approximately 50% to 75% of affected cats have peripheral eosinophilia.[41,42]

Care should be taken not to stress affected cats. The clinician should initially treat severely affected cats on the basis of clinical suspicion rather than risk stressing them while taking thoracic radiographs. Radiographs can be taken after the cat is stabilized.

A transtracheal aspirate should be taken from all cats with radiographic evidence of peribronchial disease to rule out bacterial bronchitis and *Aelurostrongylus* infection. Bacterial culture is important in ruling out a bacterial component. Eosinophils in transtracheal aspirate or bronchoalveolar lavage samples suggest allergic disease; however, care must be taken in interpreting this finding. Normal cats occasionally have eosinophils in their bronchoalveolar lavage specimens. Neutrophilic inflammation suggests an infectious process, but cats with feline asthma may also have neutrophilic inflammation.

Overt cyanosis or status asthmaticus is a medical emergency, and quick therapeutic action should be taken. Dramatic response can usually be expected within 15 to 30 minutes after initiation of therapy. Corticosteroids and bronchodilators are the cornerstone of treatment (Table V). Fast-acting parenteral glucocorticoids, such as dexamethasone sodium phosphate or prednisolone sodium succinate, are used initially. Bronchodilators, such as the methylxanthine derivatives or the β_2-adrenergic agonist terbutaline sulfate, augment the response.

ISOPROTERENOL or epinephrine is used for relief of bronchospasm in the most severely affected cats.[41] Increased parasympathetic sensitivity provides the rationale for the use of parasympatholytic agents, such as atropine. Although atropine can reduce bronchoconstriction, it is contraindicated because of the increase in viscosity of bronchial mucosal secretions. For that reason, if atropine is administered it should not be used after initial stabilization. Cats that are extremely anxious or stressed may require sedation. Ketamine hydrochloride has been shown to have a protective effect on β_2-adrenergic receptors, thus inhibiting bronchoconstriction.[43] Acepromazine maleate may have similar beneficial effects because of its α-adrenergic blocking action.[42]

Less-severely affected cats usually respond to oral corticosteroids with or without augmentation from oral bronchodilators. The dose of the glucocorticoids is slowly tapered to the lowest possible level that controls the clinical signs. As an alternative, long-acting or repository corticosteroids, such as prednisolone acetate, may provide better long-term management.

Pulmonary Thromboembolism

Pulmonary thromboembolism is the formation or lodging of thrombi in the pulmonary arterial system. The result is severe, often intractable dyspnea. The dyspnea results from ventilation–perfusion mismatch, pleural effusion, and pleuritic pain.[44] Coughing, dyspnea, hemoptysis, lethargy, anorexia, and fever are often present.[45] A split second heart sound and distended jugular pulses may be noted because of pulmonary hypertension.

The most common cause of pulmonary thromboembolism is canine and feline dirofilariasis.[46] Other causes include nephrotic syndrome, hyperadrenocorticism, autoimmune hemolytic anemia, neoplasia, bacterial endocarditis, dilative cardiomyopathy, surgery, trauma, sepsis, hyperviscosity syndrome, polycythemia, vasculitis, disseminated intravascular coagulopathy, pancreatitis, hypothyroidism, and primary hypercoagulable states.[45,47–51]

The diagnosis of pulmonary thromboembolism is supported by consistent radiographic changes in an animal

TABLE V
Drugs Used in the Treatment of Feline Allergic Bronchitis

Drug	Dose	Comments
BRONCHODILATORS		
Sympathetic amines		
Terbutaline sulfate	0.625 mg orally every 12 hours; 0.04 mg/kg intravenously	Long-term use is not recommended
Isoproterenol	0.004–0.006 mg subcutaneously	Tachycardia may occur
Epinephrine	0.5 ml of 1:10,000 dilution intramuscularly or subcutaneously	Use only in emergencies and if isoproterenol is unavailable
Methylxanthines		
Aminophylline	4 mg/kg orally or slowly intravenously every 8–12 hours	
Sustained-release theophylline	25 mg/kg orally once a day at night	
Dyphylline	4 mg/kg intramuscularly	Neutral salt of theophylline; less painful
CORTICOSTEROIDS		
Prednisolone sodium succinate	5–10 mg/kg intravenously or intramuscularly	
Dexamethasone sodium phosphate	0.2–1 mg/kg intravenously or intramuscularly	
Prednisone	1 mg/kg orally every 12 hours	Taper to lowest dose that controls signs
Methylprednisolone acetate	10–20 mg intramuscularly	Rule out infectious cause before administration
Triamcinolone	0.25–0.5 mg orally once a day	Taper to lowest dose that will control signs; once-a-week administration can often be achieved
PARASYMPATHOLYTICS		
Atropine	0.05 mg/kg subcutaneously or intramuscularly	May decrease mucociliary action

with arterial blood gases that suggest ventilation–perfusion mismatch. Radiographic changes include increased alveolar densities that are usually fluffy and indistinct but may be lobar or triangular. A hypovascular region is noted in about 50% of cases. Mild pleural effusion is also noted in some cases.[52] Heartworm-induced thromboemboli are seen in animals with moderate to severe radiographic evidence of dirofilariasis.[46] The caudal lung lobes are most commonly affected. Electrocardiographic changes depend on the presence of cardiac disease: sinus bradycardia may result from pulmonary hypertension, and T-wave abnormalities sometimes occur.

If heartworm disease is present, the diagnosis can be made from the clinical signs and radiographic appearance. A positive heartworm antigen test is confirmatory. In animals with pulmonary thromboembolism caused by other diseases, the diagnosis is usually more difficult. Selective angiography allows a definitive antemortem diagnosis of pulmonary thromboembolism but is invasive and requires general anesthesia; however, the less-invasive technique of nonselective angiography is of little use. Digital subtraction angiography has a much higher sensitivity and may be the radiographic test of choice in referral institutions with digital subtraction capabilities.[53]

Ventilation–perfusion scintigraphy is technically easier to perform than angiography in a conscious animal and has been shown to have a high sensitivity when compared with pulmonary and digital subtraction angiography.[53]

Treatment of severe pulmonary thromboembolism is difficult and often unrewarding. Oxygen and bronchodilators are initially given but may have limited efficacy in animals with severe ventilation–perfusion mismatching associated with massive thromboembolic disease. Glucocorticoids are important in the treatment of heartworm-induced disease but may be contraindicated in therapy of thromboembolism from other causes. If ongoing thrombosis resulting from a hypercoagulable state is suspected, heparin (200 U/kg intravenously followed by 50 to 100 U/kg subcutaneously every six to eight hours) or coumarin (0.1 mg/kg orally once a day) are indicated. Platelet inhibitors, such as aspirin or dipyridamole, are probably least effective for this purpose. Because of recombinant DNA technology, tissue plasminogen activator (tPA) has recently become available for use as a thrombolytic agent.[54] Acute thrombolytic effects may be seen with the administration of 0.25 to 1 mg/kg/hr for a total dose of 1 to 10 mg/kg intravenously.

Cage rest is the most critical part of treatment. If the underlying cause of thromboembolism can be determined, it is specifically treated.

The prognosis associated with heartworm-induced thromboembolism is generally fair to good with strict cage confinement and corticosteroid, oxygen, and bronchodilator therapy. The prognosis for other causes is generally guarded to poor.

PLEURAL CAVITY DISEASE

Pleural cavity disease includes restrictive conditions that decrease functional capacity of the lungs through occupation of pleural space or disruption of the functional integrity of the thoracic wall. These conditions must be differentiated from abdominal problems that compromise respiration by causing pressure on or restricting excursions of the diaphragm (e.g., ascites, gastric dilatation, intraabdominal masses or hemorrhage, pregnancy, and abdominal pain).

Pneumothorax

Pneumothorax is the accumulation of free air in the pleural cavity. As air accumulates, the resultant loss of negative pleural pressure causes the lungs to undergo elastic recoil and collapse.[55,56] Trauma is the most common cause of pneumothorax. Thoracic compression from blunt trauma may result in massive increase in pleural pressure with resultant pulmonary parenchymal or tracheobronchial rupture.[56] Penetrating injuries, as often arise from bite wounds or projectiles, allow communication of the pleural space with the atmospheric air.[33,57,58]

Leakage of air from the lungs or airways into the pleural space is usually called open pneumothorax, and leakage of air from the atmosphere through a thoracic wall defect into the pleural space is usually called closed pneumothorax. Some authors, however, reverse these terms—using the term *open pneumothorax* to refer to leakage through a thoracic wall defect and *closed pneumothorax* to refer to leakage from the lungs or airways.

Spontaneous pneumothorax sometimes develops from rupture of bullous emphysematous, neoplastic, or inflammatory lung lesions and is characteristically not associated with trauma.[59] Iatrogenic pneumothorax may follow intrathoracic surgical procedures, resuscitative efforts, and overzealous intermittent positive-pressure breathing. Animals should be watched closely for signs of pneumothorax after percutaneous transthoracic biopsy or fine-needle aspiration techniques. Rarely, severe pneumothorax may follow pneumomediastinum that resulted from trauma to the trachea or esophagus.

Tension pneumothorax is the condition in which a one-way valve effect has formed at a pleural defect. Air is drawn into the pleural space by negative pressure during inspiration but cannot be pushed out during expiration. The pleural pressure rapidly approaches or exceeds that which can be created via inspiratory efforts, thus resulting in severe pulmonary atelectasis and diminished venous return to the heart. Tension pneumothorax is a rapidly deteriorating state that must be recognized and corrected quickly. If pleural pressure is not reduced rapidly, the animal will die.

Clinical signs associated with pneumothorax vary from mild resting tachypnea to severe dyspnea and cyanosis. Tachypnea, abduction of the forelimbs, reluctance to lie down, and signs of apprehension are common observations. Diminished lung sounds on auscultation and hyperresonance on percussion may be noted during physical examination. Rib fractures, thoracic wounds, and subcutaneous emphysema may provide further evidence of trauma.

DIAGNOSIS of pneumothorax depends on demonstration of intrapleural air. This may be accomplished radiographically or via thoracocentesis. If the animal is stable and showing only mild signs of respiratory distress, thoracic radiographs are taken. Pneumothorax is evidenced by separation of the lung lobes from the ventral and dorsal thoracic wall, separation of the heart from the sternum, separation of the lung lobes from the diaphragm, and an overall increase in pulmonary density as a result of lung lobe atelectasis.[60] Total thoracic lucency is often increased because of the pleural air.

Pneumothorax may be mimicked by overexposure of the radiograph, overlying skin folds, overinflation of the lung, or hypovolemia. In patients with these conditions, pulmonary vessels normally extend to the thoracic wall margins. In cases of pneumothorax, however, a space between the thoracic wall and the end of the pulmonary vessels is apparent if the radiograph is carefully examined with a high-intensity light.

Radiography should be avoided while the animal is severely dyspneic. The stress of positioning may result in diminished ventilation and oxygen exchange, which may culminate in respiratory arrest. If pneumothorax is suspected in a severely dyspneic animal, thoracocentesis is performed first.

Thoracocentesis is indicated as treatment of pneumothorax in animals showing signs of moderate to severe respiratory distress. It may not be needed by animals that can eat, sleep, and breathe comfortably. It is important to confine these animals and observe them closely for clinical deterioration.

Thoracocentesis is best performed using a 30- to 60-ml syringe attached to a 20- to 22-gauge butterfly catheter via a three-way stopcock. A site at approximately the upper third of the seventh to ninth intercostal space is shaved and aseptically prepared. The needle end of the catheter is inserted into the pleural cavity, and a syringe is used to withdraw air from the pleural space until negative pressure is obtained. The procedure is repeated on both sides of the thorax unless radiographic evidence indicates that the pneumothorax is unilateral. If negative pressure cannot be obtained, it may be assumed that a continuous leak is present and a chest tube should be inserted.

Many cases of traumatically induced pneumothorax resolve after a single thoracocentesis. If repeated thoracocentesis procedures are required, the clinician should consider insertion of a chest tube and the use of continuous pleural drainage.

Pleural Effusion

Abnormal accumulation of fluid within the pleural space is referred to as pleural effusion. This term is not a specific diagnosis but rather describes a feature of several disease processes.[56] Normally, there is movement of fluid from the visceral and parietal pleural surfaces into the pleural space and subsequently into lymphatics and capillary drainage.[61] Abnormal types or quantities of fluid may develop from bleeding, transudation, exudation, or rupture of the thoracic duct or diaphragm.

Accumulation of pleural fluid results in restrictive disease, as seen in patients with pneumothorax. Clinical signs may not become apparent until large quantities of fluid have accumulated; however, an emergency can arise when the fluid develops acutely or when the animal is no longer able to compensate for diminished functional lung capacity. Clinical signs include tachypnea, dyspnea, orthopnea, coughing, cyanosis, and increased abdominal respiratory efforts. Clinical signs associated with the underlying cause of the pleural effusion may also be evident.

Auscultation helps differentiate pleural cavity disease from parenchymal disease. Typically, lung sounds are diminished dorsally in patients with pneumothorax and ventrally in patients with pleural effusion. Heart sounds are usually muffled bilaterally in patients with pleural effusion. Percussion reveals hyperresonance dorsally in patients with pneumothorax, particularly tension pneumothorax. Dullness ventrally may reflect pleural effusion or a diaphragmatic hernia.

Definitive diagnosis of pleural effusion is made by thoracocentesis and thoracic radiography. Pleural effusion results in loss of the cardiac silhouette and diaphragmatic shadow and displacement of the lung lobes dorsally. In such a case, thoracocentesis is attempted and the thorax is radiographed again. When a severely compromised animal is presented, thoracocentesis should be attempted because of physical findings before the stress of radiography. Thoracocentesis is performed ventrally. A sample of the fluid is submitted for cytologic examination and culture.

The appearance of the sample, its total protein, and its cytologic features are important clues to the cause of the pleural effusion.

Types of Pleural Effusion

Hemothorax is the presence of blood in the pleural space. It can result from trauma to lung parenchyma and rupture of cardiac or intrathoracic blood vessels, hemorrhage secondary to coagulopathies, bleeding neoplasms (e.g., hemangiosarcoma), or lung lobe torsion.[62] Blood should be removed from the pleural space by thoracocentesis if its presence results in dyspnea. Hemorrhagic effusions do not clot, yet blood aspirated traumatically from the intercostal or coronary arteries and heart does. If the animal is stable and bleeding is not ongoing, it is best to allow the blood to be passively absorbed. If blood loss is severe, blood transfusion should be considered.

Chylothorax is the presence of intestinal chyle within the pleural space and most often results when chyle leaks from dilated abnormal thoracic lymphatics (thoracic lymphangiectasis) into the pleural space.[63] Thoracic lymphangiectasis may be a congenital defect in the Afghan hound breed.[63] Rupture of the thoracic duct as a result of trauma is a rare cause of chylothorax. Conditions that increase thoracic-duct pressure (e.g., cranial mediastinal neoplasia, granulomatous disease, lung lobe torsion, cardiomyopathy, and dirofilariasis) may also result in chylothorax.

CHYLOUS FLUID is typically white or pinkish. A cream-colored top layer may form when a sample is left to stand. The lymphocyte is the classic cell type found in chylous fluid; but the presence of chyle or numerous thoracocentesis procedures may elicit an inflammatory response in the pleural cavity, and neutrophils can outnumber lymphocytes in cytologic specimens.[63] Definitive confirmation of chylothorax depends on demonstrating that the pleural fluid has a higher triglyceride content than serum has, while the cholesterol content is lower or equivalent to that of serum.

Pleural effusion may also result from hypoalbuminemia, heart failure and cardiomyopathy, diaphragmatic hernia, pancreatitis, pulmonary arterial thrombosis, and pleural neoplasia.[56,62] The effusions are classified as either pure transudate or modified transudate on the basis of fluid characteristics and have been generically referred to as hydrothorax.

Neoplastic effusions may result from obstruction of pleural lymphatics or invasion of the thoracic duct. Cytologic examination reveals neoplastic cells in 40% to 50% of cases,[56] but care must be taken in cytologic interpretation because reactive mesothelial cells from the pleural surface are easily confused with neoplastic cells. Lymphosarcoma, mesothelioma, and metastatic carcinomas are the most common causes of neoplastic effusions.

Inflammatory effusions may be septic or sterile. Sterile effusions may result from trauma, granulomatous or neoplastic masses, lung lobe torsion, diaphragmatic hernia, pancreatitis, pulmonary thromboembolic events, and feline infectious peritonitis. All inflammatory exudates should be cultured to rule out a septic process.

Septic inflammatory effusions (empyema or pyothorax) can arise from penetrating wounds to the thorax or esophagus; extension of infections from the lungs, mediastinum, or abdomen; hematogenous infections; or migration of foreign bodies.[56,62] The effusion is a purulent, often foul-smelling exudate. A wide variety of aerobic and anaerobic organisms (including *Actinomyces*, *Bacteroides*, *Corynebacterium*, *Propionibacterium*, *Fusobacterium*, *Nocardia*, *Pasteurella*, *Staphylococcus*, *Peptococcus*, *Streptococcus*, and *Peptostreptococcus* species) has been reported.[64] Obligate anaerobic bacteria and gram-positive filamentous organisms (e.g., *Nocardia* and *Actinomyces*) are most common in dogs, and *Pasteurella* species as well as obligate anaerobes are most common in cats.[64] Cytology may be helpful in predicting the presence of filamentous organisms. *Nocardia* species often stain partially acid-fast positive.

Emergency treatment of pyothorax includes relief of respiratory distress and reversal of shock and endotoxemia. Blood cultures are performed if septicemia is suspected. A chest tube is inserted into the pleural cavity for long-term management. Antibiotic therapy is begun while culture of the effusion is pending. An antibiotic that has a broad spectrum and is effective against anaerobic organisms should be chosen. Clindamycin, chloramphenicol, metronidazole, and the penicillins are useful. Definitive choice of an antibiotic is based on bacterial culture and sensitivity testing.

Treatment of Pleural Effusion

The major therapeutic objective in the management of the patient with pleural effusion is to evacuate all fluid from the pleural space. The animal should also be thoroughly examined for other injuries and systemic illnesses, and treatment for shock is instituted as needed.[23] Animals found in a state of collapse are intubated and oxygen therapy begun. A protocol for the management of pleural cavity disease can be found on this page.

Thoracocentesis is performed to remove fluid. In cases of pyothorax or in situations where needle thoracocentesis proves inadequate, an indwelling chest tube can be inserted[65] (Figure 2). The hair is shaved and the skin aseptically prepared on the side that radiography shows is involved or that has been the most productive during thoracocentesis. For patients that need bilateral chest tubes, both sides of the thorax should be surgically prepared. The insertion point through the skin is at about the mid thorax over the tenth or eleventh intercostal space; insertion into the thorax is through the seventh intercostal space.

Protocol for the Treatment of Pleural Cavity Disease

1. Establish patent airway; institute oxygen therapy
2. Treat for shock
3. Perform thoracic examination
   a. Auscultation
   b. Percussion
4. Bandage penetrating wounds, splint flail segments
5. Assess status of animal
   a. Severe distress
      i. Administer oxygen therapy
      ii. Perform immediate thoracocentesis
      iii. Consider insertion of chest tube
   b. Mild to moderate distress
      i. Radiograph thorax
      ii. Perform thoracocentesis
      iii. Consider insertion of chest tube
      iv. Administer oxygen therapy
   c. No to minimal distress
      i. Radiograph thorax
      ii. Prescribe cage rest
      iii. Continue to observe patient
6. Perform diagnostic workup
   a. Thoracic fluid analysis
   b. Complete blood count, biochemical profile, urinalysis
   c. Clotting survey
   d. Electrocardiography
   e. Echocardiography
   f. Pleural ultrasonography
7. Start supportive care (as indicated)
   a. Fluid therapy
   b. Antibiotics
8. Monitor patient
   a. Respiratory rate and effort (if rate exceeds 60 breaths/min, consider inserting a chest tube or increasing frequency of chest tube evacuation)
   b. Mucous membrane color; capillary refill time
   c. Patency of chest tube
   d. Serial thoracic radiographs
9. Prepare patient for surgery
   a. Herniorrhaphy
   b. Repair of wounds and rib fractures
   c. Exploratory thoracotomy
   d. Ligation of thoracic duct
   e. Lung lobectomy
10. Remove any medical causes of pleural cavity disease by appropriate therapy

---

The skin and musculature are infiltrated with a local anesthetic around both points of insertion. Dogs that are not severely depressed and most cats require sedation or general anesthesia. A stab incision is made through the skin, and the chest tube with trocar (Argyle® Trochar Catheter—Sherwood Medical) is advanced through the subcutaneous tissue cranially to the desired intercostal site. Once the seventh intercostal space is reached, the chest tube with trocar is placed perpendicular to the thoracic wall

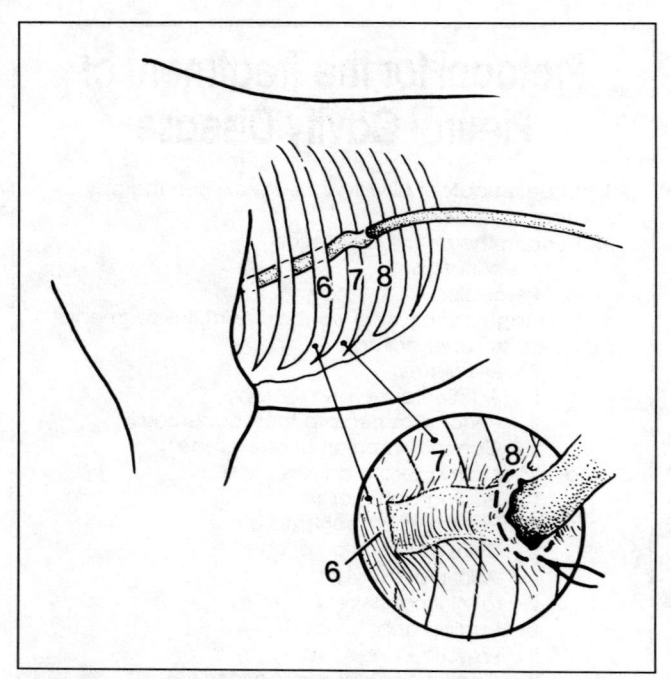

Figure 2—Technique for insertion of an indwelling chest tube. A stab incision is made one or two rib spaces caudal to the site of chest tube insertion. Magnified view shows a pursestring suture placed through the skin where the tube exits. (From Morgan RV: Surgical emergencies, in Tracy DL (ed): *Small Animal Surgical Nursing*. Chicago, Mosby–Year Book, 1983. Reproduced with permission.)

and a quick, forceful movement is used to advance it through the intercostal muscles and into the thoracic cavity. The chest tube is advanced over the trocar, the trocar is removed, the chest tube is cross-clamped, and the free end of chest tube is attached to a three-way stopcock or a continuous evacuation pump, such as the Pleur-Evac® system (Howmedica).

The clamp is released, and patency of the chest tube is ensured. A purse-string suture is placed in the skin at the point where the chest tube exits, and a cruciate suture is used to anchor the chest tube in place. In addition, the chest tube is fixed to the thorax by using a Chinese finger tie or by placing stay sutures through a tape butterfly surrounding the free end of the chest tube. A light thoracic wrap is then applied to protect the chest tube from being dislodged. Radiographs of the thorax are taken after insertion and fluid aspiration to check the position of the chest tube and possibly to establish the cause of the pleural effusion.

Supportive care with oxygen, fluid therapy, and antibiotics, as indicated, is instituted in animals with pleural effusion. Capillary refill time, mucous membrane color, and respiratory rate and effort are closely monitored. Resting respiratory rate should be less than 60 breaths/min. Respiratory rates greater than 60 breaths/min, particularly if breathing is labored, should prompt the clinician to repeat thoracocentesis or consider insertion of an indwelling chest tube. If a chest tube is already in place, it should be aspirated.

Indwelling chest tubes used to drain pleural effusion are aspirated every two to six hours or at any time the respiratory rate increases. Serial radiographs are helpful to monitor resolution of pneumothorax and pleural effusion.

DIAPHRAGMATIC HERNIA AND FLAIL CHEST
Diaphragmatic Hernia

Diaphragmatic hernia most commonly results from trauma. Blunt blows or a fall from a height can exert tremendous pressure on the peritoneal side of the diaphragm. If the glottis is open and the lungs deflate, there will be no equalizing pressure on the thoracic side of the diaphragm and the diaphragm will rupture.[33,55] If the glottis is closed, the increased pleural pressure often results in pneumothorax. Abdominal viscera can protrude into the thoracic cavity through the diaphragmatic defect. Displacement of the lungs and restriction of the respiratory bellows lead to respiratory distress. The displaced viscera may also result in pleural effusion secondary to lymphatic obstruction, venous engorgement, and inflammation.

Many of the clinical signs and physical findings in animals with diaphragmatic hernias are indistinguishable from signs associated with pleural effusion or pneumothorax. Tachypnea, dyspnea, orthopnea, cyanosis, and abdominal breathing are common. Dullness ventrally on percussion and muffled heart and lung sounds are frequently noted.[33,56,65] Abnormalities may be unilateral if only one side of the thorax is involved. Auscultation of gastrointestinal sounds within the thorax and detection of a seemingly empty abdomen on palpation should arouse suspicions of herniation of abdominal organs. Dysphagia, vomiting, and retching may occur. These signs are more common in chronic cases or patients with congenital peritoneopericardial hernias.[56] External evidence of trauma and signs of shock may be noted.

RADIOGRAPHY and ultrasonography are the most important noninvasive methods for diagnosis of diaphragmatic hernia. Radiographic findings include disruption of the diaphragmatic outline, cranial displacement of the stomach and/or duodenum, or abdominal viscera present in the thoracic cavity.[65] Concurrent pleural effusion and pulmonary contusions may make the radiographic diagnosis of diaphragmatic hernia difficult.

Treatment of diaphragmatic hernia is always surgical. The animal is treated for shock and maintained on oxygen therapy until stable. The only indication for immediate surgery is the presence of a dilated stomach within the thorax. Survival rates are variable, ranging from 50% to 90%.[66] Survival is higher if the animal is stabilized for at least 24 hours before surgical repair.[66] Survival is lower with repair of chronic hernias.

Flail Chest

Flail chest is the presence of proximal and distal fractures in several consecutive ribs so that the isolated section of chest wall moves paradoxically with respiration.[65,67] Severe respiratory compromise ensues because of an inability to establish sufficient negative pressure to expand the lungs. Decreased ventilatory capacity, as well as accompanying contusion of the underlying lung, precipitates acute respiratory distress. The animal with flail chest is severely compromised. Dyspnea and cyanosis are common. An obvious deformity that moves paradoxically with breathing is found on examination of the thoracic wall. Pain, apprehension, shock, and susceptibility to stress further complicate the situation. Flail chest may also be accompanied by pneumothorax or hemothorax.

Emergency stabilization of the flail segment can be achieved with towel clamps, orthoplast, or a splint (made from tongue depressors for a small dog or cat or from aluminum rods for a large dog). The splint material chosen is affixed to the flail segment by sutures placed around the ribs and then positioned so as to span to normal ribs on either side. Both ends of the splint are attached to the tissue overlying the normal ribs with stay sutures. The animal is stabilized until more-definitive repair can be attempted.

RESPIRATORY ARREST

Respiratory arrest, which is the cessation of breathing, may be the result of many different respiratory emergencies. Depressant drugs that affect the respiratory center and are used commonly in veterinary practice include narcotics, tranquilizers, barbiturates, and the gaseous anesthetics. These agents are major contributors to respiratory failure during anesthesia and in the immediate postoperative period.

Although a rare event, paralysis of the respiratory muscles can precipitate respiratory arrest. Myelomalacia of the cervical and thoracic spinal cord with involvement of the phrenic and intercostal nerves, myasthenia gravis, organophosphate toxicity, such ascending lower motor neuron diseases as polyradiculoneuritis, and overdose of such paralytic agents as atracurium all may cause weakness or paralysis of the respiratory muscles. Conversely, severe spasms of the respiratory muscles, such as those seen in patients with terminal tetanus, may contribute to respiratory arrest.[68]

THE SIGNS of respiratory failure are usually obvious. Hypoxemia rapidly leads to bradycardia through direct activation of the cardioinhibitory center of the brain. Hypotension follows within minutes of the bradycardia. Signs of hypoxia that must be recognized as antecedents to respiratory arrest are restlessness, anxiety, tachycardia, cardiac arrhythmias, nausea, vomiting, dilatation of the pupils, and involuntary muscle twitching.[69]

Respiratory arrest is a medical emergency that demands immediate correction and should take precedence over all other emergency care. Progressive hypotension and bradycardia can result in absence of measurable pulse within approximately 7 to 11 minutes after occlusion of the endotracheal tube in an asphyxiated canine model.[66] It is of the utmost importance that these few minutes be used to reverse respiratory arrest and stabilize the patient.

The objectives for treating respiratory arrest (see the protocol above) are to establish a patent airway, begin artificial respiration, provide oxygen therapy, and, if possible,

---

Protocol for the Treatment of Respiratory Arrest

1. Stop anesthesia
2. Establish patent airway
   a. Remove obstructions and foreign material; suction airway
   b. Intubate patient
   c. Consider tracheostomy if airway is obstructed
3. Administer artificial respiration
   a. Intubation with oxygen delivery
      i. Positive pressure—end-inspiratory pressure of 15 to 20 cm H_2O
      ii. Rate—30 to 35 breaths/min with tidal volume of 10 to 15 ml/kg
   b. Intubation with room air delivered via portable ventilator bag
      i. Positive pressure—watch for wide excursions of chest
      ii. Rate—30 to 35 breaths/min with tidal volume of 10 to 15 ml/kg
   c. Mouth-to-nostril breathing or mask respiration
      i. Attempt positive-pressure ventilation
      ii. Rates—30 to 35 breaths/min with tidal volume of 10 to 15 ml/kg
4. Call for help
5. Insert intravenous catheter—5% dextrose in water or multiple-electrolyte solution
6. Record electrocardiography
7. Eliminate depressant agents
   a. Use narcotic antagonists
      i. Naloxone hydrochloride (dogs: 0.02 to 0.04 mg/kg intravenously)
      ii. Nalorphine hydrochloride (0.1 mg/kg IV; dogs: 5 mg maximum; cats: 1 mg maximum)
8. Administer respiratory stimulants (e.g., doxapram hydrochloride (1 to 4 mg/kg intravenously))
9. Monitor patient
   a. Mucous membrane color and capillary refill time
   b. Respiratory rate and ventilation
   c. Pulse, heart rate, and rhythm
   d. Pupils
   e. Central venous pressure
   f. Arterial blood gases
10. Investigate and remove cause of respiratory failure

reestablish normal, spontaneous respiration. The animal is intubated, and 100% oxygen is administered with artificial positive-pressure breathing. A portable ventilator bag or gas anesthetic machine can be used for this purpose. The animal is ventilated at 30 to 35 breaths/min with tidal volumes of 10 to 15 ml/kg.[70] There should be little concern about the timing of breaths relative to thoracic compression if concurrent cardioresuscitation is being administered.

The positive-pressure ventilation and thoracic compression are now viewed as two unrelated events. If circumstances do not allow endotracheal intubation, mouth-to-nostril breathing or mask ventilation can be tried. If the latter techniques are used, rapid puffs and high airway pressures are avoided as they often result in gastric distension and restriction of thoracic expansion. Mask ventilatory techniques are not ideal, and endotracheal intubation should be attempted as soon as is feasible. Any mucus, vomitus, blood, or exudate is suctioned from the airway. If upper airway obstruction prevents intubation, a tracheostomy is performed.

AN INTRAVENOUS catheter is inserted, and fluid therapy with a multiple-electrolyte solution or 5% dextrose and water solution is begun. Electrocardiography is instituted, and any cardiac abnormalities are recorded. Any respiratory depressants and anesthesia are terminated as soon as respiratory arrest is noted. Narcotic agents are reversed with antagonist drugs, and respiratory stimulants may be considered. If cardiac arrest ensues, the protocol for that crisis is followed.[70]

When spontaneous respiration resumes, artificial breathing is discontinued but oxygen supplementation is maintained. Mucous membrane color and capillary refill time are monitored. Continued monitoring of the electrocardiogram is advised. As hypoxia is reversed, the pupils return to normal and the level of consciousness improves.

Once the animal is stabilized, it is closely monitored for signs of recurrence for at least 24 hours. Continued oxygen administration is needed if hypoxemia persists because of underlying respiratory disease. Stress and excessive handling should be minimized. The cause of respiratory arrest should be determined and removed if possible.

About the Authors

Dr. Taboada and Dr. Hoskins are affiliated with the Department of Veterinary Clinical Sciences of the School of Veterinary Medicine, Louisiana State University in Baton Rouge, Louisiana. Dr. Morgan is affiliated with the Rawley Memorial Animal Hospital in Springfield, Massachusetts. Drs. Taboada, Hoskins, and Morgan are Diplomates of the American College of Veterinary Internal Medicine. Dr. Morgan is a Diplomate of the American College of Veterinary Ophthalmologists.

REFERENCES

1. Vaden S, Ford RB: Medical management of upper respiratory tract disease, in Kirk RW (ed): *Current Veterinary Therapy X.* Philadelphia, WB Saunders Co, 1989, pp 337-343.
2. Meuten DJ, Calderwood-Mays MB, Dillman RC, et al: Canine laryngeal rhabdomyoma. *Vet Pathol* 22:533-539, 1985.
3. Saik JE, Toll SL, Diters RW, et al: Canine and feline laryngeal neoplasia: A 10 year survey. *JAAHA* 22:359-365, 1986.
4. Withrow SJ: Tumors of the respiratory tract, in Withrow SJ, MacEwen EG (eds): *Clinical Veterinary Oncology.* Philadelphia, JB Lippincott Co, 1989, pp 215-233.
5. Bryan RD, Frome RW: Tracheal leiomyoma in a dog. *JAVMA* 178(10):1069-1070, 1981.
6. Harvey HJ, Sykes G: Tracheal mast cell tumor in a dog. *JAVMA* 180(9):1097-1100, 1982.
7. Aron DN, Crowe DT: Upper airway obstruction: General principles and selected conditions in the dog and cat. *Vet Clin North Am [Small Anim Pract]* 15:891-917, 1985.
8. Gaber CE, Amis TC, LeCouteur A: Laryngeal paralysis in dogs: A review of 23 cases. *JAVMA* 186:377-380, 1985.
9. Greenfield CL: Canine laryngeal paralysis. *Compend Contin Educ Pract Vet* 9(10):1011-1017, 1987.
10. Aron DN: Laryngeal paralysis, in Kirk RW (ed): *Current Veterinary Therapy X.* Philadelphia, WB Saunders Co, 1989, pp 343-353.
11. Venker-van Haagen AJ, Hartman W, Goedegebuure SA: Spontaneous laryngeal paralysis in young Bouviers. *JAAHA* 14(6):714-720, 1978.
12. Venker-van Haagen AJ: Laryngeal paralysis in young Bouviers, in Kirk RW (ed): *Current Veterinary Therapy VII.* Philadelphia, WB Saunders Co, 1980, pp 290-291.
13. Venker-van Haagen AJ, Bouw J, Hartman W: Hereditary transmission of laryngeal paralysis in Bouviers. *JAAHA* 17(1):75-76, 1981.
14. Jaggy A: Neurologic manifestations of hypothyroidism in dogs. *Proc ACVIM* 8:1037-1040, 1990.
15. Schaer M, et al: Laryngeal hemiplegia due to neoplasia of the vagus nerve in a cat. *JAVMA* 174(5):513-515, 1979.
16. Hardie EM, et al: Laryngeal paralysis in three cats. *JAVMA* 179(9):879-882, 1981.
17. Dimski DS: Tracheal obstruction caused by tree needles in a cat. *JAVMA* 199:477-478, 1991.
18. Hedlund CS: Surgical diseases of the trachea. *Vet Clin North Am [Small Anim Pract]* 17:301-332, 1987.
19. Ettinger SJ, Ticer JW: Diseases of the trachea, in Ettinger SJ (ed): *Textbook of Veterinary Internal Medicine.* Philadelphia, WB Saunders Co, 1989, pp 795-815.
20. Hendricks JC, O'Brien JA: Tracheal collapse in two cats. *JAVMA* 187:418-419, 1985.
21. Fingland RB: Tracheal collapse, in Kirk RW (ed): *Current Veterinary Therapy X.* Philadelphia, WB Saunders Co, 1989, pp 353-360.
22. Tangner CH, Hobson HP: A retrospective study of 20 surgically managed cases of collapsed trachea. *Vet Surg* 11:146-149, 1982.
23. Morgan RV: Shock. *Compend Contin Educ Pract Vet* 3(6):533-539, 1981.
24. Morgan RV: Endocrine and metabolic emergencies—Part II. *Compend Contin Educ Pract Vet* 4(10):814-818, 1982.
25. Guyton AC: *Textbook of Medical Physiology.* Philadelphia, WB Saunders Co, 1981, pp 491-503.
26. Tams TR: Pneumonia, in Kirk RW (ed): *Current Veterinary Therapy X.* Philadelphia, WB Saunders Co, 1989, pp 376-384.
27. Tams TR: Aspiration pneumonia and complications of inhalation of smoke and toxic gases. *Vet Clin North Am [Small Anim Pract]* 15:971-989, 1985.
28. Tams TR, Scherding RG: Smoke inhalation injury. *Compend Contin Educ Pract Vet* 3(11):986-992, 1981.
29. Thayer GW, Robinson SK: Bacterial bronchopneumonia in the dog: A review of 42 cases. *JAAHA* 20:731-735, 1984.
30. Thayer GW: Infections of the respiratory system, in Greene CE (ed): *Clinical Microbiology and Infectious Diseases of the Dog and Cat.* Philadelphia, WB Saunders Co, 1984, pp 238-246.
31. Drolet R, Kenefick KB, Hakomki MR, et al: Isolation of group eugonic fermenter-4 bacteria from a cat with multifocal suppurative pneumonia. *JAVMA* 189:311-312, 1986.

32. Court MH, Dodman NH, Seeler DC: Inhalation therapy: Oxygen administration, humidification, and aerosol therapy. *Vet Clin North Am [Small Anim Pract]* 15:1041-1059, 1985.
33. Krahwinkel DJ: Thoracic trauma, in Kirk RW (ed): *Current Veterinary Therapy VII*. Philadelphia, WB Saunders Co, 1980, pp 268-276.
34. Spackman CJA, Caywood DD: Management of thoracic trauma and chest wall reconstruction. *Vet Clin North Am [Small Anim Pract]* 17:431-447, 1987.
35. Tamas PM, Paddleford RR, Krahwinkel DJ: Thoracic trauma in dogs and cats presented for limb fractures. *JAAHA* 21:161-166, 1985.
36. Spackman CJA, Caywood DD, Feeney DA, et al: Thoracic wall and pulmonary trauma in dogs sustaining fractures as a result of motor vehicle accidents. *JAVMA* 185:975-977, 1984.
37. Whitney WO, Mehlhaff CJ: High-rise syndrome in cats. *JAVMA* 191:1399-1403, 1987.
38. Harpster N: Pulmonary edema, in Kirk RW (ed): *Current Veterinary Therapy X*. Philadelphia, WB Saunders Co, 1989, pp 385-392.
39. Hawkins EC, Ettinger SJ, Suter PF: Diseases of the lower respiratory tract (lung) and pulmonary edema, in Ettinger SJ (ed): *Textbook of Veterinary Internal Medicine*. Philadelphia, WB Saunders Co, 1989, pp 816-866.
40. Orsher AN, Kolata RJ: Acute respiratory distress syndrome: Case report and literature review. *JAAHA* 18(1):41-46, 1982.
41. Moses BL, Spaulding GL: Chronic bronchial disease of the cat. *Vet Clin North Am [Small Anim Pract]* 15:929-948, 1985.
42. Moise NS, Spaulding GL: Feline bronchial asthma: Pathogenesis, pathophysiology, diagnostics, and therapeutic considerations. *Compend Contin Educ Pract Vet* 3(12):1091-1102, 1981.
43. Hirshman CA, Downes H, Farbood A, et al: Ketamine block of bronchospasm in experimental canine asthma. *Br J Anaesth* 51:713-718, 1979.
44. Kutty K: Pulmonary embolism: How to 'nail down' the diagnosis. *Postgrad Med* 88:72-88, 1990.
45. LaRue MJ, Murtaugh RJ: Pulmonary thromboembolism in dogs: 47 cases (1986–1987). *JAVMA* 197:1368-1372, 1990.
46. Calvert CA, Rawlings CA: Pulmonary manifestations of heartworm disease. *Vet Clin North Am [Small Anim Pract]* 15:991-1009, 1985.
47. Burns MG, Kelly AB, Hornof WJ, et al: Pulmonary artery thrombosis in three dogs with hyperadrenocorticism. *JAVMA* 178:388-393; 1981.
48. Klein MK, Dow SW, Rosychuk RAW: Pulmonary thromboembolism associated with immune-mediated hemolytic anemia in dogs: Ten cases (1982–1987). *JAVMA* 195:246-250, 1989.
49. Green RA, Russo EA, Greene RT, et al: Hypoalbuminemia-related platelet hypersensitivity in two dogs with nephrotic syndrome. *JAVMA* 186:485-488, 1985.
50. Green RA, Kabel AL: Hypercoagulable state in three dogs with nephrotic syndrome: Role of acquired antithrombin III deficiency. *JAVMA* 181:914-917, 1982.
51. Dennis JS: The pathophysiologic sequelae of pulmonary thromboembolism. *Compend Contin Educ Pract Vet* 13(12):1811-1818, 1991.
52. Fluckiger MA, Gomez JA: Radiographic findings in dogs with spontaneous pulmonary thrombosis or embolism. *Vet Radiol* 25:124-131, 1984.
53. Koblik PD, Hornof W, Harnagel SH, Fisher PE: A comparison of pulmonary angiography, digital subtraction angiography, and ^{99m}Tc-DTPA/MAA ventilation-perfusion scintigraphy for detection of experimental pulmonary emboli in the dog. *Vet Radiol* 30:159-168, 1989.
54. Pion PD, Kittleson MD: Therapy for feline aortic thromboembolism, in Kirk RW (ed): *Current Veterinary Therapy X*. Philadelphia, WB Saunders Co, 1989, pp 295-302.
55. Kagan KG, Stiff ME: Pleural diseases, in Kirk RW (ed): *Current Veterinary Therapy VIII*. Philadelphia, WB Saunders Co, 1983, pp 266-277.
56. Bauer T: Mediastinal, pleural, and extrapleural diseases, in Ettinger SJ (ed): *Textbook of Veterinary Internal Medicine*. Philadelphia, WB Saunders Co, 1989, pp 867-897.
57. Kagan KG: Thoracic trauma. *Vet Clin North Am [Small Anim Pract]* 10(3):641-653, 1980.
58. Kolata RJ: Management of thoracic trauma. *Vet Clin North Am [Small Anim Pract]* 11(1):103-120, 1981.
59. Yoshioka MM: Management of spontaneous pneumothorax in twelve dogs. *JAAHA* 18(1):57-62, 1982.
60. Burk RL, Ackerman N: *Small Animal Radiology: A Diagnostic Atlas and Text*. New York, Churchill Livingstone, 1986.
61. Creighton SR, Wilkins RJ: Pleural effusions, in Kirk RW (ed): *Current Veterinary Therapy VII*. Philadelphia, WB Saunders Co, 1980, pp 253-261.
62. Noone KE: Pleural effusions and diseases of the pleura. *Vet Clin North Am [Small Anim Pract]* 15:1069-1084, 1985.
63. Fossum TW, Birchard SJ: Chylothorax, in Kirk RW (ed): *Current Veterinary Therapy X*. Philadelphia, WB Saunders Co, 1989, pp 393-398.
64. Roudebush P: Bacterial infections of the respiratory system, in Green CE (ed): *Infectious Diseases of the Dog and Cat*. Philadelphia, WB Saunders Co, 1990, pp 114-124.
65. Gibbons G: Respiratory emergencies, in Murtaugh RJ, Kaplan PM (eds): *Veterinary Emergency and Critical Care Medicine*. Chicago, Mosby–Year Book, 1992, pp 399-419.
66. Sullivan M, Reid J: Management of 60 cases of diaphragmatic rupture. *J Small Anim Pract* 31:425-430, 1990.
67. Spackman CJA, Caywood DD: Management of thoracic trauma and chest wall reconstruction. *Vet Clin North Am [Small Anim Pract]* 17:431-447, 1987.
68. Rubin S, Faulkner RT, Ward GE: Tetanus following ovariohysterectomy in a dog: A case report and review. *JAAHA* 19:293-298, 1983.
69. Morgan RV: Respiratory emergencies. Part II. *Compend Contin Educ Pract Vet* 5(4):305-310, 1983.
70. Moses BL: Cardiopulmonary resuscitation, in Murtaugh RJ, Kaplan PM (eds): *Veterinary Emergency and Critical Care Medicine*. Chicago, Mosby–Year Book, 1992, pp 508-525.

BIBLIOGRAPHY

Harvey CE: Upper airway obstruction surgery: Overview of results. *JAAHA* 18(4):535-569, 1982.

Flail Chest: Pathophysiology, Treatment, and Prognosis

University of Missouri–Columbia
Mark Anderson, DVM
John T. Payne, DVM, MS
F. A. Mann, DVM, MS
Gheorghe M. Constantinescu, DVM, PhD

KEY FACTS

- Canine and feline patients are relatively resistant to flail chest because of the anatomic shape and resilience of the thoracic cavity.

- Clinical signs seen in veterinary patients with flail chest result from the pendulous movement of air, pulmonary contusions, pain, and other concurrent intrathoracic injuries.

- Patients must be evaluated on an individual basis before treatment of flail chest. Mechanical ventilation, medical management, and surgical treatment are good treatment options; however, none of the options is considered to be superior.

- The prognosis of veterinary patients with flail chest (with and without treatment) is unknown.

- Medical therapy for flail chest includes the judicious use of crystalloid or colloidal fluid therapy, diuretics, corticosteroids, and regional analgesics.

Flail chest is the fracture of two or more consecutive ribs in two places (ventral and dorsal); the condition causes thoracic wall instability and interferes with mechanical ventilation.[1] In 1859, Malgaigne[2] first described the paradoxic motion of the flail segment during inspiration and expiration. During inspiration, the chest wall expands and reduces the pressure in the pleural space. The reduced pressure causes the flail segment to collapse inward. Opposite movement of the flail segment occurs during expiration (Figure 1).

The most common causes of thoracic trauma that result in flail chest or rib fractures include vehicular accidents, falls from buildings, animal interactions,[3] and other forms of blunt trauma (e.g., animals kicked or bluntly traumatized by humans).[4–9] Rib fractures and other thoracic injuries are often overlooked during physical examination of traumatized patients. In one study, 79% of dogs with skeletal injuries had undetected thoracic trauma.[10] The increased resilience and anatomic shape of canine and feline thoracic cavities decrease the propensity for rib fracture; flail chest is thus relatively uncommon in these species.[4,5,8,9,11–15] Flail chest is easily diagnosed during physical examination, but concurrent intrathoracic injuries may be less obvious. Whenever thoracic trauma is suspected, clinical evaluation should include a thorough physical examination and thoracic radiographs[4,6,11,12,14,15,17–20] (Figure 2).

This article discusses the pathophysiology of flail chest and other common intrathoracic injuries that occur concomitantly with rib fractures. Methods of treatment of flail chest are evaluated, and a logical therapeutic plan is formulated for canine and feline patients. Finally, with extrapolation from the human literature, an attempt is made to determine the prognosis for dogs and cats with flail chest.

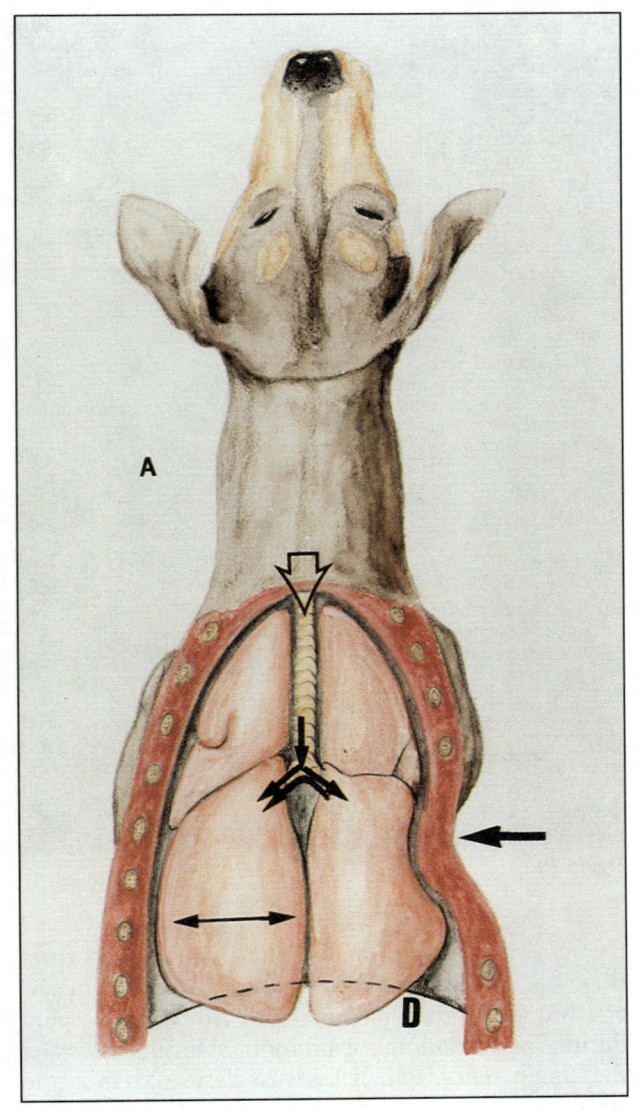

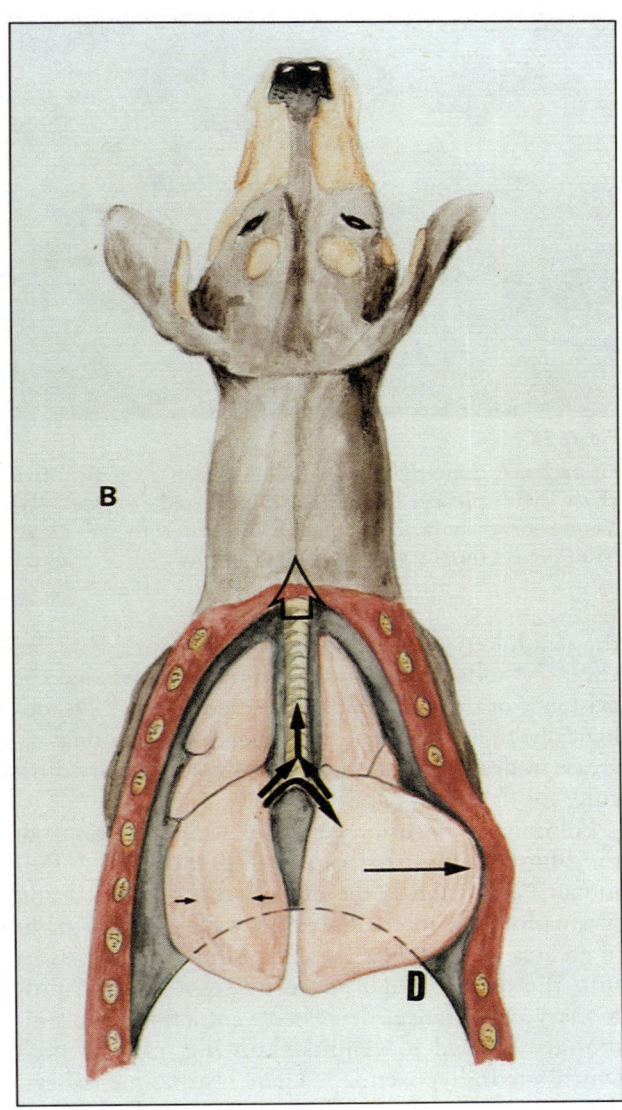

Figure 1A

Figure 1B

Figure 1—(**A**) Depiction of flail chest shows the movement of air in the trachea (*open arrow*), movement of air down the main stem bronchi (*small solid arrows*), shunting of air from the lung under the flail segment to the opposite hemithorax (*solid curved arrow*), position of the diaphragm (*D*), expansion of the lungs (*double-headed arrow*), and the movement of the flail segment (*solid arrow*) during inspiration. (**B**) Depiction of flail chest demonstrates the movement of air in the trachea (*open arrow*), movement of air out of the lungs and up the main stem bronchi (*solid arrows*), shunting of air from the lungs of the unaffected hemithorax to the lungs under the flail segment (*solid curved arrow*), position of the diaphragm (*D*), collapse of the lungs (*small arrows*), and the movement of the flail segment (*small solid arrow*) during expiration. (Drawn by Georghe M. Constantinescu, DVM, PhD, College of Veterinary Medicine, University of Missouri–Columbia)

PATHOPHYSIOLOGY

In 1909, Bauer[21] first attempted to explain the clinical signs seen with human flail chest patients. He formulated the pendelluft theory, which described the pendulous movement of air from the lungs under the flail segment to the other hemithorax (and back again) during inspiration and expiration[21] (Figure 1). Although evidence has both disproved and confirmed

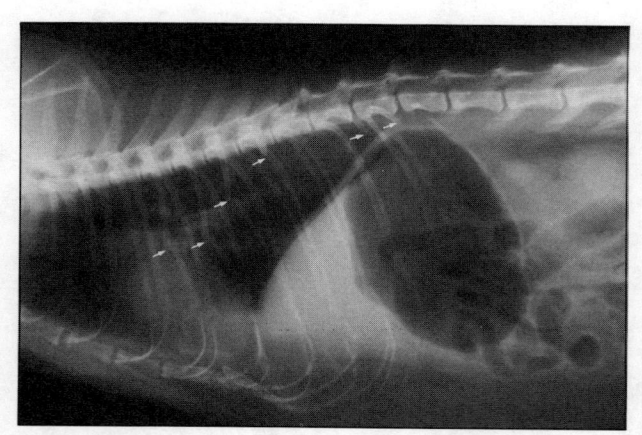

Figure 2A

Figure 2—(**A**) Lateral thoracic radiograph of a cat with flail chest. Multiple rib fractures are indicated (*arrows*). (**B**) Ventrodorsal thoracic radiograph of a cat with flail chest. Multiple rib fractures are indicated (*arrows*).

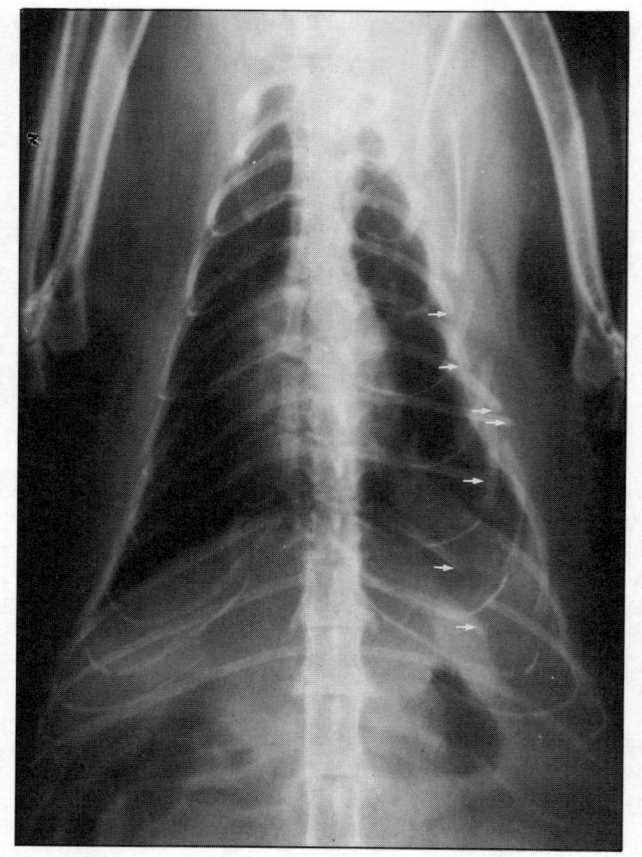

Figure 2B

the pendulous movement of air in patients with flail chest,[22,23] today most investigators acknowledge the existence of the pendulous movement of air.[24] Physiologically, this movement of air creates a functional increase in dead space, which results in respiratory difficulty for flail chest patients.[16,25–29]

Pulmonary contusion generally occurs as a result of the blunt trauma that causes flail chest.[16, 30–31] Pulmonary contusion is the extravasation of blood and plasma into the interstitial and alveolar compartment of an area of the lung.[32] Leaking of blood and plasma into the extravascular space causes decreased pulmonary compliance, decreased ventilation, and pulmonary arterial-to-venous shunting, all of which contribute to hypoxemia.[33] There is experimental evidence that gas exchange abnormalities in the lungs of patients with flail chest result from ventilation-to-perfusion (V–Q) mismatching secondary to contusion and are not secondary to intrapulmonary shunting of blood caused by pulmonary collapse.[33] The evidence that pulmonary contusion (instead of intrapulmonary shunting of blood secondary to collapse) causes the hypoxemia associated with thoracic trauma is important when a treatment protocol for pulmonary contusions associated with rib fractures is being developed.

Pain has been recognized as another cause of the clinical signs seen with human patients with flail chest injury. Rib fractures alone do not typically influence mechanical ventilation, but the pain derived from these fractures can indirectly impair ventilation in several ways.[34] Human patients with rib fractures splint during inspiration and expiration; splinting decreases the cough reflex, which leads to decreased ability to clear pulmonary secretions.[6,11,24,31,35–40] In addition, human patients with thoracic wall pain are reluctant to expand the thorax fully during inspiration; resultant hypoventilation can exacerbate the hypoxemia caused by concurrent intrathoracic injuries.[6,11,31,35,39] Finally, pain can cause inadequate ventilation of the lungs, resulting in atelectasis.[35]

The pathophysiology of respiratory distress of flail chest is complex and has many components. A few disorders that may accompany flail chest, such as pneumothorax, hemothorax, and decreased cardiac output (resulting from either direct injury to the myocardium or hypovolemia caused by hemorrhage and edema in the injured lung),[26] have also been implicat-

> It is important to realize that no superior treatment protocol exists; patients must be evaluated and treated on an individual basis.

ed as causes for respiratory distress.[4,11,13,25,30,41] Pulmonary contusions, pain, and pendulous airflow, however, are the most widely accepted causes of the ventilatory disturbances seen with flail chest.[43] The clinical signs seen with flail chest are not simply associated with rib fractures but (in general) include complicated intrathoracic injuries that must be considered when a treatment plan is being developed.

TREATMENT

In 1956, Avery[42] described the use of mechanical ventilation for the treatment of human patients with flail chest. Although this type of ventilation revolutionized the treatment of flail chest, the complication rate associated with assisted ventilation in human patients has remained between 20% and 50%.[16,24,30,43–52] Other critical care physicians have looked for alternatives and advocate use of aggressive medical management with or without surgical stabilization of the flail segment; however, the results of such management have been mixed. It is important to realize that no superior treatment protocol exists; patients (human or animal) must be evaluated and treated on an individual basis.

Mechanical Ventilation

Mechanical ventilation has been the most reliable form of treatment for flail chest in human patients. Although mechanical ventilation is generally labor intensive and cost prohibitive for veterinary patients, the increasing number of large, highly sophisticated emergency facilities may make controlled ventilation a more feasible form of treatment in the future.

Mechanical ventilation offers many advantages for treatment of flail chest and associated intrathoracic injuries. Assisted ventilation stops the paradoxic motion of the flail segment by maintaining intratracheal pressure above atmospheric level on inspiration while expiration occurs against this positive pressure.[42] By maintaining pleural pressures above atmospheric pressure, paradoxic movement of the flail segment is minimal.[42] Decreased movement of the flail segment allows better apposition of the fractured ribs, lessens the amount of pain associated with rib instability, decreases the need for narcotic analgesics,[42] and leads to more rapid healing of the ribs. Mechanical ventilation provides adequate ventilation to noncontused lungs and helps decrease the incidence of hypoxemia.[33,43] Positive end expiratory pressure with continuous positive airway pressure improves air exchange with severe contusions and decreases hypoxemia.

Complications that have occurred with use of mechanical ventilation in human patients include increased hospitalization time, increased incidence of bacterial pneumonia, barotrauma, and atelectasis resulting from the inability of the patient to ventilate spontaneously.[16,25,38,43,44,46,54–57] Although mechanical ventilation has been considered to be the panacea for treatment of flail chest, the continued high rate of complications associated with this modality make haphazard use inappropriate.[43,45,46,50,51,53,58,59]

Conservative Therapy

Conservative therapy of blunt trauma, which was at one time the mainstay for treatment of flail chest, has been repopularized in the past two decades.[16,25,36,43,44,60,61] Today, conservative management of flail chest in human patients consists of tracheostomy with intermittent suctioning of the upper airways[61]; restricted administration of fluids; and administration of diuretics, corticosteroids, and analgesics.[16] Experimental and clinical use of conservative medical management have yielded excellent results in human patients with marked parenchymal disease and flail chest.[16] For patients who have sustained more severe intrathoracic injuries and have associated hypoxemia refractory to conservative therapy, mechanical ventilation with or without continuous positive airway pressure is still the best form of treatment.[48,62]

Tracheostomy

Tracheostomy and intermittent airway suctioning have several advantages for conservative management of flail chest. Suctioning stimulates the cough reflex, which would otherwise be suppressed by the pain associated with the rib fractures.[37] Suctioning also helps remove pulmonary secretions, which may obstruct ventilation.[37] Although tracheostomy is rarely indicated for treatment of flail chest in small animals, patients with severe dyspnea may benefit from temporary tracheostomy and intermittent suctioning of the upper airways. Tracheostomy also provides a means for intermittent positive-pressure ventilation in small animal patients.

Complications from tracheostomies and suctioning of pulmonary secretions are common.[16,51,53,63,64] Disadvantages of tracheostomy include increased amount of nursing care and increased incidence of

> Fluid therapy is extremely important in treatment of the initial shock associated with blunt trauma.

bacterial pneumonia. Judicious use of tracheostomy and proper management techniques can reduce the incidence of complications.

Fluid Therapy

Fluid therapy is extremely important in treatment of the initial shock associated with blunt trauma; however, judicious administration of fluids to patients with flail chest and concurrent intrathoracic injuries is important.[6,13,14,39] Clinically, pulmonary contusions are frequently associated with thoracic trauma and flail chest. Radiographic identification of pulmonary contusions may be delayed for 24 to 48 hours after the traumatic episode.[32,65]

Experimental studies on dogs with induced pulmonary contusions from blunt trauma have shown that high flow rates (greater than 30 ml/kg/hr) of crystalloid fluids increase the size and weight of contused lungs.[66] Fluid management of patients with concomitant hypovolemic shock and flail chest is difficult because the volume of fluid necessary for shock resuscitation could result in overhydration and pulmonary edema in the contused lung lobe(s). Although central venous pressure provides an effective means for monitoring fluid loads, there is experimental evidence in dogs indicating that pulmonary contusions can increase in size, whereas central venous pressures remain within normal limits.[66]

Colloidal solutions may also be used for resuscitation of shock patients. The solutions (blood or plasma) have been infused at high flow rates with minimal changes to the contused lung(s).[66]

Thorough consideration should be given to the appropriate choice of fluid therapy for patients with hypovolemic shock and concurrent flail chest. During the initial treatment for shock, colloidal therapy (with blood or plasma) at a rate of 30 to 90 ml/kg/hr is ideal.[66] The use of low-molecular-weight dextrans should be avoided in patients with flail chest because they evidently pass through the damaged endothelium of pulmonary vessels and cause increased accumulation of extravascular fluid in pulmonary interstitial tissue.[67] High-molecular-weight dextrans have been used in endotoxic shock models where the integrity of the pulmonary vasculature was reduced.[68] Experimental results have shown that high-molecular-weight dextrans improve cardiovascular function and prevent pulmonary edema by remaining in the intravascular space. High-molecular-weight dextrans exert a hyperoncotic effect by drawing fluid from pulmonary interstitial tissue into the intravascular space.[69]

Hetastarch is a synthetic colloid that consists of heterogenous polymers. Particle size of these polymers varies greatly; however, low-molecular-weight particles can penetrate vascular endothelium and enter the interstitial space. Although experimental investigations have shown that hetastarch improves cardiac function during treatment of circulatory shock, hetastarch must be used judiciously to prevent worsening of pulmonary contusions.[70] Small volumes (4 to 5 ml/kg) of hypertonic saline solution (7% NaCl) have been demonstrated to improve hemodynamics in several species with hypovolemic shock.[68] Currently, clinical investigations of endotoxic shock have shown no beneficial effects of hypertonic saline and isotonic solutions on cardiovascular function.[69] Furthermore, hypertonic saline has been shown not to decrease pulmonary edema in association with pulmonary contusions and should thus be used cautiously.

Low-salt albumins have been used in human flail chest patients to maintain normal oncotic pressure.[16] Increasing oncotic pressure with low-salt albumins decreases leakage of intravascular fluid from pulmonary blood vessels at the site of the pulmonary contusion, thereby decreasing the size of the contusion anatomically and physiologically.[16] Low-salt albumins are not commonly used in veterinary medicine and may be cost prohibitive.

Diuretics

In 1973, Trinkle[16] provided evidence that diuretics (more specifically, the loop diuretic furosemide) decrease accumulation of fluids in contused lungs of humans. Diuretics have experimentally decreased the size of contused lungs.[67] Furosemide acts on the thick ascending loop of Henle to inhibit active chloride transport.[71] As chloride transport is inhibited, excretion of sodium is increased and rapid diuresis results. When creating this intense diuresis, furosemide decreases the plasma volume as well as the amount of plasma and blood pooling in the contused lung. This same mechanism of action has allowed diuretics to be used to shrink the size of a pulmonary contusion when used with medical management or mechanical ventilation of flail chest in dogs.[67]

Osmotic diuretics should be used cautiously in patients with flail chest that are also experiencing pulmonary contusions or have questionable pulmo-

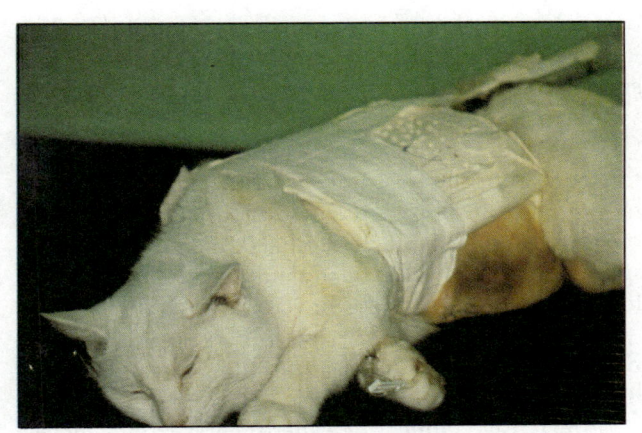

Figure 3—Postsurgical photograph demonstrating the application of splints constructed of split aluminum rods for treatment of a cat with flail chest.

nary vascular integrity. Osmotic diuretics may pass through the damaged endothelium of pulmonary vessels and increase the size of the pulmonary contusion.

Corticosteroids

Corticosteroids have been used for many years to manage pulmonary contusions associated with flail chest.[16] Methylprednisolone sodium succinate administered within the first 30 minutes of the initial blunt trauma can decrease the size and weight of contused lung lobes.[72] Dexamethasone has been shown to be ineffective for treatment of pulmonary contusions.[67] Methylprednisolone sodium succinate acts at the cellular level to stabilize cell and lysosomal membranes that prevent the release of enzymes from the lysosome.[73] The agent has been shown to increase capillary integrity in the lungs, thereby decreasing the edema in alveoli.[72] Finally, methylprednisolone sodium succinate has been proven to decrease the damage to alveolar type II cells during periods of hypoxia.[73] Alveolar type II cells are surfactant secreting cells that are sensitive to low oxygen tension.[73] Surfactant prevents the collapse of alveoli and the passage of fluid into the alveolar space, thereby preventing intraalveolar pulmonary edema.[73]

Reports of complications of corticosteroid use in pulmonary contusions have been contradictory. Some studies in human patients have shown that corticosteroids have no negative effect on pulmonary function[16,74]; another study suggests that corticosteroids increase the incidence of septicemia and bronchial in-

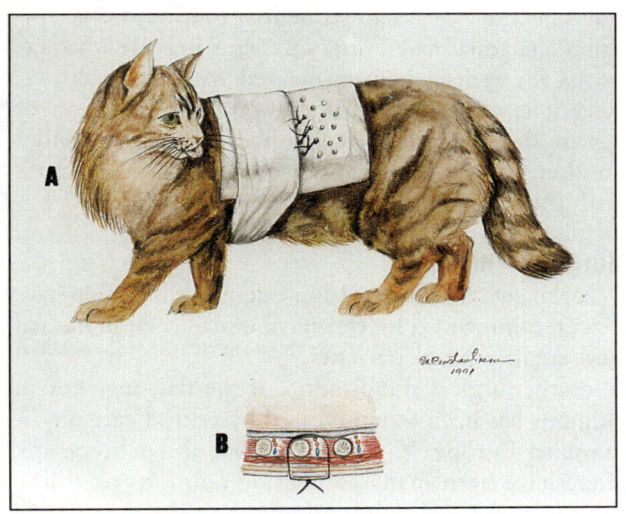

Figure 4—Depiction of the (A) application of the sutures through the splint and (B) correct placement of sutures around the ribs shown in a cross section of the thoracic wall. (Drawn by Georghe M. Constantinescu, DVM, PhD, College of Veterinary Medicine, University of Missouri–Columbia)

fections.[75] Presently, the beneficial effects of methylprednisolone sodium succinate in the treatment of pulmonary contusions far outweigh the known detrimental effects.

Analgesics

Analgesics are important in the treatment of flail chest. Parenteral narcotic analgesia (i.e., morphine sulfate) was initially used to relieve the pain associated with rib fractures in human patients; however, narcotics suppress ventilation and worsen respiratory distress.[76,77] Intercostal nerve blocks have been used successfully to alleviate flail chest pain in veterinary and human patients.[6,12–14,16,25,36,39,60,78,79] Long-acting local anesthetics, such as bupivacaine hydrochloride with epinephrine (1:2,000,000), have proven effective in veterinary patients.[13,17] Nerve blocks should be done by injecting 0.25 to 0.50 ml of 0.5% bupivacaine hydrochloride caudal to the ribs involved in the flail segment, including one rib cranial and caudal to the flail segment.[13,17] Pain relief provides better ventilation, decreases splinting, and helps prevent atelectasis.[35]

Recent research in human patients has shown that epidural injections with narcotics provide longer pain relief than intercostal nerve blocks and require only

> Pain relief provides better ventilation, decreases splinting, and helps prevent atelectasis.

one injection.[35,48,79] Consequently, routine use of epidural analgesia in veterinary patients may be advantageous for central pain associated with rib fractures. Recent research with intrapleural administration of 1.5 mg/kg 0.5% bupivacaine hydrochloride provides an alternative for administration of analgesia to dogs with thoracic wall trauma.[80]

Surgical Therapy

For many years, internal and external stabilization have been recommended for treatment of flail chest in human and small animal patients.[6,9,12–15,17,40,41,47,54,62,76–78,81–87] Recently, surgical stabilization of the flail segment in humans has been repopularized by critical care physicians in Europe.[54–57,86,88–94] In the human literature, there have been many conflicting opinions regarding the use of surgical stabilization of flail chest.

Opponents of surgical stabilization claim that the paradoxic movement of the flail segment makes an insignificant contribution to the respiratory difficulty seen with flail chest.[16,31,67,95] Consequently, immobilizing the flail segment should not alleviate respiratory difficulty. Excellent clinical results have, however, been reported after surgical stabilization in human patients with paradoxic rib movement, impaired ventilation, and inability to cough.[41,47,93] Although the flail segment does not contribute to a significant decrease in mechanical ventilation, surgical stabilization decreases pain and has been noted to result in decreased respiratory rate, increased tidal volume, and increased vital capacity.[94]

Internal and external forms of fixation of rib fractures have been used in veterinary medicine.[6,9,11–15,17,19,40,76,87,96] Krahwinkel[9] described the use of internal surgical fixation with Kirschner wires with or without orthopedic wire; however, when the increased risk of anesthesia precludes internal fixation, external stabilization is the recommended approach. In cases of acute injury, towel clamps can be placed around the ribs of the flail segment and held under traction; lack of patient cooperation may preclude the use of this technique without anesthesia.[6,15,76,96] Long-term stabilization techniques include splints constructed of split aluminum rods[12,14,15,76,40] and malleable plastic frames that conform to the thoracic wall[13,14,87] (Figure 3).

Many forms of external splintage for rib fractures can be applied with local anesthesia.[13] When such forms of rib stabilization are used, it is important to pass sutures (nylon or polypropylene) around the ribs in more than two places to prevent pivoting around a single row of sutures[13] (Figure 4). External splints should remain in place for two to four weeks.[12,14,87] Osseous union of rib fractures will not be complete at this point, but the fractures should be adequately immobilized from fibrous tissue formation.[12] Restrictive types of external stabilization (e.g., sandbags and tape splints) impede ventilation and are not recommended for fixation of rib fractures in veterinary patients.[13]

Recommendations for Treatment in Veterinary Patients

No extensive clinical or experimental studies have been done to support any one treatment protocol as the most appropriate in animals. Because the pathophysiology of flail chest is complicated and there are many other intrathoracic injuries associated with this form of blunt trauma, all treatment modalities for flail chest should be selected on an individual basis. Some suggested guidelines for treatment of flail chest include (1) medical management if the patient is stable and can adequately oxygenate or has minor injuries associated with the flail chest,[16,60,97] (2) immediate internal stabilization if there is concurrent intrathoracic injury requiring repair (e.g., diaphragmatic hernia) or paradoxic movement and pain that significantly impair the patient's ability to ventilate and cough,[24,47,54,57,59,86,93,94,98] and (3) assisted ventilation (arterial PO_2 [oxygen partial pressure] <60 mm Hg)[16,65,97,99] in hypoxemic patients that are unconscious or in shock[16,44,53,79] as well as in patients experiencing severe respiratory distress.[16,25,44,48,79,99]

Medical management of a patient in shock should include restricted colloidal infusions (30 to 90 ml/kg/hr), aggressive pulmonary toilet (e.g., cuppage of the chest), furosemide (1 to 2 mg/kg intravenously every 8 to 12 hours), methylprednisolone sodium succinate (5.5 to 11 mg/kg intravenously within the first 30 minutes), and intercostal nerve blocks or intrapleural blocks as needed for pain.[16]

PROGNOSIS

There is very little information describing the morbidity and mortality of thoracic trauma in the veterinary literature. The survival rate in small animal patients is probably lower than that of humans because mechanical ventilation and other complex forms of treatment for thoracic trauma are cost prohibitive for most veterinary patients. Animals with thoracic trauma should always be considered at high risk for life-threatening complications and should be treated as aggressively as possible.

Long-term disabilities associated with flail chest in humans include chest wall pain, dyspnea or tightness of the chest, and chest wall deformities.[43,45] If an animal survives acute thoracic injury, the long-term complications are probably similar to those seen in humans but are noticed less frequently because of the difficulty in evaluating pain. Long-term complications, such as anatomic deformation, are often not considered when a treatment plan is being established because of the severity of the thoracic trauma and the priority given to life-saving measures. Consequently, veterinary patients surviving acute injuries may have long-term complications similar to humans.

CONCLUSION

Flail chest is a complicated injury with many aspects, and the appropriate treatment may not be obvious. At present, no retrospective studies in the veterinary literature have evaluated the prognosis for survival associated with different treatment protocols of flail chest. Information is presently extrapolated from the human literature for possible treatments and prognostic evaluation but may not be accurate. A controlled study using different therapeutic plans is needed for veterinarians to be able to better understand a particular treatment plan and associated prognosis when treating flail chest and other concurrent intrathoracic injuries.

About the Authors

Drs. Anderson, Payne, and Mann are affiliated with the Department of Veterinary Medicine and Surgery, and Dr. Constantinescu is with the Department of Veterinary Biomedical Sciences, College of Veterinary Medicine, University of Missouri–Columbia, Columbia, Missouri. Drs. Payne and Mann are Diplomates of the American College of Veterinary Surgeons.

REFERENCES

1. Suter PF: Trauma to the thorax and cervical airways. *Thoracic Radiology of the Dog and Cat.* Switzerland, PF Suter, 1984, pp 130–151.
2. Malgaigne JF: *A Treatise on Fracture Repair.* Philadelphia, JB Lippincott Co, 1859.
3. McKiernan BC, Adams WM, Huse DC: Thoracic bite wounds and associated internal injury in 11 dogs and 1 cat. *JAVMA* 184:959–964, 1984.
4. Spackman CJA, Caywood DD, Feeney DA, et al: Thoracic wall and pulmonary trauma in dogs sustaining fractures as a result of motor vehicle accidents. *JAVMA* 185:975–977, 1984.
5. Tamas PM, Paddleford RR, Krahwinkel DJ Jr: Thoracic trauma in dogs and cats presented for limb fractures. *JAAHA* 21:161–166, 1985.
6. Zaslow IM: Initial management of wounds and injuries to the chest, in Zaslow IM (ed): *Veterinary Trauma and Critical Care.* Philadelphia, Lea & Febiger, 1984, pp 245–285.
7. Kolata RJ, Kraut NH, Johnston DE: Pattern of trauma in urban dogs and cats: A study of 1000 cases. *JAVMA* 174:499–502, 1974.
8. Kolata RJ, Johnston DE: Motor vehicle accidents in urban dogs: A study of 600 cases. *JAVMA* 167:938–941, 1975.
9. Krahwinkel DJ Jr: Lower respiratory tract trauma, in Kirk RW (ed): *Current Veterinary Therapy. VI.* Philadelphia, WB Saunders Co, 1977, pp 278–291.
10. Selcer BA, Buttrick M, Barstad R: The incidence of thoracic trauma in dogs with skeletal injury. *J Small Anim Pract* 28:21–27, 1987.
11. Hunt CA: Chest trauma-specific injuries. *Compend Contin Educ Pract Vet* 1(8):624–632, 1979.
12. Bjorling DE, Kolata RJ, DeNova RC: Flail chest: A review, clinical experience and new method of stabilization. *JAAHA* 18:269–276, 1982.
13. Spackman CJA, Caywood DD: Management of thoracic trauma and chest wall reconstruction. *Vet Clin North Am Small Anim Pract* 17:431–447, 1987.
14. Kolata RJ: Management of thoracic trauma. *Vet Clin North Am Small Anim Pract* 11:103–120, 1984.
15. Dixon JS: Use of a slab traction splint to stabilize canine flail chest. *VM SAC* 77:601–604, 1982.
16. Trinkle JK, Richardson JD, Franz JL, et al: Management of flail chest without mechanical ventilation. *Ann Thorac Surg* 19:355–363, 1975.
17. Kagan KG: Thoracic trauma. *Vet Clin North Am Small Anim Pract* 10:641–653, 1980.
18. Spencer CP, Ackerman N: Thoracic and abdominal radiography of the trauma patient. *Vet Clin North Am Small Anim Pract* 10:541–559, 1980.
19. Short CE: Management of thoracic trauma in the cat. *Feline Pract* 12:11–20, 1982.
20. Berkwitt L, Berzon JL: Thoracic trauma. *Vet Clin North Am Small Anim Pract* 15:1031–1039, 1985.
21. Bauer L: Erfahunger und uberlegungen zur lungenkollapstherapie. *Beitr Klin Tuberk* 12:49, 1909.
22. Maloney JV Jr, Schmutzer KJ, Raschke E: Paradoxical respiration and "pendelluft." *J Thorac Cardiovasc Surg* 41:291–298, 1961.
23. Harada K, Saoyama N, Izumi K, et al: Experimental pendulum air in the flail chest. *Jpn J Surg* 13:219–226, 1983.
24. Myllynen P, Kivioja A, Wilppula E, et al: Flail chest—Pathophysiology, treatment and prognosis. *Ann Chir Gynaecol* 72:43–46, 1983.
25. Carpintero JL, Diez AR, Elvira JR, et al: Methods of management of flail chest. *Intensive Care Med* 6:217–221, 1980.
26. Moseley RV, Vernick JJ, Doty DB: Response to blunt injury: A new experimental model. *J Trauma* 10:673–683, 1970.

27. Craven KD, Oppenheimer L, Wood LDH: Effects of contusion and flail chest on pulmonary perfusion and oxygen exchange. *J Appl Physiol* 47:729–737, 1979.
28. Garzon AA, Seltzer B, Karlson KE: Physiopathology of crushed chest injuries. *Ann Surg* 168:128–136, 1968.
29. James OF, Moore PG: Respiratory failure after chest injury: The development of effective treatment. *Ann R Coll Surg Engl* 64:253–255, 1982.
30. Schaal MA, Fischer RP, Perry JF: The unchanged mortality of flail chest injuries. *J Trauma* 19:492–496, 1979.
31. Cullen P, Modell JH, Kirby RR, et al: Treatment of flail chest. *Arch Surg* 110:1099–1103, 1975.
32. Greene R: Lung alterations in thoracic trauma. *J Thorac Image* 2:1–11, 1987.
33. Oppenheimer L, Craven KD, Forkert L, et al: Pathophysiology of pulmonary contusions in dogs. *J Appl Physiol* 47:718–728, 1979.
34. Karlson K: Physiological changes in crushed chest injuries. *NY State J Med* 68:2880–2882, 1968.
35. MacKersie RC, Shackford SR, Hoyt DB, et al: Continuous epidural fentanyl analgesia: Ventilatory function improvement with routine use in treatment of blunt chest injury. *J Trauma* 27:1207–1212, 1987.
36. Miller HAB, Taylor GA, Harrison AW, et al: Management of flail chest. *Can Med Assoc J* 129:1104–1107, 1983.
37. Jensen NK: Recovery of pulmonary function after crushing injuries of the chest. *Dis Chest* 22:319–346, 1952.
38. Ginsberg RJ, Kostin RF: New approaches to the management of flail chest. *Can Med Assoc J* 116:613–615, 1977.
39. Hunt CA: Chest trauma—The approach to the patient with chest injuries. *Compend Contin Educ Pract Vet* 1(7):537–541, 1979.
40. Houlton JEF: Thoracic wall injuries. *Vet Annu* 27:257–263, 1987.
41. McDowell A Jr, Dykes J, Paulsen GA: Early reconstruction of the crushed chest. *Dis Chest* 41:618–623, 1962.
42. Avery EE, Morch ET, Benson DW: Critically crushed chest. *J Thorac Cardiovasc Surg* 32:291–311, 1956.
43. Landercasper J, Cogbill TH, Lindesmith LA: Long-term disability after flail chest injury. *J Trauma* 24:410–414, 1984.
44. Richardson JD, Adams L, Flint LM: Selective management of flail chest and pulmonary contusions. *Ann Surg* 196:481–487, 1982.
45. Beal SL, Oreskovich MR: Long-term disability associated with flail chest injury. *Am J Surg* 150:324–326, 1985.
46. Landercasper J, Cogbill TH, Strutt PJ: Delayed diagnosis of flail chest. *Crit Care Med* 18:611-613, 1990.
47. Moore BP, Grillo HC: Operative stabilization of nonpenetrating chest injuries. *J Thorac Cardiovasc Surg* 70:619–630, 1975.
48. Shackford SR, Virgilio RW: Selective use of ventilator therapy in flail chest injury. *J Thorac Cardiovasc Surg* 81:194–201, 1981.
49. Roscher R, Bittner R, Stackmann U: Pulmonary contusion. *Arch Surg* 109:508–510, 1974.
50. Relihan M, Litwin MS: Morbidity and mortality associated with flail chest injury: A review of 85 cases. *J Trauma* 13:663–671, 1973.
51. Sankaran S, Wilson RF: Factors affecting prognosis in patients with flail chest. *J Thorac Cardiovasc Surg* 60:402–410, 1970.
52. As Van AWW, Zwi S: Respiratory treatment of crushed chest injury. *S Afr Med J* 43:409–413, 1969.
53. Fleming WH, Bowen JC: Early complications of long-term respiratory support. *J Thorac Cardiovasc Surg* 64:729–738, 1972.
54. Thomas AN, Blaisdell FW, Lewis Jr FR, et al: Operative stabilization for flail chest after blunt trauma. *J Thorac Cardiovasc Surg* 75:793–801, 1978.
55. Manzano JL, Balanos J, Lubillo S, et al: Internal costal fixation of fractured ribs in a 6-year-old patient. *Crit Care Med* 10:67–68, 1982.
56. Tscharner C, Schupbach P, Meier P, et al: Zur operativen be handlung des instabilen thorax bei respiratorischer insuffizienz. *Helv Chir Acta* 55:711–717, 1988.
57. Haasler GB: Open fixation of flail chest after blunt trauma. *Ann Thorac Surg* 49:993–995, 1990.
58. Tzelepis GE, Mecool FD, Hoppin FG: Chest wall distortion in patients with flail chest. *Am Rev Respir Dis* 140:31–37, 1989.
59. Majeski JA: Management of flail chest after blunt trauma. *South Med J* 74:848–849, 1981.
60. Dittmann M, Steenblock U, Kranzlin M, et al: Epidural analgesia or mechanical ventilation for multiple rib fractures? *Intern Care Med* 8:89–92, 1982.
61. Kaunitz VH: Flail chest. *J Thorac Cardiovasc Surg* 82:463–464, 1981.
62. Youmans CG, McMinn M, Jenicek J, et al: Recognizing and managing flail chest. *Postgrad Med* 48:87–93, 1970.
63. Reid JM, Baird WLM: Crushed chest injury: Some physiological disturbances and their correction. *Sr Med J* 24:1105–1109, 1965.
64. Mulder DS, Rubush JL: Complications of tracheostomy: Relationship to long ventilatory assistance. *J Trauma* 9:389–402, 1969.
65. Crowe DT Jr: Traumatic pulmonary contusions, hematomas, pseudocysts, and acute respiratory distress syndrome: An update—Part I. *Compend Contin Educ Pract Vet* 5(5):396–404, 1983.
66. Richardson JD, Franz JL, Grover FL, et al: Pulmonary contusion and hemorrhage-crystalloid versus colloid replacement. *J Surg Res* 16:330–336, 1974.
67. Trinkle JK, Furman RW, Hinshaw MA, et al: Pulmonary contusion. *Ann Thorac Surg* 16:568–573, 1973.
68. Allen DA, Schertel ER, Muir WM, et al: Hypertonic saline/dextran resuscitation of dogs with experimentally induced gastric dilatation-volvulus shock. *Am J Vet Res* 52:92–96, 1991.
69. Kristensen J, Modig J: Ringer's acetate and dextran-70 with or without hypertonic saline in endotoxin-induced shock in pigs. *Crit Care Med* 18:1261–1268, 1990.
70. Rackow EC, Falk JL, Fein IA, et al: Fluid resuscitation in circulatory shock: A comparison of the cardiorespiratory effects of albumin, hetastarch, and saline solutions in patients with hypovolemic and septic shock. *Crit Care Med* 11:839–850, 1983.
71. Keene BW, Rush JE: Therapy of heart failure, in Ettinger SJ (ed): *Textbook of Veterinary Internal Medicine*. Philadelphia,

WB Saunders Co, 1989, pp 939–975.
72. Franz JL, Richardson JD, Grover FL, et al: Effect of methylprednisolone sodium succinate on experimental pulmonary contusions. *J Thorac Cardiovasc Surg* 68:842–844, 1974.
73. Wilson JW: Treatment or prevention of pulmonary cellular damage with pharmacological doses of corticosteroids. *Surg Gynecol Obstet* 134:675–681, 1975.
74. Svennevig JL, Bugge-Asperheim B, Geniran O, et al: High-dose corticosteroids in thoracic trauma. *Acta Scand Chir* 526:110–119, 1985.
75. Richardson JD, Woods D, Johanson WG Jr, et al: Lung bacterial clearance following pulmonary contusion. *Surgery* 86:730–735.
76. Houlton J: Acute trauma in small animals 2: Thoracic injuries. *In Pract* 8:152–162 1986.
77. Robertson R: Crushing injuries of the chest. *J Thorac Surg* 15:324–335, 1946.
78. Gardner Jr CE: Chest injuries. *Surg Clin North Am* 26:1082–1094, 1946.
79. Glinz W: Problems caused by the unstable thoracic wall and by cardiac injury due to blunt trauma. *Injury* 17:322–326, 1986.
80. Thompson SE, Johnson JM: Analgesia in dogs after intercostal thoracotomy: A comparison of morphine, selective intercostal nerve block, and intrapleural regional analgesia with bupivacaine. *Vet Surg* 20:73–77, 1991.
81. Hudson TR, McElvenny RT: Chest wall stabilization by soft tissue traction. *JAMA* 156:768–769, 1954.
82. Cohen EA: Treatment of the flail chest by towel clip traction. *Am J Surg* 90:517–521, 1955.
83. Jaslow IA: Skeletal traction in the treatment of multiple fractures of the thoracic cage. *Am J Surg* 72:753–755, 1946.
84. Jones TB, Richardson EP: Traction on the sternum in the treatment of multiple fractured ribs. *Surg Gynecol Obstet* 42:283–285, 1926.
85. Heroy WW, Eggleston FC: A method of skeletal traction applied through the sternum in steering wheel injury of the chest. *Ann Surg* 133:135–138, 1951.
86. Schmit-Neuerburg KP, Weiss H, Labitzke R: Indications for thoracotomy and chest wall stabilization. *Injury* 14:26–34, 1982.
87. Brasmer TH: The thoracic wall, in Bojrab MJ (ed): *Current Techniques in Small Animal Surgery*. Philadelphia, Lea & Febiger 1975, pp 198–202.
88. Sanchez-Lloret J, Letang E, Mateu M, et al: Indications and surgical treatment of the traumatic flail chest syndrome. An original technique. *Thorac Cardiovasc Surg* 30:294–297, 1982.
89. Borrelly J, Grosdidier G, Wack B: Notre experience de cing ans d'utilisation d'un nouveau materiel d'osteosynthese thoracique: lattelle-agrafe a glissieres (AAG). *Ann Chir* 39:465–470, 1985.
90. Borrelly J, Grosdidier G, Wack B: The stabilization of flail chest by sliding staples. *Revue Chir Orth* 71:241–250, 1985.
91. Menard A, Testart J, Philippe JM, et al: Treatment of flail chest with Judet's struts. *J Thorac Cardiovasc Surg* 86:300–305, 1983.
92. Graeber GM, Cohen DJ, Patrick DH, et al: Rib fracture healing in experimental flail chest. *J Trauma* 25:903–908, 1985.
93. Hellberg K, de Vivie ER, Fuchs K, et al: Stabilization of flail chest by compression osteosynthesis—Experimental and clinical results. *J Thorac Cardiovasc Surg* 29:275–281, 1981.
94. Ali J, Harding B, Ch B, et al: Effect of temporary external stabilization on ventilator weaning after sternal resection. *Chest* 95:472–473, 1989.
95. Fulton RL, Peter ET: Physiologic effects of fluid therapy after pulmonary contusion. *Am J Surg* 126:773–777, 1973.
96. Colville TP: First aid for epistaxis, respiratory obstructions, rib fractures, diaphragmatic hernia, bloat in ruminants and gastric dilatation in dogs. *Mod Vet Pract* 67:378–379, 1986.
97. Trinkle JK: Management of major thoracic wall trauma. *Curr Surg* 42:181–183, 1985.
98. Hankins JR, Shin B, McAslan TC, et al: Management of flail chest: An analysis of 99 cases. *Am J Surg* 45:176–181, 1979.
99. Lee RB, Morris JA Jr: Current concepts in the management of flail chest. *J Tenn Med Assoc* 81:631–633, 1988.

UPDATE

Flail chest has been infrequently reported in the veterinary literature over the past few years. Our article provided a comprehensive discussion of the pathogenesis, treatment, and prognosis of the veterinary patient sustaining multiple rib fractures; however, several new ideas on the management of flail chest have been described recently. While McNaulty, et al described the use of tongue depressors as an effective means of noninvasive external coaptation of rib fractures,[1] other methods of external coaptation have been described in the past.[2,3]

Since surgical and medical therapies for the treatment of rib fractures have been sporadic, the authors would like to comment on the use of colloidal therapy in the resuscitation of the veterinary patient after thoracic trauma. Although we briefly described the use of hetastarch and pentastarch in fluid resuscitation of the patient in shock, we caution against the use of these fluids in dogs or cats with early onset of pulmonary edema occurring concomitantly with flail chest. As described in our article, particle size of these polymers varies greatly. In situations where the vascular endothelium is vasodilated, low molecular-weight particles in hetastarch and pentastarch may escape the vascular space, drawing fluid with them.[4] As a consequence, the pulmonary edema may be exacerbated.

Finally, the authors believe that as the methods of monitoring trauma patients become more sophisticated (i.e., pulse oximetry, continuous ECG, and direct or indirect blood pressure), a better classification system to categorize the severity of flail chest may be developed. As a consequence, this may assist the veterinarian in predicting patient response to therapy.

Editor's Note: For further updated information on fluid therapy, refer to "Use of Hypertonic Saline Solutions in Hypovolemic Shock" (Duval, D.) in this volume.

REFERENCES

1. McNaulty JF: A simplified method for stabilization of flail chest injuries in small animals. *JAAHA* 31:137-141, 1995.
2. Kolata RJ: Management of thoracic trauma. *Vet Clin North Am Small Anim Pract* 11:103-120, 1984.
3. Bjorling DE, Kolata RF: Flail chest: A review, clinical experience and a new method of stabilization. *JAAHA* 18:269-276, 1982.
4. Rackow EC, Falk JL, Fein IA, et al: Fluid resuscitation in circulatory shock: A comparison of the cardiorespiratory effects of albumin, hetastarch, and saline solutions in patients with hypovolemic and septic shock. *Crit Care Med* 11:839-850, 1983.

Heatstroke in Dogs

KEY FACTS

- Heatstroke occurs commonly during forced confinement or exercise in hot, humid environments.
- As environmental temperature approaches body temperature, evaporative cooling through panting is the primary mechanism of heat loss.
- A selective loss of splanchnic vasoconstriction is a key event in the pathogenesis of heatstroke.
- At body core temperatures above 43°C, severe internal organ damage occurs; this increases mortality in dogs with heatstroke.
- To lower the core temperature, ice-water immersion techniques are inferior to immediate cooling via evaporative techniques and selective placement of ice packs over large superficial veins.

40th GAINES CYCLE
SYMPOSIUM 1992
Sponsor by Gaines® Cycle®

University of Melbourne, Australia
Steven A. Holloway, BVSc, MVS

EACH SUMMER in the United States, dogs are presented to veterinarians for treatment of heatstroke. Heatstroke is defined as the state of extreme hyperthermia that occurs when excess heat (generated by body metabolism, exercise, and/or environmental conditions) exceeds the body's ability to dissipate heat.[1] Although heatstroke is encountered sporadically in veterinary practice, it is a life-threatening emergency that requires quick therapeutic intervention and recognition of dangerous sequelae to avoid death of the patient.

In comparison with the large amount of information on heatstroke in the human medical literature, there is a paucity of information in the veterinary literature concerning canine heatstroke. Because relatively few veterinary case reports have been published recently,[2-6] much of the information contained in this article is gleaned from the human medical literature and from experimental studies of heatstroke in dogs. The discussion is prefaced by a review of thermoregulation and is followed by a description of pathophysiologic processes, clinical signs, and treatment modalities.

THERMOREGULATION

Because of the process of thermoregulation, the temperature of the deep tissues of the body (the core temperature) remains almost constant under various environmental conditions.[7] The core temperature represents the balance between heat gain and heat loss. Heat gain can be of endogenous (metabolism and exercise) or exogenous (environmental) origins. Heat loss from the body can occur by convection, conduction, radiation, or evaporation (Figure 1).

At ambient temperatures below 32°C (89.5°F), convection, conduction, and radiation contribute to the maintenance of normothermia. As environmental temperature increases and approaches body temperature, evaporative heat loss becomes an increasingly important defense mechanism of normothermia. In humans, evaporative heat loss occurs through the process of sweating; in dogs, evaporative heat loss occurs through panting.[7]

The panting response is initiated by neurogenic signals relayed from the hypothalamus to the panting center, which is closely related to the pneumotaxic center of the pons. When the core temperature increases, the blood supplying the hypothalamus is overheated; this initiates the neurogenic signals to decrease body temperature. Panting brings large quantities of air into contact with the mucosal surfaces of the mouth and nose. In addition, dogs drool saliva when they overheat, thus providing a large amount of water for evaporative cooling. As water evaporates from the mucosal surfaces of the mouth and nose, cooling of the mucosal blood supply and lowering of body core temperature occur.

In situations of abnormally increased ambient temperature and humidity, evaporative heat loss mechanisms are hindered and the core temperature increases. The increased core temperature causes an increase in metabolic rate and

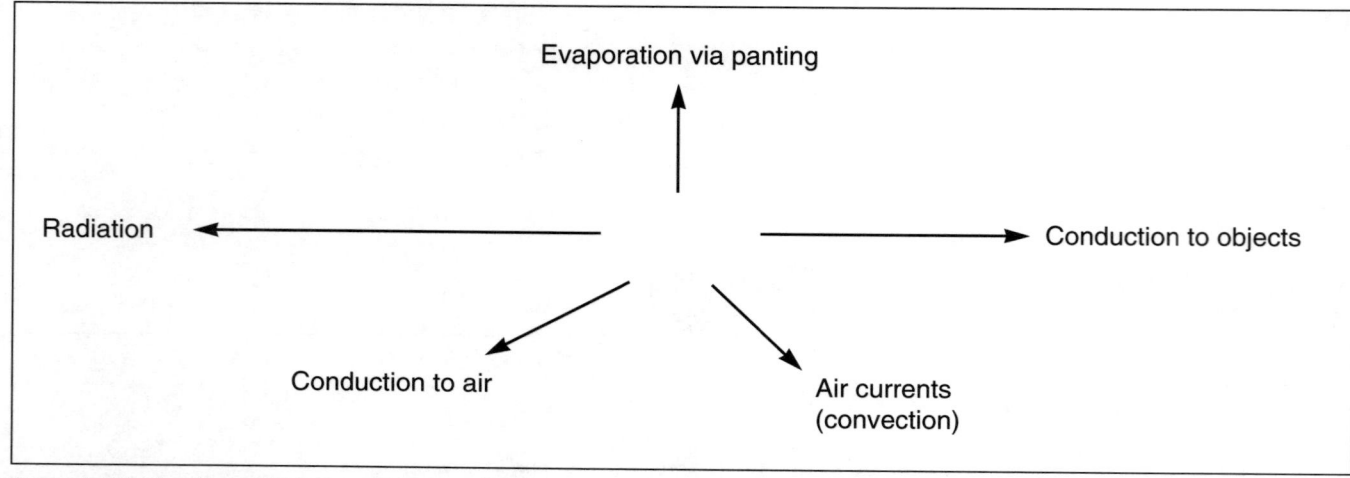

Figure 1—Mechanisms of heat loss from the body.

endogenous heat production; a vicious cycle is initiated.[8] The core temperature continues to increase and culminates in the clinical syndrome of heatstroke. As the core temperature exceeds 43°C (109°F) in dogs, severe organ damage occurs and mortality increases markedly.[9]

PATHOPHYSIOLOGY

Heatstroke occurs in exertional and nonexertional (classic) types. There may be increased endogenous heat production (exertional heatstroke), increased exogenous heat load (classic heatstroke), or a combination of the two types.[8,10]

Exertional heatstroke in dogs is uncommon but may occur during forced exercise in hot and/or humid environments. This is particularly true in highly motivated greyhounds training or racing in the southern United States. In studies conducted at the University of Florida College of Veterinary Medicine, rectal temperatures of racing greyhounds often exceeded 42°C after a 400-meter race.[11] Although these temperatures are not life threatening for short periods, a lack of shade and a cooling-down period after a race may produce exertional heatstroke. I am aware of two dogs that developed exertional heatstroke after forced exercise (running next to an owner riding a bike) in a hot environment without adequate fluid intake or a cooling-down period.

During the initial stages of experimental heatstroke, panting causes minimal changes in alveolar ventilation. With continuing heat stress, panting becomes more forceful and respiratory minute volume and alveolar ventilation increase; marked respiratory alkalosis develops.[10,12] In such cases, arterial pH may increase to 7.7 to 7.8 while PCO_2 decreases to approximately 8 to 10 mm Hg.[10,13] Despite these changes, hyperthermia overrides the effects of cerebrospinal fluid hypocapnia and alkalosis on the respiratory center of the brain stem; panting continues, becoming slower and deeper.[13] With ongoing hyperthermia, respiratory alkalosis is modified within three to four hours by metabolic acidosis.

In exertional heatstroke, combined respiratory alkalosis and metabolic acidosis may be evident on initial evaluation of arterial or venous blood gas values. Metabolic acidosis develops in exercising animals because of the production of lactic acid by working muscle cells.

In classic heatstroke, metabolic acidosis develops after the onset of severe hypotension (systolic pressure less than 50 mm Hg) and lactic acid production. With continuing hyperthermia, hypotension and metabolic acidosis worsen; cerebral edema, decreased respirations, and eventually apnea develop. Death occurs shortly thereafter.[10]

DURING the early stages of heat stress, cardiac output is markedly increased as a result of decreased peripheral vascular resistance after cutaneous vasodilation and the displacement of blood to active muscles during exercise.[13] To compensate for decreased vascular resistance, splanchnic blood flow is decreased to maintain normal blood pressure and circulating plasma volume. As the core temperature continues to increase, however, skin blood flow increases. At this stage, splanchnic arterioles are unable to constrict enough to prevent venous pooling, and blood pressure and cardiac output are decreased.[13] With the decline in cardiac output, circulating plasma volume decreases and heat dissipation mechanisms fail; the results are a spiral increase in temperature and the onset of heatstroke.[14,15]

These findings suggest that the selective loss of splanchnic vasoconstriction is a key point in the pathogenesis of heatstroke; this is further supported by experimental studies in hyperthermic laboratory animals.[14,15] Alternatively, myocardial injury and a marked increase in pulmonary vascular resistance have been proposed as a cause of decreased cardiac output in humans with heatstroke.[16,17] A similar increase in pulmonary vascular resistance in dogs has not been reported.

Irreparable organ damage occurs at core temperatures above 43°C.[9] At this temperature, oxidative phosphorylation is uncoupled, cellular membrane function is impaired, and critical enzymes are denatured.[18] Organ failure may occur following widespread cellular death, even after the core temperature has returned to normal.

Acute renal failure is a common complication of heatstroke.[6,9,13,19–22] Renal failure occurs because of direct thermal injury to the renal tubular epithelium, decreased renal blood flow and hypotension, and thrombosis associated with disseminated intravascular coagulation (DIC).[21]

THE INCIDENCE of heatstroke-induced hepatic damage in canine patients is unknown. Hepatic damage has been documented in case reports and experimental studies of canine heatstroke.[6,9,13] In one case report, increased hepatic transaminase values occurred in two of three dogs in the 24-hour period after treatment for heatstroke.[6] Further, thrombosis and hemorrhage were present on histopathologic examination of hepatic tissue from dogs experimentally subjected to heatstroke. In comparison, liver specimens in humans with heatstroke exhibited cholestasis, centrilobular necrosis, and vascular degeneration.[23] Heatstroke-induced hepatic damage results from the effects of direct thermal injury to hepatocytes and prolonged splanchnic hypotension.

In the digestive tract, the effects of profound hypotension and exposure to thermal injury may cause widespread gastrointestinal epithelial damage; massive hematemesis and hemorrhagic stools may result.[8,19] With disruption of the intestinal mucosal barrier, gram-negative bacteremia and septic shock may further complicate heatstroke.[19]

During heatstroke, the occurrence of widespread endothelial damage and cell necrosis may cause the consumption of platelets and coagulation factors; hemorrhagic diathesis caused by disseminated intravascular coagulation results.[9,19,24,25] In addition, platelets may become thermally inactivated after exposure to abnormally high body temperature; this may further complicate bleeding during recovery from heatstroke.[26]

Direct thermal damage to neurons is a consequence of prolonged exposure to core temperatures above 43°C. Thermal damage to vascular endothelium may produce brain hemorrhage and edema, thrombosis, and infarction of cerebral tissue with subsequent coma or seizures.[9] The potential for reversal of cerebral edema is related to the length of exposure of neurons to abnormal temperatures. Coma is often reversible in humans if early cooling is initiated. With prolonged exposure to high temperatures, neuron death occurs and results in permanent brain damage.[19]

Respiratory complications of canine heatstroke have not been reported. In humans with heatstroke, cor pulmonale, pulmonary edema, and adult respiratory distress syndrome may complicate recovery.[7,17,22,27] Causal factors include direct thermal injury to pulmonary vascular endothelium, myocardial dysfunction, and the return of a large volume of plasma to the central circulation after cooling-induced vasoconstriction.

CLINICAL FINDINGS

The initial findings in dogs with heatstroke include rapid panting, tachycardia, hyperdynamic arterial pulse, and hyperemic and dry mucous membranes.[9,10,12] In patients presented at a late stage of heatstroke, physical examination demonstrates signs of profound depression, prostration, and vasocollapse. Clinically, these signs in the presence of severe hyperthermia (core temperature greater than 43°C) and marked respiratory effort strongly indicate heatstroke.

As heatstroke worsens, the femoral pulse weakens and the mucous membranes become pale to ashen in color (signaling inadequate cardiac output). At this stage, vomiting and diarrhea ensue and suggest the presence of severe gastrointestinal damage. Dogs presented in the terminal stages of heatstroke may have shallow respirations and tend toward apnea. Seizures or coma can develop terminally.[9,10,13]

If successful cooling measures are instituted, clinical signs related to the presence of disseminated intravascular coagulation and renal, hepatic, and gastrointestinal damage may occur as long as three to five days after apparent recovery. These signs include oliguria, vomiting and/or bloody diarrhea, icterus, dyspnea, and bleeding tendencies.

DIAGNOSIS

In most cases, a history of confinement in a hot environment together with the clinical signs of heatstroke is sufficient for diagnosis. Similarly, if increased environmental temperature and humidity coincide with clinical evidence of heatstroke associated with a history of forced exercise, a diagnosis of exertional heatstroke should be considered.

If there is no historical evidence of confinement or exercise during hot weather, the differential diagnosis includes meningitis, encephalitis, and other inflammatory or infectious diseases. Space-occupying lesions that involve the hypothalamic thermoregulatory center also may cause marked hyperthermia. Malignant hyperthermia should be considered in dogs that are exposed to inhalational anesthetic agents (e.g., halothane).

LABORATORY FINDINGS

Serum chemistry findings in patients with heatstroke reflect major organ damage. Increased blood urea nitrogen and serum creatinine, together with an increased number of renal tubular casts, may occur with acute tubular necrosis. Similarly, increased hepatic transaminase enzymes (aspartate transaminase [AST] and alanine transaminase [ALT]) and increased serum bilirubin suggest liver damage.[6,9,13]

> **Initial Management of Heatstroke**
>
> Transportation to a cooled environment
> Immediate cooling using evaporative techniques augmented by ice packs over axillary and inguinal regions and neck
> Placement of an intravenous catheter (preferably in a large vein)
> Meticulous fluid therapy for hemodynamic stabilization
> Continuous monitoring of rectal temperature
> Insertion of a Foley urinary catheter to monitor urine output
> Baseline laboratory tests (including complete blood and platelet count, blood urea nitrogen, creatinine, glucose, liver enzymes, coagulation profile, and urinalysis)

TABLE I
Treatment of Complications of Heatstroke

Complication	Treatment
Coma	Cooling to reverse coma
Hypotension	Cooling and cautious fluid administration
Seizures	Intravenous diazepam (0.5 mg/kg)
Oliguria or anuria	Intravenous furosemide (1 mg/kg every two hours) and dopamine (2.5 µg/kg/min)
Disseminated intravascular coagulation	Subcutaneous heparin (100 to 150 units/kg every eight hours) plus fresh plasma transfusion
Liver failure	Fluid therapy, correction of hypoglycemia, and broad-spectrum antibiotic prophylaxis

Heatstroke-induced rhabdomyolysis causes markedly increased serum creatine phosphokinase (CK) and aspartate transaminase values.[19]

The presence of thrombocytopenia, hypofibrinogenemia, increased fibrin split products, and prolonged prothrombin times (PT) and partial thromboplastin times (PTT) indicates the onset of disseminated intravascular coagulation. These abnormal values often presage terminal hemorrhagic diathesis.

Hemoconcentration caused by volume depletion may be severe in heatstroke, with the packed cell volume increasing more than 30% above normal values.[10] Serum sodium and chloride levels also increase. Dogs with heatstroke frequently develop mild hyperkalemia. In comparison, humans affected by heatstroke commonly develop hypokalemia.[10,20,28] In dogs that develop oliguric renal failure and/or concomitant rhabdomyolysis, however, marked hyperkalemia may occur.

TREATMENT

The goals of treatment are threefold: to manage hyperthermia (see Initial Management of Heatstroke), to provide intensive cardiovascular support, and to treat complications (Table I).

Initial management of heatstroke depends on early diagnosis and lowering of the core temperature. Cooling must be undertaken immediately because any delay in treatment increases the possibility of secondary complications and death.[8,19,29] In field conditions, a heatstroke-affected dog should be moved immediately to a shaded area; the coat is thoroughly soaked with cool water. The application of cold packs to the inguinal, axillary, and jugular vein areas will cool central venous blood and lower body core temperature without causing vasoconstriction.[30,31] Immediately after initial treatment, the patient should be transferred to a veterinary hospital.

Various methods of lowering the core temperature have been suggested.[8,19,29,30–38] Ice-water baths are traditionally used to treat heatstroke, but this may be difficult in a collapsed or comatose patient. Such baths have the disadvantage of promoting cutaneous vasoconstriction, which impairs heat loss and induces shivering.[8,29] Furthermore, experimental studies demonstrate that cool tap water is as effective as ice-water immersion in lowering body temperature.[35] In humans, the most successful and commonly used technique is to saturate the skin with cool water (17.2°C [63°F]) and circulate air over the patient to promote evaporative cooling.

Other techniques described include administration of chilled intravenous fluids, iced gastric lavage, and cold water enemas.[33–37] These techniques lower the core temperature without causing cutaneous vasoconstriction. In an experimental study of hyperthermic dogs, cold peritoneal lavage lowered body temperature better than iced slush and room-air evaporative cooling techniques.[36]

Contrary to these findings, another experimental study in hyperthermic dogs demonstrated evaporative cooling via tap water to be superior to iced gastric lavage in terms of rate of cooling and return to baseline cardiac indexes.[37] In conscious dogs, peritoneal lavage and iced gastric lavage are more difficult to perform than evaporative cooling techniques. Regardless of the cooling method used, the overall goal is a reduction of the core temperature to approximately 39°C (102°F) in 30 to 60 minutes. The use of a high rectal thermistor probe instead of a clinical thermometer (which only measures up to 42.5°C [108°F]) helps in monitoring the effects of cooling procedures.

Once the body temperature reaches 39°C, cooling measures should be discontinued because further decreases in the core temperature induce shivering and heat production.[8] Although the administration of phenothiazine tranquilizers to prevent shivering has been recommended, I do not recommend them because of their hypotensive effects and their ability to further depress consciousness in a critically ill patient.[10] In some patients, the core temperature may continue to decline after the cooling procedures; monitoring of temperature thus is extremely important, and warming may be necessary in order to maintain core temperature at 39° to 39.5°C (102° to 103°F).

PATIENTS with hemoconcentration and hypotension should be treated cautiously with intravenous fluids. In cases of heatstroke, the actual fluid deficit may be modest. The central venous pressure, pulse strength, capillary refill time, urine output, and respiratory rate should be closely monitored during treatment for hypotension and circulatory shock.

The use of glucocorticoids has not been found to be valuable in treating heatstroke in humans[8] and should be reserved for specific complications (e.g., cerebral edema and septic shock). Similarly, I do not recommend the use of nonsteroidal antiinflammatory agents in treating shock associated with heatstroke because of their potential for exacerbating heatstroke-induced renal damage and their ability to promote gastric ulceration.

In many cases, hypotension improves with cooling measures alone because cutaneous vasoconstriction directly increases the circulating blood volume. Overzealous parenteral fluid administration during initial treatment thus should be avoided in order to prevent the onset of pulmonary edema. If serum electrolyte and acid–base parameters are unavailable, lactated Ringer's solution should be used initially.

After successful temperature-lowering treatment measures, the dangerous sequelae to heatstroke should be considered. If acute tubular necrosis and oliguric renal failure occur, intravenous furosemide (1 mg/kg every two hours) and dopamine (2 to 5 µg/kg/min) may be given to improve urine production. Euhydration must be restored before any form of diuresis is attempted. Persistently oliguric or anuric patients require peritoneal dialysis to maintain metabolic homeostasis; the prognosis in this circumstance is guarded to grave.

Patients with disseminated intravascular coagulation are treated with transfusions of fresh-frozen plasma, to provide coagulation factors, and low-dose heparin (100 to 150 units/kg) given subcutaneously three times daily.[38] The use of heparin should be restricted in the presence of hemorrhagic diathesis.

Treatment of liver failure and severe gastroenteric disease is mainly supportive and is coupled with maintenance of fluid and electrolyte balance, correction of hypoglycemia, and use of antiemetics if required. The presence of severe gastrointestinal damage may be associated with bacteremia; empirical therapy with broad-spectrum nonnephrotoxic antibiotics should be administered. Cerebral edema is treated with intravenous dexamethasone (1 to 2 mg/kg).[10] Seizures are initially treated with intravenous diazepam (0.5 mg/kg).

Antipyretics (e.g., aspirin and dipyrone), which work by lowering the body's thermoregulatory set point, are ineffective and potentially dangerous.[8] Similarly, dantrolene sodium, which reduces endogenous heat production, lacks efficacy in managing heatstroke.[39-41]

PREVENTION

For dogs that are confined in hot environments, prevention requires education of owners concerning the risk of confining and exercising dogs in such environments. To prevent exertional hyperthermia, exercise should be undertaken during the cooler periods of the day. In particular, greyhound racing should be scheduled for early morning or evening, when the temperature is cooler. Furthermore, only well-conditioned dogs should be subjected to vigorous exercise in hot environments. Adequate shade and intake of fluids before, during, and after exercise are essential.

SUMMARY

Heatstroke may occur when dogs are forced to exercise or are confined in a hot environment. In normal conditions of temperature and humidity, the body's core temperature is maintained by the process of evaporative cooling via panting. In severe heat stress, heat gain exceeds heat loss via panting and the core temperature increases. At body core temperatures approaching 43°C, a selective loss of splanchnic vasoconstriction occurs; hypovolemia, a failure of thermoregulation, and the clinical signs of heatstroke result.

Treatment by means of a combination of evaporative cooling techniques and ice packs placed over large superficial veins should be started as soon as possible. A patient's chances of survival are improved by recognition and treatment of the dangerous sequelae to heatstroke.

ACKNOWLEDGMENT

The author thanks Michael Schaer, DVM, of the Department of Veterinary Clinical Sciences, College of Veterinary Medicine, University of Florida, for his assistance in the preparation of this article.

About the Author

Dr. Holloway, who is a Diplomate of the American College of Veterinary Internal Medicine, is affiliated with the Department of Veterinary Science at the University of Melbourne, Australia.

REFERENCES

1. Shapiro Y, Seidman DS: Field and clinical observations of exertional heat stroke patients. *Med Sci Sports Exerc* 22(1):6–12, 1990.
2. Meyer HP: A case of heat shock. *Tijdschr Diergeneesk* 115(23):1118–1122, 1990.

3. Caird JJ, Mann N: Fatal heat stroke in a dog. *Vet Rec* 121(3):72, 1987.
4. Heat stroke in a dog (letter). *Vet Rec* 121(6):135–136, 1987.
5. Clutton RE: Atropine and the control of heat stroke (letter). *Vet Rec* 121(13):311–312, 1987.
6. Krum SH, Osborne CA: Heat stroke in the dog. A polysystemic disorder. *JAVMA* 170(5):531–535, 1977.
7. Guyton AC: *Textbook of Medical Physiology*, ed 8. Philadelphia, WB Saunders Co, 1991, pp 801–804.
8. Louzon H: Heat illness, in May H (ed): *Emergency Medicine*, ed 2. New York, John Wiley & Sons, 1992, pp 425–430.
9. Shapiro Y, Rosenthal T, Sohar E: Experimental heatstroke, a model in dogs. *Arch Intern Med* 131:688–692, 1973.
10. Schall WD: Heat stroke, in Kirk RW (ed): *Current Veterinary Therapy*, ed 8. Philadelphia, WB Saunders Co, 1983, pp 183–185.
11. Rose RJ, Bloomberg MS: Responses to sprint exercise in the greyhound: Effects on hematology, serum biochemistry, and muscle metabolism. *Res Vet Sci* 47:212–218, 1989.
12. Hales JRS, Bligh J, Maskrey M: Cerebrospinal fluid acid-base balance during respiratory alkalosis in the panting animal. *Am J Physiol* 219(2):468–473, 1970.
13. Hales JRS, Bligh J: Respiratory responses of the conscious dog to severe heat stress. *Experiment* 25(8):818–819, 1969.
14. Horowitz M, Nadel ER: Effect of plasma volume on thermoregulation in the dog. *Pflugers Arch* 400:211–213, 1984.
15. Kregel KC, Wall TP, Gisolfi CV: Peripheral vascular responses to hyperthermia in the rat. *J Appl Physiol* 64(6):2582–2588, 1988.
16. O'Donnel TF, Clowes GHA: The circulatory abnormalities of heat stroke. *N Engl J Med* 287:734–737, 1972.
17. Clowes GHA, O'Donnel TF: Current concepts: Heat stroke. *N Engl J Med* 291(1):564–567, 1974.
18. Hubbard RW: Heatstroke pathophysiology: The energy depletion model. *Med Sci Sports Exerc* 22(1):19–28, 1990.
19. Shibolet S, Lancaster MC, Danon Y: Heat stroke: A review. *Aviat Space Environ Med* 47(3):280–301, 1976.
20. Knochel JP, Beisel WR, Herndon EG, et al: The renal, cardiovascular, hematologic and serum electrolyte abnormalities of heat stroke. *Am J Med* 30(1):299–308, 1961.
21. Schrier RW, Hano J, Keller HI, et al: Renal, metabolic and circulatory responses to heat and exercise. *Ann Intern Med* 73(2):213–223, 1970.
22. Chao TC, Sinniah R, Parkiam JE: Acute heat stroke deaths. *Pathology* 13(1):145–156, 1981.
23. Rubel LR: Hepatic injury associated with heatstroke. *Ann Clin Lab Sci* 14(2):130–136, 1984.
24. Reed WA, Manning RT, Hopkins LT: Effect of hypoxia and hyperthermia on hepatic tissue of the dog. *Am J Physiol* 206:1304–1308, 1957.
25. Rosenthal T, Shapiro Y, Seligsohn V, et al: Disseminated intravascular coagulation in experimental heat stroke. *Thromb Diath Haemor* 26:417–425, 1971.
26. White JG: Effects of heat on platelet structure and function. *Blood* 32(2):324–335, 1968.
27. El-Kassimi FA, Al-Mashadanni S, Akhtar J: Adult respiratory distress syndrome and disseminated intravascular coagulation complicating heat stroke. *Chest* 90(4):571–574, 1986.
28. Spurr GB, Barlow G: Tissue electrolytes in hyperthermic dogs. *J Appl Physiol* 28(1):13–17, 1970.
29. Tek DA, Olshaker JS: Hyperthermia, pulmonary edema and disseminated intravascular coagulation in a military recruit. *Ann Emerg Med* 19(6):715–722, 1990.
30. Costrini A: Emergency treatment of exertional heatstroke and comparison of whole body cooling techniques. *Med Sci Sports Exerc* 22(1):15–18, 1990.
31. Hanson PG: Treatment of heatstroke (letter). *West J Med* 134:167, 1981.
32. Syverud SA, Barber WJ, Amsterdam JT, et al: Iced gastric lavage for treatment of heatstroke—Efficacy in a canine model. *Ann Emerg Med* 14(5):424–432, 1985.
33. Bynum G, Patton J, Bowers W, et al: Peritoneal lavage cooling in an anesthetized dog heat stroke model. *Aviat Space Environ Med* 49(6):779–784, 1978.
34. Barker WJ, Falls-Church V, Amsterdam JT, et al: High frequency jet ventilation cooling in a canine hyperthermia model. *Ann Emerg Med* 15(6):680–684, 1986.
35. Magazanik A, Epstein Y, Udassin R, et al: Tap-water, an efficient method for cooling heatstroke victims—A model in dogs. *Aviat Space Environ Med* 51(9):864–867, 1980.
36. Graham BS, Lichenstein MJ, Hinson JM, et al: Non-exertional heat stroke. Physiologic management and cooling in fourteen patients. *Arch Intern Med* 146(1):87–90, 1986.
37. White JD, Riccobene E, Nicci R, et al: Evaporation versus iced gastric lavage treatment of heatstroke: Comparative efficacy in a canine model. *Crit Care Med* 15(8):748–750, 1987.
38. Greene CE: Management of DIC and thrombosis, in Kirk RW (ed): *Current Veterinary Therapy*, ed 8. Philadelphia, WB Saunders Co, 1983, pp 401–405.
39. Syverud SA, Barker WJ, Amsterdam JT: Dantrolene sodium for treatment of heatstroke. Lack of efficacy in a canine model. *Crit Care Med* 12(3):243, 1986.
40. Murphy RJ: Heat illness in the athlete. *Am J Sports Med* 12(4):258–261, 1984.
41. Beyer CB: Heat stress and the young athlete, recognizing and reducing the risks. *Postgrad Med* 76(1):109–112, 1984.

Hypothermia in Dogs and Cats

Tufts University
Nishi Dhupa, BVM, MRCVS

KEY FACTS

- Hypothermia can occur in any healthy animal exposed to severe cold.

- Impairment of thermoregulatory mechanisms (behavioral and metabolic) will predispose an animal to hypothermia.

- Animals with moderate to severe hypothermia are at risk of developing cardiac arrhythmia.

- Rewarming techniques depend on the degree of hypothermia; aggressive core rewarming methods are reserved for animals with severe hypothermia.

- Prolonged hypothermia may result in multiorgan system dysfunction, including cardiac dysfunction, respiratory compromise, and coagulopathy.

Hypothermia is defined as a state of body temperature that is below normal in a homeothermic organism.[1] Hypothermia develops in healthy animals as a result of an inability to maintain thermal homeostasis after prolonged or intense exposure to cold. In more moderate environmental conditions, hypothermia may be a manifestation of disease processes that alter normal thermoregulation[2] or may develop inadvertently when anesthetic agents[3] or other drugs are used. In this article, mild hypothermia will be defined as a core body temperature ranging from 32°C to 37°C (90°F to 99°F), moderate hypothermia as a range from 28°C to 32°C (82°F to 90°F), and severe hypothermia as any temperature below 28°C (82°F).

THERMOREGULATION

Normal body temperature is a function of the balance between heat loss from the skin and lungs and heat production in the skeletal muscle and liver.[4] Body temperature is controlled by the thermoregulatory center in the hypothalamus; this center is responsive to changes in blood and skin temperature. In dogs and cats, heat loss to the environment occurs mainly through convection and conduction. An animal exposed to a cold environment will attempt to conserve heat through behavioral means (e.g., seeking shelter or curling up) as well as through reflex physiologic responses, including piloerection and peripheral vasoconstriction. The trapping of a layer of air next to the skin as well as the shunting of blood away from the periphery of the body creates thermal insulation.[4] Heat production involves voluntary muscle activity (i.e., shivering) and an increase in cellular metabolic rate. The failure of these protective mechanisms results in hypothermia.

PREDISPOSING FACTORS

Hypothermia can occur in any healthy, conscious animal exposed to severe cold. It also may occur at relatively moderate environmental temperatures in animals with impaired heat production and conservation mechanisms. Factors that predispose animals to hypothermia are listed in Table I and described in the following section.

Small animals are more susceptible to hypothermia because of the greater surface area:mass ratio. Neonates and geriatric animals may not respond appropriately to changes in the environment.[4] In addition, neonates (as well as cachectic animals) have reduced reserves of muscle, glycogen, and fat, which

TABLE I
Factors that Predispose to Hypothermia

Decreased Heat Production	Increased Heat Loss
Neonates	Burns
Trauma	Trauma
Immobility (e.g., as a result of unconsciousness, leg hold traps, or debility)	Immobility (e.g., as a result of unconsciousness, leg hold traps, or debility)
Anesthesia	Exposure to the environment (e.g., as a result of immersion in cold water)
Cachexia	General anesthesia
Cardiac disease	Surgery
Impaired thermoregulation	Increased surface area: mass (as occurs in small dogs and cats and in young animals)
Endocrine disorders (e.g., hypothyroidism, hypopituitarism, adrenal insufficiency, or hypoglycemia)	Exposure to toxic agents (e.g., ethylene glycol or barbiturates)
Neuromuscular disorders	

are required for heat production.

Animals that have experienced major trauma also are at increased risk of developing hypothermia because of forced immobility and compromised body surfaces. Animals with burns over a large portion of the body are at risk of having large evaporative losses and severe underlying illness. Immersion in cold water poses special dangers because the high thermal conductivity of water results in rapid cooling.

Impairment of central metabolic control can seriously affect the response of the body to hypothermic stimuli. Hypothyroidism can result in depressed core body temperature (even in the absence of adverse environmental conditions) and inefficient metabolic and shivering responses.[5] Hypoglycemia may facilitate hypothermia by lowering cerebral intracellular glucose concentrations and impairing hypothalamic function.[6] Panhypopituitarism and adrenal insufficiency, although infrequent causes of hypothermia, blunt the response of the body to the stress of cold.[7,8] Central nervous system disorders and carbon monoxide poisoning also can produce hypothermia by impairment of hypothalamic function.

Iatrogenic hypothermia can occur as a result of general anesthesia or surgery. General anesthesia can lead to impaired thermoregulation, depression of metabolism, and elimination of the shivering response. During surgery, direct losses of heat can occur from exposed body surfaces.

Other predisposing factors to hypothermia include toxicity associated with consumption of alcohol, ethylene glycol, barbiturates, and phenothiazines. Such toxicity results in peripheral vasodilatation and increased heat loss as well as impairment of the shivering mechanism.[8,9]

PATHOPHYSIOLOGY

When body temperature is between 32°C (90°F) and 37°C (99°F), compensatory mechanisms work to restore normothermia. The initial response of the homeothermic animal is an increase in sympathetic release, muscular activity (shivering), vasoconstriction, oxygen consumption, respiratory rate, pulse rate, blood pressure, and cardiac output.[10–12] The result is a decrease in heat loss and an increase in endogenous heat production. As cooling progresses from 32°C (90°F) to approximately 28°C (82°F), thermoregulation begins to fail. Shivering stops, muscles become rigid, and mental depression becomes obvious. Pupillary light reflexes are decreased. Sinus bradycardia, depressed respiration, and hypotension are observed.[13] Increased blood viscosity and increased afterload secondary to peripheral vasoconstriction and capillary sludging reduce cardiac output. The physiologic changes associated with hypothermia are listed in Table II.

Changes seen on an electrocardiogram include lengthening of the PR, QRS, and QT intervals. In humans, the Osborn J wave is pathognomonic for severe hypothermia. This electrocardiographic abnormality, which is a secondary, positive wave that follows the S wave, is seen more prominently in the avL, avF, and all left chest leads. The Osborn J wave has rarely been recognized in small animals.[14,15]

Atrial irritability is a feature of early hypothermia. As body temperature decreases, ventricular irritability increases and the animal is predisposed to such dysrhythmias as premature ventricular contractions and ventricular tachycardia. When body temperature is below 28°C (82°F), ventricular fibrillation is very common and tends to be unresponsive to electrical defibrillation.[10,16,17]

As body temperature decreases, the most obvious central nervous system change is a decreased level of consciousness, which culminates in coma. Signs of hypothermia that are related to the central nervous and cardiovascular systems depend on the rate at which cooling occurs in an individual animal and how the particular animal acclimates to cold.

An animal with severe hypothermia may seem dead. Under such conditions, an animal is protected against anoxia because of a decrease in cellular metabolism. The decreased cellular metabolism allows the animal to meet the metabolic demands of the body for a short period, even in the presence of profound bradycardia, asystole, or ventricular fibrillation. In

TABLE II
Physiologic Changes Associated with Hypothermia

Core Temperature	Physiology	Signs
32°C–37°C (90°F–99°F) (Mild)	Increased basal metabolic rate; increased oxygen consumption; vasoconstriction; sympathetic release	Heat-seeking ataxia; shivering; tachypnea, tachycardia; diuresis
28°C–32°C (82°F–90°F) (Moderate)	Decreased basal metabolic rate; decreased oxygen consumption; decreased cerebral blood flow; fluid shifts and hypovolemia; alkalosis and acidosis	Loss of shivering; muscle rigidity; mental obtundation; cardiac dysrhythmias; hypotension
<28°C (<82°F) (Severe)	Loss of thermoregulation; vasodilatation; decreased conduction; slowed nerve conduction; increased cardiac irritability; decreased cardiac output and asystole; apnea; suspended central nervous system activity	Stupor or coma; fixed dilated pupils; bradycardia; loss of reflexes; ventricular fibrillation; lack of pulse and hypotension; appearance of death

dogs, oxygen consumption is decreased to 50% of normal when body temperature is 30°C (86°F)[10] and 16% of normal at a body temperature of 23°C (73°F).[18] Oxygen delivery is also slowed by a combination of alveolar hypoventilation, decreased dissociation of oxyhemoglobin, and sludging of blood. Cellular function can still be maintained under these circumstances.[19]

Laboratory evaluation of hypothermic animals may reveal multiple abnormalities. Metabolic acidosis, if present, is caused by lactic acid accumulation. This accumulation is the result of decreased tissue perfusion, increased muscle use in shivering, and decreased liver metabolism. In animals with mild hypothermia, tachypnea may result in mixed respiratory alkalosis and metabolic acidosis. As body temperature decreases, consciousness is depressed and the resultant reduction in respiratory rate may lead to respiratory acidosis. Respiratory function may become impaired further as fluid shifts into the alveoli and interstitium of the lung begin to limit oxygen diffusion. Limited oxygen diffusion and decreased dissociation of oxygen from oxyhemoglobin result in decreased oxygen delivery to tissue. Bronchial secretions become thick and tenacious and may predispose to infections.

The renal effects of hypothermia include diuresis resulting in part from reduced tubular reabsorption[20] and depressed production of antidiuretic hormone. These events are a direct consequence of increased blood volume caused by early vasoconstriction. After the initial diuresis, renal blood flow and glomerular filtration rate decrease as cardiac output decreases.

Cellular metabolism increases in animals with mild hypothermia, thereby producing osmotically active metabolites in the intracellular space. The osmotic forces that are generated create significant intracellular shifts. There is also an increase in transcapillary fluid loss into the extravascular space. Increases in hematocrit reflect the resultant hemoconcentration.

Electrolyte changes are unpredictable and should be evaluated on an individual basis. As hypothermia progresses, the concentration of serum sodium tends to decrease and the concentration of serum potassium to increase, probably because enzymatic activity of the cell membrane sodium–potassium pump is decreased.[21] Total body sodium and potassium concentrations, however, may be close to normal.

Hypothermia has complex effects on blood coagulation. Splenic sequestration induced by hypothermia results in reduced white blood cell and platelet counts.[22] Disseminated intravascular coagulation also may occur in severe cases.[8,23] Hypothermia has been shown to cause platelet dysfunction that can be reversed by rewarming to a normal body temperature.[24] Experimental studies in hypothermic dogs have demonstrated variable alterations in clotting factor levels.[25,26] Hypothermia also has been shown to prolong the coagulation times (activated partial thromboplastin time [APTT] and prothrombin time [PT]) of human plasma that contains normal levels of coagulation factors.[27] In clinical laboratories, standard kinetic tests of coagulation are routinely performed at 37°C (99°F); therefore, results will not reflect the effects of low body temperature on the enzymes of the clotting cascade.[27]

Exocrine and endocrine pancreatic function are depressed when an animal is exposed to cold. The major result is decreased insulin production. Hyperglycemia sometimes occurs, but because of the shivering associated with mild hypothermia, glucose utilization increases and the animal may remain normoglycemic.

DIAGNOSIS

Severe hypothermia can be easily overlooked, because standard rectal thermometers can measure body temperatures only as low as 34°C (93°F). Rectal or esophageal probes, low-recording thermometers, or indirect tympanic thermometers should be used to identify and monitor body temperature in animals with moderate to severe hypothermia. A history that reveals exposure to cold, disappearance from home, trauma, or underlying illness may be helpful. Signs of hypothermia may be misleading. Early signs are vague and include mental depression, impaired gait, and lethargy. Animals with moderate hypothermia may have considerable muscle stiffness without shivering. Animals with severe hypothermia may be mistaken for being dead, because respiration may be difficult to detect, heart sounds inaudible, and the pupils fixed and dilated. A cold animal should not be pronounced dead until serious attempts have been made to detect vital signs. Such attempts include performing electrocardiography or checking respiratory activity.

A complete physical examination should be done on hypothermic animals. Vital signs (i.e., airway, ventilation, and circulation) and core body temperature should be assessed. An electrocardiogram may reveal the presence of cardiac arrhythmias. A minimum data base consisting of a hematocrit, total plasma solids, blood urea nitrogen, blood glucose, serum sodium, serum potassium, and urinalysis should be conducted. More complete testing may involve a complete blood count, platelet count, coagulation panel, fibrinogen level, serum biochemistry profile, basal thyroid hormone levels, and blood gas analysis.

Traditionally, all blood gas values are adjusted to the body temperature of the animal before evaluation.[28] This adjustment is based primarily on the general concept that pH values at normal temperatures are also appropriate at lower temperatures. Recent reports in the human literature indicate that unadjusted values may be more useful in assessing the acid-base status of patients.[29–31] In homeothermic animals, the temperature and pH of blood perfusing the skin may fall to 25°C (77°F) and pH 7.6. There seems to be a temperature-dependent shift in the pH of blood. This shift is similar to the alpha-stat regulation seen in ectothermic animals.[32] The ectothermic strategy for preserving the optimum (alkaline) environment at a lower temperature has been shown to improve function of the canine myocardium,[33,34] to preserve Donnan ratios and cell volume,[35] and to optimize the function of a number of enzymes in hypothermic dogs.

The fact that chilled blood returns to normal values at normothermic temperatures indicates that appropriate pH will be present at lower temperatures. As reference values are only available within the normothermic temperature range, it is best to measure the pH and Pco_2 values of a hypothermic animal at 37°C (99°F) (uncorrected for body temperature). Treatment is aimed at maintaining the patient's pH at 7.4 and Pco_2 at 40 torr when measured at 37°C. An animal with a marked metabolic acidosis at 37°C may benefit from a lowering of the Pco_2 through ventilation or by the cautious administration of bicarbonate. It should be noted that correction of arterial blood gases for body temperature is still essential for assessment of pulmonary function.

TREATMENT

Animals with moderate to severe hypothermia usually are critically ill. Several factors may cause death after treatment has been started. First, unnecessary movement may precipitate lethal dysrhythmias in the cold, irritable myocardium. Second, body temperature may continue to decline after the animal has been removed from a cold environment. This phenomenon (known as afterdrop) may be caused by the continuing conduction of heat from the warmer core to colder surface layers as well as the return of cold blood from peripheral vessels to the core during rewarming.[36–38] Third, the metabolic burden of rewarming together with the vasodilatation that is created may overwhelm the compromised circulatory system.[39] These events, coupled with the influx of cold resuscitation fluids or return to the heart of cold peripheral blood, can contribute to sudden death (known as rewarming shock).

Treatment of hypothermic animals is directed toward supporting vital organ systems, preventing further heat loss, rewarming, and preventing further complications. Airway management is of primary importance. If the airway is patent and the animal is breathing spontaneously at greater than 4 to 10 breaths/min., oxygen that is warm and humidified should be supplied by mask. If the respiratory rate is slower or the patient is hypoventilating, intubation and ventilation with warm oxygen are necessary. Intravenous access should be achieved as soon as possible because volume resuscitation is essential. Most isotonic, balanced electrolyte solutions can be used. Lactated Ringer's solution should be avoided in animals that are very cold and that have reduced hepatic metabolism of lactate. Fluid solutions should be warm, which will prevent additional heat loss. Sup-

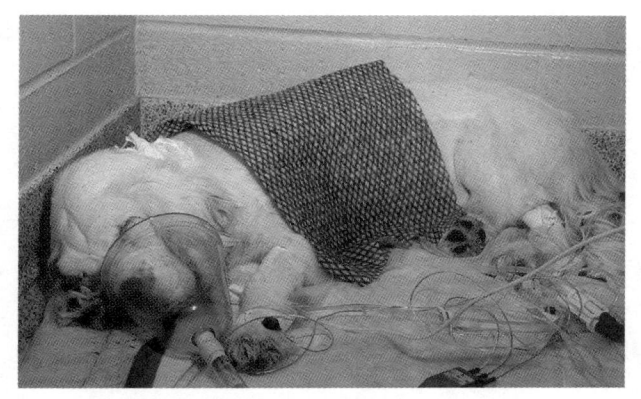

Figure 1—Active external rewarming (using a recirculating water blanket wrapped around the chest) and oxygen supplementation by face mask.

plementation with dextrose is recommended because dextrose provides a substrate for energy production to meet increased metabolic demands. Continuous electrocardiogram and blood pressure monitoring is recommended for critical patients.

An accurate reading of core body temperature will serve as a guide to subsequent therapy. A patient with a temperature of greater than 28°C (82°F) should be handled gently; cardiopulmonary resuscitation, if necessary, should be instituted promptly. Cardiopulmonary resuscitation should be avoided in a patient with severe hypothermia and a perfusing cardiac rhythm because of the risk of inducing ventricular dysrhythmia.[40] A cardiopulmonary resuscitation protocol is indicated in patients with severe hypothermia and a nonperfusing arrest rhythm. At temperatures below 28°C (82°F), the heart will be refractory to atropine, antiarrhythmic agents, and electroconversion therapy.[40] Because a degree of protection is provided by the decrease in cell metabolism in patients with severe hypothermia, it is advisable to continue the cardiopulmonary resuscitation protocol until the patient is normothermic. Cardiopulmonary resuscitation can be performed at half the normal rate because of the decreased perfusion needs at lower temperatures. Ventilation rates should not exceed 8 to 12 breaths/min.

Rewarming methods are divided into three classes: passive rewarming, active external rewarming, and core rewarming. Passive rewarming is appropriate for stable, adult patients with mild hypothermia (temperature greater than 32°C [90°F]). Passive rewarming involves providing insulation with blankets and allowing the patient's intrinsic heat production mechanisms, such as shivering, to correct the hypothermia. The result is greatly increased oxygen consumption.

Moderate hypothermia (28°C to 32°C [82°F to 90°F]) requires more active rapid external rewarming.

The patient is exposed to an exogenous heat source, such as hot water bottles, recirculating water blankets (Figure 1), heating pads, and radiant heat. Problems seen with active external rewarming and peripheral vasodilatation include afterdrop, intravascular volume depletion, and hypotension. Heat should be applied only to the thorax; the extremities should be kept cool. Such action allows the body's core to warm selectively until the heart is better able to perfuse the cool extremities; rewarming shock, therefore, is prevented. External heat sources should not be in direct contact with the patient's skin because animals that are cold and that have vasoconstricted vessels are unable to conduct heat away and are prone to burns. Radiant heat sources should be placed at least 29 inches from the patient.

Severe hypothermia mandates the most aggressive therapy. Core rewarming options available in human medicine include thoracic, peritoneal, and gastric lavage; airway rewarming; extracorporeal continuous arteriovenous or venovenous rewarming; and cardiopulmonary bypass. Although more complex to perform, core rewarming allows rapid rewarming and avoids the problems of afterdrop and rewarming shock. In emergency veterinary medicine, airway rewarming and peritoneal or gastric lavage are the best options. Warm water enemas and bladder lavage are other possibilities.

Airway rewarming involves supplying warm, humidified air through either a face mask or endotracheal tube. Airway rewarming is considered to be less effective than peritoneal or gastric lavage[41] but may be a useful adjunct to therapy. The heart and lungs may be rewarmed preferentially, thus reducing the risk of dysrhythmias. Thermal stimulation of the respiratory ciliary mechanism also may facilitate the clearance of tracheobronchial secretions.

Gastrointestinal rewarming consists of the use of warm intragastric irrigation via a stomach tube. Heat applied to the gastrointestinal tract has the advantage of selectively warming the liver and potentially improving the metabolism of drugs and lactate. Gastrointestinal perforation and the induction of cardiac dysrhythmias during placement of the stomach tube are potential risks.

Peritoneal irrigation involves the use of one or two peritoneal dialysis catheters and a stock dialysate solution. In a practice situation, Foley catheters and any balanced electrolyte solution can be used.[42] Dialysate should be warmed in a water bath or microwave oven to 45°C (113°F) and allowed to flow into the peritoneal cavity by gravity flow (50 ml/kg/exchange).[43] With rapid instillation and immediate removal of dialysate, return to normothermia should be accomplished in six to eight exchanges.[44] Extremely rapid rewarming occurs because of the heat capacity of the volume of fluid and the large peritoneal surface area available for heat exchange. Spontaneous hyperthermia occurs for several hours unless rewarming is discontinued before normal body temperature is reached.[45]

Common complications seen during correction of severe hypothermia relate to rewarming shock, cardiac dysrhythmias, and sudden death. Coagulopathies and disseminated intravascular coagulation may be seen. Rewarming results in an increase in fibrinolytic activity in dogs.[46] It is important to fully understand the nature of the coagulopathy in a hypothermic patient before beginning therapy. Prolongation of the activated partial thromboplastin time and prothrombin time evaluated at 37°C (99°F) indicates a coagulation factor deficiency, which may be helped by the administration of fresh frozen plasma. In a patient that is bleeding and that has normal activated partial thromboplastin and prothrombin time values evaluated at 37°C, rewarming may be of more benefit in correcting the coagulopathy because increasing body temperature may correct functional coagulation factor abnormalities.[27]

During rewarming, the return of blood from peripheral vessels may produce metabolic acidosis as well as an increase in serum potassium concentration as a result of the potassium ion–hydrogen shift. Metabolic acidosis, if present, should be treated cautiously because the right shift of the oxyhemoglobin dissociation curve from metabolic acidosis partially compensates for the left shift in the dissociation curve resulting from hypothermia.

Pulmonary complications after rewarming are common and include pneumonia, pulmonary edema, and acute respiratory distress syndrome.[47–49] Fluid shifts into the lungs because of capillary leakage during hypothermia. Infections and sepsis are major causes of death after rewarming. The increased susceptibility to infection is probably multifactorial and may include bacterial translocation across ischemic regions of intestine and skin; cold-induced granulocytopenia[22]; and impaired phagocytosis and migration as well as reduced half-life of polymorphonuclear cells.[50] Animals may be predisposed to pneumonia because of an increase in atelectasis resulting from hypoventilation and thickening of tracheobronchial secretions.

Patients that become increasingly unresponsive as rewarming continues may have cerebral edema. Increased intracranial pressure may be secondary to a combination of edema, osmotic gradients associated with changing glucose levels, or ischemic injury.[21] Treatment consists of administering osmotic diuretics and corticosteroids. Pancreatitis[48,49,51] and acute renal tubular necrosis[52] also may develop and have been associated with shock and ischemia. Rhabdomyolysis as well as electrolyte and glucose disturbances also may be seen. Continued monitoring and support are essential.

CONCLUSION

Hypothermia is seen by veterinarians in emergency rooms, operating rooms, and intensive care units. Prolonged hypothermia may result in multiorgan system dysfunction. Severely hypothermic patients require aggressive early management involving rapid rewarming and life support. Careful monitoring for potential complications, especially malignant cardiac arrhythmias, is recommended.

About the Author
Dr. Dhupa, who is a Diplomate of the American College of Veterinary Emergency and Critical Care and American College of Veterinary Internal Medicine, is a staff veterinarian in emergency and critical care at Tufts University Foster Hospital for Small Animals, North Grafton, Massachusetts.

REFERENCES

1. Virtue RW: *Hypothermic Anesthesia*, ed 1. Springfield, IL, Charles C Thomas, 1955, p 3.
2. Ferguson J, Epstein F, Van de Leuv J: Accidental hypothermia. *Emerg Med Clin North Am* 1:619–637, 1983.
3. Waterman A: Accidental hypothermia during anesthesia in dogs and cats. *Vet Rec* 96:308–313, 1975.
4. Adams T: Carnivores, protection against hypothermia, in Whittow GC (ed): *Comparative Physiology of Thermoregulation*. New York, Academic Press, 1971, pp 158–171.
5. Feldman EC, Nelson RW: *Canine and Feline Endocrinology and Reproduction*. Philadelphia, WB Saunders Co, 1987, p 55.
6. Freinkel N, Metzger BE, Harris E, et al: The hypothermia of hypoglycemia: Studies with 2-deoxy-D-glucose in normal human subjects and mice. *N Engl J Med* 287:841–847, 1972.
7. Davidson M, Grant E: Accidental hypothermia: A community hospital perspective. *Postgrad Med* 70:42–52, 1981.
8. Reuler JB: Hypothermia: Pathophysiology, clinical setting, and management. *Ann Intern Med* 89:519–527, 1978.
9. Danzl DF, Pozos RS, Auerbach PS, et al: Multicenter hypothermia survey. *Ann Emerg Med* 16:1042–1055, 1987.
10. Bigelow WG, Lindsay WK, Harrison RC, et al: Oxygen transport and utilization in dogs at low body temperatures. *Am J Physiol* 160:125, 1950.
11. Penrod KE: Oxygen consumption and cooling rates in immersion hypothermia in the dog. *Am J Physiol* 157:436–443, 1949.
12. Prec O, Rosenman R, Braun K, et al: Cardiovascular effects in acutely induced hypothermia. *J Clin Invest* 28:193–196, 1949.
13. Harari A, Regnier B, Rapin M, et al: Hemodynamic study of prolonged deep accidental hypothermia. *Eur J Intern Care Med* 1:65–70, 1975.
14. Chastain CB, Graham CL, Riley MG: Myxedema coma in two dogs. *Canine Pract* 9:20–34, 1982.

15. Bussadori C, Vercelli C: The Osborn wave in a dog with hypothermia. *Boll Assoc Ital Vet Piccoli Anim* 26:97–100, 1987.
16. Elenbass RM, Mattson K, Cole H, et al: Bretylium in hypothermia-induced ventricular fibrillation in dogs. *Ann Emerg Med* 13:994–999, 1984.
17. Orts A, Alcarez C, Delaney KA, et al: Bretylium tosylate and electrically induced cardiac arrhythmias during hypothermia in dogs. *Am J Emerg Med* 10(4):311–316, 1992.
18. Churchill-Davidson HG, McMillan IK, Melrose DG, et al: Hypothermia; experimental study of surface cooling. *Lancet* 2:1011–1015, 1953.
19. Morray JP, Pavlin EG: Oxygen delivery and consumption during hypothermia and rewarming in the dog. *Anesthesiology* 72:510–516, 1990.
20. Segar WE, Riley PA, Barlla TG: Urinary composition during hypothermia. *Am J Physiol* 185:528–532, 1956.
21. Shoemaker WC: *Textbook of Critical Care*. Philadelphia, WB Saunders Co, 1989, pp 105–108.
22. Villalobos TJ, Adelson E, Riley PA, et al: A cause of the thrombocytopenia and leukopenia that occurs in dogs during deep hypothermia. *J Clin Invest* 37:1–7, 1958.
23. Carr ME, Wolfert AI: Rewarming by hemodialysis for hypothermia: Failure of heparin to prevent DIC. *J Emerg Med* 6:277–280, 1988.
24. Valeri CR, Cassidy G, Khuri S, et al: Hypothermia-induced reversible platelet dysfunction. *Ann Surg* 205:175–181, 1987.
25. Villalobos TJ, Adelson E, Barlla TG: Hematologic changes in hypothermic dogs. *Proc Soc Exp Biol Med* 89:192–196, 1955.
26. Willson JT, Miller WR, Eliot TS: Blood studies in the hypothermic dog. *Surgery* 43:979–989, 1958.
27. Reed RL II, Bracey AW Jr, Hudson JD, et al: Hypothermia and blood coagulation: Dissociation between enzyme activity and clotting factor levels. *Circ Shock* 32:141–152, 1990.
28. Kelman GR, Nunn JF: Normograms for correction of blood pO_2, pCO_2, pH, and base excess for time and temperature. *J Appl Physiol* 21:1484–1490, 1966.
29. Ream AK, Reitz BA, Silverberg G: Temperature correction of $PaCO_2$ and pH in estimating acid-base status: An example of the emperor's new clothes? *Anesthesiology* 56(1):41–44, 1982.
30. Swain JA: Hypothermia and blood pH: A review. *Arch Intern Med* 148:1643–1646, 1988.
31. White FN: A comparative physiological approach to hypothermia. *J Thorac Cardiovasc Surg* 82:821–831, 1981.
32. Reeves RB: An imidazole alpha-stat hypothesis for vertebrate acid base regulation: Tissue carbon dioxide content and body temperature in bullfrogs. *Respir Physiol* 14:219–236, 1972.
33. McConnel DM, White FN, Nelson RL, et al: Importance of alkalosis in maintenance of ideal blood pH during hypothermia. *Surg Forum* 26:263–266, 1975.
34. Becker H, Vinten-Johansen J, Buchberg GD, et al: Myocardial damage caused by keeping pH 7.40 during systemic deep hypothermia. *J Thorac Cardiovasc Surg* 82:810–815, 1982.
35. Reeves RB: Temperature-induced changes in blood acid-base status: Donnan ratio and red cell volume. *J Appl Physiol* 40:762–765, 1976.
36. Hayward JS, Eckerson JD, Kenna D: Thermal and cardiovascular changes during 3 methods of resuscitation from mild hypothermia. *Resuscitation* 11:1–2, 1984.
37. Webb P: Afterdrop of body temperature during rewarming: An alternative explanation. *J Appl Physiol* 60:385–390, 1986.
38. Savard GK, Cooper KE, Veale WL, et al: Peripheral blood flow during rewarming from mild hypothermia in humans. *J Appl Physiol* 58:4–13, 1985.
39. Lloyd EL: Hypothermia: The cause of death after rescue. *Alaska Med* 26:74–76, 1984.
40. Bigelow WG, Callaghan JC, Hoopes JA: General hypothermia for experimental intracardiac surgery: The use of electrophrenic respirations, an atrial pacemaker for experimental cardiac standstill and radiofrequency rewarming in general hypothermia. *Ann Surg* 132:531–539, 1950.
41. Otto RJ, Metzler MH: Rewarming from experimental hypothermia: Comparison of heated aerosol inhalation, peritoneal lavage, and pleural lavage. *Crit Care Med* 16:869–875, 1988.
42. Murtaugh RJ, Kaplan PM: *Veterinary Emergency and Critical Care Medicine*. Philadelphia, Mosby Year Book, 1992, p 199.
43. Zenoble RD: Accidental hypothermia, in Kirk RW (ed): *Current Veterinary Therapy. VIII*. Philadelphia, WB Saunders Co, 1983, pp 186–187.
44. Patton JF, Doolittle WH: Core rewarming by peritoneal dialysis following induced hypothermia in the dog. *J Appl Physiol* 33(6):800–804, 1972.
45. Behnke AR, Yaglou CP: Physical responses of man to chilling in ice water and to slow and fast rewarming. *J Appl Physiol* 3:591, 1951.
46. Yoshihara H, Yamamoto T, Mihara H: Changes in coagulation and fibrinolysis occurring in dogs during hypothermia. *Thromb Res* 37:503–512, 1985.
47. Moss J: Accidental severe hypothermia. *Surg Gynecol Obstet* 162:501–513, 1986.
48. Mant AK: Autopsy diagnosis of accidental hypothermia. *J Forensic Med* 16:126–129, 1969.
49. Fitzgerald FT, Jessop C: Accidental hypothermia: A report of 23 cases and review of the literature. *Adv Intern Med* 27:128–135, 1982.
50. Bohn D, Baker C, Kent G, et al: Accidental and induced hypothermia: Effects of neutrophil migration in vivo. *Crit Care Med* 129:112–120, 1984.
51. Maclean D, Murison J, Griffiths PD: Acute pancreatitis and diabetic ketoacidosis in accidental hypothermia and hypothyroid myxoedema. *Br Med J* 4:757–763, 1973.
52. Kugelberg J, Schuller H, Berg B, et al: Treatment of accidental hypothermia. *Scand J Thorac Cardiovasc Surg* 1:142–148, 1967.

Fluid and Electrolyte Metabolism During Heat Stress

Martin J. Fettman, DVM, MS, PhD
Diplomate, ACVP
Comparative Nephrology Unit
Department of Pathology
College of Veterinary Medicine and
Biomedical Sciences
Colorado State University
Fort Collins, Colorado

Heat stress is a multifaceted syndrome that occurs when an individual's capacity for heat dissipation is exceeded by the heat load acquired through excessive exposure to high environmental temperatures. Predisposition to heat stress is increased by increased environmental humidity and by sustained physical exertion under this environmental condition.[1,2] Heat exchange occurs between an individual and its environment by conduction, convection, radiation, and evaporation. The former three modalities are limited by high environmental temperature; while the latter, even in environments of moderate humidity, is limited by an individual's capacity to maintain adequate fluid and electrolyte balance during sustained periods of intense perspiration.

The term *heat stress* is applied to a group of clinical entities observed most often in humans undergoing intensive military or athletic training in hot environments or in heat-exposed individuals predisposed to fluid imbalance or cardiovascular system failure, such as atherosclerosis, congestive heart disease, or multiple sclerosis.[3,4] Inadequate conditioning to exercise, lack of environmental acclimatization, and confinement with poor ventilation likewise may predispose an animal to heat stress in a hot environment.[5,6]

Although several of the clinical signs of heat stress may be related to the direct pathologic effects of hyperpyrexia and thermal denaturation within the body, most pathophysiologic changes can be attributed to imbalances in fluid and electrolyte metabolism. These imbalances develop secondary to circulatory adjustments and water and salt losses induced by profuse sweating and evaporative losses from the respiratory surfaces (Figure 1).[6-8]

Alterations in Metabolic Profile Associated with Heat Stress
Early Metabolic Changes

The first in a sequence of metabolic changes during exercise in a hot environment involves development of mild hyperkalemia and lactic acidosis attributed to the release of potassium and lactic acid from working muscle cells.[9] The release of potassium by contracting muscle cells is believed to be responsible, in part, for local vasodilation and the muscular hyperemia associated with exercise.[10] When an individual's heat load exceeds the capacity for heat elimination (particularly by evaporation), hyperpyrexia follows and hyperventilation may occur (Figure 1). The latter leads to development of respiratory alkalosis characterized by alkalemia, decreased carbon dioxide par-

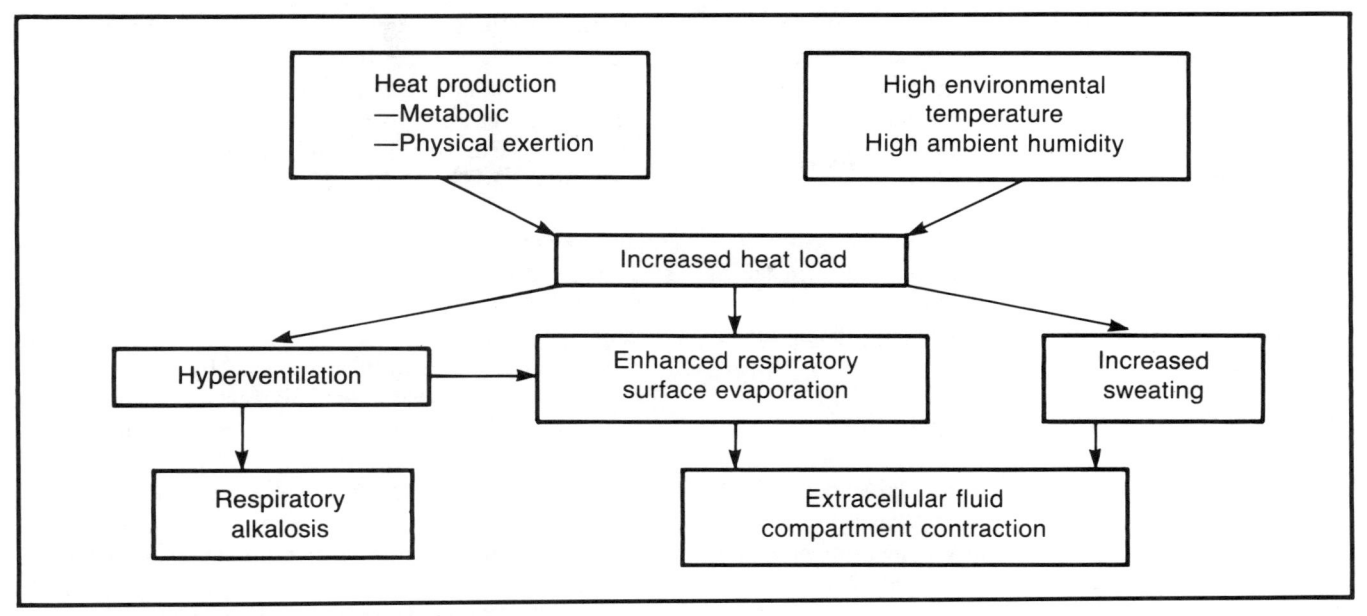

Figure 1—Scheme 1 in the pathogenesis of heat stress.

tial pressure (pCO_2) in blood, and (following extracellular potassium exchange for intracellular protons) hypokalemia.[7,11] Dogs and cats are capable of producing little sweat; and, in these animals, hyperventilation may enhance the evaporative heat loss from the tongue, upper respiratory system, and alveolar surfaces of the lungs.[12] The alterations in acid-base status associated with hyperventilation are identified with the very early clinical signs of heat exhaustion, including syncope, tetany, and muscle cramps.[2,11]

Metabolic Responses to Continued Heat Stress

As an animal continues to lose fluid and electrolytes through perspiration and evaporation in response to a high ambient temperature and continuing metabolic heat production, more severe derangements of electrolyte balance will occur. In dogs and cats, losses of water in excess of solute with upper and lower respiratory evaporation may result in hypertonic dehydration and contraction of the extracellular fluid compartment.[12] In ruminants and humans, sweat is a hypotonic fluid relative to the blood plasma[13]; and, in combination with evaporative water losses, hypertonic dehydration may result. Unlike humans and ruminants, sweat produced by Equidae is extremely hypertonic relative to blood plasma.[14] Despite significant evaporative water losses, heat stress may result in hypotonic dehydration in these species.[14,15] Not surprisingly, if heat stress is accompanied by water deprivation, hypertonic dehydration will occur or be considerably aggravated.[15]

In response to water and sodium losses, especially from plasma volume reductions, the cardiac output, renal arteriolar perfusion, and glomerular filtration rate are reduced sufficiently to elicit renin secretion by the juxtaglomerular apparatus of the kidneys (Figure 2).[9,16,17] This release initiates a cascade of events leading to secretion of aldosterone by the adrenal cortex. Aldosterone mediates increased sodium retention by cells of the distal renal tubules, small intestine, and sweat glands and thereby helps the body to conserve sodium and water in the face of continued perspiratory and evaporative losses.

Although control of sodium excretion by the renal tubules may exhibit *mineralocorticoid escape* following prolonged periods of aldosterone stimulation, urinary potas-

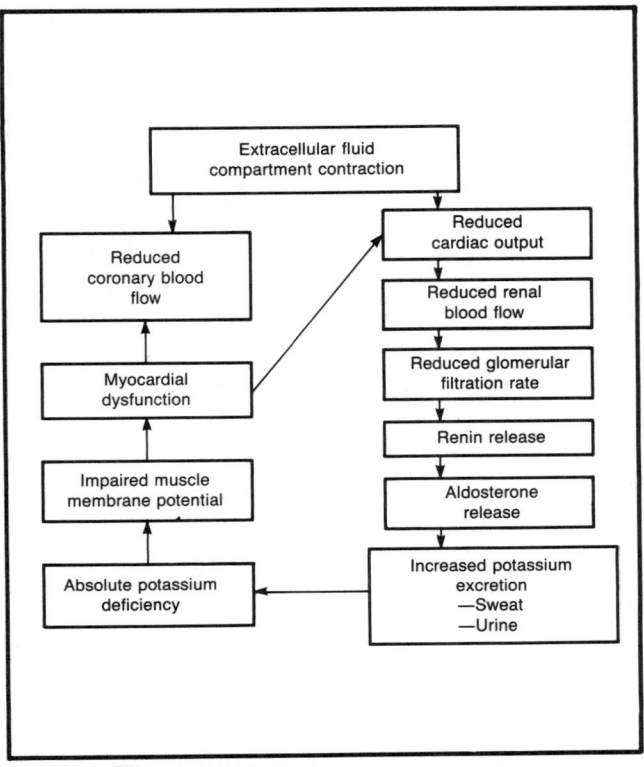

Figure 2—Scheme 2 in the pathogenesis of heat stress.

sium excretion does not and may continue at high rates under the influence of aldosterone.[16] In addition, the sweat glands exhibit no refractoriness to long-term mineralocorticoid stimulation; and aldosterone-mediated sweat modification may continue with prolonged heat exposure.[16,18]

Potassium concentrations in sweat have been reported as high as 92 mM/L in ruminants[13] and 62 mM/L in horses[14] and thus may represent a substantial route for body potassium loss (Figure 2). Despite adequate dietary intake of potassium, a profound body potassium deficit may be incurred and may result in several pathophysiologic alterations throughout the body.[9,16]

Adverse Effects of Potassium Depletion

Modified membrane potentials induced by potassium redistribution and loss may diminish vascular smooth muscle responsiveness to catecholamines, thereby resulting in peripheral vasodilation and circulatory compartment expansion in excess of available fluid volume (Figure 3).[16,19] This reduction in relative blood volume, and hence diastolic filling volume and pressure, imposes an additional burden on the heart, whose function is already compromised by the hypokalemia and increased oxygen demand associated with hyperpyrexia.[2,19]

Hypokalemia of sufficient duration may have a direct pathologic effect on the renal nephrons, leading to reduction in the glomerular filtration rate as well as vacuolar changes and coagulative necrosis of distal tubular cells (Figure 3).[20-22] Body potassium depletion also may blunt the muscular response to work, during which potassium release by contracting muscle elements modifies capillary circulatory dynamics to increase blood flow for exercise. Therefore, with combined volume and potassium depletion, failure to increase tissue perfusion with exercise may contribute to ischemic degeneration of musculature and rhabdomyolysis, after which there is a release of increased amounts of lactic acid, muscle enzymes (creatine phosphokinase, lactate dehydrogenase, and aspartate transaminase), myoglobin, and purine catabolites (Figure 3).[10,20,23] The latter two substances may by themselves have potentially toxic effects; heme pigments and hypoxanthine are particularly nephrotoxic in conjunction with reduced renal blood flow and acidic urine.[2,20,24] Thus, reduced renal perfusion, hypokalemia, myoglobinuria, and xanthinuria all may contribute to the development of acute renal failure during heat stress (Figure 3). In terminal cases, acute renal failure has been associated with "fulminating hyperkalemia," leading to cardiac failure and convulsions.[2,20]

Additional Acid-Base Disturbances

Reduced peripheral tissue perfusion resulting from volume contraction and failure of exercise hyperemia leads to increased rates of anaerobic glycolysis and lactic acidosis.[10,23,25] Subsequent deterioration of renal function may include impaired proximal tubular bicarbonate reclamation and decreased distal tubular proton secretion, thus reducing

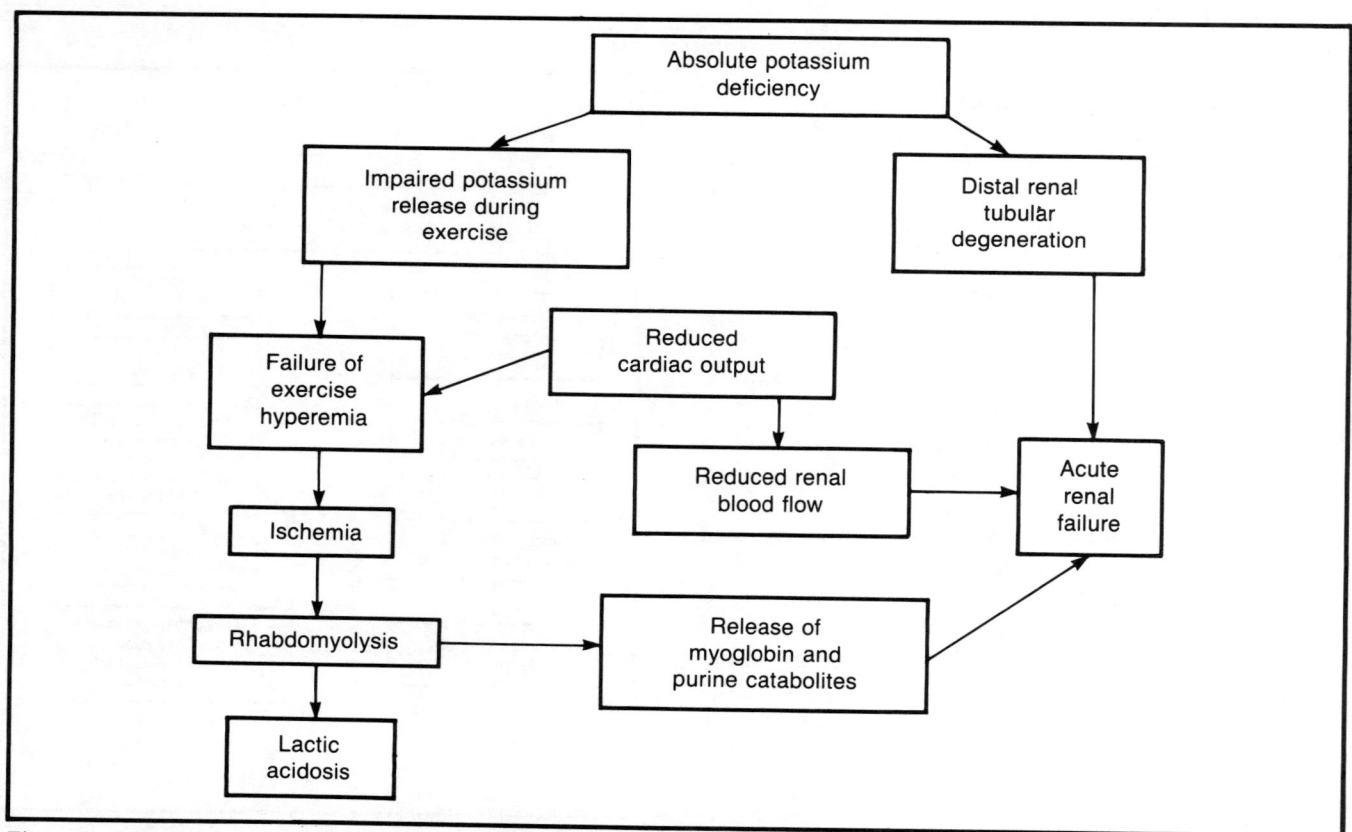

Figure 3—Scheme 3 in the pathogenesis of heat stress.

net urinary acid elimination.[20-22] Therefore, early respiratory alkalosis may be followed later by metabolic acidosis during prolonged heat stress.

In conditioned, heat-stressed endurance horses, a hypochloremic, hypokalemic metabolic alkalosis may supervene over the lactic acidemia (resulting from exercise) because of secretion of a hypertonic sweat high in chloride and potassium.[25,26] Metabolic alkalosis is a common manifestation of body depletion of chloride and potassium.[27] Because of the limited availability of chloride, tubular sodium resorption is preferentially coupled to bicarbonate retention in the proximal tubules as well as proton or potassium secretion in the distal tubules of the kidneys. When potassium depletion progresses to a point that secretion of potassium by the distal nephron is limited, protons are substituted, paradoxically acidifying the urine and thus compounding the systemic metabolic alkalosis.[27]

Alterations in Calcium and Phosphorus Metabolism

Additional electrolyte abnormalities may include early hypophosphatemia and, later, hypocalcemia. Respiratory alkalosis, induced by hyperventilation accompanying early heat stress, may result in preferential alkalization of intracellular fluids as a result of the rapid extracellular diffusivity of carbon dioxide. This change, in combination with reduced rates of aerobic respiration from volume contraction and ischemia, may result in increased rates of glycolytic enzyme activity and accumulation of phosphorylative glycolytic intermediates, thus trapping more phosphorus intracellularly.[28,29] Hypocalcemia does not usually develop for several days and may occur after serum phosphorus levels have corrected spontaneously. This change has been attributed to calcium phosphate and calcium carbonate deposits in injured skeletal musculature.[28,29]

Clinical signs attributable to hypocalcemia (muscle cramps and tetany), however, typically are seen early in heat stress, when total serum calcium concentrations are normal; but respiratory alkalosis has reduced ionized calcium levels.[2,30] Similarly, it is more likely that the hypocalcemia observed later in heat stress, particularly when muscle damage is minimal and clinical signs are absent, is (in addition to losses in sweat)[14] attributable to an adaptive response to increased ionized calcium levels induced by metabolic acidosis, which results from tissue ischemia (lactic acidosis) and renal dysfunction (impaired urinary acidification).[30]

Additional Complications of Fluid and Electrolyte Imbalances

Carbohydrate Intolerance

Primary and secondary hyperaldosteronism and hypertension have been associated with impaired carbohydrate tolerance.[18,31,32] Heat-stressed individuals also demonstrate impaired responsiveness to a carbohydrate challenge, which has been attributed to a defect in pancreatic islet β-cell secretory capability in the potassium-depleted state.[2,31-33] Optimum pancreatic β-cell response to insulin secretagogue requires a change in membrane potential, which is mediated, in part, by an abrupt increase in intracellular potassium.[34] Experiments with hyperaldosteronemic patients transfused intravenously with potassium solutions have demonstrated that the carbohydrate intolerance associated with the previously mentioned conditions is attributed to body potassium depletion and not to the glucocorticoid effects of the mineralocorticoids. In these experiments, potassium administration resulted in stimulation of increased mineralocorticoid release by the adrenal glands, except with simultaneous improvement in pancreatic β-cell responsiveness and carbohydrate tolerance.[31]

Pulmonary Edema

Humans who are less tolerant to exercise in heat and who find it difficult to become heat-acclimated are often less responsive to changes in solute and water distribution among the fluid compartments of the body.[35] These heat-intolerant persons apparently are less able to mobilize extravascular protein reserves required for adequate plasma volume expansion during heat acclimatization. This disability was attributed to differences in extravascular free-protein reserves and decreased capillary permeability.[35] It also points out a potential problem, even in heat-tolerant individuals, of maintaining normal transvascular oncotic pressures in the face of sodium and water imbalances during prolonged heat exposure. Regardless of the tolerance level, inability to maintain adequate vascular oncotic pressure is only one of several factors that may contribute to the development of edema, particularly in the lungs, in the later stages of heat exhaustion. Other causative factors include preexisting cardiac insufficiency, hyperpnea-induced depression of intraalveolar pressures, left ventricular failure secondary to reduced venous blood return and coronary blood flow, and cardiac failure from direct thermal myocardial damage.[16]

Postural Hypotension and Heat Syncope

These transient conditions are related to both the hypokalemia and the hypovolemia associated with heat stress. Impaired vascular responsiveness to catecholamines resulting from hypokalemia, postural pooling of blood, diminished venous return to the heart, and reduction in cardiac output results in transient cerebral ischemia and syncopic attacks.[1,2] Spontaneous recovery is common, and subsequent attacks may be prevented by replacement of both fluid and potassium.

Hypotonic Dehydration, Heat Cramps, and Heat Exhaustion Following Primary Salt Depletion

Hypoosmolal hypovolemia may result when heat-stressed horses and hypotonically dehydrated individuals of other species are allowed to replace water deficits in excess of the salt lost through sweating. Mild to moderate hyponatremia results in intermittent muscular cramping. This may be attributed to inhibition of the sarcoplasmic reticulum Na/Ca-ATPase, which is normally responsible for reaccumulation and sequestration of calcium between muscle cell contractions.[2] Severe hyponatremia may result in the more profound signs characteristic of heat exhaustion: fatigue, disorientation, anorexia, nausea, emesis, diarrhea, and pronounced muscle spasms.[2] These signs are presumably caused by the direct effects of electrolyte imbalances on cardiac and muscular function and on fluid distribution in the central nervous system.

Summary and Therapeutic Considerations

The severity of clinical signs associated with an animal's response to heat stress is determined by both the initial fluid and electrolyte losses sustained through perspiration and evaporation and the degree to which the cardiovascular and endocrine systems are able to compensate for these insults before cardiopulmonary, muscular, and renal deterioration begin to occur. The sooner that hyperpyrexia, a given history, and the progression of clinical and ancillary signs are linked together, the sooner that a diagnosis of heat stress can be made.

Treatment of heat-stress–related disorders primarily involves the immediate replacement of fluid and electrolyte deficits and, if the body temperature is abnormal, ice water or alcohol baths to return the temperature to normal. It is particularly important to monitor the cardiovascular, respiratory, and renal functions continuously and to be aware of the potential polysystemic complications that may occur after spontaneous return to normal body temperature.

One potential, but frequently unrecognized, endocrine-induced complication that is important in the treatment of heat-stressed animals is the continued cellular response to aldosterone up to eight hours after discontinuation of its secretion (a result of the biologic half-life and persistence of subcellular effects).[16-20] Even following initial fluid and electrolyte therapy, aldosterone-induced sodium retention and potassium excretion may continue, thereby exaggerating the potential for pulmonary edema and allowing potassium losses to continue. Diuretics are presently used in cases involving heat edema and in the prophylaxis and treatment of acute renal failure in order to relieve excess fluid accumulation, to maintain renal tubular perfusion, and to promote urine formation. The more potent loop diuretics (furosemide, ethycrynic acid), however, increase renal potassium wasting, which would be contraindicated in a heat-stressed patient.[36] While oral and parenteral potassium supplementation may replace much of this deficit, modification of renal potassium excretion would be beneficial. More routine use of a potassium-sparing diuretic (such as spironolactone or triamterene) in combination with a loop diuretic has the therapeutic advantage of modifying postsecretory mineralocorticoid effects and promoting a prophylactic diuresis against fluid retention and acute renal failure in a heat-stressed individual.[36]

References

1. Knochel JP: Environmental heat illness. *Arch Intern Med* 133:841-864, 1974.
2. Knochel JP: Clinical physiology of heat exposure, in Maxwell MH, Kleeman CR (eds): *Clinical Disorders of Fluid and Electrolyte Metabolism*, ed 3. New York, McGraw-Hill Co, 1980, pp 1519-1562.
3. Knochel JP, Beisel WR, Herndon EG, et al: The renal, cardiovascular, hematologic, and serum electrolyte abnormalities of heat stroke. *Am J Med* 30:299-399, 1961.
4. O'Donnell TF: Acute heat stroke: Epidemiologic, biochemical, renal, and coagulation studies. *JAMA* 234:824-828, 1975.
5. Johnson KE: Pathophysiology of heatstroke. *Compend Contin Educ Pract Vet* 4(2):141-144, 1982.
6. Krum SH, Osborne CA: Heatstroke in the dog: A polysystemic disorder. *JAVMA* 170:531-535, 1977.
7. Sprung CL, Protocarrero CJ, Fernaine AV, et al: The metabolic and respiratory alterations of heat stroke. *Arch Intern Med* 140:665-669, 1980.
8. Clowes GHA, O'Donnell TF: Heat stroke. *N Engl J Med* 291:564-567, 1974.
9. Coburn JW, Reba RC, Craig FN: Effect of potassium depletion on response to acute heat exposure in unacclimatized man. *Am J Physiol* 211:117-124, 1966.
10. Knochel JP, Schlein EM: On the mechanism of rhabdomyolysis in potassium depletion. *J Clin Invest* 51:1750-1758, 1972.
11. Boyd AE, Beller GA: Heat exhaustion and respiratory alkalosis. *Ann Intern Med* 83:835, 1975.
12. Hanneman GD, Higgins EA, Price GT, et al: Transient and permanent effects of hyperthermia in dogs: A study of a simulated air transport environmental stress. *Am J Vet Res* 38:955-958, 1977.
13. Singh SP, Newton WM: Acclimation of young calves to high environmental temperatures: Composition of blood and skin secretions. *Am J Vet Res* 39:799-801, 1978.
14. Kerr MG, Snow DH: Composition of sweat of the horse during prolonged epinephrine infusion, heat exposure, and exercise. *Am J Vet Res* 44:1571-1577, 1983.
15. Carlson GP, Rambaugh GE, Harrold D: Physiologic alterations in the horse produced by food and water deprivation during periods of high environmental temperatures. *Am J Vet Res* 40:982-985, 1979.
16. Knochel JP, Dotin LN, Hamburger RJ: Pathophysiology of intense physical conditioning in a hot climate. *J Clin Invest* 51:242-255, 1972.
17. Streeten DHP, Conn JW, Louis LH, et al: Secondary aldosteronism: Metabolic and adrenocortical responses of normal men to high environmental temperatures. *Metabolism* 9:1071-1092, 1960.
18. Conn JW: Aldosteronism in man. Some clinical and climatological aspects. *JAMA* 183:775-781, 1963.
19. Biglieri EG, McIlroy MB: Abnormalities of renal function and circulatory reflexes in primary aldosteronism. *Circulation* 33:78-86, 1966.
20. Schrier RW, Henderson HS, Tisher CC: Nephropathy associated with heat stress and exercise. *Ann Intern Med* 67:356-376, 1967.
21. Relman AS, Schwartz WB: The kidney in potassium depletion. *N Engl J Med* 254:764-781, 1958.
22. Schwartz WB, Relman AS: Effect of electrolyte disorders on renal function. *N Engl J Med* 276:383-389, 1967.
23. Van Horn G, Drori JB, Schwartz FD: Hypokalemic myopathy and elevation of serum enzymes. *Arch Neurol* 22:335-341, 1970.
24. Paller MS, Hoidal JR, Ferris TF: Oxygen free radicals in ischemic acute renal failure in the rat. *J Clin Invest* 74:1156-1164, 1984.
25. Carlson GP, Ocen PO, Harrold D: Clinicopathologic alterations in normal and exhausted endurance horses. *Theriogenology* 6:93-104, 1976.
26. Carlson GP, Mansmann RA: Serum electrolyte and plasma protein alterations in horses used for endurance rides. *JAVMA* 165:262-264, 1974.
27. Fettman MJ, Chase LE, Bentinck-Smith JB, et al: Effects of dietary

chloride restriction in lactating dairy cows. *JAVMA* 185:167-172, 1984.
28. Mason J, Thomas E: Rhabdomyolysis from heat hyperpyrexia: Severe hypocalcemia and hypophosphatemia as complicating factors. *JAMA* 235:633-634, 1976.
29. Knochel JP, Caskey JH: The mechanism of hypophosphatemia in acute heat stroke. *JAMA* 238:425-426, 1977.
30. Pedersen KO: Binding of calcium to serum albumin. II. Effect of pH via competitive hydrogen and calcium ion binding to the imidazole groups of albumin. *Scand J Clin Lab Invest* 29:75-83, 1972.
31. Conn JW: Hypertension, the potassium ion, and impaired carbohydrate tolerance. *N Engl J Med* 273:1135-1143, 1965.
32. Rowe JW, Tobin JD, Rosa RM, et al: Effect of experimental potassium deficiency on glucose and insulin metabolism. *Metabolism* 29:498-502, 1980.
33. Gardner LJ, Talbot NB, Cook CD, et al: The effect of potassium deficiency on carbohydrate metabolism. *J Lab Clin Med* 35:592-602, 1950.
34. Kalkhoff RK, Siegesmund KA: Fluctuations of calcium, phosphorus, sodium, potassium, and chlorine in single alpha and beta cells during glucose perfusion of rat islets. *J Clin Invest* 68:517-524, 1981.
35. Senay LC, Kok R: Body fluid responses of heat-tolerant and intolerant men to work in a hot wet environment. *J Appl Physiol* 40:55-59, 1976.
36. Kaloyanides GJ: Pathogenesis and treatment of edema with special reference to the use of diuretics, in Maxwell MH, Kleeman CR (eds): *Clinical Disorders of Fluid and Electrolyte Metabolism*, ed 3. New York, McGraw-Hill Co, 1980, pp 647-701.

The Veterinarian's Responsibility: Assessing and Managing Acute Pain in Dogs and Cats. Part I

KEY FACTS

- Managing pain in dogs and cats is a four-part process.
- First, veterinarians must acknowledge that pain exists and that as professionals, they have an inherent responsibility to treat pain.
- Second, veterinarians must know those stimuli that are likely to result in pain, must recognize the signs exhibited by an animal in pain, and must continually improve veterinary skills in assessing pain.
- Third, veterinarians must be aware of the agents available to manage pain in dogs and cats.
- Fourth, veterinarians must know how and when to use these agents and how to assess their effectiveness.

Allpets Clinic
Boulder, Colorado
Janna M. Johnson, DVM

RECENTLY there has been a heightened awareness on behalf of the veterinary profession with regard to pain in animals. This increased interest is at least partially attributable to a call by the public for accountability with respect to animal care. One would hope that this interest was spawned within the veterinary profession itself as an obligatory response to correct a heretofore overlooked area of veterinary medicine that has profound effects on patients.

In Part I of this two-part presentation, the ethical implications and veterinarian responsibilities with regard to animal pain are considered, followed by a discussion of the definition, classifications, and signs of animal pain. In Part II, the agents available to manage acute pain in dogs and cats are presented, including how and when to use these agents and how to assess their effectiveness.

ANIMAL PAIN: ETHICAL IMPLICATIONS AND VETERINARIAN RESPONSIBILITIES

The veterinary profession's understanding and management of pain is yet in its infancy, but it has left the dark ages of the early 1900s as evidenced in this 1906 surgery text: "Anesthesia in veterinary surgery today is a means of restraint and not an expedient to relieve pain. So long as an operation can be performed by forcible restraint ... the thought of anesthesia does not enter into the proposition...."[1]

The AVMA's 1987 Panel Report on the *Colloquium on Recognition and Alleviation of Animal Pain and Stress* has set the groundwork for the veterinary profession with regard to the responsibility of all veterinarians in providing effective management of pain in their patients. "The Veterinarian's Oath charges graduates to use their skills and knowledge for the relief of animal suffering. This charge is no longer an option but is clearly a defined obligation."[2] The time has come for veterinarians to act on the words of this oath. The charge has been made by the leaders of the veterinary profession; all involved as researchers, practitioners, and future practitioners must become equipped to fulfill it.

Managing pain in dogs and cats is a four-part process. If veterinarians are to minimize pain and suffering in patients, careful attention must be paid to each step; otherwise treatment will be rendered at best ineffective and at worst dangerous, regardless of whether the patient is undertreated, overtreated, or inappropriately treated.

First, veterinarians must acknowledge that pain exists and that as professionals, they have an inherent responsibility to treat it. If one lacks personal conviction, compassion, or a moral obligation to alleviate pain, pursuit of the next three phases is of no practical importance.

Second, veterinarians must know those stimuli that are likely to result in pain, must recognize the signs exhibited by an animal in pain, and must continually improve veterinary skills in assessing pain.

Third, veterinarians must be aware of the agents available to manage pain in dogs and cats.

Fourth, veterinarians must know how and when to use these agents and how to assess their effectiveness.

PAIN IS best understood and managed when scientific data, behavioral data, and anthropomorphism are integrated and a rational approach is used. It is now conceded that anthropomorphism plays a vital role in the veterinarian's ability to identify and treat pain,[2-7] as scientific data have shown that in response to pain, animals "exhibit the same motor behaviors and physiologic responses as do human beings in response to such stimulation. Such behaviors include simple withdrawal reflexes, more complex unlearned behaviors such as vocalization, and learned behaviors such as pressing a bar to avoid further exposure to a noxious stimulation."[8] Neuroanatomy, physiology, and behavioral data indicate there are many more similarities in pain perception in humans and animals than there are differences. The differences that do exist are attributed to alternative pathways rather than a presence or absence of them.[3-6] Human and animal pain detection threshold data indicate that animals begin to escape noxious stimulation at approximately the same intensity as humans.[3,7] Therefore, veterinarians cannot disregard their own understanding of human pain when clinically assessing an animal in pain or in anticipating when pain might be expected to occur after certain stimuli.

Extrapolation of data from one species to another is not always reliable; however, one can assume when a stimulus causes pain in humans it is likely to cause pain in animals.[2] This therapeutic approach may infrequently result in overtreatment; but if practitioners are to err, let them err in favor of the patient.[2,9] One should remember that "pain and suffering may actually constitute the only situation in which one should go ahead and treat, even if in doubt."[10]

Many veterinarians believe that pain is beneficial and that it provides a reminder to the patient not to move so that further injury might be avoided. This belief is invalid on at least two counts. First, it assumes that analgesia is complete—it is not. Second, it assumes there is no other way to prevent movement and avoid further injury. Confinement to a kennel and the use of analgesics with or without the addition of a tranquilizer will accomplish the same end, but in a humane manner. Finally, in recognizing the existence of pain, veterinarians must recognize its deleterious effects. Pain, in and of itself, could result in the death of the patient if the physiologic derangements initiated by the perception of severe, acute pain were severe enough. Pain also leads to prolonged, unpredictable tissue healing in animals and "prolonged catabolic reactions in the postoperative period"[11] in humans. The same also is likely true for animals.

PAIN: DEFINITION, CLASSIFICATIONS, AND SIGNS

Before beginning the discussion of the presenting signs of pain, a definition of pain and its classification is in order.

Pain has been defined by the International Association of the Study of Pain as "an unpleasant sensory and emotional experience associated with actual or potential tissue damage, or described in terms of such damage."[11] Pain is further divided into three categories based on its onset and duration: acute pain, cancer pain, and chronic pain.[12] Acute pain is seen when a stimulus results in injury to the body regardless of whether that stimulus be traumatic, surgical, or infectious. The onset usually is well-defined and abrupt and is associated with physical signs of autonomic nervous system activity.[10,12] Acute pain usually is alleviated by the use of analgesics and by healing of injured tissue. Cancer pain usually also presents with a well-defined onset and is best classified as acute recurrent pain.[12] It is responsive to analgesics, but long-term control leads to drug tolerance and addiction. Chronic pain is the least understood of the three types and is the most difficult type of pain to manage. Pain is considered chronic when it persists for longer than six months.[3] The onset of chronic pain often is not easily defined; there is no autonomic nervous system response, and chronic pain often is unresponsive to pharmacologic treatment directed at the underlying cause of the pain.[12]

ACUTE PAIN can be the most dangerous in its effects, and yet it is the easiest of the different classifications of pain to manage. Acute pain is the type of pain discussed in the remainder of this article.

Acute pain is further classified into two groups based on its site of origin: somatic or visceral.[5] Somatic pain arises from superficial structures, such as skin or subcutaneous tissue, or from deeper structures of the body wall.[3,5] Superficial pain is subdivided into first pain and second pain.

First pain is the initial, sharp, stabbing, well-localized pain associated with tissue injury. Second pain is the delayed pain that is considered dull, burning, and diffuse in character.[3] Visceral pain, on the other hand, arises from the abdominal or thoracic viscera and is associated primarily with serosal irritation.[3,5,10]

Although a comprehensive study of the neural pathways involved in pain perception is beyond the scope of this article, a few basic concepts must be dealt with to enhance therapeutic success. In general, pain is initiated by response of nociceptors (pain receptors) to noxious stimuli. Nerve impulses will then be generated if stimulation intensity reaches threshold.[7] Nerve impulses travel to the brain stem or spinal cord, the thalamus, and then the cerebral cortex for sensory processing.[3] Low-level stimulation of nociceptors may not result in the perception of pain. The lowest stimulus intensity perceived as painful or that results in a pain response is considered the pain detection threshold. The pain tolerance threshold differs from the pain detection threshold in that the former is the highest stimulus intensity that an animal will tolerate voluntarily. The pain tolerance threshold may vary, especially in patients that have experienced previous and repeated pain, as they tend to have higher pain tolerance thresholds.[2,7] The pain tolerance threshold also varies depending on the type of pain present; for example, dull pain is more easily tolerated than sharp pain.[7]

When considering the subject of pain, distress and suffering also must be considered. Distress is defined as "a state in which the animal is unable to adapt to an altered environment or to altered internal stimuli."[2] Suffering is defined as "a severe emotional state that is extremely unpleasant, that results from physical pain, emotional pain, and/or discomfort at a level not tolerated by the individual, and that results in some degree of physiologic distress."[9]

Distress can be pain-free, for example, distress following separation from the owner or being placed in an unfamiliar environment. It is important to attempt to differentiate pain-induced stress from fear- or anxiety-induced stress when considering therapeutic intervention. Non-pain–induced stress should be treated with a tranquilizer or sedative. Neither classification of drug is analgesic in and of itself. If a nonsedative analgesic is given to a pain-free distressed animal, dysphoria, excitement, and hyperactivity can result. On the other hand, treating an animal in pain with a sedative alone can result in hysteria or delirium.[13]

Humans exposed to pain above the tolerance threshold can exhibit intense emotional reactions that are associated with suffering. In humans, low-intensity, dull pain is said to be an unpleasant, tolerable situation that usually is not considered overly disruptive and does not evoke an intense emotional response. This is the mechanism by which dogs and cats adapt after such procedures as ovariohysterectomy or castration. Although the animal is uncomfortable the day after surgery, it is able to tolerate the dull pain with minimal disruption in its emotional reactivity.[7]

By understanding the classification system of pain, it becomes easier to establish an index of suspicion for those noxious stimuli that are likely to result in pain and the pain level and duration they are expected to induce. Table I is a useful generalization of expected postoperative pain response. The expected pain level can be extrapolated to nonsurgical trauma and systemic disease (e.g., meningitis, pleuritis, necrotizing pancreatitis, dissolving saddle thrombi, osteosarcomas, or metabolic bone disease).

TABLE I
Expected Postsurgical Pain Response[a]

Surgery	Expected Pain Level
Head, ear, throat, dental	Moderate to high
Anorectal	Moderate to high
Ophthalmologic	High
Orthopedic	Moderate to high (upper axial segments, e.g., shoulder/humerus and hip/femur, are very painful)
Amputation	High (transection of large muscle masses and nerves)
Thoracotomy	High (sternal); moderate to high (lateral)
Celiotomy	Mild to high (varies with duration of procedure and procedures associated with major pathologic changes)
Cervical spine	High
Lumbar and thoracic spine	Moderate

[a]Compiled from Crane SW: Perioperative analgesia: A surgeon's perspective. JAVMA 191:1254–1257, 1987; Wright EM, Marcella KL, Woodson JF: Animal pain: Evaluation and control. Lab Anim May/June:20–36, 1985; Haskins SC: Use of analgesics postoperatively and in a small animal intensive care setting. JAVMA 191:1266–1268, 1987; and the author's experience.

EXPECTATIONS of the clinician as to the severity of pain that is likely elicited from a given noxious stimulus based on human pain perception standards often is all the clinician has to form a subjective evaluation of pain intensity. It must be remembered that evolution has made pain recognition in animals difficult, as those animals displaying pain, weakness, or distress become prey.[10] Therefore, stoicism persists in many breeds of dogs, such as the sporting and working breeds, and the majority of cats.[5] The clinician must be aware of the possibility of nonexpressed pain. To disregard analgesia therapy in a stoic animal in the face of tissue injury is wrong.[5]

In evaluating the common signs of acute pain, it must be remembered that great individual variability exists, for example, the stoic animal or the animal too weak and systemically ill to respond to painful stimuli even though it is less able to tolerate pain. Also, young animals and males tend to be less tolerant of pain.[10]

A dog or cat in pain may exhibit none to many of the following signs. The animal may vocalize (moan, groan, whimper, or cry), attempt escape, or become aggressive when the painful region is approached or manipulated. A dog or cat often will attempt to guard or protect the area or may self-mutilate the affected area by biting, scratching, or licking it. Lameness, limb disuse, unusual body posture, restlessness (pacing, continuously getting up and down), prolonged recumbency, rolling, thrashing, and turning its head toward the stimulus are each indicative of pain. An animal may move slowly and stiffly, decrease its activity, or have a diminished appetite. The dog or cat may appear anxious, nervous, or trembling. Any change in normal behavior should be considered as a possible response to pain. Animals with abdominal pain will tend to splint their abdominal muscles, and animals with chest pain tend to breathe shallowly and abduct their elbows. If an animal has experienced pain over several days, it may not display overt painful reactions but may just become quiet and withdrawn. The contributions of pain to shock and the masking of any overt signs of pain by altered states of consciousness must also be considered, especially after surgery or acute trauma.[3-5,7,9,10,12,14]

Physiologic responses to pain may include tachypnea or panting, sinus tachycardia, ventricular premature contractions, atrial premature contractions, mydriasis, ptyalism, hyperglycemia, hypotension or hypertension, and pallor.[3-5,9,12,14,15]

ACKNOWLEDGMENT

The author thanks Leo K. Bustad, DVM, PhD, Professor and Dean Emeritus, College of Veterinary Medicine, Washington State University, for his interest, advice, and support.

About the Authors

Dr. Johnson is staff surgeon and dentist at Allpets Clinic in Boulder, Colorado.

REFERENCES

1. Merillat LA: *Veterinary Surgery. Volume II. The Principles of Veterinary Surgery*. Chicago, Alexandar Eger, 1906, p 225.
2. Kitchen H, Aronson AL, Bittle JL, et al: Panel report on the colloquium on recognition and alleviation of animal pain and stress. *JAVMA* 191:1186-1191, 1987.
3. Kitchell RL: Problems in defining pain and peripheral mechanisms of pain. *JAVMA* 191:1195-1199, 1987.
4. Haskins SC: Control of pain and suffering. *Proc 55th Annu AAHA Meet Vet Tech Prog*:18-22, 1988.
5. Crane SW: Perioperative analgesia: A surgeon's perspective. *JAVMA* 191:1254-1257, 1987.
6. Morton DB: Epilogue: Summarization of colloquium highlights from an international perspective. *JAVMA* 191:1292-1296, 1987.
7. Sawyer DC: Understanding animal pain and suffering. *Proc 55th Annu AAHA Meet Vet Tech Prog*:1-6, 1988.
8. Dubner R: Research on pain mechanisms in animals. *JAVMA* 191:1273-1276, 1987.
9. Spinelli JS, Markowitz H: Clinical recognition and anticipation of situations likely to induce suffering in animals. *JAVMA* 191:1216-1218, 1987.
10. Wright EM, Marcella KL, Woodson JF: Animal pain: Evaluation and control. *Lab Anim* May/June:20-36, 1985.
11. Schecter NL: An approach to the child with pain. *Patient Care* March 30:116-133, 1988.
12. Pain R, Max M, Inturrisi C, et al: Principles of analgesic use in the treatment of acute pain and chronic cancer pain. *Syllabus Commit Meet Amer Pain Soc Brd Dir*:1-9, 1986.
13. Benson J: The recognition and alleviation of animal pain and suffering: Opioid analgesics. *Proc 55th Annu AAHA Meet Vet Tech Prog*:7-17, 1988.
14. Haskins SC: Use of analgesics postoperatively and in a small animal intensive care setting. *JAVMA* 191:1266-1268, 1987.
15. Willis WD, Chung JM: Central mechanisms of pain. *JAVMA* 191:1200-1202, 1987.

The Veterinarian's Responsibility: Assessing and Managing Acute Pain in Dogs and Cats. Part II

Allpets Clinic
Boulder, Colorado
Janna M. Johnson, DVM

KEY FACTS:

❏ Controlling pain involves pharmacologic, physical, environmental, and behavioral management.

❏ Three classes of analgesics are used in management of pain: (1) opioids, (2) nonopioids (nonsteroidal antiinflammatory drugs and acetaminophen), and (3) adjuvant analgesics.

❏ Opioid analgesia is postoperatively indicated to relieve pain, especially during the first 48 hours.

❏ When choosing an analgesic for treatment of the patient in pain, the veterinarian should consider the level of pain expected and leave alternatives to provide greater analgesia if needed.

In Part I of this two-part presentation, the ethical implications and veterinarian responsibilities with regard to animal pain were considered; the definition, classifications, and signs of animal pain also were discussed. In Part II, the different classes of agents available to manage acute pain in dogs and cats are described, including how and when to use these agents and how to assess their effectiveness.

ANALGESIA AND ANALGESICS

In the simplest terms, analgesia is defined as relief of pain without unconsciousness.[1] Prevention is the ideal method of pain alleviation; however, this often is not possible, thereby necessitating other forms of intervention to provide analgesia.[2]

Controlling pain involves pharmacologic, physical, environmental, and behavioral management.[3] Treatment of pain is best accomplished by identifying and treating the cause of pain; drug therapy is the primary means of control for acute pain.[3,4] Contributory factors, such as environmental and behavioral management, are important adjuncts to drug therapy. For example, the patient's environment should not be too hot or cold or be too humid or dry. Adequate padding should be provided, and monitoring cables should be attached comfortably. Providing adequate rest and sleep, compassionate care, and visitation from the owners also is important to the psychologic well-being of the patient and enables the patient to tolerate its painful state better.[5] Adjunct physical management of acute injury and inflammation may include immobilization and the application of ice to the affected area.[1] Three classes of analgesic drugs are used in management of pain: (1) opioids, (2) nonopioids (nonsteroidal antiinflammatory drugs and acetaminophen), and (3) adjuvant analgesics.[4]

Opioid Analgesics

Opioids act by binding opiate receptors and thus activate central nervous system endogenous pain suppression systems; they are classified into three groups: (1) full agonists, (2) mixed agonist-antagonists, and (3) full antagonists. These divisions are based on the actions of the opioid at receptor sites.[1] Three major opiate receptors, the μ-, κ-, and ς-receptors, are found within the central nervous system, muscle, and gastrointestinal tract.[1,6] Opioids bind with receptors, induce a conformational change, and an effect results. The ability of opioids to produce this effect is known as intrinsic activity or efficacy, which has no relationship to the potency of the opioid or affinity for the receptor.[6] Agonist opioids have high affinity and high intrinsic activity. Opioid antagonists have high receptor affinity but no intrinsic activity. Agonist-antagonists have high affinity for the receptors but less intrinsic activity than the agonists.[6]

Binding at the μ-receptor with intrinsic activity produces supraspinal analgesia, euphoria, respiratory depression, mydriasis and/or miosis, hypothermia, bradycardia, sedation, physical dependence, and abuse potential.[1,6,7] Intrinsic activity at the κ-receptor results in spinal analgesia, miosis, moderate sedation, mild respiratory depression, and dysphoria. Sigma receptors mediate excitement (i.e., restlessness, mental anxiety, hallucinations, hyperkinesia, mydriasis, and respiratory and circulatory stimulation).[1,7] Some species respond with opioid-induced excitement (cats, horses) rather than depression (dogs, primates). As previously explained, analgesia and excitement are mediated by different receptors and effects occur concurrently but are drug- and dose-related. Low-dose therapy or concomitant administration of a major tranquilizer (e.g., acepromazine or droperidol) prevents excitation and makes opioid use extremely acceptable in cats.[6,7]

Different opioids have greater affinity at different receptors. Opioid agonists exhibit greatest affinity at the μ-receptors and are considered to be narcotics because they have the potential for causing physical dependence or abuse.[1] Potent narcotic agonists include morphine, oxymorphone, hydromorphone, methadone, etorphine, fentanyl, carfentanyl, sulfentanil, alfentanil, and lofentanil. Moderate agonists are codeine, dihydrocodeine, meperidine, and propoxyphene.[5,8,9] Common opioid agonist-antagonists are butorphanol, pentazocine, buprenorphine, and nalorphine.[8] The common antagonist is naloxone.[1,9] The appropriate analgesic doses and routes of administration are listed in Table I. The systemic effects that can occur after opioid administration are addressed in the following sections.

Central Nervous System. Opioids act on the central nervous system (CNS) to alter pain perception and relieve anxiety and distress. Although they create drowsiness and clouded mentation, the animal generally is arousable. Cats given higher doses demonstrate excitatory signs. A decreased response to blood CO_2 results in respiratory center depression; thus, opioids are contraindicated in patients suffering from respiratory depression caused by brain stem trauma unless ventilatory support can be provided.[6] Cough center depression occurs as well as stimulation of the chemoreceptive trigger zone, thereby resulting in possible emesis. Miosis occurs in dogs, and mydriasis occurs in cats.

Cardiovascular System. There are few major direct effects on the cardiovascular system at usual doses. In human medicine, large doses of narcotics often are substituted for inhalant anesthetics in patients with significant heart disease or in those who are critically ill.[10,11] The heart rate may initially increase and then decrease because of vagal influences. Hypotension could occur in some instances, possibly resulting from histamine release or central depression of the vasomotor center. Venous tone also is decreased, thereby reducing cardiac preload; this effect can be beneficial in managing congestive heart failure.[9]

Gastrointestinal Tract. Salivation, emesis, and defecation may occur immediately after administration of a potent agonist but this is followed, especially with repetitive administration, by an increase in gastric motility, decreased hydrochloric acid secretion, increased resting tone of the small and large intestine, and a reduction in amplitude of the nonpropulsive contraction of the small and large intestines resulting in constipation. Spasm of the biliary and pancreatic ducts also can occur.[9]

Urogenital Tract. Decreased urinary output can occur as a result of increased vasopressin release and decreased renal plasma flow. Ureteral smooth muscle spasm, increased bladder tone, and decreased uterine tone may occur.[9]

Pharmacokinetic Disposition of Opioids. Opioids are highly lipophilic, well absorbed parenterally, and penetrate tissue readily. They are metabolized by hepatic enzymes and often are conjugated with glucuronic acid. Opioid metabolism can be impaired in neonates, the aged, or patients with liver disease or reduced hepatic blood flow.[9]

A high degree of tolerance develops to analgesia as well as euphoria or dysphoria, mental clouding, sedation, respiratory depression, antidiuresis, nausea, vomiting, and cough suppression after repeated administration of agonist opioids. In humans, tolerance to morphine develops

TABLE I
Doses and Administration Routes of the Common Analgesics, Antagonists, and Adjuvants[a]

Agent	Dose and Route[b]
Morphine	Dog: 0.1–1.1 mg/kg IM or SC prn Cat: 0.1 mg/kg IM or SC prn
Meperidine	Dog/Cat: 1.0–4.0 mg/kg IM
Fentanyl	Dog: 0.04–0.08 mg/kg SC, IV, or IM
Oxymorphone	Dog/Cat: 0.025–0.05 mg/kg IM or IV prn
Codeine	Dog: 1.0–2.0 mg/kg PO every 6 hours
Pentazocine	Dog/Cat: 1.0–4.0 mg/kg IM every 4 hours
Butorphanol	Dog/Cat: 0.2–0.6 mg/kg IM, IV, or SC every 4 hours
Buprenorphine	Dog/Cat: 0.005–0.02 mg/kg IM every 10–14 hours
Naloxone	Dog/Cat: 0.5–1.0 µg/kg IV, IM, or SC
Aspirin	Dog: 10 mg/kg PO every 12 hours Cat: 10 mg/kg PO every 48 hours
Phenylbutazone	Dog: 15 mg/kg IV every 8 hours Dog: 22 mg/kg PO every 8 hours
Meclofenamic acid	Dog: 2.2 mg/kg PO daily
Diazepam	Dog/Cat: 0.2 mg/kg IM
Bupivacaine	Dog/Cat: 0.5 ml/site (0.5%) for selective intercostal nerve block every 6–8 hours 1.5 mg/kg (0.5% with 1:100,000 epinephrine) interpleurally every 3–12 hours

[a]Compiled from Haskins SC: Control of pain and suffering. *Proc 55th Annu AAHA Meet Vet Tech Program*:18–22, 1988; Haskins SC: Use of analgesics postoperatively and in a small animal intensive care setting. *JAVMA* 191:1266–1268, 1987; Miller JN: Anesthesiology. *Sci Am* 252:124–131, 1985; Schultz CS: Formulary 1987; Veterinary Hospital Pharmacy, Washington State University. Pullman, WA, W.S.U. Press, 1987; Thompson SE, Johnson JM: Postoperative analgesia in dogs after intercostal thoracotomy: A comparison of morphine, selective intercostal nerve block, and pleural regional analgesia with bupivacaine. *Vet Surg*, in press; and Muir WW: *Postoperative Pain: Surgical Fixation of Fractures and Nonunions*. The Ohio State University, A Course in AO/ASIF Techniques, 19th Annual Canine Basic Course, 1988.
[b]IM = intramuscular; IV = intravenous; PO = oral; prn = as needed; SC = subcutaneous.

in approximately two to three weeks. Physical dependence develops in approximately 25 days unless the drug is given continuously, in which case physical dependence begins to occur after 48 hours.[9,10] The fear of patients becoming addicted to narcotics is unwarranted. In a study of 12,000 human patients given narcotics, in which those with histories of addiction were eliminated, only four patients became addicted to the drugs they received.[10a]

Agonists

Morphine, oxymorphone, meperidine, codeine, and fentanyl are the more commonly used agonists in veterinary medicine. Their effects are reversible with naloxone or agonist-antagonists such as butorphanol.

Morphine

Morphine is the prototypic opioid agonist with which all other opioids are compared.[10] It has been used extensively in veterinary and human medicine and provides apparent pain relief for approximately four to six hours in dogs.[5,12] With intramuscular (IM) administration, the onset of effect of morphine occurs within 15 to 30 minutes; peak effects occur within 20 to 45 minutes.[3,10] Morphine can be given subcutaneously (SC) or intramuscularly in dogs and cats; intravenous (IV) administration is not recommended because morphine may initiate histamine release.[5,8] Morphine as an analgesic has no ceiling effect; therefore, increasing the dose increases the analgesic effect. Increasing the dose, however, may lead to profound respiratory depression. The elimination half-life of morphine in humans is 114 minutes.[10] With higher doses of morphine, nausea and vomiting occur in humans and animals that are capable of vomiting.[9,10] Miosis, hypoventilation, and coma are suggestive of an opioid overdose, and ventilation and administration of naloxone should be initiated.[10] The margin of safety for morphine in dogs is wide. Fatal subcutaneous or intravenous doses range from 22.7 to 45.5 mg/kg. Doses from 400 to 500 mg/kg have been given and, if convulsions are controlled with sodium pentobarbital, death does not result.[13]

Meperidine

Meperidine is less potent than morphine and provides apparent pain relief for approximately 45 minutes,[14] making it useful only as a preanesthetic. Meperidine also causes histamine release, and its pharmacologic effects are similar to those of morphine. Nausea and vomiting are less likely to be induced by meperidine.

Fentanyl

Fentanyl is used primarily in clinical practice in combination with droperidol for neuroleptanalgesia. Fentanyl is a more effective analgesic than morphine; fentanyl has a more rapid onset but a shorter duration of action, thereby making it impractical for long-term pain relief.[3] Fentanyl currently best lends itself to use in neuroleptanalgesia and as an adjuvant to inhalant anesthesia for intraoperative pain control. Fentanyl does not induce histamine release, but its depressant effects on the respiratory center are greater than those of morphine.[3,10]

Oxymorphone

Oxymorphone also has been used extensively in veterinary medicine and provides apparent pain relief for two to four hours and does not initiate histamine release. Oxymorphone causes less stimulation of the vomiting center than morphine but causes auditory hypersensitivity in some patients as well as bradycardia.[3,8]

Codeine

Codeine is often used as an antitussive in veterinary medicine and is very useful as an analgesic (with or without aspirin carrier) for oral use in the relief of mild to moderate pain.

Agonist-Antagonist Opioids

The agonist-antagonist opioids are analgesic. These opioids have decreased tendency to produce respiratory and central nervous system depression in the patient and minimal tendency to produce constipation as well as a minimal abuse potential.[5,8] The common agonist-antagonists include pentazocine, butorphanol, and buprenorphine.[8] These mixed opioids bind to μ-receptors. In other words, they have affinity for μ-receptors but have either limited or no intrinsic activity at the μ-receptors. Agonist-antagonist opioids do, however, have affinity and intrinsic activity at the κ-receptors and provide analgesia and varying degrees of sedation. Of the agonist-antagonists, some have greater agonistic activities; for example, butorphanol has strong agonist activity, whereas nalbuphine has stronger antagonistic activity.[1] Agonist-antagonists have greater affinity and/or potency for their receptors than the pure agonists and can therefore be used to reverse the effects of agonists by displacing them at their receptor sites. Unlike the agonists, the agonist-antagonists demonstrate a ceiling effect. In other words, increasing the dose does not produce increased analgesia or respiratory depression. The agonistic effects of agonist-antagonists are reversible with naloxone.

Pentazocine

Pentazocine is an inadequate drug for the treatment of severe pain. Pentazocine can be used for relief of mild to moderate pain, especially in old or debilitated patients.[3,10]

Butorphanol

Butorphanol is a more effective analgesic than pentazocine. It provides effective relief of mild to moderate pain, and its duration of analgesia is about one to four hours.[15]

Buprenorphine

Buprenorphine is a long-acting agonist-antagonist. This increased duration of effect may be attributable to slow dissociation from μ-receptors. Buprenorphine is effective in relieving moderate to severe pain; however, the duration of its respiratory depression effects may be prolonged, and it is resistant to antagonism by naloxone. Doxapram may be required to maintain adequate ventilation in patients under the influence of this drug.[10]

Opioid Antagonists

Naloxone and naltrexone are the two antagonists used to reverse effects of agonists and agonist-antagonists. Antagonists attach competitively to all opioid receptors and displace opioid agonists, but antagonists excite no intrinsic activity of their own.[1,9] The primary use of antagonists is to reverse respiratory depression that can occur after agonist administration. Naloxone has a shorter duration of action than the agonists (30 to 45 minutes); therefore, repeated doses of naloxone often are necessary for sustained antagonism. Naltrexone is effective orally and offers sustained antagonism for up to 24 hours.[10]

When an antagonist or an agonist-antagonist is used to reverse opioid-induced respiratory depression, reversal of analgesia occurs as well.[9,10] It is best to attempt to titrate the dose of naloxone so that respiratory depression is relieved partially to an acceptable level while partial analgesia is maintained. Alternatively, butorphanol can be used to reverse the respiratory depression and sedation while maintaining analgesia. With abrupt cessation of analgesia and onset of pain, tachycardia, hypertension, pulmonary edema, and cardiac dysrhythmias (including ventricular fibrillation) may occur due to increased sympathetic nervous system activity.[10] Titration of naloxone at 0.5 to 1.0 µg/kg intravenously helps reverse sedation and maintain analgesia.[16]

Nonopioid Analgesics

The two major classes of nonopioid analgesics are (1) nonsteroidal antiinflammatory drugs (NSAIDs [cyclooxygenase inhibitors]) and (2) paraaminophenol derivatives (acetaminophen). Nonsteroidal antiinflammatory drugs produce analgesia and suppress the inflammatory response, thereby relieving pain of low to moderate intensity, especially if the pain is associated with inflammation or prostaglandin release. Nonsteroidal antiinflammatory drugs are most effective against pain of somatic or integumental origin.[9] These drugs are of little use in treating acute, severe, or postoperative pain in dogs and cats during the first 48 hours.[6] Opioid analgesics and nonsteroidal antiinflammatory drugs may act synergistically and potentiate analgesic effects.[9] Nonopioids are believed to exert analgesic effects at the nociceptor level in tissue by impairing impulse generation or conduction that results in pain perception. Nonsteroidal antiinflammatory drugs are readily absorbed from the gastrointestinal tract, metabolized by the liver, and excreted in urine.[9] Nonopioid analgesics have no ceiling effect and do not produce tolerance or dependence.[4]

Nonsteroidal antiinflammatory drugs that have been used in dogs include aspirin, flunixin, ibuprofen, naproxen, meclofenamic acid, and phenylbutazone. The side effects of most nonsteroidal antiinflammatory drugs are many and common. Gastric and intestinal ulceration, hemorrhage, and/or perforation; impaired platelet adhesion; renal failure in the face of preexisting renal disease; hypersensitivity; and occasional blood dyscrasias are known to occur.[5,9] Agents that are least likely to produce untoward gastrointestinal side effects are aspirin, phenylbutazone, and meclofenamic acid.[8]

Acetaminophen inhibits prostaglandin synthesis centrally but not peripherally and is therefore a poor visceral and somatic analgesic. Although acetaminophen does not induce impaired platelet function or gastrointestinal tract ulceration, it can produce a hepatotoxic metabolite in the face of an overwhelmed glutathione scavenging system. This is especially true in cats. Use of acetaminophen is contraindicated in dogs and cats.[5]

Adjuvant Analgesics

The adjuvant analgesics form a miscellaneous group of pharmacologic agents that may potentiate narcotic analgesics or produce independent analgesic effects.[4] This group includes such agents as xylazine, diazepam, phenothiazines, and local anesthesia.

Xylazine

Xylazine is an aminothiazine, sedative-analgesic that acts on central and peripheral α-2 receptors. This agent is rapidly eliminated as a result of extensive biotransformation and has a plasma half-life of 1.2 to 6 minutes in dogs after intravenous administration. It often is used in combination with an opioid for neuroleptanalgesia as both are completely reversible.[6,7]

Diazepam

Diazepam is a minor tranquilizer that acts as a muscle relaxant and possibly has some inherent analgesic properties in animals. Diazepam can be combined with an analgesic to treat postsurgical pain, and it produces minimal respiratory and cardiovascular effects.[15]

Phenothiazines

Phenothiazines may potentiate analgesia.[3,4] They are beneficial as antiemetics in combination with narcotics, and they provide muscle relaxation. Caution must be exercised in their use because they enhance sedation and can produce hypotension.[3]

Local Anesthesia

Local field blocks and regional blocks using long-acting local anesthetics, such as bupivacaine, can be useful adjuvants to analgesic therapy. In the case of multiple trauma, incipient shock, metabolic damage, and highly altered homeostasis, organ function may be further compromised by pain. Under such circumstances, systemic analgesia may be less than desirable, while local or regional analgesia via bupivacaine infiltration may be a powerful therapeutic adjuvant.[17]

Intercostal nerve blocks have been shown to aid in the relief of early postsurgical and/or posttraumatic pain of the thorax in humans and dogs.[8] Selective intercostal nerve blocks may improve postoperative ventilation by providing analgesia without the negative effect of central respiratory tract depression. Selective intercostal nerve blocks provide relief from somatic pain, which is the major component of postthoracotomy pain. Intercostal nerve blockage results in analgesia and paralysis of the intercostal muscles. Several nerves must be blocked to provide adequate pain relief. Respiratory muscle paralysis does produce a small decrease in ventilation, but this is considered insignificant in the face of the improvement seen in ventilation with selective intercostal nerve blocks. Epinephrine can be added to the bupivacaine to decrease systemic absorption and extend the duration of analgesia.[18]

An alternative to selective intercostal nerve blocks that also provides postsurgical and/or posttraumatic pain relief of the thorax is interpleural regional analgesia. Bupivacaine hydrochloride (0.5% with 1:100,000 epinephrine) administered interpleurally at a dose of 1.5 mg/kg of bupivacaine provided effective analgesia for 3 to 12 hours in dogs in one study.[19] Interpleural regional analgesia is superior to selective intercostal nerve blocks in that multiple nerve blocks are not required because bupivacaine diffuses across the pleura and blocks intercostal nerves. In interpleural regional analgesia, bupivacaine can be administered through an indwelling thoracic catheter or by a single interpleural injection.[19] Interpleural bupivacaine tends to be ineffective in cases with severe pleural effusion in which dilution of the local anesthetic occurs.[20]

Regional anesthesia and analgesia also can be obtained in the forelimb with a brachial plexus block. Using sterile technique, lidocaine hydrochloride or bupivacaine hydrochloride is injected with a spinal needle medial to the shoulder joint, parallel to the vertebral column, and directed toward the costochondral junction. This will provide anesthesia and analgesia from the distal part of the foot to the elbow. Lidocaine hydrochloride used at 4 to 6 mg/kg will take 20 minutes to become effective and has a duration of 120 minutes. A bupivacaine hydrochloride (0.5%) dose of 1.5 mg/kg is used for bilateral blocks and 2 mg/kg is used for unilateral blocks. The duration of effect is 180 to 300 minutes.[20a]

Epidural blocks, which diminish the need for systemic analgesics, provide anesthesia and analgesia caudal to the umbilicus and are effective in providing long-term analgesia for dogs and cats with pelvic or hindlimb fractures, tail or hindlimb amputation, anal or perianal surgery, or abdominal surgery. After surgical preparation, a spinal needle is placed in the lumbosacral epidural space for injection of a local anesthetic and/or opioid. Alpha$_2$-adrenergic agonists also can be used alone or concomitantly with opioids. Lidocaine hydrochloride (2%) provides effective analgesia within five minutes and lasts for 60 to 90 minutes, while bupivacaine hydrochloride (0.5%) has an onset of action of 20 to 30 minutes and lasts several hours. Both local anesthetics are dosed at 0.22 ml/kg and provide motor and sensory blockade.[20a]

Epidurally administered morphine has no effect on motor or sympathetic activity, but provides analgesia for 12 to 24 hours. Morphine (0.1 mg/kg) is diluted with 0.9% saline to a volume of 0.3 ml/kg with a maximum volume of 6 milliliters.

WHEN TO USE ANALGESICS

The following statement by D. M. Ross, a prominent authority on human pain, holds true for animals as well: "...severe acute pain in the postoperative period, or after burns or after accidental injury, has no useful function, and if not adequately relieved produces serious abnormal physiologic and psychologic reactions which often cause complications."[21]

Opioid analgesia is postoperatively indicated to relieve pain, especially during the first 48 hours.[4] Practitioners often choose to wait until an animal is showing profound signs of postoperative pain before treatment is initiated because they want to ensure that the patient is experiencing pain. This is an ineffective means of treatment because some animals in pain do not show overt signs; the most effective way to alleviate pain is to treat it before it happens. When using an opioid, analgesic effects are most prominent when it is administered before the pain stimulus occurs.[10] Two appropriate times to begin administering a postoperative analgesic are (1) when surgery is nearing completion and the vaporizer is turned off (in the case of halothane and isoflurane) or (2) when the animal starts to show signs of recovery, such as initiation of swallowing, presence of a strong palpebral reflex, or just before extubation. If an analgesic is administered after extubation, intramuscular administration is indicated.[22]

If analgesics are given before recovery, sharp pain is alleviated and a dull pain situation is produced. With dull pain, opioid analgesics become more effective and the animal can more readily adjust and begin to accept the discomfort. Analgesics given to a crying, screaming patient require large doses, repeated doses, and often potentiation with tranquilizers.[22]

An animal under the effects of an analgesic should be monitored for recurring signs of pain, and the analgesic dose should be repeated according to dosage intervals recommended for the respective drug. Clinicians often are reluctant to use the Schedule II narcotics for relief of pain in animals. Extra quantities of paperwork and the required safeguarding of narcotics should not deter a clinician from using the most effective means of treatment. Morphine provides uniform, effective analgesia with the least number of side effects of any of the agonists and agonist-antagonists. Morphine is inexpensive and produces profound visceral and somatic analgesia[10]; it is reversible, has no ceiling effect, and it can be potentiated with tranquilizers.[22]

When choosing an analgesic for treating a patient in pain, the clinician should consider the level of pain expected and leave alternatives to provide greater analgesia if needed. It is not important which agent is chosen if analgesia is achieved. Administering an agent and believing analgesia is created without assessing whether the drug has been effective is inappropriate and dangerous therapy. After analgesic administration, animals should be able to sleep comfortably yet remain arousable and should demonstrate minimal physical and physiologic signs of pain. If the chosen agent is ineffective, an increase in the dose (if there is no ceiling effect), an increase in the frequency of the dose, potentiation with an adjuvant, or a change to another analgesic is indicated.

Opioid analgesia is indicated for moderate to severe pain, but mild pain should not be overlooked. Aspirin and other nonsteroidal antiinflammatory drugs can be very effective in relieving mild pain. Some animals require opioid analgesia for mild pain, especially if other factors (such as concomitant disease and mild injury) occur or if there are other stressors that might enhance what would normally be considered mild pain. Butorphanol also is available in tablet form as an antitussive agent, and an animal that requires analgesia at home greater than that afforded by the nonsteroidal antiinflammatory drugs can be treated with butorphanol as an analgesic or codeine phosphate or aspirin with codeine, which provide more effective analgesia. Nonsteroidal antiinflammatory therapy can be used after cessation of opioid therapy to provide continued analgesia during the healing phase.

Current concepts in pain include neuroplasticity, in which nociceptive traffic transmission and processing are considered an activity-dependent, dynamic, and plastic phenomenon where adaptive and maladaptive sensitization of peripheral afferents and central pathways occurs. Acute pain is currently classified as physiologic or clinical pain. Physiologic pain is the high threshold; well localized and transient pain we consider to be a "protective system." Clinical pain includes inflammatory pain associated with peripheral tissue damage (e.g., surgery) and neuropathic pain associated with damage to the nervous system. Clinical pain produces a pathologic hypersensitivity by two mechanisms: Peripheral sensitization and central sensitization. Peripheral sensitization is the hyperalgesia that follows peripheral tissue injury and is caused by an increase in sensitivity of primary afferent nociceptors in the vicinity of injury.

Central sensitization is triggered by nociceptive afferent inputs and manifests as a prolonged reduction in the threshold, an expansion of the extent, and an increase in the responsiveness of the cutaneous receptive fields of dorsal horn neurons. Central sensitization is precipitated by a phenomenon known as windup. Windup is a progressive increase in the number of action potentials elicited per stimulus that occurs in dorsal horn neurons where C afferent fibers are repetitively stimulated.[22a, 22b]

The stress response to acute surgical injury and critical illness induces neural, endocrine, metabolic, and inflammatory changes that initiate peripheral and central sensitization. With the exception of high dose narcotic techniques or regional anesthesia, general anesthesia minimally moderates the surgical stress response. The goal of analgesia is to minimize or eliminate peripheral and central sensitization by treating pain in advance of its manifestation. This concept is termed preemptive analgesia. Preemptive analgesia can be directed at the periphery, at inputs along sensory axons, and at central neurons by using NSAIDs, local anesthetics, and opioids either alone or in combination and applied intermittently to establish balanced analgesia. The benefits of preemptive analgesia in people include decreased pain, earlier mobilization, decreased hospital stay, prevention of intraoperative hemodynamic reactions, and a reduction of respiratory complications.[22a, 22b] The use of preemptive analgesia should produce the same effects in our veterinary patients.

The final word in assessing and managing animals in pain is *compassion*. Dr. Leo Bustad's comments are most appropriate: "As things are now it may well be that the survival of the species will depend upon our ability to foster a boundless capacity for compassion. Compassion, compassionate love, and concern may save us. It is our last great hope.... Compassion is suffering with, having empathy with, and feeling for...an awareness of the mutuality of all living things. The bond is not only between people but also with people and animals.... Compassion is not merely feeling and sentiment, however, but active relief of pain and suffering in others...Compassion is a way of treating all life...It involves seeing, feeling, and acting!"[23]

ACKNOWLEDGMENT

The author thanks Leo K. Bustad, DVM, PhD, Professor and Dean Emeritus, College of Veterinary Medicine, Washington State University, for his interest, advice, and support.

About the Authors

Dr. Johnson is a staff surgeon and a staff dentist at Allpets Clinic in Boulder, Colorado.

REFERENCES

1. Sawyer DC: Understanding animal pain and suffering. *Proc 55th Annu AAHA Meet Vet Tech Program*:1–6, 1988.
2. Kitchen H, Aronson AL, Bittle JL, et al: Panel report on the colloquium on recognition and alleviation of animal pain and stress. *JAVMA* 191:1186–1191, 1987.
3. Wright EM, Marcella KL, Woodson JF: Animal pain: Evaluation and control. *Lab Anim* May/June:20–36, 1985.
4. Pain R, Max M, Inturrisi C, et al: Principles of analgesic use in the treatment of acute pain and chronic cancer pain. *Syllabus Committ Meet Am Pain Soc Brd Dir*:1–9, 1986.
5. Haskins SC: Control of pain and suffering. *Proc 55th Annu*

AAHA Meet Vet Tech Program:18–22, 1988.
6. Benson GJ: The recognition and alleviation of animal pain and suffering: Opioid analgesics. *Proc 55th Annu AAHA Meet Vet Tech Program*:7–17, 1988.
7. Benson GJ, Thurman JC: Species differences: A consideration in alleviation of animal pain and distress. *JAVMA* 191:1227–1230, 1987.
8. Haskins SC: Use of analgesics postoperatively and in a small animal intensive care setting. *JAVMA* 191:1266–1268, 1987.
9. Jenkins WL: Pharmacologic aspects of analgesic drugs in animals: An overview. *JAVMA* 191:1231–1240, 1987.
10. Stoeting RK: *Pharmacology and Physiology in Anesthetic Practice.* Philadelphia, JB Lippincott Co, 1987, pp 69–101.
10a. Allis S: Less pain, more gain. *TIME* October 19, 1992, pp 61, 64.
11. Miller JN: Anesthesiology. *Sci Am* 252:124–131, 1985.
12. Willis WD, Chung JM: Central mechanisms of pain. *JAVMA* 191:1200–1202, 1987.
13. Lumb WV, Jones EW: *Veterinary Anesthesia.* Philadelphia, Lea & Febiger, 1984, p 177.
14. Schultz CS: Formulary 1987, Veterinary Hospital Pharmacy, Washington State University. Pullman, WA, W.S.U. Press, 1987.
15. Sawyer DC: Use of narcotics and analgesics for pain control. *Proc 52nd Annu AAHA Meet*:7–11, 1985.
16. Muir WW: *Postoperative Pain. Surgical Fixation of Fractures and Nonunions.* The Ohio State University, A Course in AO/ASIF Techniques, 19th Annual Canine Basic Course, 1988.
17. Crane SW: Perioperative analgesia: A surgeon's perspective. *JAVMA* 191:1254–1257, 1987.
18. Berg RJ, Orton EC: Pulmonary function in dogs after intercostal thoracotomy: Comparison of morphine, oxymorphone, and selective intercostal nerve block. *Am J Vet Res* 47:471–474, 1986.
19. Thompson SE, Johnson JM: Postoperative analgesia in dogs after intercostal thoracotomy: A comparison of morphine, selective intercostal nerve block, and pleural regional analgesia with bupivacaine. *Vet Surg* 20:73–77, 1991.
20. Seltzer JL, Larijani GE, Goldberg ME, et al: Intrapleural bupivacaine: A kinetic and dynamic evolution. Anesthesiology 67:798–800, 1987.
20a. Quandt JE, Rawlings CR: Reducing postoperative pain for dogs: Local anesthetic and analgesic techniques. *Compend Contin Educ Pract Vet* 18:101–140, 1996.
21. Ross DM, Ross SA: *Childhood Pain: Current Issues, Research, and Management.* Baltimore, MD, Urban & Schwarzenburg, 1988, p 19.
22. Sawyer DC, Benson GJ, Hawkins SC: Animal technician lecture series: Pain panel discussion. *Proc 55th Annu AAHA Meet*:1988.
22a. Woolf CJ, Mun-Seng C: Preemptive analgesia—treating postoperative pain by preventing the establishment of central sensitization. *Anesth Analg* 77:362–379, 1993.
22b. Brown DL, Mackey DC: Subspecialty clinics: Anesthesiology management of postoperative pain: Influence of anesthetic and analgesic choice. *Mayo Clin Proc* 68: 768–777, 1993.
23. Bustad LK: *Equipping God's People for Monday's Ministries.* Address at Pacific Lutheran University, Tacoma, WA, 1986.

Life-Threatening Bacterial Infection

North Carolina State University
Elizabeth M. Hardie, DVM, PhD

KEY FACTS

❑ Early recognition of infection, before the generalized release of inflammatory mediators, is associated with successful treatment.

❑ The major elements in the treatment of severe bacterial infection are appropriate antibiotic therapy, aggressive cardiovascular support, and surgical removal of infected matter.

❑ Death in appropriately treated animals is the result of the effects of the systemic inflammatory response.

❑ For the survival rate to increase in patients with severe bacterial infection, treatments that modify the host response to infection must be developed.

Scientific knowledge about the pathophysiology of severe bacterial infection is exploding—computerized reviews of the subject often yield hundreds of articles each month. Despite the rapid increase in understanding of a highly complex phenomenon, the mortality for human patients with severe bacterial infection has changed very little over the past 10 years.[1] Numerous clinical trials have tested therapies that work in the laboratory but fail to increase survival in hospital patients. The reason for the disparity is becoming apparent. The clinical disease is much more heterogenous than was first suspected, and therapies that are successful in models of gram-negative infection may not be effective when used as treatments for the disease clinicians call sepsis.[1]

SYSTEMIC INFLAMMATORY RESPONSE SYNDROME

To understand the heterogenous nature of clinical sepsis, one must separate the concept of infection from the concept of host response to infection.[2,3] Infection is the confirmed presence of a pathogenic organism in tissue. The host response to infection is a continuum from a local, limited response to a condition of generalized shock. Superimposed on the large range of host responses are species differences, preexisting differences in immune status, and concurrent diseases. In the laboratory, a tightly standardized infection or bacterial toxin injection is used to produce a standardized host response. In the hospital, the clinician sees the host response first; infection may or may not be confirmed at some time in the future. Careful studies of human patients and increasing understanding of the inflammatory response have resulted in the following concepts[1-3]:

1. What has been called *sepsis*, *septic syndrome*, or *septic shock* in the past is now being renamed *systemic inflammatory response syndrome* (SIRS), because similar host responses can be elicited by gram-negative organisms, gram-positive organisms, fungi, viruses, parasites, rickettsial organisms, yeasts, pancreatitis, ischemia, severe trauma and tissue injury, hemorrhagic shock, immune-mediated organ injury, or administration of such exogenous mediators as tumor necrosis factor. Patients entered into human clinical trials with the suspected diagnosis of bacterial sepsis eventually proved to have the following spectrum of disease: positive blood culture in less than half the patients, gram-negative infections in 21% to 37% of patients, gram-positive infections in 9% to 17% of patients, fungal infec-

tions in 1% to 3% of patients, and no organisms cultured at any site in 15% of patients.[1]
2. If severe infection is untreated, infection is the major determinant of mortality. In healthy experimental animals, as the number of bacteria or the amount of endotoxin increases, a trigger point at which the inflammatory response shifts from a local reaction to an uncontrolled systemic reaction is reached.[4] Without treatment, death rapidly ensues.

   If infection is treated but the patient has major ongoing pathophysiologic abnormalities resulting from severe disease (as is the case with the human intensive care unit population), SIRS can develop as a result of minor opportunistic infections.[2] In such situations, the trigger for SIRS is irrelevant—it is the host response that kills.

3. Treatment affects the outcome of the organism–host interaction only if it is begun before the onset of irreversible changes associated with the host response. Once endogenous mediators have been released and SIRS is present, even optimal treatment fails to increase survival rates higher than 60%.[1] In an older study of human patients with sepsis, mortality was 12% if treatment was begun when fever and leukocytosis were present, 65% if treatment was initiated when either organ dysfunction or shock was present, and 88% if shock and organ dysfunction were present.[5] More recently, mortality of human patients with SIRS has been shown to be remarkably constant: 22% to 28% at 14 days and 41% to 43% at 30 days, regardless of whether or not infection or shock (i.e., hypotension not responsive to fluid therapy) was present.[1]

   If one assumes that severe bacterial infection in most veterinary patients is recognized after mediator release and before the onset of refractory shock, a reasonable goal would be a 50% to 60% survival rate. Survival rates range from 29% to 69% in various veterinary studies of confirmed bacterial infection associated with severe systemic signs.[6–10] In a canine model of lethal peritonitis, a survival rate of 50% was reached when both antibiotics and cardiovascular support were provided.[11]

4. Treatment for severe bacterial infection continues to rely on three main tools: surgery, antibiotics, and aggressive cardiovascular support.[2,11] The effects of such therapy are synergistic. In the previously mentioned model of peritonitis, treatment with either antibiotics or cardiovascular support alone increased the survival rate to only 13%.[11] Once a survival rate of 50% to 60% is reached, however, the only way to increase survival further is to block the development of SIRS.[1] It is easy to block SIRS in the laboratory, where the trigger for SIRS is defined and the time course of mediator release is known. The challenge for the future is to develop ways to block the development of SIRS associated with a variety of triggering events (not just endotoxin) or to modify the host response after mediators have been released.[1]

TABLE I
Bacterial Infections Often Associated with Systemic Inflammatory Response Syndrome

Disease	Typical Organisms
Pyothorax	Mixed anaerobic infection
Peritonitis	Anaerobes; gram-negative enteric organisms
Pyometra	*E. coli*, anaerobes, *Staphylococcus* species; *Streptococcus* species
Prostatic abscess	*E. coli* and other gram-negative enteric organisms; *Staphylococcus* species; *Streptococcus* species
Liver abscess; biliary tract infection	Anaerobes; gram-negative enteric organisms
Renal abscess	*E. coli* and other gram-negative enteric organisms; *Staphylococcus* species; *Streptococcus* species
Epididymitis; orchitis	Studies lacking; probably similar to urinary tract infection
Mastitis	Anaerobes; gram-negative enteric organisms
Wound infections	*Staphylococcus intermedius*; nosocomial pathogens; *Pseudomonas* species
Bacterial endocarditis	*Staphylococcus intermedius*; *Streptococcus* species; *E. coli*; *Erysipelothrix rhusiopathiae*; *Corynebacterium* species
Bacteremia Associated disease	
Urinary tract infection	*Staphylococcus intermedius*; *Streptococcus* species; *E. coli* and other gram-negative enteric organisms
Pyoderma	*Staphylococcus intermedius*; *Streptococcus* species
Severe enteritis	*E. coli*
Severe gingivitis	Anaerobes; gram-negative organisms
Neoplasia	Enterobacteriaceae
ICU patients	46% gram-negative bacilli; 30% gram-positive cocci; 31% anaerobes; 15% polymicrobial

CLINICAL SIGNS

Bacterial infections known to be associated with

> **Definition of Systemic Inflammatory Response Syndrome**
>
> **Humans**
> The presence of two or more of the following clinical conditions:
> - Body temperature >38°C or <36°C
> - Heart rate >90 beats/min
> - Respiratory rate >20 breaths/min or $PaCO_2$ <32 mm Hg
> - White blood cell count >12,000/mm³ or <4,000/mm³ or >10% immature (band) forms
>
> **Proposed for Dogs**
> The presence of two or more of the following clinical conditions:
> - Body temperature >40°C or <38°C
> - Heart rate >120 beats/min in calm, resting dog
> - Hyperventilation or $PaCO_2$ <30 mm Hg
> - White blood cell count >18,000/mm³ or <5,000/mm³ or >5% immature (band) forms
>
> **Proposed for Cats**
> The presence of two or more of the following clinical conditions:
> - Body temperature >40°C or <38°C
> - Heart rate >140 beats/min in calm, resting cat
> - Respiratory rate >20 breaths/min or $PaCO_2$ <28 mm Hg
> - White blood cell count >18,000/mm³ or <5,000/mm³ or >5% immature (band) forms

SIRS are listed in Table I. Physical examination findings associated with severe bacterial infection can be vague.[6,7,12] As stated in the definition of SIRS (see the box), fever or hypothermia, tachycardia, and hyperventilation are the hallmarks of this syndrome. The frequency with which each sign is present varies. In a study of dogs with bacteremia, 75% had fever, whereas in a study of dogs with surgically confirmed infection, 40% had fever and 3% had hypothermia.[7,12] In a prospective study of intensive care unit patients, fever was most likely to be present with gram-positive or polymicrobial bacteremia and least likely to be present with anaerobic bacteremia.[6] Overt tachycardia (i.e., heart rate greater than 160 beats per minute) was found in only 21% of dogs with severe postsurgical infection, but 47% had rate increases of 20% or greater from hospital admission values.[7] Tachypnea has not been documented in clinical patients but is always present in experimental canine and feline SIRS models. Additional clinical signs of severe bacterial infection include lethargy, depression, anorexia, vomiting and/or diarrhea, pain associated with the site of infection, and generalized pain.

Early SIRS is associated with brick-red mucous membranes, tachycardia, high cardiac output, normal or low systemic arterial blood pressure, and low systemic vascular resistance.[7,11,13] Animals with inadequate intravascular volume (usually due to massive fluid shifts into the peritoneum or interstitium) have pale mucous membranes, cold extremities, tachycardia, low cardiac output, low systemic arterial blood pressure, and high systemic vascular resistance.[7,11,13] The provision of adequate amounts of intravenous fluids usually results in clinical signs similar to those of early SIRS.[11] If refractory hypotension is present, no response will be seen with fluid and inotropic therapy. Blood pressure in patients with refractory hypotension cannot be increased, because fluid leakage through the vascular endothelium prevents expansion of intravascular volume, generalized vasodilatation unresponsive to pressor therapy is present, and/or myocardial depression limits cardiac output.[4,14]

The order of organ dysfunction associated with SIRS varies with species. In dogs, the order is usually the gastrointestinal tract, liver, kidney, and then lung.[13,15] Gram-positive bacteremia is associated with a high incidence of thromboembolism, which may result in organ dysfunction independent of the development of SIRS.[16] Clinical signs of gastrointestinal dysfunction include anorexia, vomiting, diarrhea, and mucosal sloughing (manifested by vomiting or diarrhea containing blood and obvious mucosal remnants). Hepatic dysfunction leads to anorexia, vomiting, and icterus. Anuria due to renal dysfunction is rare. Anuria is usually associated with hypotension and shock, and correction of hemodynamic status resolves the problem. Lung dysfunction is associated with the development of pulmonary edema (pink-tinged frothy fluid is seen coming from the mouth and nostrils) and hypoxemia and rarely occurs before refractory shock.

In cats, the pattern of organ failure is different, and respiratory dysfunction occurs early in the course of SIRS.[17] Tachypnea in cats should thus be presumed to be associated with hypoxemia from pulmonary dysfunction.

Depression of cardiac function occurs early in the course of SIRS, but unless highly sensitive measures of cardiac function are used, overt biventricular failure will not be noted until the later stages of disease.[18,19] Myocardial dysfunction is rarely severe enough to affect cardiac output, even early in the course of SIRS.[20]

LABORATORY FINDINGS

The primary laboratory finding associated with SIRS is an abnormal leukogram.[6,12] Leukocytosis or leukopenia, an increased concentration of immature neutrophils (left shift), and monocytosis occur. Platelet counts tend to be decreased.[21]

Hemoconcentration occurs following fluid losses from the intravascular space.[22,23] Total serum solids decrease as a result of decreased synthesis (the liver shifts to synthesis of acute-phase proteins) and increased movement of protein from blood to the tissues. Serum biochemical abnormalities associated with SIRS reflect vascular leakage and organ dysfunction.[7,12,13] Hypoalbuminemia, hypoglycemia or hyperglycemia, and increased serum alkaline phosphatase activity are seen most often. Bilirubinemia is caused by intrahepatic cholestasis, which may occur in the absence of other forms of hepatic dysfunction.[24] Increased serum alanine transaminase concentration indicates probable hepatocellular necrosis. The presence of two or more serum biochemical abnormalities has been shown to be correlated with increased mortality.[12]

The clotting status of SIRS patients can range from a hypercoagulable state to overt disseminated intravascular coagulation (DIC).[13] Evidence of DIC (i.e., low fibrinogen, low antithrombin III, prolonged prothrombin and activated partial thromboplastin times, increased fibrin degradation products) should be regarded as evidence of advanced SIRS.[25] If organ dysfunction and/or cardiovascular collapse are also present, irreversible shock is likely. The presence of low platelet numbers alone should not be used as evidence of DIC, because thrombocytopenia can occur independently from DIC in patients with SIRS.[21]

Metabolic acidosis with respiratory compensation is usually present in dogs with SIRS.[22] Hypoxemia is not seen in awake dogs with severe gram-negative infection but may become apparent in sedated or anesthetized dogs that cannot control the depth and rate of respiration.[26] Blood gas changes have been measured in endotoxic but not infected cats.[17] Hypoxemia, hypercapnia, and metabolic acidosis develop rapidly.

Blood lactate concentrations are increased in patients with SIRS because of poor oxygen delivery to the tissues and impaired cellular oxidative respiration.[27,28] If lactate values are not available, dogs in endotoxic shock with high anion gap metabolic acidosis due to lactic acidosis have been shown to have the following approximate relationship between anion gap and lactic acid concentration[29]: [lactate] = (0.27 × anion gap) − 1.46.

INSTRUMENTATION

Several intravenous lines (including one central line) should be placed to supply fluids, administer drugs, and withdraw blood samples. If venous access cannot be rapidly accomplished in severely hypoten-

TABLE II
Monitoring Variables for Animals with Systemic Inflammatory Response Syndrome

Variable	Goal
Core temperature	38°C–40°C
Core/toe-web temperature differential	<4°C
Heart rate (beats/min)	70–120 (dogs) 100–140 (cats)
Capillary refill time (seconds)	<2
Systemic arterial blood pressure (mm Hg)	mean >90; >120/80
Central venous pressure (cm H_2O)	5–15
Urine output (ml/kg/hr)	2–5
Hematocrit (%)	30–35
Total solids (mg/dl)	3.5–5.0
Arterial oxygen tension, PaO_2 (mm Hg)	100–120
Base excess (mM/L)	−2–+2
Central venous oxygen saturation, SvO_2 (%)	>70
Arterial-venous O_2 content[a] difference[b] (ml of O_2/dl)	3–5
Arterial-venous CO_2 tension difference[b] (mm Hg)	<6
Blood lactate concentration (mg/dl)	<1
Blood glucose concentration (mEq/dl)	70–150
Albumin (g/dl)	2.5–4.5
Potassium (mEq/L)	4–5
Blood urea nitrogen (mg/dl)	<30

[a]Oxygen content = (hemoglobin concentration × 1.34 × oxygen saturation) + (0.003 × oxygen tension).
[b]Subtract the venous value of the variable from the arterial value. The venous value may be obtained from blood drawn through a central venous catheter, but a value from mixed venous blood drawn from a pulmonary arterial catheter is preferred.

sive patients, a bone marrow needle must be placed to administer fluids into the marrow cavity of the humerus or femur.[30] An indwelling urinary catheter allows monitoring of urine output. Systemic arterial blood pressure can be measured using indirect methods, but a direct arterial line allows more accurate monitoring of systemic arterial blood pressure.

Core and toe-web thermometers should be placed to assess peripheral vasoconstriction and flow.[31] Baseline values must be obtained for a complete blood count, serum chemistry profile, clotting profile, blood lactate concentration, and room-air arterial blood gas analysis to determine the severity of SIRS and to monitor the progress of treatment (Table II).

TABLE III
Antibiotics Used to Treat Severe Bacterial Infection in Dogs and Cats

Drug	Dosage
Enrofloxacin	5 mg/kg/12 hr, IV
Gentamicin	6 mg/kg/24 hr, IV
Amikacin	10 mg/kg/8 hr, IV
Tobramycin	2–4 mg/kg/8 hr, IV
Ampicillin	20–40 mg/kg/8 hr, IV
Clindamycin	11 mg/kg/8 hr, IV
Metronidazole	10 mg/kg/8 hr, IV
Cefazolin	20 mg/kg/8 hr, IV
Cefoxitin	30 mg/kg/5 hr, IV
Imipenem	2–5 mg/kg/8 hr, IV

IV = intravenously.

TABLE IV
Additional Cardiovascular Therapeutic Goals for Animals with Systemic Inflammatory Response Syndrome and with a Pulmonary Arterial Catheter in Place

Variable	Goal
Mixed venous oxygen tension, P_{VO_2} (mm Hg)	>40
Pulmonary artery pressure (mm Hg)	>25/10
Pulmonary wedge pressure (mm Hg)	<18
Systemic vascular resistance (dyne × sec/cm^{-5} × m^2)	>1450
Pulmonary vascular resistance (dyne × sec/cm^{-5} × m^2)	45–250
Oxygen extraction (%)	22–30
Cardiac index (L/min × m^2)	>4.5
Oxygen delivery (ml/min × m^2)	>600
Oxygen consumption (ml/min × m^2)	>170

A sterile urine sample should be saved so that a culture can be performed if urinalysis reveals evidence of infection.

ANTIBIOTICS

Broad-spectrum intravenous antibiotic therapy (Table III) must be initiated early. For dogs, therapy should be effective against gram-negative organisms (particularly *Escherichia coli* and *Klebsiella pneumoniae* subspecies); gram-positive organisms (*Staphylococcus intermedius*, *Streptococcus* species, and *Enterococcus* species); anaerobes (particularly *Clostridium perfringens*); and *Rickettsia rickettsii* (if tick exposure is a possibility).[3,12,32] For cats, therapy should be particularly effective against gram-negative organisms (*Escherichia coli*, *Klebsiella pneumoniae* subspecies, and *Salmonella* species) and resistant anaerobes (*Propionibacterium acnes* and *Bacteroides* species).[6]

For dogs, a combination of enrofloxacin and ampicillin will provide broad-range coverage.[33,34] The obvious omissions in this combination are efficacy against resistant enterococci and anaerobes. Thus, in cats and in dogs with known intraabdominal infection, such combinations as amikacin–clindamycin or amikacin–metronidazole should be used.[33] If renal function is compromised and rickettsial infection unlikely, a first-generation cephalosporin (cefazolin) will be effective against most gram-positive organisms associated with bacteremia in dogs.[35] If a gram-negative, anaerobic infection is suspected, a second-generation cephalosporin (cefoxitin) may be used.[35] Imipenem, a carbepenam, has the widest spectrum of any beta-lactam antibiotic and is the drug of choice for the SIRS patient with renal compromise and a documented resistant bacterial infection.[35]

Regardless of the initial choice of antibiotic, rapid identification of the causal organism(s) and antibiotic sensitivities are needed, because knowledge of organism type and antibiotic sensitivities often results in a change of therapy.[6] Samples for blood culture[36] should be taken directly from a vein after sterile preparation of the skin overlying the vein. If necessary, cultures can be aseptically taken from a catheter that was recently placed using aseptic technique. Depending on the size of the animal, 5 to 10 milliliters of blood are drawn into the syringe and directly inoculated into the culture bottle. The cultures should be processed for isolation of both aerobic and anaerobic bacteria, because as many as 30% of pathogens that cause bacteremia can be anaerobes. Ideally, two to three blood samples, taken at least one hour apart, should be obtained for culture. If fever is following a known pattern, blood samples should be drawn immediately before the predicted fever spikes.

CARDIOVASCULAR SUPPORT

The goal of cardiovascular support in patients with SIRS is supranormal oxygen delivery to the tissues, sufficient to meet the needs of stressed hypermetabolic patients.[37] Oxygen delivery and consumption can be directly measured if a pulmonary arterial catheter is in place or if an indirect calorimeter is available (Table IV). Although less effective, goals can be set using indirect measurements of cardiovascular function, tissue blood flow, oxygen delivery, and oxygen extraction[27,38] (Table II).

TABLE V
Drugs Used to Treat Animals with Systemic Inflammatory Response Syndrome

Metabolic Derangement	Dose Regimen	Use and/or Frequency
Hypovolemia		
Hypertonic crystalloids		
7.5% NaCl solution (70 ml 23.4% NaCl in 180 ml 0.9% NaCl or 6% dextran 70)	4 ml/kg, IV	Once
Colloids		
Plasma	Maximum: 20 ml/kg/24 hr, IV	As needed
Hetastarch 120	Maximum: 20 ml/kg/first 24 hr, then 10 ml/kg/24 hr, IV (slow infusion)	As needed
Dextran 70	Maximum: 20 ml/kg/first 24 hr, then 10 ml/kg/24 hr, IV (slow infusion)	As needed
3% Albumin (12 ml 25% human albumin in 488 ml lactated Ringer's solution)	20 ml/kg, IV	Resuscitation
Isotonic crystalloids		
Lactated Ringer's solution	90–270 ml/kg, IV 10–20 ml/kg/hr, IV	Resuscitation To meet ongoing needs
Cardiac Dysfunction and Hypotension (inotropic and pressor agents)		
Dopamine	1–30 µg/kg/min, IV	As needed; monitor the animal closely and titrate the agent to obtain optimal oxygen delivery
Dobutamine	5–20 µg/kg/min, IV	
Norepinephrine	0.01–0.4 µg/kg/min, IV	
Altered Clotting Function		
Heparin (low dosage)	75–100 units/kg, SC	Every 6–8 hr
Heparin-activated plasma (incubate 5–10 units/kg heparin with 1 unit fresh plasma for 30 minutes)	10 ml/kg, IV	Every 3 hr, based on clotting function
Metabolic Dysfunction		
KCl	0.125–0.25 mEq/kg/hr, IV; do not exceed 0.5 mEq/kg/hr	As needed
Glucose	50–500 mg/kg/hr, IV	As needed
$NaHCO_3^-$	Base excess × 0.3 × body weight in kg = mEq needed to correct deficit, IV (slow infusion)	As needed
Gastrointestinal Tract Dysfunction		
Cimetidine	5–10 mg/kg, IV, IM, PO	Every 6–8 hr
Ranitidine	2 mg/kg, IV, IM, PO	Every 8–12 hr
Omeprazole	0.7 mg/kg, PO	Every 24 hr
Misoprostol	3 µg/kg, PO	Every 24 hr
Sucralfate	250 mg (cats), PO 500 mg (dogs <20 kg), PO 1 gram (dogs >20 kg), PO	Every 8–12 hr Every 8–12 hr Every 8–12 hr

TABLE V (continued)
Drugs Used to Treat Animals with Systemic Inflammatory Response Syndrome

Metabolic Derangement	Dose Regimen	Use and/or Frequency
Kaolin/pectin	1–2 ml/kg, PO	Every 6–8 hr
Metoclopramide	0.2–0.5 mg/kg, SC	Every 6–8 hr
Renal Dysfunction		
Mannitol	0.25–1 g/kg, IV	Once (slow bolus)
Furosemide	1–2 mg/kg, IV	If no effect, repeat in 2 hours and increase dose by 1 mg/kg
Dopamine	1–3 µg/kg/min, IV	As needed until urine production consistently >2 ml/kg/hr

IV = intravenously, SC = subcutaneously, IM = intramuscularly, and PO = orally.

Crystalloid fluid volumes needed to restore intravascular volume in patients with SIRS are high (90 to 270 ml/kg) but can be reduced by concomitant administration of colloids or hypertonic crystalloids[11,39] (Table V). Administration of hypertonic saline solutions results in rapid restoration of cardiovascular function, but the effect is transient and the development of hyperchloremic acidosis worsens preexisting acidosis.[40,41] Species-matched plasma directly replaces fluid and protein losses to extravascular spaces, but adequate amounts are rarely available. The two major synthetic colloids, hetastarch 120 and dextran 70, are equally efficacious in producing volume expansion.[39,42]

Hetastarch is a polymer made from a waxy starch consisting mainly of amylopectin; dextran 70 is a glucose polymer with an average molecular weight of 70,000. Hetastarch has no antigenic properties, does not interfere with blood typing or crossmatching, and is stable at widely fluctuating temperatures. Dextran 70 is antigenic, rarely causes anaphylaxis, interferes with blood typing and crossmatching due to rouleaux formation, interferes with blood glucose measurements, and must be stored at stable temperatures (25°C) to prevent the formation of precipitates. At high doses (20 ml/kg), both solutions result in increased clotting times due to decreased platelet function and altered fibrin clot structure.

Human albumin can be administered to maintain plasma protein levels and does not affect clotting function.[43] Disadvantages of albumin administration are high cost and the potential for antigenic reactions after repeated administration.

A suggested protocol for resuscitation is as follows. A synthetic colloid solution (7 ml/kg) and a replacement crystalloid solution (15 ml/kg) should be administered. Bolus administration of this combination should be continued until therapeutic goals (Tables II and IV) are met. If the limiting dose of colloid solution occurs before restoration of circulatory function, additional amounts of crystalloid solution should be administered until goals are met or until fluid administration is limited by central venous pressure (>15 cm H_2O) or hemodilution. If packed cell volume is below 20% or total serum solids are below 3.5 mg/dl, blood, plasma, or albumin should be administered (as needed) to raise values to acceptable levels.

Once initial resuscitation is accomplished, ongoing crystalloid fluid requirements of the animal remain high (10 to 20 ml/kg/hr if peritonitis is present).[11,43] Unless maximal doses of synthetic colloid were used during resuscitation, the colloid administration rate is set to deliver 20 ml/kg in the first 24 hours. On subsequent days, the colloid rate is set to deliver 10 ml/kg/24 hr. Hypokalemia and hypoglycemia often occur, and fluids should be supplemented to maintain serum values within normal ranges.

In the absence of sophisticated monitoring equipment, it is much safer for the clinician to err on the side of giving too much, rather than too little, fluids.[37] Complications of massive fluid administration, such as hemodilution, pulmonary edema, and peripheral edema, are easily remedied, whereas a lethal oxygen debt cannot be treated. If crystalloid fluids alone must be used for maintenance of vascular volume, the clinician should be aware that (1) peripheral edema will probably occur[11] and (2) no matter how much fluid is administered, the improvement in oxygen delivery and consumption obtained will not equal that achieved by administration of colloid and crystalloid mixtures.[44]

If cardiovascular goals are not met with fluid therapy, inotropic and pressor therapy may be used (Table V). In patients with acceptable blood pressure values, dobutamine is recommended; experimental and clinical studies document increased oxygen delivery and consumption in patients that received dobutamine rather than dopamine therapy.[45] If acceptable values are not reached with fluids and dobutamine administration, low dosages of dopamine can be used to increase urine output.[46] If it is likely that volume expansion will be limited by hemodilution or hypoproteinemia, the clinician may elect to use dopamine rather than dobutamine, because more fluids must be given with dobutamine than with dopamine to maintain a given cardiac-filling pressure.[45] In extremely hypotensive patients, titrated doses of either dopamine or norepinephrine can be used to raise blood pressure,[46] but pressure should only be increased until evidence of improved tissue blood flow (as evidenced by increased urine output or a decreased core/toe-web temperature differential) is seen. Constriction beyond that point will result in organ hypoxia.

Newer inotropic agents, such as dopexamine and amrinone, are currently being investigated in SIRS models but are not routinely used in patients with SIRS.[47] Nitric oxide inhibitors have been suggested as a method of reversing severe hypotension, because nitric oxide is a major mediator of vasodilatation.[48] These inhibitors cannot be recommended at this time, because evidence is accumulating that the presence of nitric oxide prevents severe vasoconstriction in such key vascular beds as the kidney.[49]

Acid–base abnormalities should be corrected by cardiovascular resuscitation and provision of respiratory support, if indicated. Sodium bicarbonate therapy is controversial but may be given if life-threatening acidemia (pH <7.1) is present.[50]

SURGERY

As soon as an animal has received resuscitative treatment, a search should be made for any surgically correctable source of infection. Physical examination will reveal superficial disease, but peritoneal aspiration or lavage (Table VI), pleural aspiration, urinalysis, radiographs, and/or ultrasonography may be needed to identify sources within body cavities.[51,52] When using peritoneal lavage to diagnose abdominal infection, clinicians should be aware that intraabdominal leukocyte counts do not increase until two to three hours after peritoneal contamination.

The principles of surgical therapy are straightforward. The source of infection should be removed, if possible; accumulations of exudate should be removed or drained; and adjuvant substances, such as bile, blood, and fluid, should be removed.[53] The exact method used to achieve these goals seems to be less important than host factors in determining outcome. In a recent study of human patients with peritonitis,[54] there was no difference in outcome between various open- and closed-abdomen techniques.

TABLE VI
Peritoneal Lavage Values that Indicate Peritonitis[a]

Test	No History of Recent Surgery	History of Recent Surgery[b]
Color	Turbid or cloudy indicates peritonitis	Turbid fluid will be present
White blood cell count	>1000/μl = mild to moderate irritation	7000/μl = mild to moderate irritation
	2000/μl = marked peritonitis	>9000/μl = marked peritonitis
Cytology	Toxic neutrophils, bacteria, vegetable fibers, and organic debris indicate peritonitis	Toxic neutrophils, bacteria, vegetable fibers, and organic debris indicate peritonitis

[a]The values presented are obtained when the abdomen is infused with isotonic crystalloid fluids (20 ml/kg).
[b]Values given in the column are from Bjorling DE, et al.[52]

Mortality was correlated with severe disease (high APACHE II score), low serum albumin level, and decreased cardiac reserve (high New York cardiac function status). Samples of infected matter, if not collected previously, should be collected during surgical treatment of the animal.

If the source of infection is within the abdomen, a jejunal feeding tube should be placed, because patients with SIRS tolerate jejunal feeding significantly earlier than they tolerate gastric feeding.[55] If the need for parenteral nutrition support is anticipated, a large-gauge central catheter should be aseptically placed.

TREATMENT OF CLOTTING ABNORMALITIES

If clotting times and platelet counts are normal at the time of presentation, measures should be taken to prevent activation of intravascular clotting. Synthetic colloids, which the animal may already be receiving, are effective in preventing activation of intravascular clotting.[42] If crystalloid fluids alone are being used, low-dosage heparin administration (Table V) may be indicated to prevent activation of clotting cascades and to maintain blood flow in the microcirculation.[56] If platelet counts are low and clotting times are prolonged, platelets and clotting factors should be replaced before initiating heparin therapy.[25,57] In human patients with SIRS, severe depletion of antithrombin III is highly predictive of death; trials with antithrombin III replacement are ongoing.[25]

SUPPORT OF ORGAN DYSFUNCTION

Increased oxygen delivery to the tissues is critical for both resolution of infection and SIRS.[37,58,59] Supple-

TABLE VII
Enteral Feeding Recommendations for Animals with Systemic Inflammatory Response Syndrome

1. Calculate resting energy requirement (RER):
    For animals that weigh between 2 kg and 45 kg:
        $30 \times$ body weight in kg $+ 70 =$ RER (kcal/day)
    For animals that weigh <2 kg or >45 kg:
        $70 \times$ (body weight in kg)$^{0.75} =$ RER (kcal/day)
2. For the first several days, calculate total daily calories as follows: $(0.5 - 1.0) \times$ RER. Gradually increase the amount fed to meet increased caloric needs due to hypermetabolism or increased movement. For dogs, calculate total daily calories (kcal/day) as follows: $(1.25 - 1.50) \times$ RER. For cats, calculate total daily calories (kcal/day) as follows: $(1.1 - 1.2) \times$ RER.
3. Choose a diet that meets the protein requirement of the animal and supplies other nutrients needed during stress (see the table below).
4. Calculate the volume of diet required: (kcal/day)/(kcal/ml) = ml of formula/day.
5. Calculate the volume of each feeding: (ml of formula/day)/(number of feedings/day). Because duodenal and jejunal feedings are continuous, calculate ml/hr for small bowel feeding.

Species	Condition	Protein Requirement (g/100 kcal)	Example Diets	Calories (kcal/ml)	Protein (g/100 kcal)
Dog	Standard	4.0–8.0	312 g Prescription Diet® a/d®[a] + 50 ml water	1.0	9
			CliniCare® Canine[b]	0.9	5.5
	Hepatic or renal dysfunction	<4.0	Blenderized 224 g Prescription Diet® Canine k/d®[a] + 284 ml water	0.6	3.1
			RenalCare™ Canine[b]	0.8	2.8
	Protein loss	>8.0	312 g Prescription Diet® a/d®[a] + 50 ml water	1.0	9
			237 ml Sustacal®[c] + 24 g ProBalance® Max Stress Feline[d]	1.2	8.8
Cat	Standard	6.0–9.0	Blenderized 224 g Prescription Diet® Feline p/d®[a] + 170 ml water	0.9	9.3
			50 ml Sustacal®[c] + 50 ml Pulmocare®[e] + 4.8 g ProBalance® Max Stress Feline[d]	1.3	6.4
	Hepatic or renal dysfunction	<6.0	Blenderized 224 g Prescription Diet® Feline k/d®[a] + 284 ml water	0.9	4.4
			100 ml Pulmocare®[e] + 50 ml water + 4.8 g ProBalance® Max Stress Feline[d]	1.3	5.3
	Protein loss	>9.0	312 g Prescription Diet® a/d®[a] + 50 ml water	1.0	9
			237 ml Sustacal®[c] + 24 g ProBalance® Max Stress Feline[d]	1.2	8.8

[a]Hill's Pet Nutrition, Inc., Topeka, KS.
[b]PetAg, Hampshire, IL.
[c]Bristol-Meyers Squibb, Princeton, NJ.
[d]Pfizer Animal Health, Exton, PA.
[e]Ross Laboratories, Columbus, OH.

mental oxygen should be supplied through a nasal oxygen catheter, and transition to a respirator is indicated if lung dysfunction is present. If PaO_2 is not maintained >70 mm Hg or the animal has obvious signs of respiratory distress, lung dysfunction is occurring. Gastrointestinal dysfunction results in a high risk of ulcer formation, and drugs should be administered to reduce the risk of severe gastrointestinal hemorrhage (Table V).[60] In patients with SIRS, there is no direct therapy for hepatic dysfunction beyond adequate oxygen delivery and optimal nutritional support. Renal dysfunction associated with SIRS is initially treated with aggressive cardiovascular resuscitation. If anuria persists despite adequate intravascular volume expansion, furosemide, mannitol, and low-dose dopamine (Table V) should be administered.[61]

NUTRITIONAL SUPPORT

After a single, life-threatening episode of shock, patients undergo a period of hypermetabolism and catabolism of skeletal muscle protein lasting 7 to 10 days.[62] In the presence of continuing injury or inflammation, hypermetabolism will progress to severe metabolic dysfunction. During the hypermetabolism stage, carbohydrate intolerance develops[62] and caloric needs must be met by supplying a mixture of carbohydrate, fat, and protein. Progression to metabolic failure is associated with an increased reliance on amino acids as an oxidative fuel source and a decreasing tolerance of lipid. Originally, it was believed that nutritional therapy could prevent these changes, but because the changes are mediator-induced, provision of large quantities of nutrients will not reverse them.[63] Current goals of nutritional therapy are (1) preservation of gut function and integrity, (2) improved immunocompetence, and (3) provision of sufficient nutrients to improve patient outcome without increasing mortality related to complications associated with overfeeding.[63,64]

The safest, most effective route of feeding human patients with SIRS is to use direct small-bowel food administration through a nasoduodenal or jejunostomy tube.[55] Gastric tube-feeding can be used, but bacterial contamination of stomach contents, pneumonia, and tolerance of only small volumes of food are encountered.[55] Small-bowel and gastric tube-feeding have been shown to be practical in veterinary intensive care unit patients. Clinicians should follow current recommendations for supplying nutrients until additional information is available from large-scale studies in humans, which may provide evidence for modifying the currently used formulas[64,a] (Table VII).

MEDIATOR BLOCKERS

The future treatment of SIRS will undoubtedly involve modification of mediator cascades, and human trials with several mediator blockers are currently underway.[65] At present, however, there are no mediator blockers that have been convincingly proven to increase survival in clinical patients beyond that achieved with conventional therapy.

SUMMARY

Bacterial infection continues to be a significant cause of mortality in veterinary patients. If signs of SIRS are present, mortality may be as high as 50%. The clinician should be vigilant to recognize the early stages of SIRS. Aggressive cardiovascular support and the administration of appropriate antibiotics are the main elements of treatment. Surgical drainage or removal of the source of infection is used when possible. Future increases in survival will be achieved with modification of the inflammatory response.

About the Author

Dr. Hardie is affiliated with the Department of Companion Animal and Special Species, College of Veterinary Medicine, North Carolina State University, Raleigh, North Carolina. Dr. Hardie is a diplomate of the American College of Veterinary Surgeons.

REFERENCES

1. Bone RC: Toward an epidemiology and natural history of SIRS (systemic inflammatory response syndrome). *JAMA* 268:3452–3455, 1992.
2. Marshall J, Sweeney D: Microbial infection and the septic response in critical surgical illness. *Arch Surg* 125:17–23, 1990.
3. American College of Chest Physicians—Society of Critical Care Medicine Consensus Conference: Definitions for sepsis and organ failure and guidelines for the use of innovative therapies in sepsis. *Chest* 101:1644–1655, 1992.
4. Creasey AA, Stevens P, Kenney J, et al: Endotoxin and cytokine profile in plasma of baboons challenged with lethal and sublethal *Escherichia coli*. *Circ Shock* 33:84–91, 1991.
5. Macheido GW, Suval WD: Detection of sepsis in the postoperative patient. *Surg Clin North Am* 68:215–228, 1988.
6. Dow SW, Curtis CR, Jones RL, et al: Bacterial culture of blood from critically ill dogs and cats: 100 cases (1985–1987). *JAVMA* 195:113–117, 1989.
7. Hardie EM, Rawlings CA, Calvert CA: Severe sepsis in selected surgical patients. *JAAHA* 22:33–41, 1986.
8. Greenfield CL, Walshaw R: Open peritoneal drainage for treatment of contaminated peritoneal cavity and septic peritonitis in dogs and cats: 24 cases (1980–1986). *JAVMA* 191:100–105, 1987.
9. Woolfson JM, Dulish ML: Open abdominal drainage in the treatment of generalized peritonitis in 25 dogs and cats. *Vet Surg* 15:27–32, 1986.
10. Hosgood G, Salisbury SK: Generalized peritonitis in dogs: 50 cases. *JAVMA* 193:1448–1450, 1988.
11. Natanson C: A canine model of septic shock. *Ann Intern Med* 113:231–235, 1990.
12. Calvert CA, Greene CE, Hardie EM: Cardiovascular infections in dogs: Epizootiology, clinical manifestations, and prognosis. *JAVMA* 187:612–616, 1985.
13. Sugarman JH, Newsome HH, Greenfield W: Hemodynamics, oxygen consumption and serum catecholamine changes in progressive, lethal peritonitis in the dog. *Surg Gynecol Obstet* 154:8–12, 1982.
14. Martin C, Saux P, Eon B, et al: Septic shock: A goal-directed therapy using volume loading, dobutamine and/or norepinephrine. *Acta Anaesthesiol Scand* 34:413–417, 1990.
15. Gilbert RP: Mechanisms of the hemodynamic effects of endotoxin. *Physiol Rev* 40:245–279, 1960.
16. Shilin H, Hinshaw L, Emerson T, et al: Comparison of pathogenesis between *Escherichia coli* and *Staphylococcus aureus* infusion-induced shock in baboons. *Circ Shock* 37:28, 1992.
17. Parratt JR, Sturgess RM: The effects of the repeated administration of sodium meclofenamate, an inhibitor of prostaglandin 54 synthetase, in feline endotoxin shock. *Circ Shock* 2:301–310, 1975.
18. Stahl TJ, Alden PB, Ring WS, et al: Sepsis-induced diastolic dysfunction in chronic canine peritonitis. *Am J Physiol* 258:H625–H633, 1990.
19. Parker MM: Right ventricular dysfunction and dilatation,

---

[a]Davenport D: Personal communication, Mark Morris Associates, Topeka, KS, 1995.

similar to left ventricular changes, characterize the cardiac depression of septic shock in humans. *Chest* 97:126–131, 1990.
20. Jardin F, Brun-Ney D, Auvert B, et al: Sepsis-related cardiogenic shock. *Crit Care Med* 18:1055–1060, 1990.
21. Sugarman HJ, Hylemon P, Greenfield W: Thrombocytopenia in progressive lethal canine peritonitis. *Surg Gynecol Obstet* 154:193–196, 1982.
22. Hardie EM, Kolata EM, Rawlings CA: Canine septic peritonitis: Treatment with flunixin meglumine. *Circ Shock* 11:159–173, 1983.
23. Ba ZF, Wang P, Tait SM, et al: Correlation between circulating blood volume (CBV) and plasma lactate in sepsis. *Circ Shock* 37:16, 1992.
24. Taboada J, Meyer DJ: Cholestasis associated with extrahepatic bacterial infection in five dogs. *J Vet Intern Med* 3:216–221, 1989.
25. Fourrier F, Chopin C, Goudemand J, et al: Septic shock, multiple organ failure, and disseminated intravascular coagulation. *Chest* 101:816–823, 1992.
26. Hardie EM, Rawlings CA, Shotts EB, et al: *Escherichia coli*-induced lung and liver dysfunction in dogs: Effects of flunixin treatment. *Am J Vet Res* 48:56–62, 1987.
27. Schertel ER, Muir WW: Shock: Pathophysiology, monitoring, and therapy, in Kirk RW (ed): *Current Veterinary Therapy. X.* Philadelphia, WB Saunders Co, 1989, pp 316–330.
28. Schaefer CF, Lerner MR, Biber B: Dose-related reduction of intestinal cytochrome a,a3 induced by endotoxin in rats. *Circ Shock* 33:17–25, 1991.
29. Hauptman JG, Tvedlen H: Osmolal and anion gaps in dogs with acute endotoxic shock. *Am J Vet Res* 487:1671–1673, 1986.
30. Otto CM, Kaufman GM, Crowe DT: Intraosseus infusion of fluids and therapeutics. *Compend Contin Educ Pract Vet* 11(4):421–431, 1989.
31. Kolata RJ: The clinical management of circulatory shock based on pathophysiological patterns. *Compend Contin Educ Pract Vet* 2(4):314–322, 1980.
32. Keenan KP, Buhles NC, Huxsoll DL, et al: Studies on the pathogenesis of *Rickettsia rickettsii* in the dog: Clinical and clincopathologic changes of experimental infection. *Am J Vet Res* 38:851–856, 1977.
33. Haskins SC: Management of septic shock. *JAVMA* 200:1915–1924, 1992.
34. Breitschwerdt EB, Davidson MG, Aucoin DP, et al: Efficacy of chloramphenicol, enrofloxacin, and tetracycline for treatment of experimental Rocky Mountain spotted fever in dogs. *Antimicrob Agents Chemother* 35:2375–2381, 1991.
35. Donowitz GR, Mandell GL: Beta-lactam antibiotics. *N Engl J Med* 318:490–500, 1988.
36. Calvert CA, Dow SW: Cardiovascular infections, in Greene CE (ed): *Infectious Diseases of the Dog and Cat*. Philadelphia, WB Saunders Co, 1990, pp 97–113.
37. Shoemaker WC, Appel PL, Kram HB, et al: Hemodynamics and oxygen transport monitoring to titrate therapy in septic shock. *New Horizons* 1:127–137, 1993.
38. Bakkers L, Coffernils M, Leon M, et al: Blood lactate levels are superior to oxygen-derived variables in predicting outcome in human septic shock. *Chest* 99:956–962, 1991.
39. Astiz ME, Gabra-Santiago A, Rachow EC: Intravascular volume and fluid therapy for severe sepsis. *New Horizons* 1:127–137, 1993.
40. Luypaert P, Vincent JL, Domb M, et al: Fluid resuscitation with hypertonic saline in endotoxic shock. *Circ Shock* 20:311–320, 1986.
41. Kramer GC, Moon P, Drace C, et al: Hyper-chloremic acidosis induced after resuscitation with hypertonic saline dextran. *Circ Shock* 37:19, 1992.
42. McEvoy GK (ed): Replacement preparations. AHFS Drug Information 91, Bethesda, MD, American Society of Hospital Pharmacists, pp 1500–1516, 1991.
43. Emerson TE: Unique features of albumin: A brief review. *Crit Care Med* 17:690–694, 1989.
44. Linko K, Makelainen A: Cardiorespiratory function after replacement of blood loss with hydroxyethyl starch 120, dextran 70, and Ringer's acetate in pigs. *Crit Care Med* 17:1031–1035, 1989.
45. Vincent JL, Van der Linden P, Domb M: Dopamine compared with dobutamine in experimental septic shock: Relevance to fluid administration. *Anesth Analg* 66:565–571, 1987.
46. Lawson N: Therapeutic combinations of vasopressors and inotropic agents. *Semin Anesthesia* 9:270–287, 1990.
47. Vincent JL, Preiser J-C: Inotropic agents. *New Horizons* 1:137–144, 1993.
48. Vallance P, Moncada S: Role of endogenous nitric oxide in septic shock. *New Horizons* 1:77–86, 1993.
49. Shultz PJ, Raij L: Endogenously synthesized nitric oxide prevents endotoxin-induced glomerular thrombosis. *J Clin Invest* 90:1718–1725, 1992.
50. Biebuyck JF: Sodium bicarbonate in the treatment of subtypes of acute lactic acidosis: Physiologic considerations. *Anesthesiology* 72:1064–1076, 1990.
51. Hunt CA: Diagnostic peritoneal paracentesis and lavage. *Compend Contin Educ Pract Vet* 2(6):449–453, 1980.
52. Bjorling DE, Latimer KS, Rawlings CA, et al: Diagnostic peritoneal lavage before and after abdominal surgery in dogs. *Am J Vet Res* 44:816–820, 1983.
53. Hardie EM: Peritonitis from urogenital conditions. *Probl Vet Med* 1:36–49, 1989.
54. Christou NV, Barie PS, Dellinger EP, et al: Surgical Infection Society Intra-abdominal Infection Study, prospective evaluation of management techniques and outcome. *Arch Surg* 128:193–199, 1993.
55. Montecalvo MA, Steger KA, Farber HW, et al: Nutritional outcome and pneumonia in critical care patients randomized to gastric verus jejunal tube feedings. *Crit Care Med* 20:1377–1387, 1992.
56. Rana MW, Singh G, Wang P, et al: Heparin administration before or after hemorrhagic shock protects microvascular patency. *Circ Shock* 31:59, 1990.
57. Ruehl W, Mills C, Feldman BF: Rational therapy in disseminated intravascular coagulation. *JAVMA* 181:76–78, 1982.
58. Seigel JH: Through a glass darkly: The lung as a window to monitor oxygen consumption, energy metabolism, and severity of critical illness. *Clin Chem* 36:1585–1593, 1990.
59. Knighton DR, Fiegel VD, Halverson T, et al: Oxygen as an antibiotic. *Arch Surg* 125:97–100, 1990.
60. Papich MG: Antiulcer therapy. *Vet Med Rep* 1:309–320, 1989.
61. Linder A, Culter RE, Goodman WG: Synergism of dopamine plus furosemide in preventing acute renal failure in the dog. *Kidney Int* 16:158–166, 1979.
62. Cerra FB: Metabolic manifestations of multiple systems organ failure. *Crit Care Clin* 5:119–129, 1989.
63. Cerra FB, Lehmann S, Konstantinicles N, et al: Improvement in immune function in ICU patients by enteral nutrition supplemental with arginine, RNS, and menhaden oil is independent of nitrogen balance. *Nutrition* 7:193–199, 1991.
64. Abood SK, Dimski DS, Buffington CA, et al: Enteral nutrition, in DiBartola SP (ed): *Fluid Therapy in Small Animal Practice*. Philadelphia, WB Saunders Co, 1992, pp 419–435.
65. Lowry SF: Anticytokine therapies in sepsis. *New Horizons* 1:120–126, 1993.

UPDATE

TABLE I
Updated Antibiotic Doses for Use in Life-Threatening Infection

Drug	Intravenous Dose
Cefotetan	30 mg/kg q 8 hr
Imipenam	0.7–1.1 mg/kg q 8 hr
Vancomycin	15 mg/kg q 8 hr
Gentamicin	6 mg/kg q 24 hr. To minimize renal toxicity, keep patient hydrated and limit use to 5 days.
Amikacin	15 mg/kg q 24 hr. To minimize renal toxicity, keep patient hydrated and limit use to 5 days.
Enrofloxacin	up to 25 mg/kg q 12 hr
Metronidazole	15 mg/kg q 12 hr. Severe CNS toxicity reported if dose > 50 mg/kg/day.

SYSTEMIC INFLAMMATORY RESPONSE SYNDROME

A study of dogs and cats with peritonitis[1] has confirmed that tachycardia, hyper- or hypothermia, and leukocytosis were almost always present at the time of presentation. Hypotension was common. Tachypnea was not documented at the time of presentation, suggesting that this clinical sign was either difficult to recognize or absent. The proposed heart rate limit of 140 beats/min in the cat is probably too low to indicate SIRS. Additional experience with cats in the intensive care unit has demonstrated that heart rates greater than 200 beats/min are common in cats with SIRS.

The development of organ failure was followed closely in the animal peritonitis study.[1] In addition to previously recognized organ dysfunction, respiratory dysfunction and pancreatitis were common. It was unclear whether respiratory dysfunction was due to thromboembolism, silent aspiration of gastric contents, edema, or other causes. In our experience, aspiration pneumonia is a common complication in this patient population. Pancreatitis in the peritonitis patients was associated with marked peritoneal effusion, resulting in extensive fluid loss in patients undergoing peritoneal drainage procedures.[1]

Recent experimental studies have confirmed that the gastrointestinal tract is a target organ during SIRS in the dog.[2] In a model in which dogs were subjected to endotoxin infusion, followed by resuscitation with dextran, resuscitation increased cardiac output above normal and restored systemic oxygen delivery and uptake to normal values. The resuscitated dogs had normal muscle tissue PO_2. Gut PO_2 and gut oxygen delivery and uptake remained low, while gut lactate production remained high.

LABORATORY FINDINGS

Two additional facts on the laboratory findings associated with SIRS emerged from the peritonitis study.[1] First, the presence of band neutrophils was rare. Only 2/22 animals had a higher than normal number of band neutrophils. Second, hypernatria was present in 3/22 animals at presentation and developed in 6 more animals during treatment.

ANTIBIOTICS

Correct empirical choice of antibiotics remains critical in life-threatening infection. In a study of human patients with peritonitis, a major determinant of survival was selection of an antibiotic(s) to which the organisms eventually cultured were sensitive.[3] In the study of animals with peritonitis, 4/5 dogs treated with inappropriate antibiotics did not survive.[1] The use of dual or triple antibiotic combinations has been shown to have no benefits over the use of a single broad-spectrum antibiotic such as cefoxitin or cefotetan.[3] Doses of antibiotics often need to be increased in patients with shock due to altered pharmacokinetics.[4]

Updated antibiotic dosage regimens are presented in Table I.[5] In particular, the once-a-day dosing of aminoglycosides may decrease toxicity yet preserve the efficacy of these drugs. Older doses of enrofloxicin do not achieve adequate plasma levels to effectively inhibit many gram-negative pathogens, thus higher doses are needed in patients with severe infection.

CARDIOVASCULAR SUPPORT

Studies continue to confirm the need for aggressive cardiovascular support in these patients. Rapid cardiovascular response to volume support indicates a good prognosis. The need for inotrope and vasopressor use to maintain cardiovascular function worsens the prognosis, while unresponsive hypotension indicates that death is near.[1] A study of human patients demonstrated that patients pushed with inotropes to an oxygen delivery of > 600 mL/min/m had a 14% mortality rate.[2] Those patients allowed to remain at a normal oxygen delivery had a 67% mortality rate, which was equivalent to the 62% mortality rate in patients who failed to respond to inotropes.[6] Early use of plasma, rather than albumin, to maintain plasma proteins improves survival.[7]

MEDIATOR BLOCKERS

Human trials with various endotoxin and mediator blockers continue to be disappointing.[8] Shock and/or organ failure may be ameliorated by these agents, but 30-day mortality rates are not affected by all agents tested to date.

REFERENCES

1. King LG: Postoperative complications and prognostic indicators in dogs and cats with septic peritonitis: 23 cases (1989–1992). *JAVMA* 204:407–414, 1994.
2. Vallet B, Lund N, Curtis SE, et al: Gut muscle tissue PO_2 in endotoxemic dogs during shock and resuscitation. *J Appl Physiol* 76:793–800, 1994.
3. Mosdell DM, Morris DM, Voltura A, et al: Antibiotic treatment for surgical peritonitis. *Ann Surg* 214:543–549, 1991.
4. Livingston DH, Shumate CR, Polk HC, et al: More is better, antibiotic treatment after hemorrhagic shock. *Ann Surg* 208:451–459, 1988.
5. Rosin E: Rational use of antibiotics in small animal surgery. *Proceedings of the 1993 ACVS Veterinary Symposium*, p 229.
6. Yu M, Takanishi D, Myers SA, et al: Frequency of mortality and myocardial infarction during maximizing oxygen delivery: A prospective randomized trial. *Crit Care Med* 23:1025–1032, 1995.
7. Busand R, Konning G, Lindsetmo RO, et al: The effects of plasma and albumin infusion on organ function and sepsis markers in experimental gram-negative sepsis. *Shock* 2:402–407, 1994.
8. Fink MP: Another negative clinical trial of a new agent for the treatment of sepsis: Rethinking the process of developing treatments for serious infection. *Crit Care Med* 23:989–991, 1995.

Diagnosis and Symptomatic Therapy of Acute Gastroenteritis

Iowa State University
Albert E. Jergens, DVM, MS

KEY FACTS

❏ The acute onset of vomiting and/or diarrhea is a common clinical complaint that has numerous potential causes.

❏ Diagnosis of acute gastrointestinal diseases is largely based on patient history and performance of a thorough physical examination.

❏ The principal goals of symptomatic therapy are resting the alimentary tract and restoring fluid and electrolyte balance.

❏ Animals with self-limiting gastroenteritis require minimal diagnostic testing and readily respond to symptomatic therapy.

❏ Life-threatening causes of acute gastroenteritis necessitate detailed diagnostic evaluation, aggressive management of clinical signs, and treatment geared to the underlying cause.

Acute vomiting and diarrhea are common gastrointestinal signs in dogs and cats and are frequent presenting complaints encountered by small animal clinicians. In most instances, these clinical signs represent minor gastrointestinal disturbances that may be self-limiting or that readily resolve after appropriate symptomatic therapy is initiated. Other causes, such as parvoviral enteritis and hemorrhagic gastroenteritis, are more fulminant and potentially life-threatening.

The diagnosis of acute gastrointestinal diseases is largely based on patient history and thorough physical examination. Although the specific cause of acute gastrointestinal signs is seldom identified, rational symptomatic therapy is often indicated to ameliorate clinical signs and expedite recovery. This article provides an overview of the diagnosis and therapy of acute gastrointestinal diseases in dogs and cats.

SIGNALMENT AND HISTORY

A wide variety of disorders and numerous stimuli may cause acute vomiting and/or diarrhea in small animals[1] (see Common Causes of Acute Gastroenteritis). A problem-oriented approach to diagnosis facilitates identification of problems, assesses their severity, establishes rule-outs for each problem, and assists in designing a plan to diagnose or treat each problem. A thorough medical history, based on careful client interviews, helps to determine whether vomiting or diarrhea is due to a primary gastrointestinal disease or is secondary to organ dysfunction.

The patient profile should include information concerning the signalment, environment, diet, current medications, and potential exposure to toxins and infectious agents. Young animals are prone to gastroenteritis of dietary, infectious, and parasitic causes. An acute onset of vomiting or diarrhea in unvaccinated puppies or kittens should alert the clinician to the possibility of infectious diseases, such as parvoviral or canine distemper gastroenteritis. Infectious causes should be considered if the patient has a

Common Causes of Acute Gastroenteritis

Diet
- Abrupt dietary change
- Overeating
- Indiscretions (garbage, foreign material)
- Food intolerance or allergy

Gastrointestinal Inflammation
- Acute gastritis
- Parasitism (helminths, protozoa)
- Bacterial enteritis (*Salmonella* species,[a] *Campylobacter jejuni*, *Clostridium* species)
- Viral enteritis (parvovirus,[a] coronavirus)
- Salmon poisoning disease[a]
- Hemorrhagic gastroenteritis[a]
- Erosions or ulcers[a]

Neurologic Disorders
- Vestibular disease
- Psychogenic factors (fear, excitement, pain)

Drugs and Toxins
- Antiinflammatory agents
- Antimicrobial agents
- Antineoplastic drugs[a]
- Heavy metals or organophosphates[a]
- Ethylene glycol[a]

Functional or Mechanical Ileus
- Electrolyte disturbances (potassium, calcium)
- Gastric dilatation–volvulus[a]
- Intussusception[a]
- Gastrointestinal foreign bodies[a]

Extraintestinal Disorders
- Acute pancreatitis[a]
- Liver disease[a]
- Kidney disease[a]
- Hypoadrenocorticism[a]
- Pyometra[a]
- Peritonitis[a]
- Diabetic ketoacidosis[a]

[a]Potentially life-threatening.

---

recent history of exposure to animals with vomiting or diarrhea. Vomiting or diarrhea in adult animals should cause the clinician to suspect metabolic, systemic, and gastrointestinal permeability derangements. Breed predispositions for gastroenteritis include acute pancreatitis in miniature schnauzers,[2] parvoviral enteritis in rottweilers,[3] and gastric dilatation-volvulus syndrome in Great Danes.[4]

Animals that roam in an unconfined environment are more likely to develop parasitic, toxic, and infectious gastroenteritis. Gastrointestinal parasitism is much more common in animals kept outdoors than in house pets. Acute vomiting and diarrhea due to poisoning should be suspected if there are clinical signs referable to other body systems. The list of potential intoxicants that cause gastrointestinal upset is extensive and includes caustic chemicals, plant products, heavy metals, ethylene glycol, and pesticides that contain carbamates or organophosphates.[5] Environmental stress may precipitate acute intermittent large-bowel diarrhea in such performance animals as police dogs, guide dogs, and field-trial dogs.[6]

Dietary problems (e.g., adverse reactions to foods and ingestion of spoiled foods or indigestible material) are prominent causes of acute diarrhea. Dietary indiscretion is common in dogs, and owners should be asked about the type of diet fed, the amount and frequency of feeding, and whether there have been recent dietary changes that might involve offending nutrients. A previous response to dietary manipulation is useful historical information. Diarrhea that persists after food is withheld for 24 to 36 hours is characteristic of inflammatory and secretory disturbance; diarrhea that resolves with fasting suggests a primary osmotic cause. Owners may report that fecal consistency improves when low-fat diets are fed, suggesting that the diarrhea is of small-bowel rather than large-bowel origin.

After the patient's dietary history has been considered, the history taking should include questions concerning current medications that are being administered. These medications may include preparations prescribed for the immediate clinical signs or as treatment for other disorders. Drugs that may precipitate acute clinical signs of gastroenteritis include antibiotics, cardiac glycosides, aspirin, and such other nonsteroidal antiinflammatory drugs as flunixin meglumine and phenylbutazone.[7–9]

In many cases, a description of the vomiting and/or diarrhea episodes yields important information. It is essential to distinguish clearly between regurgitation and vomiting; failure to do so often results in misdiagnosis. Regurgitation denotes the passive, retrograde movement of ingesta from the oral cavity or esophagus. Vomiting is an active process characterized by salivation, retching, and the expulsion of gastrointestinal contents. The timing of vomiting episodes and the physical characteristics of the vomitus provide important clues. Vomiting shortly after eating suggests dietary indiscretion, food intolerance, stress, or excitement. Undigested food in the vomitus implies a gastric cause. Bilious vomiting indicates bile reflux into the stomach. Blood in the vomitus (i.e., hematemesis) implies a breach in the upper gastrointestinal barrier.

Similarly, a description of the physical appearance of the feces helps in characterizing the nature of the diarrhea. Loose or watery feces that contain undigested food, melena, and various colors suggest small-bowel diarrhea. Loose to semisolid feces that contain excess mucus and fresh blood indicate large-bowel diarrhea.

PHYSICAL EXAMINATION

In evaluating patients with acute gastroenteritis, a thorough physical examination is extremely important because it provides valuable information concerning the origin of the vomiting and/or diarrhea and the severity of the illness. A systematic evaluation of all body systems should be performed, including examination under the tongue for string (linear) foreign bodies and digital examination of the rectum. Acute gastrointestinal disease may cause derangements in the fluid, electrolyte, and nutritional status; these parameters should be critically assessed.

Although physical examination findings are often normal, signs of mild to moderate dehydration (loss of lumbar skin turgor, dry mucous membranes, and prolonged capillary refill time) may be observed. Careful abdominal palpation should be performed to assess for pain (focal or diffuse), organ distention, foreign bodies, or intussusception. Fluid-distended small-bowel loops are often palpable in patients with acute enteritis. Digital examination of the rectal canal allows collection of fresh feces for parasitic and cytologic testing for infectious agents or antigens. Feces should be visually inspected for consistency, evidence of melena or fresh blood, and the presence of foreign material.

At the completion of the physical examination, the clinician should be able to classify acute gastroenteritis as self-limiting or potentially life-threatening. Warning signs of serious gastrointestinal disease include fever; severe vomiting; severe dehydration; abdominal pain; recumbency; mucous membrane pallor, congestion, or icterus; and bloody diarrhea. Any of these signs indicate the need to expedite appropriate diagnostic and therapeutic strategies (Figure 1).

DIAGNOSTIC EVALUATION

Extensive diagnostic evaluation is seldom required because most animals with acute gastroenteritis have mild, self-limiting disease. Determination of packed

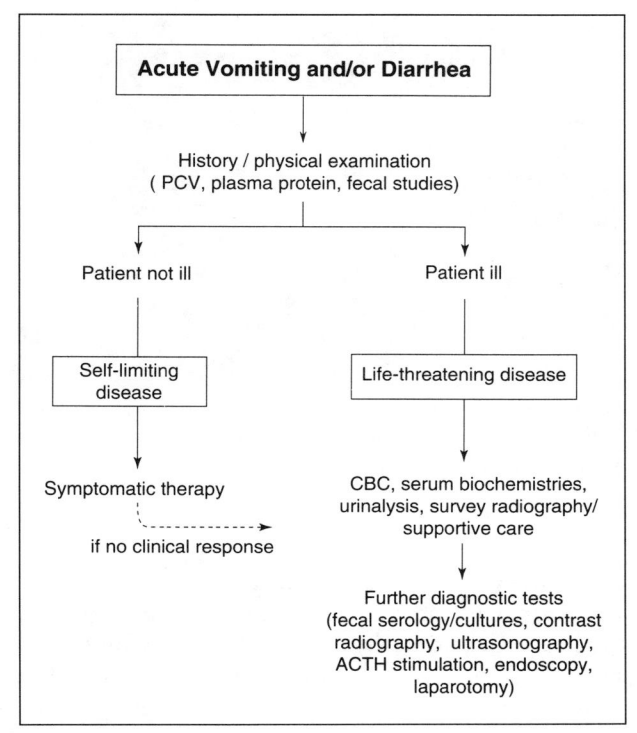

Figure 1—Simplified diagnostic approach to acute gastroenteritis (*PCV* = packed cell volume, *CBC* = complete blood count, *ACTH* = adrenocorticotropic hormone).

cell volume and total plasma protein concentration help in assessing the patient's hydration status. Fecal flotation for parasitic ova and direct fecal smears for protozoa should be performed to eliminate parasitism as a cause of the clinical signs. Multiple zinc sulfate fecal flotation examinations may be necessary to detect *Giardia* infestation.[10] Fecal cytology is especially useful in identification of *Clostridium* spores or fecal leukocytes associated with some inflammatory causes of acute large-bowel diarrhea (Figures 2 and 3). Patients that may have an infectious cause for vomiting or diarrhea should be tested for the presence of canine parvovirus antigen in the feces[11] or should have fecal cultures performed to identify enteropathogenic bacteria, such as *Campylobacter jejuni*,[12] *Salmonella* species,[13] or *Clostridium perfringens*.[14]

Additional testing in animals with life-threatening gastroenteritis should include a complete blood count, serum biochemistry profile (including lipase and electrolytes), urinalysis, direct and indirect fecal examinations, and survey abdominal radiographs. This data base helps to rule out infectious, metabolic, or endocrine causes of acute vomiting or diarrhea. Serum biochemistry is useful in assessing fluid, electrolyte, and acid–base homeostasis. Abdominal radiographs may detect radiopaque foreign bodies, obstructive lesions, extraalimentary structures, and

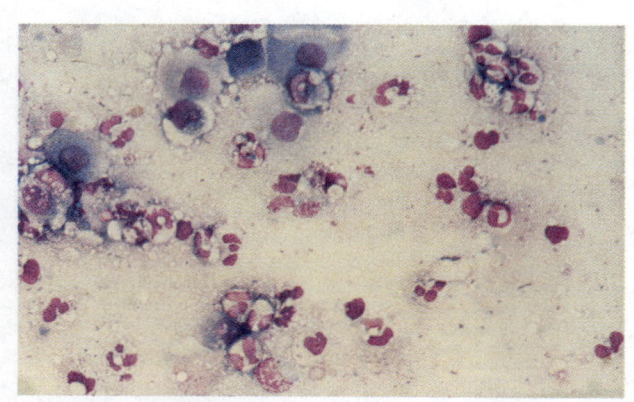

Figure 2—Fecal cytology demonstrating increased fecal leukocytes in a four-month-old puppy with *Campylobacter jejuni* infection (Wright's stain).

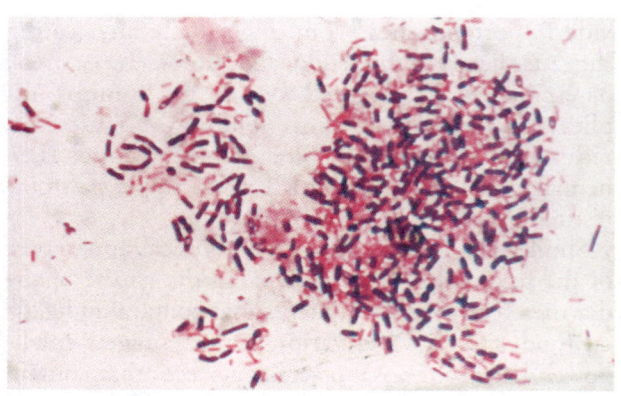

Figure 3—Fecal cytology demonstrating vegetative cells of *Clostridium* species in a five-year-old dog with hematochezia and mucoid stools (Gram's stain, original magnification ×100).

organomegaly. Additional diagnostic studies (e.g., abdominal ultrasonography, contrast radiography, adrenocorticotropic hormone [ACTH] stimulation test, endoscopy, or laparotomy) may be indicated in some patients.

SYMPTOMATIC THERAPY

In most situations, acute vomiting and diarrhea are easily resolved. Symptomatic therapy is primarily supportive because the cause for these clinical signs is often undetermined. The principal goals of symptomatic therapy are restoration of fluid and electrolyte balance and resting of the alimentary tract. Additional therapy may include the use of drugs to alter gut motility, antimicrobial therapy, and the selective use of antiemetic drugs (Table I).

Fluid Therapy

Fluid therapy is the most critical component of supportive care in patients with acute gastroenteritis. This is particularly true if food and water must be withheld. The goals of fluid therapy are correction of dehydration and acid–base derangements, replacement of electrolyte deficits, and provision for maintenance requirements and ongoing losses.[15] The metabolic consequences of diarrhea and vomiting vary; however, predictable depletions in sodium, potassium, chloride, and water are observed in most animals because of the loss of gastrointestinal secretions. Mildly affected patients often have normal acid–base status.

Metabolic acidosis may occur in patients with severe vomiting or watery diarrhea as a consequence of intestinal bicarbonate loss, hypovolemia, and lactic acidosis caused by poor capillary perfusion.[15,16] Less commonly, metabolic alkalosis, hyponatremia, and hypochloremia occur in dogs and cats with vomiting secondary to pyloric outflow obstruction. The choice of fluid, route of administration, and rate of delivery are largely dictated by the clinical examination and serum electrolyte levels. Hydration status should be correlated with laboratory evidence of dehydration (e.g., increased packed cell volume, increased total protein concentration, and prerenal causes of elevations in serum urea nitrogen and creatinine).

Oral rehydration therapy that involves isotonic glucose–electrolyte solutions may be useful in mildly dehydrated animals that can ingest oral fluids.[17,18] Oral fluid therapy is based on the observation that glucose stimulates small intestinal sodium absorption, creating a concomitant osmotic gradient for water absorption. Use of these solutions is primarily indicated in patients with secretory diarrhea in which the gut mucosa is preserved.[19] Definitive recommendations for the use of oral rehydration therapy in animals are limited.

Patients that are mildly dehydrated may be managed with subcutaneous fluid therapy. The intravenous route is preferred for the rapid replacement of significant fluid deficits. Because vomiting precludes oral intake, fluid therapy for vomiting patients requires parenteral administration. A balanced electrolyte solution, such as lactated Ringer's solution, is usually effective in correcting mild to moderate metabolic acidosis. The solution also provides a small amount of potassium and a large amount of sodium chloride. The volume of rehydration fluid used to correct initial fluid deficits should be calculated accurately and given during a four- to six-hour period (see Calculation of Fluid Replacement Requirements). After replenishment of fluid deficits, additional fluids are given to match the patient's maintenance requirements and ongoing losses from vomiting or diarrhea.

After rehydration, potassium chloride supplemen-

TABLE I
Potential Pharmacotherapy for Patients with Acute Gastroenteritis

Drug	Dosage and Route	Comments
Narcotic Analgesics		
Paregoric (with kaolin–pectin)	0.25–0.5 ml/kg every 8 hours, orally	Opioids not used in cats. Contraindicated in cases of infectious diarrhea.
Diphenoxylate	0.1–0.2 mg/kg every 8 hours, orally	
Loperamide	0.1–0.2 mg/kg every 8 hours, orally	
Antimicrobial Agents		
Erythromycin	10 mg/kg every 8 hours, orally	Treatment for patients with *Campylobacter jejuni* infection.
Enrofloxacin	2.5–5.0 mg/kg every 12 hours, orally	Treatment for patients with invasive salmonellosis.
Trimethoprim–sulfonamide	15 mg/kg every 12 hours, orally	Treatment for patients with severe mucosal injury.
Metronidazole	10–20 mg/kg every 8–12 hours, orally	Treatment for patients with *Clostridium* species infection.
Ampicillin sodium	10–20 mg/kg 6–8 hours, orally, intramuscularly, intravenously, or subcutaneously	Treatment for patients with sepsis.
Antiemetics		
Prochlorperazine	0.1–0.5 mg/kg every 6–8 hours subcutaneously	Phenothiazines may cause hypotension or sedation.
Chlorpromazine	0.5 mg/kg every 6–8 hours subcutaneously	
Metoclopramide hydrochloride	0.2–0.4 mg/kg every 6 hours subcutaneously	Also has gastrointestinal prokinetic activity.
Antisecretory or Protectant Agents		
Bismuth subsalicylate	1.0 ml/kg initially orally, then decrease dosage	Used cautiously in cats because of salicylate fraction.
Sucralfate	100–500 mg every 8 hours, orally	Used in patients with gastric erosions.

tation is usually indicated and should be guided by the measurement of serum potassium concentration. If electrolyte analysis is unavailable, the addition of 10 to 15 mEq potassium chloride per liter of lactated Ringer's solution during maintenance fluid administration is generally safe. Intravenous flow rates of potassium chloride should not exceed 0.5 mEq/kg/hr. The adequacy of fluid therapy in correcting fluid deficits is assessed by repeated physical examination, measurement of body weight, evaluation of packed cell volume and total protein, and estimation of urine output.

Nutritional Management

Traditional dietary recommendations for dogs and cats with acute gastroenteritis include withholding food for at least 24 hours. Potential benefits are decreased loss of mucosal epithelium because of the abrasive action of ingesta, reduced risk of dietary hypersensitivity, minimized colonization of the enteric flora by foreign bacteria, restoration of intestinal brush-border disaccharidase activity, and reduction of gastric acid secretion.[7] After clinical signs resolve, small quantities of a bland diet should be offered four to six times a day. Initially, the quantity fed should supply one third of the amount needed to meet daily caloric requirements. The caloric intake is then gradually increased during the next three to five days.

The ideal diet is highly digestible; is relatively hypoallergenic; contains adequate protein of high biologic value; is reasonably palatable; and contains a minimum of fat, lactose, and additives. Rice, the preferred carbohydrate in dogs, is more completely digested than are the corn or wheat flours in most commercial foods. This higher digestibility reduces the allergenicity of the diet and minimizes bacterial overgrowth, which can alter gut motility and cause secretory diarrhea.

The dietary protein content should be minimized to reduce gastric acid secretion and the development of acquired dietary hypersensitivity (which may delay clinical recovery).[20] Suitable protein sources include

> **Calculation of Fluid Replacement Requirements**
>
> 1. Replacement requirement
>   Body weight (kg) × Percentage dehydration = Fluid deficit (liters)
> 2. Maintenance requirement
>   40 to 60 ml/kg/day
> 3. Contemporary (ongoing) losses
>   - Secondary to diarrhea
>   - Secondary to vomiting
>
> The sum of 1, 2, and 3 equals 24-hour fluid requirement.

cottage cheese, chicken, and lamb. Low-fat diets are recommended to hasten gastric emptying and to minimize colonic secretions (which might exacerbate diarrhea). Feeding diarrheic cats a diet rich in digestible fat rather than carbohydrates may lessen the severity of the diarrhea.[21] In dogs, high-fiber diets may improve clinical signs of acute large-bowel diarrhea caused by *C. perfringens* enterotoxicosis.[22]

Various protein-selected commercial diets are currently available. A convenient homemade diet for dogs consists of cottage cheese (4 ounces) and boiled white rice (8 ounces); rice baby cereal (5 ounces) and diced chicken (5 ounces) are palatable to most cats.[20] These diets provide approximately 400 kcal and can be nutritionally balanced by the addition of a vitamin and mineral supplement. Most cases of acute gastroenteritis require three to five days of feeding the controlled diet; the patient is then slowly reintroduced to the normal diet.

Antimicrobial Therapy

Routine use of antibiotics is rarely indicated in treating patients with acute gastroenteritis. Antibiotic use is justified in animals with severe mucosal injury and a high risk of septicemia, as in cases of parvoviral enteritis, hemorrhagic gastroenteritis, and salmon poisoning disease.[23,24] Evidence of mucosal invasion by bacteria includes hemorrhagic diarrhea, increased fecal leukocytes, severe leukopenia, leukocytosis with a left shift, positive blood cultures, or clinical indications of sepsis (e.g., fever, depression, or shock). Antibiotics are also indicated if specific bacterial pathogens (e.g., *Salmonella* species, *C. jejuni*, or *Clostridium* species) are suspected.

The appropriate choice of an antibacterial drug is dictated by such factors as the suspected causative organism, antimicrobial spectrum of activity, host immunocompetence, and potential disruptive effects of the antibiotic on the host microflora. In managing animals with severe hemorrhagic diarrhea or compromised immune status, bactericidal drugs are preferable to bacteriostatic drugs. Parenteral administration is recommended in vomiting animals and in individuals with disseminated bacterial infections. If possible, the results of bacterial culture and antibiotic susceptibility testing should be obtained before antimicrobial therapy is initiated. Patients with positive fecal cultures for specific enteric pathogens should be treated according to the susceptibility pattern of the isolated bacteria. Because of the suppressive effects on the normal host microflora and the risk of promoting resistant strains of bacteria, empirical use of antibiotics in patients with uncomplicated acute gastroenteritis is not recommended.[24]

Motility-Modifying Drugs

Narcotic analgesics (opioids) are the most effective motility-modifying drugs for symptomatic treatment of intractable acute diarrhea in dogs.[25] These drugs include paregoric, loperamide, and diphenoxylate. The antidiarrheal effects of these agents are attributed to the pharmacologic actions on intestinal motility and on fluid and electrolyte transport. Opioids directly increase rhythmic segmentation and decrease propulsive contractions of the intestinal smooth muscle.[26] The net effect is inhibition of the flow of ingesta.

Some opioids also inhibit intestinal secretion and increase mucosal absorption of fluids, electrolytes, and glucose.[19,27] These agents are most appropriate in treating patients with secretory diarrhea; use of the drugs should be limited to less than seven days.[19] Because they are available as liquids, loperamide and paregoric are most conveniently used in small dogs (weighing less than 10 kilograms). Loperamide is quite palatable and reportedly has a faster onset of action and greater antisecretory effect than does diphenoxylate.

Narcotic analgesics should be administered carefully. Because opioids are narcotics, they may produce central nervous system depression in dogs if used inappropriately. Opioids are not recommended for use in cats because safe, effective dosages have not been verified. The agents are also contraindicated in animals with diarrhea caused by infection with invasive or enterotoxigenic bacteria. In these cases, drug-induced decreases in intestinal transit facilitate microbial proliferation, mucosal invasion, and absorption of bacterial toxins.

Anticholinergic drugs, such as atropine, have no useful role in the symptomatic therapy of patients with acute gastroenteritis. The agents reduce peristaltic and segmental contractions in the intestinal tract and thus reduce resistance to the flow of ingesta. Because of their generalized suppression of bowel motility, anticholinergic drugs can precipitate ileus and subsequently promote bacterial overgrowth of the small intestine.

Antiemetics

Because most vomiting episodes cease after food and water are withheld for 24 hours, antiemetic drugs are not frequently required in the management of patients with acute vomiting. The use of antiemetic drugs should be reserved for patients with persistent vomiting that results in distress or for instances in which control of vomiting is required to maintain fluid, electrolyte, and acid–base homeostasis.[28] Injudicious use of antiemetics must be avoided because the drugs do little to correct the primary cause of vomiting. Furthermore, intractable vomiting may signal the presence of serious gastrointestinal disease, which may necessitate a more aggressive diagnostic and therapeutic strategy. Empirical use of antiemetics in these instances may prevent the recognition of life-threatening causes of vomiting and the need for further evaluation.

The reflex pathway of vomiting is mediated via neural activity in the chemoreceptor trigger zone and/or the vomiting center in the brain. Antiemetics inhibit activation of these central pathways or inhibit vomiting by acting on peripheral sites of input to these higher centers. The promazine hydrochloride derivatives (chlorpromazine and prochlorperazine) are highly effective centrally acting antiemetics. These drugs may be administered by parenteral means. Prochlorperazine can also be administered as a rectal suppository. Because of their potential to induce vasodilation and hypotension, dehydration should be corrected before these drugs are used. The agents also lower the seizure threshold and may exacerbate seizure activity in animals.

Metoclopramide hydrochloride has centrally acting (via inhibition of dopamine in the chemoreceptor trigger zone) and peripheral antiemetic properties.[29] Peripherally, metoclopramide hydrochloride acts as a prokinetic agent to stimulate gastric and proximal duodenal motility.[30] These stimulatory actions on gastrointestinal smooth muscle inhibit the vomiting reflex and are believed to contribute to the antiemetic effects. In contrast with the phenothiazines, metoclopramide hydrochloride does not inhibit vomiting that is mediated directly through the vomiting center. This selective pharmacologic action coupled with the short serum half-life make metoclopramide hydrochloride an imperfect first-choice antiemetic for use in dogs and cats. The agent is contraindicated in patients with gastrointestinal obstruction.

Miscellaneous Therapeutic Agents

Various intestinal protectant and absorbent agents (including kaolin, pectin, activated charcoal, and barium sulfate) reportedly act locally in the gut by coating the intestinal wall and absorbing various bacteria and toxins. Clinical confirmation of the efficacy of these agents is lacking, and their use is not recommended. Bismuth subsalicylate may be an effective agent for treating patients with acute, nonspecific diarrhea.[31] This drug has antienterotoxic, antisecretory, and antiinflammatory actions, which are probably mediated through antiprostaglandin mechanisms. The agent should be used cautiously in cats because of their low tolerance for salicylates.

Sucralfate may be administered to patients with possible gastric erosions or ulceration. The drug has various mucosal cytoprotective functions, including increased mucous and bicarbonate production, the promotion of epithelial cell renewal, and increased gastric mucosal blood flow.[32] A therapeutic trial with an appropriate anthelmintic agent is indicated in dogs and cats that may have acute gastroenteritis associated with a parasitic cause.[33]

SUMMARY

Acute vomiting and diarrhea are common clinical signs that prompt the presentation of dogs and cats to small animal clinicians. On the basis of history and physical examination findings, most cases of acute gastroenteritis can be classified as self-limiting or potentially life-threatening. Patients with self-limiting disease readily respond to symptomatic fluid therapy, temporary restriction of oral intake, and selected use of pharmacologic agents. The prognosis for full recovery in these patients is excellent.

Patients that fail to respond to symptomatic therapy and those with life-threatening causes of gastroenteritis require more in-depth diagnostic evaluation and more aggressive supportive therapy. In these instances, definitive diagnosis should be postponed until symptomatic management (consisting of vigorous intravenous fluid therapy and withholding food, water, and oral medication) has been instituted.

About the Author

Dr. Jergens, who is a Diplomate of the American College of Veterinary Internal Medicine, is affiliated with the Department of Veterinary Clinical Sciences, College of Veterinary Medicine, Iowa State University, Ames, Iowa.

REFERENCES

1. Sherding RG: Diseases of the small bowel, in Ettinger SJ (ed): *Textbook of Veterinary Internal Medicine*. Philadelphia, WB Saunders Co, 1983, pp 1278–1346.

2. Rogers WA, Donovan EF, Kociba GJ: Idiopathic hyperlipoproteinemia in dogs. *JAVMA* 166:1087–1091, 1975.
3. Glickman LT, Domanski LM, Patronek GJ, et al: Breed-related risk factors for canine parvovirus enteritis. *JAVMA* 187: 589–594, 1985.
4. Muir WW: acid–base and electrolyte disturbances in dogs with gastric dilatation–volvulus. *JAVMA* 181:229–231, 1982.
5. Osweiler GD: A brief guide to clinical signs of toxicosis in small animals, in Kirk RW (ed): *Current Veterinary Therapy. IX.* Philadelphia, WB Saunders Co, 1986, pp 132–135.
6. Strombeck DR, Guilford WG: Motility disorders of the bowel, in Strombeck DR, Guilford WG (eds): *Small Animal Gastroenterology.* Davis, CA, Stonegate Publishing Co, 1990, pp 422–428.
7. Strombeck DR, Guilford WG: Classification, pathophysiology, and symptomatic treatment of diarrheal diseases, in Strombeck DR, Guilford WG (eds): *Small Animal Gastroenterology.* Davis, CA, Stonegate Publishing Co, 1990, pp 279–295.
8. Moreland KJ: Ulcer disease of the upper gastrointestinal tract in small animals: Pathophysiology, diagnosis, and management. *Compend Contin Educ Pract Vet* 10(11):1265–1279, 1988.
9. Greene CE, Ferguson DC: Antibacterial chemotherapy, in Greene CE (ed): *Infectious Diseases of the Dog and Cat.* Philadelphia, WB Saunders Co, 1990, pp 461–493.
10. Zimmer JF, Burrington DB: Comparison of four techniques of fecal examination for detecting canine giardiasis. *JAAHA* 22:161–167, 1986.
11. Mathys A, Mueller R, Pederson NC, et al: Comparison of hemagglutination and competitive enzyme-linked immunoabsorbent assay procedures for detecting canine parvovirus in feces. *Am J Vet Res* 44:151–154, 1983.
12. Fox, JG, Krakowka S, Taylor NS: Acute-onset *Campylobacter*-associated gastroenteritis in adult beagles. *JAVMA* 187: 1268–1271, 1985.
13. Nation PN: *Salmonella dublin* septicemia in two puppies. *Can Vet J* 25:324–326, 1984.
14. Kruth SA, Prescott JF, Welch MK, et al: Nosocomial diarrhea associated with enterotoxigenic *Clostridium perfringens* infection in dogs. *JAVMA* 195:331–334, 1989.
15. Twedt DC, Grauer GF: Fluid therapy for gastrointestinal, pancreatic, and hepatic disorders. *Vet Clin North Am Small Anim Pract* 12:463–485, 1982.
16. Cornelius LM, Rawlings CA: Arterial blood gas and acid–base values in dogs with various diseases and signs of disease. *JAVMA* 178:942–949, 1981.
17. Zenger E, Willard MD: Oral rehydration therapy in companion animals. *Comp Anim Pract* 19:6–10, 1989.
18. Johnson SE: Fluid therapy for gastrointestinal, pancreatic, and hepatic disease, in DiBartola SP (ed): *Fluid Therapy in Small Animal Practice.* Philadelphia, WB Saunders Co, 1992, pp 507–528.
19. Willard MD: Newer concepts in treatment of secretory diarrheas. *JAVMA* 186:86–88, 1985.
20. Guilford WG: Nutritional management of gastrointestinal tract diseases. *Proc 12th ACVIM Forum* 12:102–105, 1994.
21. Lewis LD, Morris ML, Hand MS: Gastrointestinal, pancreatic and hepatic diseases, in Lewis LD, Morris ML, Hand MS (eds): *Small Animal Clinical Nutrition. III.* Topeka, KS, Mark Morris Associates, 1987, pp 7-1–7-65.
22. Twedt DC: *Clostridium perfringens*–associated enterotoxicosis in dogs, in Kirk RW, Bonagura JD (eds): *Current Veterinary Therapy. XI.* Philadelphia, WB Saunders Co, 1992, pp 602–604.
23. Dillon R: Therapeutic strategies involving antimicrobial treatment of the gastrointestinal tract in small animals. *JAVMA* 185:1169–1171, 1984.
24. Jergens AE: Rational use of antimicrobials for gastrointestinal disease in small animals. *JAAHA* 30:123–131, 1994.
25. DeNovo RC: Therapeutics of gastrointestinal diseases, in Kirk RW (ed): *Current Veterinary Therapy. IX.* Philadelphia, WB Saunders Co, 1986, pp 862–872.
26. Stewart JJ, Weisbrodt NW, Burks TF: Central and peripheral actions of morphine on intestinal transit. *J Pharmacol Exp Therap* 205:547–555, 1978.
27. Fedorak RN, Field M: Antidiarrheal therapy. Prospects for new agents. *Dig Dis Sci* 32:195–205, 1987.
28. Leib MS: Acute vomiting: A diagnostic approach and symptomatic management, in Kirk RW, Bonagura JD (eds): *Current Veterinary Therapy. XI.* Philadelphia, WB Saunders Co, 1992, pp 583–587.
29. Albibi R, McCallum RW: Metoclopramide: Pharmacology and clinical application. *Ann Intern Med* 98:86–95, 1983.
30. Burrows CF: Metoclopramide. *JAVMA* 183:1341–1343, 1983.
31. Dupont HL, Sullivan P, Evans DG, et al: Prevention of traveler's diarrhea (emporiatric enteritis) by prophylactic administration of subsalicylate bismuth. *JAMA* 243:237–241, 1980.
32. Nagashima R: Development and characteristics of sucralfate. *J Clin Gastroenterol* 3:103–110, 1981.
33. Cornelius LM, Robertson EL: Treatment of gastrointestinal parasitism, in Kirk RW (ed): *Current Veterinary Therapy. IX.* Philadelphia, WB Saunders Co, 1986, pp 921–924.

UPDATE

New clinical briefs that may enhance the clinician's ability to diagnose potentially life-threatening causes for acute gastroenteritis include the following:

ABDOMINAL ULTRASONOGRAPHY

This technique is extremely useful in detecting foreign bodies, intussusception, and acute causes for adynamic ileus of varied causes. Sonographic diagnosis of acute pancreatitis provides definitive information concerning the extent of parenchymal involvement and the presence of regional effusion, pancreatic cysts, and abscesses.[1] The pancreas is usually enlarged and hypoechoic with moderate to severe parenchymal inflammation. Hyperechoic peripancreatic mesentery may also be visible. Ultrasound-guided aspirates or biopsies are particularly helpful when a diagnosis of abscess or necrosis is suspected.

GASTRIC DILATATION-VOLVULUS

New information[2] suggests that risks for the development of GDV include increasing breed size, being a purebred, increased age, and a large thoracic depth to width ratio. This latter variable is consistent with the theory that anatomic factors, such as conformational defects to the gastroesophageal sphincter, gastric retention of ingesta, or laxity of the gastric ligaments[3], may contribute to the development of the disease. The five breeds at increased risk in this ret-

(continues on page 361)

Acute Renal Failure. Part I. Risk Factors, Prevention, and Strategies for Protection

University of Prince Edward Island,
Charlottetown, Prince Edward Island,
Canada
India F. Lane, DVM, MS

Colorado State University
Gregory F. Grauer, DVM, MS
Martin J. Fettman, DVM, MS, PhD

KEY FACTS

❏ Acute renal failure may be prevented in patients that are at risk in a hospital setting by identifying such patients and adjusting clinical monitoring and therapy.

❏ Early recognition of impending acute renal failure and therapeutic intervention are facilitated by careful monitoring of urine output and urine characteristics.

❏ Acute renal failure occurs as a result of renal hemodynamic changes or tubular damage caused by nephrotoxic or ischemic insult.

❏ Vasodilators, calcium channel blockers, atrial natriuretic peptide, free radical scavengers, adjustments to diet, and other therapeutic measures show promise for future use in the prevention and treatment of acute renal failure.

Acute renal failure (ARF) is a sudden, severe reduction in renal function. It may be caused by prerenal, postrenal, or intrinsic renal insult. Intrinsic renal insult is generally ischemic or toxic in nature; it can occur as a result of a variety of systemic diseases, injuries, or therapeutic manipulations. Ischemic intrinsic renal insult is the most common cause of acute renal failure in humans; in dogs and cats, intrinsic renal insult resulting from nephrotoxic agents is the most common cause.[1] Acute renal failure carries a guarded prognosis and, despite many years of study and many advances in medical therapy, the overall outcome for patients with the disease has not changed significantly. Before dialysis became available, the mortality rate for humans with acute renal failure exceeded 90%[2-3]; today, with dialytic therapy widely available, the mortality rate is still greater than 50%.[4-6] Because of the potentially devastating results of established acute renal failure, prevention, early recognition, and early intervention are important.

Part I of this two-part series discusses the pathophysiology of acute renal failure, examines the factors that place certain patients at risk, and details methods of early recognition and intervention. Part II discusses diagnosis, management, and prognosis of acute renal failure.

PATHOPHYSIOLOGY

Intricacies of the pathogenesis of ischemic and toxic renal injury are yet to be completely explored. An understanding of these intricacies holds the key to successful intervention in and prevention of cases of acute renal failure.

The general mechanisms of acute renal failure can be categorized as vascular or tubular. Several mechanisms are usually involved in each case of renal dysfunction.[1,7] There are six specific sites of impairment. *Afferent arteriolar vasoconstriction* disrupts glomerular blood flow. Such vasoconstriction is often a physiologic response to decreased effective blood volume caused by

> **Selected Causes of Acute Renal Failure**[1,7]
>
> **Vascular or Ischemic**
> Dehydration
> Hemorrhage
> Shock
> Hypotension
> Anesthesia
> Surgery
> Sepsis
> Heart failure
> Arrhythmia
> Cardiac arrest
> Trauma
> Renal vascular occlusion
> Thromboembolism
> Hypertension
> Vasculitis
> Extensive burns
> Hyperthermia
> Disseminated intravascular coagulation
> Hyperviscosity
>
> **Nephrotoxic**
> Ethylene glycol
> Hydrocarbons
> Heavy metals
> Antimicrobial agents
> Angiotensin-converting-enzyme inhibitors
> Chemotherapeutic agents
> Nonsteroidal antiinflammatory drugs
> Thiacetarsamide
> Radiocontrast agents
> Anesthetic agents
> Hemoglobinemia
> Myoglobinemia
> Hypercalcemia
> Snake venom
>
> **Other**
> Glomerulonephritis
> Pyelonephritis
> Urinary tract obstruction
> Leptospirosis
> Amyloidosis
> Diabetes mellitus

largely modulated by mesangial cell contraction, which can be affected by ischemia, humoral agents, or toxicants. Glomerular permeability may be reduced by toxicant or immunologic injury to podocytes or endothelial architecture.

Decreased glomerular capillary pressure and filtration forces result from *vasodilation of the efferent arteriole*. Damage to tubular epithelial cells disrupts the integrity of the tubular lining and may result in *tubular backleak* of filtrate into the peritubular capillaries and interstitium. Tubular damage also creates cellular casts and debris, which can cause *obstruction of tubular flow*. Tubular flow may be further reduced by interstitial edema and cellular swelling; increased intratubular pressure may exacerbate existing backleak and filtration failure.

Ischemic Injury

Ischemic injury occurs when renal blood flow is attenuated by decreased blood pressure or by renal vasoconstriction. Conditions that result in volume depletion, depressed cardiac output, or sustained systemic hypotension can result in ischemic renal injury (see Selected Causes of Acute Renal Failure).[1,7] Decreased renal blood flow causes a reduction in the amount of oxygen and metabolic substrates available to tubular cells, and this cellular starvation initiates a complicated cycle of events (Figure 1). The adenosine triphosphate (ATP) energy pool is depleted rapidly. Cellular transport mechanisms are affected, particularly the sodium-potassium and sodium-calcium adenosinetriphosphatase (ATPase) pumps.

Increased intracellular concentrations of sodium cause extraction of plasma water and cell swelling, which occludes vascular and tubular lumens.[8] Membrane damage results in excessive calcium influx into renal tubular epithelial cells.[9] The depletion of energy sources depresses calcium efflux from the cell by calcium–adenosinetriphosphatase (Ca–ATPase) dependent transport; calcium processing by mitochondria and the endoplasmic reticulum is subsequently overwhelmed.[9–13] Increased intracellular calcium activates phospholipases, disrupts oxidative phosphorylation in mitochondria, and further constricts renal blood vessels.[11] Thus, intracellular calcium overload acts to perpetuate membrane damage, vasoconstriction, and energy depletion initiated by the ischemic event (Figure 2).

Persistent vasoconstriction and cell swelling create vascular stasis and platelet and red blood cell aggregation.[8] Red blood cells are trapped in the vascular space, occluding as much as 30% of the blood supply to the renal cortex, thereby creating further ischemic injury. Energy substrate delivery remains impaired; adenosine triphosphate restoration cannot occur. De-

dehydration, systemic hypotension, or fluid loss.[1,7] Excessive neurogenic or humoral response to vascular disease, trauma, or systemic injury is also implicated, although involvement of the renin–angiotensin axis is controversial.[7]

Reduced glomerular capillary surface area and *altered intrinsic glomerular filtration properties* also cause dysfunction. Surface area and filtration characteristics are

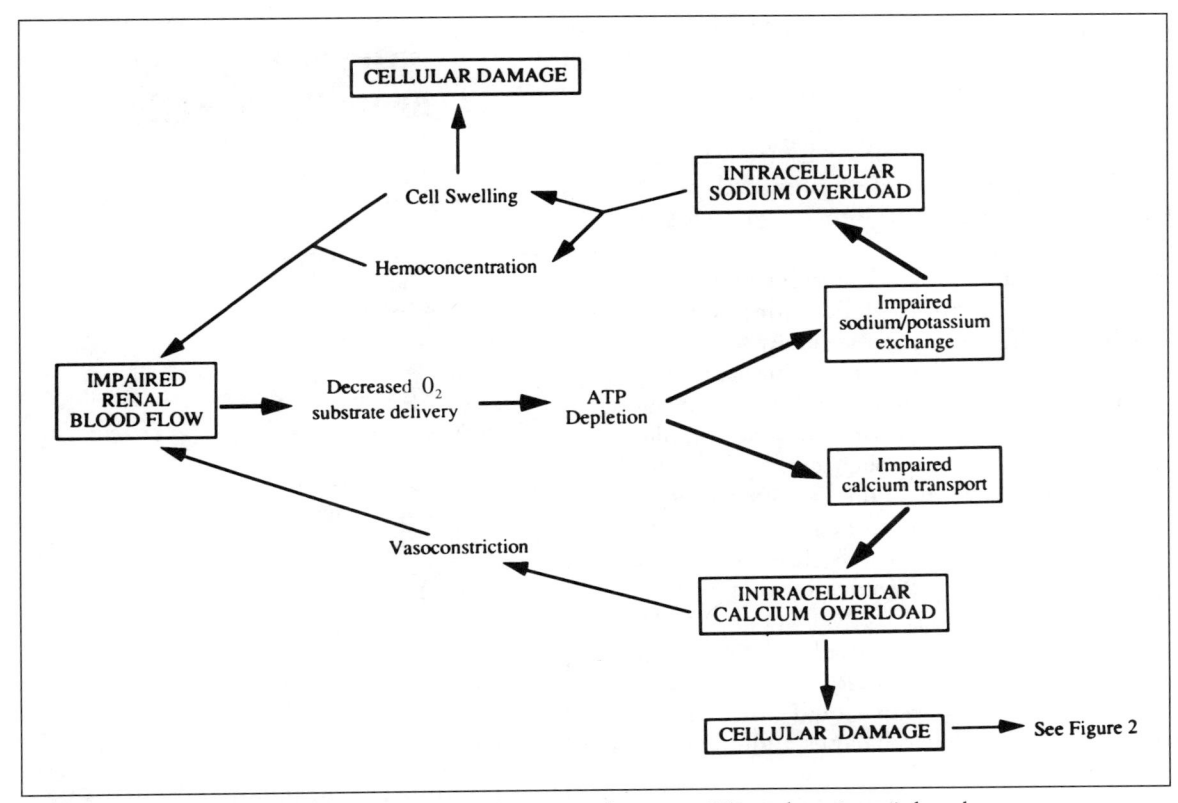

Figure 1—Circulatory and cellular events of ischemic renal injury. *ATP* = adenosine triphosphate.

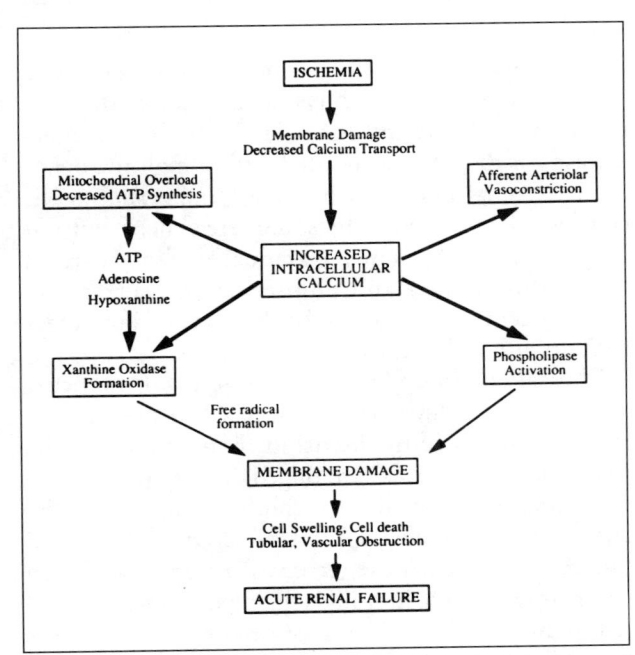

Figure 2—Schematic representation of the role of increased intracellular calcium in ischemic renal injury. *ATP* = adenosine triphosphate.

creased energy production results in membrane damage and oxygen free radical formation. Free radical scavengers are rapidly depleted; damage caused by free radicals contributes to membrane and cellular defects. Leukotrienes, thromboxane A_2, and other chemotactic factors cause infiltration by inflammatory cells and generation of additional inflammatory mediators and vasoactive chemicals.[8]

Nephrotoxic Injury

The kidneys are particularly susceptible to toxic injury for several reasons. They receive 20% of cardiac output, and therefore receive a relatively high proportion of blood-borne toxicants. Each kidney's large glomerular capillary surface area provides a large area for toxicant–endothelial interaction. In the proximal tubule and thick ascending loop of Henle, transport functions and a high metabolic rate make the epithelial cells especially sensitive to toxicants that disrupt energy sources or membrane functions. Tubular epithelial cells may also actively resorb toxicants, allowing such toxicants to accumulate to dangerous levels. The countercurrent mechanism and tubular concentrating functions result in increasing concentrations of toxic substances in the distal portions of the nephron. Finally, biotransformation activity of the kidney may result in local production of metabolites that are more toxic than parent compounds, as is the case with intrarenal oxidation of ethylene glycol.[14,15]

Nephrotoxic injury to the glomerulus can be direct

or immune mediated. Direct nephrotoxic injury includes destruction of capillary surface area by such substances as aminoglycosides; disruption of endothelial integrity and surface barriers by cationic substances, such as doxorubicin hydrochloride, probenecid, and protamine; and mesangial cell proliferation and hypertrophy caused by such substances as azathioprine and penicillamine.

Immunologic injury to the glomerulus occurs secondary to immune complex deposition, systemic lupus-like injury with antinuclear antibody formation, or other hypersensitivity reactions. In humans, such drugs as penicillin, penicillamine, gold salts, and sulfadiazine have been associated with immune complex disease, and procainamide, probenecid, hydralazine, and isoniazid can result in lupus-like syndromes.[14] Immune-complex deposition secondary to other antigens (e.g., *Dirofilaria immitis*) is, however, more common in small animals. Toxicants that disrupt tubular function may also indirectly affect glomerular function. They do so because tubular damage may trigger tubuloglomerular feedback mechanisms and local production of angiotensin II and other mediators that can precipitate hemodynamic and mesangial cell alterations.

Nephrotoxicant-induced tubular injury usually is caused by the effect of a toxicant on epithelial cells. Toxicants attach at luminal or basolateral membrane sites or to intracellular organelles.[1] Cellular function is then disrupted as a result of membrane and transport system damage, interference with energy production and cellular respiration, calcium influx, cell swelling, and cell death.[14]

Nonoliguric Acute Renal Failure

Urine production in cases of acute renal failure is variable. Although oliguria is considered the hallmark of acute renal failure, in many instances urine production is preserved or increased. Nonoliguric acute renal failure may be caused by exposure to such nephrotoxicants as aminoglycosides and cisplatin, or it may occur as a result of milder ischemic events.[16] Impaired tubular responses to antidiuretic hormone (ADH) can contribute to polyuric acute renal failure. Depressed responsiveness to antidiuretic hormone results from reduced medullary hypertonicity or from agents that impair concentrating ability, such as *E. coli* endotoxins, glucocorticoids, and diuretics.[17]

RISK FACTORS

Although prevention of accidental exposure to such nephrotoxic agents as ethylene glycol outside the hospital relies on client education and environmental control, prevention of iatrogenic acute renal failure is aided by the identification of patients at risk (see Risk

Risk Factors for Acute Renal Failure

Preexisting Disease
Renal insufficiency
Pancreatitis
Hepatic insufficiency
Diabetes mellitus
Cardiovascular disease
Multiple myeloma
Trauma
Extensive burns
Increasing age

Clinical Conditions
Volume depletion
Electrolyte abnormalities
Hypoalbuminemia
Systemic hypotension
Systemic hypertension
Fever
Sepsis
Anesthesia
Surgery
Radiocontrast media
Nonsteroidal antiinflammatory drugs
Nephrotoxic drugs

Factors for Acute Renal Failure). Trauma, extensive burns, pancreatitis, cardiovascular disease, diabetes mellitus, multiple myeloma, and preexisting renal disease are disorders associated with a high incidence of acute renal failure in humans.[7] Increasing age is considered a risk factor by some researchers[7] but not by others.[18] In humans, a gradual decline in renal blood flow (RBF) and glomerular filtration rate (GFR) occurs with age, probably placing some older patients at increased risk.[19]

Clinical conditions that increase the risk for acute renal failure include dehydration, electrolyte abnormalities, systemic hypotension, hypoalbuminemia, vasculitis, fever, sepsis, prolonged surgery or anesthesia, administration of radiographic contrast media, and use of potentially nephrotoxic agents.[19,20] Surgical procedures in which the renal vasculature is occluded or disrupted result in a high incidence of acute renal failure in humans.[4,7] The most important risk factors in small animals are volume depletion, electrolyte imbalances, anesthesia and surgery, and use of potentially nephrotoxic drugs. Risk factors are additive, and almost any complication occurring in a high-risk patient increases the potential for development of acute renal failure.

Volume depletion is the most significant factor

predisposing patients to acute renal failure, and it is often the only factor that can be prevented or corrected.[7,20] Volume depletion results from renal hypoperfusion, a decreased volume of distribution of nephrotoxic drugs, and decreased tubular flow. Decreased tubular flow potentiates tubular reabsorption, which can increase the intratubular and intracellular concentration of nephrotoxicants.[14] Rapid repletion of circulating blood volume and maintenance of adequate blood pressure in acutely ill or critically ill patients are important. Volume can be replaced by isotonic fluids or colloids. Pressor agents may be used in cases in which severe hypotension does not respond to volume replacement; improved systemic pressure may, however, affect renal vasoconstriction and result in reduced renal blood flow.

With high-risk patients, anesthetic protocols should be adjusted to prevent hypotension or possible nephrotoxicosis. Volume replacement and blood-pressure monitoring are critical. Renal autoregulation can maintain glomerular capillary pressure for short periods, but renal blood flow is compromised when systolic pressure drops below 80 mm Hg for sustained periods.[1] Anesthesia with methoxyflurane occasionally results in acute renal failure in humans if the duration of exposure is prolonged. Nephrotoxicity of methoxyflurane is enhanced by dehydration or concurrent use of nephrotoxic drugs.[21] Dogs seem to be resistant to the effects of methoxyflurane if exposed for only a short time[22]; however, the administration of flunixin meglumine with methoxyflurane anesthesia has been shown to result in acute tubular necrosis.[23]

Electrolyte imbalances, particularly sodium or potassium disturbances, also increase the risk of acute renal failure. Hyponatremia potentiates contrast-media induced acute renal failure in dogs and humans.[24] Hypokalemia, hypocalcemia, hypomagnesemia, and metabolic acidosis enhance gentamicin nephrotoxicity in dog and rat experimental models.[25,26] Electrolyte status should be routinely monitored in high-risk patients and corrected before anesthesia, surgery, contrast imaging procedures, or use of potentially nephrotoxic drugs.

Other specific risk factors for gentamicin nephrotoxicity include old age; dehydration; preexisting renal disease; prolonged duration of therapy; and the concurrent use of cytotoxic drugs, other nephrotoxic agents, or prostaglandin inhibitors.[27] In high-risk patients, the potential dangers of aminoglycoside therapy must be weighed against the benefits. When aminoglycosides are used, therapeutic-drug monitoring allows the clinician to tailor individual dose regimens. Nephrotoxicity increases with elevated trough serum levels (greater than 2 µg/ml for gentamicin; greater than 5 µg/ml for amikacin).[14]

Trough levels can be reduced by decreasing the dose or increasing the dose interval.[27] Recent investigations suggest that increasing the dose interval by a factor arithmetically related to serum creatinine or creatinine clearance values is the most effective way to reduce nephrotoxicity.[28,29] Frequent dosing of gentamicin (every eight hours) may be less efficacious and potentially more nephrotoxic, however, than an equivalent total daily dose given in 12-hour intervals.[29] Other mechanisms of protection in gentamicin therapy are discussed below.

Nonsteroidal antiinflammatory drugs (NSAIDs) may act as nephrotoxicants; administration of such drugs may increase the risk of acute renal failure. Used long term and given in single doses, nonsteroidal antiinflammatory drugs inhibit renal prostaglandin synthesis and decrease urinary prostaglandin excretion by inhibiting cyclooxygenase activity. Prostaglandins, particularly of the E and I series, serve important vasodilatory functions in the kidney; and they influence glomerular filtration rates and solute excretion.[30,31] Prostaglandins also modulate renin release, tubular ion transport, and water balance.[31]

Inhibition of prostaglandin synthesis in the normal kidney does not significantly impair renal function because other regulatory mechanisms compensate for the loss of prostaglandin influence. In diseased kidneys or with the addition of volume depletion or other stressors, however, the vasoconstrictor influences predominate and normal prostaglandin counter-response is required[30] (Figure 3). Anesthesia, surgery, sodium or volume depletion, sepsis, congestive heart failure, nephrotic syndrome, and hepatic disease cause renal function to become more dependent on prostaglandin synthesis; therefore, in such cases, susceptibility to nonsteroidal antiinflammatory drugs is increased.[30] Dogs seem to be particularly sensitive to newer nonsteroidal antiinflammatory drugs, such as ibuprofen or naproxen; reaction may include gastrointestinal ulceration and renal failure.[32] Acute interstitial nephritis and papillary necrosis have also been reported secondary to administration of nonsteroidal antiinflammatory drugs.[30-33]

EARLY RECOGNITION OF RENAL DYSFUNCTION

Acute renal failure occurs in three distinct phases: (1) the induction phase, in which the insult occurs and azotemia, oliguria, or polyuria develop; (2) the maintenance phase, in which established loss of function occurs; and (3) the recovery phase, during which resolution of azotemia, nephron repair, and functional compensation occur.[1] Because therapeutic intervention is most successful when initiated in the induction phase of acute renal failure (which can be very short in duration), early recognition of renal dysfunction can save the patient's life.

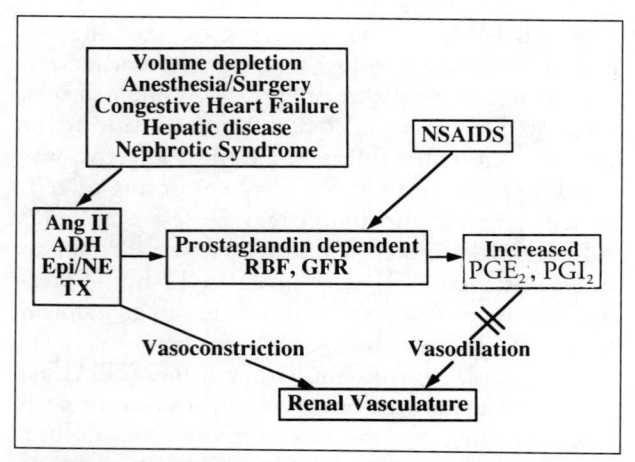

Figure 3—Influence of nonsteroidal antiinflammatory drugs (*NSAIDs*) in conditions in which renal vascular resistance is highly prostaglandin dependent. *Ang II* = angiotensin II, *ADH* = antidiuretic hormone, *Epi/NE* = epinephrine/norepinephrine, *TX* = thromboxane, *RBF* = renal blood flow, *GFR* = glomerular filtration rate, PGE_2 = prostaglandin E_2, PGI_2 = prostaglandin I_2 (prostacyclin).

In humans, acute renal failure has been defined as an increase in serum creatinine of 0.5 mg/dl/day for two consecutive days.[7] Such relatively small changes are probably often missed or overlooked in veterinary patients. Frequent monitoring of serum creatinine in high-risk patients may allow earlier detection of prerenal or renal azotemia. Monitoring other patient criteria, however, may help to detect renal damage and dysfunction before the development of azotemia.

Physical examination of the patient at risk for acute renal failure should include observation of cardiac rate, rhythm, and pulse quality and assessment of hydration status. Pulse quality and hydration characteristics are outward indexes of hemodynamic status. Frequent recording of body weight, packed cell volume, and plasma total solids helps to detect subtle changes in hydration status. In critically ill patients, direct or indirect monitoring of blood pressure can help to identify hypotension and hypertension, conditions which increase the risk of renal damage. Palpation of the abdomen and kidneys is also important. Kidneys may become enlarged or painful if acute dysfunction and intracapsular swelling occur.

Urine output of critically ill patients should be monitored; it should also be objectively quantified in high-risk patients, using a metabolic cage, intermittent catheterization, or a closed indwelling collection system. Normal urine output should be 1 to 2 ml/hr/kg body weight; significant increases or decreases from normal output may signal acute renal failure. Oliguria (<0.27 ml/hr/kg) or anuria (<.08 ml/hr/kg)[34] requires prompt attention and treatment.

Urine should be assessed at each collection for turbidity or the presence of blood; the urine sediment should be examined daily for red blood cells, white blood cells, casts, renal epithelial cells, and cellular debris. The presence of low–molecular-weight proteins in the urine that normally are freely filtered and then reabsorbed in the proximal tubules is an early marker of acute renal failure. Beta$_2$-microglobulin and retinol binding protein assays have been used in humans as early indicators of proximal tubular damage.[35] In practice, the onset of proteinuria detected by semiquantitative (dipstick or turbidimetric) or quantitative (urine protein/creatinine ratio) methods may indicate early glomerular or tubular damage.

Urinary enzyme activity is a sensitive method of detecting early tubular damage. In cases of tubular damage or necrosis, enzymes such as γ-glutamyl transpeptidase and N-acetyl-β-D-glucoaminidase (NAG) are not filtered normally by the glomerulus but, instead, increase in the urine.[36] Urinary γ-glutamyl transpeptidase originates from the proximal tubular brush border; N-acetyl-β-D-glucoaminidase is present in the proximal tubule lysosomes.[36,37] Urinary γ-glutamyl transpeptidase activity was the earliest known marker of toxicosis reported in studies of gentamicin nephrotoxicity in a dog model.[36] In cases of early gentamicin nephrotoxicity, urinary N-acetyl-β-D-glucoaminidase activity is increased in proportion to tubular damage. Urinary N-acetyl-β-D-glucoaminidase has also been investigated as an early marker for diabetic nephropathy in humans.[37] In a study of experimental organonitrile nephrotoxicity in rats, increases in urinary N-acetyl-β-D-glucoaminidase correlated well with renal morphologic lesions that developed before the onset of azotemia.[38]

Urinary amylase, lysozyme, β-glucuronidase, lactic dehydrogenase, and aspartate transaminase activities also have been investigated in nephrotoxic models.[39–41] False-positive results can occur with severe glomerular damage that results in abnormal filtration into the urine; false-negative results can occur after chronic damage and depletion of enzyme stores.[36] The development of glucosuria or alterations in the fractional excretion of other electrolytes are other early signals of tubular dysfunction.[42]

MECHANISMS OF PROTECTION AND EARLY INTERVENTION

Methods designed to protect the kidneys from acute insults (Table I) attempt to prevent or interrupt the pathophysiologic events that result in acute renal failure. Goals of protective maneuvers are to (1) preserve or restore renal hemodynamics, (2) increase solute excretion, (3) minimize intratubular obstruction, (4) enhance cellular recovery, and (5) reduce toxicity of nephrotoxic agents.[20] Dietary manipulations, va-

TABLE I
Protective Agents in Cases of Acute Renal Failure

Agent	Type of Injury[a]	Timing[a]	Possible Mechanisms
Sodium[42–46]	Toxicant	Prior	Causes volume expansion Increases natriuresis Suppresses RAAS Reduces TGF
Mannitol[55–59]	Toxicant Ischemic	Prior/Post	Causes volume expansion Increases tubular flow, GFR Causes vasodilation Acts as a free radical scavenger
Furosemide[60,62,63]	Toxicant	Prior/Post	Increases renal blood flow Increases tubular flow More effective when used with dopamine
Low-protein diets[46–51]	Toxicant Ischemic	Prior	Reduces renal work Reduces tubular uptake
Atrial natriuretic peptide[24,65–67]	Ischemic	Initiation	Causes Aa vasodilation May cause Ea vasoconstriction Causes diuresis, natriuresis
Calcium channel blockers[10,12,68–71]	Ischemic Transplant	Prior/Init	Causes Aa vasodilation Prevents calcium overload Prevents membrane damage Prevents reperfusion injury
Free radical scavengers[72,73]	Toxicant Ischemic	Init/Post	Reduces reperfusion injury
ATP-magnesium chloride[76,78]	Ischemic	Initiation	Supplies energy substrate Reduces adenosine accumulation May supply magnesium
Theophylline, Aminophylline[75,77]	Toxicant	Prior	Acts as adenosine receptor blockade
Thyroxin[80]	Toxicant	Initiation	Stimulates renal tubular gluconeogenesis Restores sodium-potassium transport pumps
Thromboxane inhibitors[83]	Ischemic	Init/Post	Reduce vasoconstrictive influence

[a] Type of injury and timing of administration represent best results in experimental models. Selected references are listed for each agent. ATP = adenosine triphosphate, RAAS = renin-angiotensin-aldosterone system, TGF = tubuloglomerular feedback, GFR = glomerular filtration rate, Aa = afferent arteriole, Ea = efferent arteriole.

sodilatory compounds, diuretics, and cytoprotective agents are some treatments that may protect the kidneys from acute renal failure.

Dietary Factors
Sodium

Low-sodium diets have been shown to enhance gentamicin nephrotoxicity.[43] Oral sodium–loading strategies have been beneficial in reducing mortality and cortical gentamicin concentrations in rats.[43] The benefits of sodium loading may involve suppression of intrarenal and plasma renin activity and attenuation of early renin–angiotensin responses. Other manipulations to block renin or angiotensin effects, however, are not uniformly protective after acute renal failure is established.[20] Volume expansion secondary to sodium retention may protect the renal vasculature and may increase the volume of distribution of nephrotoxic drugs, thus reducing their effective serum and tissue concentrations.[43]

Increasing natriuresis, urine volume, and solute excretion before a potential renal insult may also be important to prevent acute renal failure.[44] Saline diuresis has been helpful before the administration of some nephrotoxic agents (cisplatin,[45] amphotericin B[46]) because it results in volume expansion and increased natriuresis. Although sodium loading does not consistently protect against acute renal failure, it is clear that sodium depletion and hyponatremia should be avoided in patients at high risk for acute renal failure.

Protein

The effects of dietary protein on chronic renal disease have been investigated for many years. Recently, however, conditioning with reduced dietary protein has been shown to improve renal function and survival rates in rats subjected to acute ischemic insults[47,48] and uranyl nitrate-,[49] puromycin-[50] and gentamicin-induced[51] acute renal failure. In a model of ischemia, 88% of rats receiving a 5% protein diet and all rats receiving a 0% protein diet survived, whereas only 31% and 7% of rats receiving diets with an average or high level of protein, respectively, survived.[47] Preconditioning with reduced-protein diets had to occur for at least one week before insult to be effective; dietary manipulation immediately after the insult was not protective.[47,48]

In one study in which rats were given nephrotoxic doses of gentamicin, animals that were preconditioned with a low-protein diet showed improved creatinine clearance, decreased enzymuria, and decreased renal cortical concentrations of gentamicin compared with animals that received diets with an average or high protein content.[51] In another study, low-protein conditioning again improved survival in rats treated with gentamicin; however, significant protection was also provided by preconditioning the rats with a high-protein diet, and then switching them to a low-protein diet at the time of gentamicin administration.[52]

Low protein intake may downshift renal work by reducing renal blood flow and glomerular filtration rate. A low-protein diet reduces tubular metabolic work, thus perhaps decreasing tubular uptake of gentamicin. In one study in dogs, however, conditioning with a high-protein (26%) diet before and during gentamicin administration reduced nephrotoxicity[53] and enhanced gentamicin clearance[54] compared with such functions in dogs fed diets that were 13% or 9% protein.

The effects of dietary protein conditioning on susceptibility to renal failure may depend on the nephrotoxicant involved, because high protein intake is protective in models of mercuric chloride toxicity, even with short-term conditioning.[55] Evaluation of dietary protein conditioning in dogs before and after renal ischemia or nephrotoxicant-induced renal injury may have important clinical implications.

Diuretics and Vasodilators

Diuretics have long been used in cases of acute renal failure to combat oliguria. Mannitol, an osmotic diuretic, serves to increase intravascular volume, increase tubular fluid flow, and prevent tubular obstruction and collapse. Mannitol also acts as a renal vasodilator, improving renal blood flow and glomerular filtration rate, if given early in acute renal failure.[56–58] The vasodilatory effects of mannitol may be mediated by renal prostaglandins[57] or by the release of atrial natriuretic hormone.[58] Hypertonic mannitol solutions help reduce cellular swelling in cases of acute renal failure and thus prevent tubular obstruction and cell death. Cellular protection may also be afforded by the free radical scavenging properties of mannitol and its influence on prevention of mitochondrial calcium accumulation.[57]

Experimentally, mannitol has proven protective against acute renal failure in ischemic models[59,60] and toxicant-induced models including glycerol, methemoglobin, cisplatin, and amphotericin B.[57] Mannitol is used in humans to protect against acute renal failure during high-risk surgeries, radiocontrast procedures, and use of amphotericin B and cisplatin.[57]

Furosemide also acts to increase renal blood flow and tubular flow, but it does not significantly influence glomerular filtration rate. Enhanced diuresis created by furosemide may resolve oliguria, but it does not seem to affect recovery or survival.[57] Furosemide seems to be more effective in inducing diuresis when it is used in combination with dopamine infusion.[61] The intravenous infusion of dopamine at low dosages (1 to 3 µg/kg/min) acts via renal dopaminergic receptors to increase renal blood flow, glomerular filtration rate, and sodium excretion in normal kidneys. Low-dose dopamine alone may also improve renal function in cases of acute renal failure.[62] Furosemide has been protective in some models of ischemia,[63–65] but mixed results have been obtained from its use with nephrotoxicants. Both furosemide and dopamine are most effective when administered soon after onset of renal failure. Furosemide in combination with gentamicin actually enhances nephrotoxicity, probably by creating volume depletion.[65]

Atrial Natriuretic Peptide

Atrial natriuretic peptide (ANP) counterbalances the vasoconstrictive activity of catecholamines and angiotensin II. Atrial natriuretic peptide release results in vasorelaxation, diuresis, and natriuresis.[66] It seems to preserve renal blood flow and glomerular filtration rate during ischemia and volume depletion by causing afferent arteriolar vasodilation and, possibly, efferent arteriolar vasoconstriction.[67]

In a canine model of norepinephrine-induced acute

renal failure, atrial natriuretic peptide infusion resulted in better protection of renal blood flow and creatinine clearance than did dopamine infusion; elevations in systemic blood pressure and total vascular resistance were attenuated.[66] Natriuretic peptide, used in a model of ischemia in rats, improved glomerular capillary pressure and afferent arteriolar blood flow resulting from a decrease in afferent arteriolar resistance were documented.[68] In another study, atrial natriuretic peptide preserved renal function in dogs with congestive heart failure receiving iodinated radiocontrast media.[24] Atrial natriuretic peptide infusion was not found, however, to be significantly more protective than mannitol in a clinical trial of humans at high risk of acute renal failure during angiography procedures.[58]

Calcium Channel Blockers

Increased intracellular calcium concentrations secondary to ischemic or nephrotoxicant-induced injury cause membrane and cytoskeletal damage, deranged cellular metabolism, and sustained vasoconstriction in the injured kidney.[10,12] Calcium channel blockers (CCBs, calcium-entry blockers) exert a cytoprotective and vasodilatory effect if given before or early in the course of ischemia.[10–12]

In a normal animal, calcium channel blockers increase renal blood flow, glomerular filtration rate, urine flow, and electrolyte excretion.[10] Hemodynamic alterations result from a decrease in afferent arteriolar resistance and are accentuated if preexisting vascular tone is high.[10]

The protective mechanisms of calcium channel blockers in acute renal failure may involve preservation of renal blood flow or cytoprotective effects, including the prevention of mitochondrial calcium overload and reperfusion injury.[10,13,69,70] An interaction between calcium channel blockers and tissue magnesium also seems to be important. In a model of ischemic injury in guinea pigs in which verapamil infusion was protective, the significant difference between treated and untreated animals was the preservation of tissue magnesium levels.[71] Interfering with the effects of calcium may preserve membrane integrity and therefore prevent loss of tissue magnesium.[71]

Calcium channel blockers have been protective in models of ischemic acute renal failure in dogs.[72] Calcium channel blockers have also improved glomerular filtration rate in transplanted kidneys in dogs, and they are used clinically to help prevent acute renal failure in transplanted kidneys in humans.[69] It seems that calcium channel blockers improve graft function slightly and may protect transplanted kidneys from cyclosporine toxicity,[10] but improved graft survival has not been demonstrated.[69] Protection in ischemic acute renal failure models was best when calcium channel blockers were administered via intraarterial or intrarenal infusion before and after the insult,[10,69] a frequency that may limit their practicality and effectiveness in clinical cases of acute renal failure. Finally, although promising results have been observed in many experimental models, infusion of calcium channel blockers may have systemic hypotensive and cardiodepressant effects that could decrease renal blood flow.

Free Radical Scavengers

Hypoxia, membrane damage, adenosine triphosphate degradation, and reperfusion can result in free radical formation, which creates further membrane damage.[8,9,73] During ischemia, tissue adenosine triphosphate is used rapidly and adenosine degradation to hypoxanthine occurs. Xanthine dehydrogenase is converted to xanthine oxidase, which preferentially metabolizes hypoxanthine to free radicals. Xanthine oxidase formation is also enhanced by elevated intracellular calcium concentration. When oxygen reappears, a burst of free radical production occurs. Intermediates of oxygen, including superoxides, hydroxyl radicals, and singlet oxygen, are toxic to mitochondria and cell membranes.[73]

Free radical scavengers have been protective in ischemic, aminoglycoside-induced, and glycerol-induced acute renal failure models.[75] In one study, increased lipid peroxidation and depressed glutathione peroxidase activity occurred after renal ischemia in rats fed a diet deficient in vitamin E and selenium—both natural free radical scavengers.[75] Superoxide dismutase, which metabolizes hydroxyl radicals to hydrogen peroxide, and allopurinol, which inhibits xanthine oxidase and reduces peroxide formation, have been shown to be protective by reducing reactive oxygen metabolites in some models.[75] Superoxide and hydroxyl radical scavengers, however, did not attenuate renal dysfunction in a recent model of endotoxin-induced acute renal failure in rats.[74]

Adenosine Nucleotides

Elevations in tissue adenosine concentrations occur after adenosine triphosphate degradation in renal ischemia, and infusion of adenosine into the interstitium of rat kidneys has resulted in decreased glomerular filtration rate.[76] Adenosine may be responsible for tubuloglomerular feedback and renal vasoconstriction after ischemia.[77] Adenosine receptor blockade with theophylline[76] or aminophylline[78] has been shown to reverse the effects of adenosine.

Postischemic infusion of adenine nucleotides (adenosine triphosphate, adenosine diphosphate, and adenosine monophosphate) combined with magnesium chloride in rats enhanced renal recovery, possibly by reducing adenine catabolism and adenosine production.[77] Adenosine triphosphate with magnesium chloride may also protect the kidney from ischemia by promoting prostaglandin synthesis or by acting as an intracellular energy source; the influence of magnesium may, again, be important. In one study involving dogs, however, adenosine triphosphate with magnesium chloride actually enhanced toxicity of cisplatin.[79]

Other Mechanisms

The effect of many other vasodilatory and cytoprotective agents in cases of acute renal failure are being investigated. Magnesium apparently plays a role in the protection afforded by calcium channel blockers, and it may have an influence on the effects of adenosine triphosphate-magnesium chloride infusion.[71,77] High magnesium intake is also protective against gentamicin toxicity.[80] Magnesium and calcium compete with gentamicin for binding sites at the renal tubular brush border.[80,81] Magnesium and calcium will probably be important components in dietary protection against acute renal failure. Attention to plasma magnesium levels is warranted with the use of aminoglycosides. Thyroxin administration has been protective in several toxicant-induced acute renal failure models in rats, possibly because of its role in the stimulation of gluconeogenesis and restoration of sodium-potassium pumps in renal tubular epithelial cells.[82] Vasodilatory substances, such as β-adrenergic antagonists,[83] synthetic vasodilatory prostaglandins,[84] and thromboxane synthetase inhibitors,[84] may also prove to be useful in the intervention of acute renal failure.

About the Authors

Dr. Lane is affiliated with the Department of Companion Animals, Atlantic Veterinary College, University of Prince Edward Island, Charlottetown, Prince Edward Island, Canada. Dr. Grauer is affiliated with the Department of Clinical Science and Dr. Fettman is affiliated with the Department of Pathology at the College of Veterinary Medicine and Biomedical Sciences, Colorado State University, Fort Collins, Colorado.

REFERENCES

1. Chew DJ, Dibartola SP: Diagnosis and pathophysiology of renal disease, in Ettinger SJ (ed): *Textbook of Veterinary Internal Medicine*, ed. 3. Philadelphia, WB Saunders Co, 1989, pp 1893–1961.
2. Byrick RJ, Rose DK: Pathophysiology and prevention of acute renal failure; the role of the anaesthetist. *Can J Anaesth* 37:457–467, 1990.
3. Guly UM, Turney JH: Post-traumatic acute renal failure, 1956–1988. *Clin Nephrol* 34:79–83, 1990.
4. Cioffi WG, Ashikaga T, Gamelli RL: Probability of surviving postoperative acute renal failure; development of a prognostic index. *Ann Surg* 200:205–211, 1984.
5. Maher ER, Robinson KN, Scoble JE, et al. Prognosis of critically ill patients with acute renal failure; APACHE II score and other predictive factors. *Q J Med* 72:857–866, 1989.
6. Liano F, Garci-Martin F, Gallego A, et al. Easy and early prognosis in acute tubular necrosis: A forward analysis of 228 cases. *Nephron* 51:307–313, 1989.
7. Wilkes BM, Mailloux LU: Acute renal failure; pathogenesis and prevention. *Am J Med* 80:1129–1136, 1986.
8. Mason J: The pathophysiology of ischemic acute renal failure; a new hypothesis about the initiation phase. *Renal Physiol* 9:129–147, 1986.
9. Weinberg J: The cell biology of ischemic renal injury. *Kidney Int* 39:476–500, 1991.
10. Chan L, Schrier RW: Effects of calcium channel blockers on renal function. *Annu Rev Med* 41:289–302, 1990.
11. Hume HD: Role of calcium in pathogenesis of acute renal failure. *Am J Physiol* 250:F579–F589, 1986.
12. Schrier RW, Arnold PE, Van Putten VJ, Burke TJ: Cellular calcium in ischemic acute renal failure: Role of calcium entry blockers. *Kidney Int* 32:313–321, 1987.
13. Schrier RW: Role of calcium channel blockers in protection against experimental renal injury. *Am J Med* 90 (Suppl 5A):21S–25S, 1991.
14. Brown SA, Engelhardt JA: Drug-related nephropathies. Part I. Mechanisms, diagnosis, and management. *Compend Contin Educ Pract Vet* 9(2):148–160, 1987.
15. Weening JJ: Mechanisms leading to toxin-induced impairment of renal function, with a focus on immunopathology. *Toxicol Lett* 46:205–211, 1989.
16. Anderson RJ, Linsa SL, Berns AS, et al: Nonoliguric acute renal failure. *N Engl J Med* 296:1134–1138, 1977.
17. Anderson RJ, Schrier RW: Clinical spectrum of oliguric and nonoliguric acute renal failure, in Brenner BM, Stein H (eds): *Acute Renal Failure*. New York, Churchill Livingstone, 1980, pp 3, 4.
18. Rasmussen HH, Pitt EA, Ibels LS, McNeil DR: Prediction of outcome in acute renal failure by discriminant analysis of clinical variables. *Arch Intern Med* 145:2015–2018, 1985.
19. Cowgill LD: Acute renal failure, in Bovee KC (ed): *Canine Nephrology*. Media, PA, Harwal Publishing Co, 1984, pp 405–438.
20. Mandal AK, Lightfoot BO, Treat RC: Mechanisms of protection in acute renal failure. *Circ Shock* 11:245–253, 1983.
21. Mazze RI: Methoxyflurane nephropathy. *Environ Health Perspect* 15:111–119, 1976.
22. Pedersoli WM: Serum flouride concentration, renal and hepatic function test results in dogs with methoxyflurane anesthesia. *Am J Vet Res* 38:949–953, 1977.
23. Mathews K, Doherty T, Dyson D, Wilcock B: Renal failure in dogs associated with flunixin meglumine and methoxyflurane anesthesia. *Vet Surg* 16:323, (abstract) 1987.
24. Margulies KB, McKinley LJ, Cavero PG, Burnett JC: Induction and prevention of radiocontrast-induced nephropathy in dogs with heart failure. *Kidney Int* 38:1101–1108, 1990.
25. Brinker KR, Bulger RE, Dolgan DC, et al: Effect of potassium depletion on gentamicin nephrotoxicity. *J Lab Clin Med* 98:292–301, 1981.
26. Hsu CH, Kurtz TW, Easterling RE, Weller JM: Potentiation of gentamicin nephrotoxicity by metabolic acidosis. *Proc Soc Exp Biol Med* 46:894–897, 1974.
27. Cooper K, Bennett WM: Nephrotoxicity of common drugs used in clinical practice. *Arch Intern Med* 147:1213–1218, 1987.
28. Rogers RA, Hanna AY, Riviere JE: Dose response studies of

gentamicin nephrotoxicity in rats with experimental renal dysfunction. III. Effects of dosage adjustment method. *Res Commun Chem Path Pharm* 57:301–311, 1987.
29. Frazier DL, Riviere JC: Gentamicin dosing strategies for dogs with subclinical renal dysfunction. *Antimicrob Agent Chemother* 31:1929–1934, 1987.
30. Patrono C, Dunn MJ: The clinical significance of inhibition of renal prostaglandin synthesis. *Kidney Int* 32:1–12, 1987.
31. Clive DM, Stoff JS: Renal syndromes associated with nonsteroidal antiinflammatory drugs. *N Engl J Med* 310:563–571, 1984.
32. Spyridakis LK, Bacia JJ, Barsanti JA, Brown SA: Ibuprofen toxicosis in the dog. *JAVMA* 189:918–919, 1986.
33. Rubin SI: Nonsteroidal antiinflammatory drugs, prostaglandins, and the kidney. *JAVMA* 188:1065–1068, 1986.
34. English PB: Acute renal failure in the dog and cat. *Aust Vet J* 50:384–392, 1974.
35. Roberts DS, Haycock GB, Dalton RN, et al: Prediction of acute renal failure after birth asphyxia. *Arch Dis Child* 65:1021–1028, 1990.
36. Greco DS, Turnwald GH, Adams R, et al: Urinary gamma-glutamyl transpeptidase activity in dogs with gentamicin-induced nephrotoxicity. *Am J Vet Res* 46:2332–2335, 1985.
37. Stolarek I, Howey JE, Fraser CG. Biological variation of urinary N-acetyl-β-D-glucosaminidase: Practical and clinical implications. *Clin Chem* 35:560–563, 1989.
38. Gould DH, Fettman MJ, Daxenbichler ME, Bartuska BM: Functional and structural alterations of the rat kidney induced by the naturally occurring organonitrile 25-1-cyano-2-hydroxy-3,4 epithiobutane. *Toxicol Appl Pharmacol* 78:190–201, 1985.
39. Aderka D, Tene M, Graff E, Levo Y: Amylase-creatinine clearance ratio: A simple test to predict gentamicin nephrotoxicity. *Arch Intern Med* 148:1093–1096, 1988.
40. Szczech GM, Carlton WW, Lund JE: Determination of enzyme concentrations in urine for diagnosis of renal damage. *JAAHA* 10:1093–1096, 1974.
41. Hardy ML, Hsu RC, Short CR: The nephrotoxic potential of gentamicin in the cat; enzymuria and alterations in urine concentrating ability. *J Vet Pharmacol Ther* 8:382–392, 1985.
42. Garry F, Chew DJ, Hoffsis GF: Urinary indices of renal function in sheep with induced aminoglycoside nephrotoxicosis. *Am J Vet Res* 51:420–427, 1990.
43. Bennett WM, Hartnett MN, Gilbert D, et al: Effect of sodium intake on gentamicin nephrotoxicity in the rat. *Proc Soc Exp Biol Med* 151:736–738, 1976.
44. Vari RC, Natarajan LA, Whitescaver SA, et al: Induction, prevention and mechanisms of contrast media induced acute renal failure. *Kidney Int* 33:699–707, 1988.
45. Ogilvie GK, Krawiec DR, Gelberg HB, et al: Evaluation of a short-term saline diuresis protocol for the administration of cis-platinum. *Am J Vet Res* 49:1076–1078, 1988.
46. Gerkens JF, Branch RA: The influence of sodium status and furosemide on canine acute amphotericin B nephrotoxicity. *J Pharmacol Exp Ther* 214:306–311, 1980.
47. Andrews PM, Bates SB: Dietary protein prior to renal ischemia dramatically affects postischemic kidney function. *Kidney Int* 30:299–303, 1986.
48. Andrews PM, Bates SB: Dietary protein prior to renal ischemia and postischemic kidney function. *Kidney Int* 32(Suppl 22):576–580, 1987.
49. Andrews PM, Bates SB: Effects of dietary protein on uranyl-nitrate-induced acute renal failure. *Nephron* 45:296–301, 1987.
50. Marinides GN, Groggel GC, Cohen AH, Border WA: Enalapril and low protein diet reverse chronic puromycin aminonucleoside nephropathy. *Kidney Int* 37:749–757, 1990.
51. Whiting PH, Power DA, Petersen J, et al: The effect of dietary protein restriction on high dose gentamicin nephrotoxicity in rats. *Br J Exp Path* 69:35–41, 1988.
52. Andrews PM, Bates SB: Dietary protein as a risk factor in gentamicin nephrotoxicity. *Renal Failure* 10:153–159, 1987–1988.
53. Grauer GF, Behrend EN, Greco DS, et al: Effects of dietary protein conditioning on gentamicin-induced nephrotoxicity in dogs. *J Am Soc Nephrol* 3:724, (abstract) 1992.
54. Behrend EN, Grauer GF, Greco DS, et al: Effects of dietary protein conditioning on gentamicin pharmokinetics in dogs. *J Am Soc Nephrol* 3:720, (abstract) 1992.
55. Andrews PM, Chung EM: High dietary protein regimens provide significant protection from mercury nephrotoxicity in rats. *Toxicol Field Pharmacol* 105:288–304, 1990.
56. Finn WF: Diagnosis and management of acute tubular necrosis. *Med Clin North Am* 74(4):873–892, 1990.
57. Burnier M, Schrier RW: Protection from acute renal failure. *Adv Exp Med Biol* 212:275–283, 1986.
58. Kurnik BR, Weisberg LS, Cuttler IM, Kurnik PB: Effects of atrial natriuretic peptide versus mannitol on renal blood flow during radiocontrast infusion in chronic renal failure. *J Lab Clin Med* 116:27–35, 1990.
59. Johnston PA, Bernard DB, Perrin NS, et al: Prostaglandins mediate the vasodilatory effect of mannitol in the hypoperfused rat kidney. *J Clin Invest* 68:127–133, 1981.
60. Burke TJ, Cronin RE, Duchin KL, et al: Ischemia and tubule obstruction during acute renal failure in dogs: Mannitol in protection. *Am J Physiol* 238:F305–F314, 1980.
61. Lindner A: Synergism of dopamine and furosemide in diuretic-resistant, oliguric acute renal failure. *Nephron* 33:121–126, 1983.
62. Parker S, Carlon GC, Isaacs M, et al: Dopamine administration in oliguria and oliguric renal failure. *Crit Care Med* 9:630–632, 1981.
63. DeTorrente A, Miller PD, Cronin RE, et al: Effects of furosemide and acetylcholine in norepinephrine-induced acute renal failure. *Am J Physiol* 235:F131–F136, 1978.
64. Kramer HJ, Schuurmann J, Wasserman C, Dusing R: Prostaglandin-independent protection by furosemide from oliguric ischemic renal failure in conscious rats. *Kidney Int* 17:455–464, 1980.
65. Adelman RD, Spangler WL, Beasom F, et al: Furosemide enhancement of experimental gentamicin nephrotoxicity: Comparison of functional and morphological changes with activities of urinary enzymes. *J Infect Dis* 140:342–352, 1979.
66. Aikawa N, Wakabayashi GO, Masakazu U, Shinozawa Y: Regulation of renal function in thermal injury. *J Trauma* 30:S174–S178, 1990.
67. Flier JS, Underhill LH: Atrial natriuretic hormone, the renin-aldosterone axis, and blood pressure electrolyte homeostasis. *N Engl J Med* 315:1330–1340, 1985.
68. Conger JD, Falk SA, Yuan BH, Schrier RW: Atrial natriuretic peptide and dopamine in a rat model of ischemic acute renal failure. *Kidney Int* 35:1126–1132, 1989.
69. Russell JD, Churchill DN: Calcium antagonists and acute renal failure. *Am J Med* 87:306–315, 1989.
70. Blau A, Shulman L, Eliahou HE: Calcium channel blockers and experimental acute renal failure. *Isr J Med Sci* 26:334–336, 1990.
71. Widener LL, Mela-riker LM: Verapamil pretreatment preserves mitochondrial function and tissue magnesium in the

ischemic kidney. *Circ Shock* 13:27–37, 1984.
72. Burke TJ, Arnold PE, Gordon JA, et al: Protective effect of intrarenal calcium membrane blockers before or after renal ischemia; functional, morphological and mitochondrial studies. *J Clin Invest* 74:1830–1841, 1984.
73. Canavese C, Stratta P, Vercellone A: The case for oxygen free radicals in the pathogenesis of ischemic acute renal failure. *Nephron* 49:9–15, 1988.
74. Nath KA, Paller MS: Dietary deficiency of antioxidants exacerbates ischemic injury in the rat kidney. *Kidney Int* 38:1109–1117, 1990.
75. Walker PD, Shah SV: Reactive oxygen metabolites in endotoxin-induced acute renal failure in rats. *Kidney Int* 38:1125–1132, 1990.
76. Pawlowska D, Granger JP, Knox FG: Effects of adenosine infusion into renal interstitium on renal hemodynamics. *Am J Physiol* 252:F678–F682, 1987.
77. Siegel NJ, Glazier WB, Chaudry IH, et al: Enhanced recovery from acute renal failure by the postischemic infusion of adenine nucleotides and magnesium chloride in rats. *Kidney Int* 17:338–349, 1980.
78. Gerkens JF, Heidemann HT, Jackson EK, Branch RA: Effect of aminophylline on amphotericin B nephrotoxicity in the dog. *J Pharmacol Exp Ther* 224:609–613, 1983.
79. Hardie EM, Pose RL, Hoopes PJ: ATP–MgCl$_2$ increases cisplatin toxicity in the dog and rat. *J Appl Toxicol* 12:369–375, 1992.
80. Wong NL, Magil AB, Dirks JH: Effect of magnesium diet in gentamicin-induced acute renal failure in rats. *Nephron* 51:84–88, 1989.
81. Humes HD, Sastrasinh M, Weinberg JM: Calcium is a competitive inhibitor of gentamicin-renal membrane binding interactions and dietary calcium supplementation protects against gentamicin nephrotoxicity. *J Clin Invest* 73:134–147, 1984.
82. Siegel NJ, Gaudio KM, Katz LA, et al: Beneficial effect of thyroxin on recovery from toxic acute renal failure. *Kidney Int* 25:906–911, 1984.
83. Chevalier RL, Finn WF: Effects of propranolol on postischemic acute renal failure. *Nephron* 25:77–81, 1980.
84. Grekas D, Kalekou H, Tourkantonis A: Effect of prostaglandin E$_2$ (PGE$_2$) in the prevention of acute renal failure in anesthetized dogs; in situ renal preservation. *Renal Failure* 11:27–31, 1989.
85. Benabe JE, Klahr S, Hoffman MK, et al: Production of thromboxane A$_2$ by the kidney in glycerol induced acute renal failure in the rabbit. *Prostaglandins* 19:333–347, 1980.

UPDATE

Angiotensin converting enzyme (ACE) inhibitors such as captopril, enalapril, and lisinopril are now widely used in the management of congestive heart failure in dogs. As an inhibitor of the production of the potent vasopressor angiotensin II (which stimulates the secretion of aldosterone, a hormone that prompts water and sodium retention), the ACE agent fosters balanced vasodilation and enhances sodium and water excretion. In the glomerulus, angiotensin II blockade can cause preferential dilation of the efferent arteriole, a loss of glomerular capillary pressure, and a reduction in the glomerular filtration rate.[1] This vasodilatory effect is most prominent in diseased or poorly perfused kidneys. Poor renal perfusion is a common complication among heart failure patients, particularly those receiving diuretics. Progression of azotemia or acute renal failure may be observed. Renal function should be monitored following the initiation of ACE inhibitor therapy in dogs. Adjusting the dosage of the ACE inhibitor and/or diuretic agent(s) administered usually is sufficient to attenuate azotemia; more intensive support is required in some cases. Azotemia that develops early in the course of enalapril therapy may resolve over time in some cases, presumably because of improvements in peripheral perfusion.[2]

In dogs, acute renal failure has also been described as a significant component of some infectious diseases, including bacterial endocarditis and rickettsial diseases.[3,4] Bacterial endocarditis may cause renal thrombosis or infarction, or inflammatory lesions such as glomerulonephritis or pyelonephritis.[4] Rickettsial organisms (e.g., the etiologic agents in Rocky Mountain spotted fever or canine ehrlichiosis) create a variety of clinical signs, including those associated with the consequences of diffuse vasculitis. Direct or immune-mediated damage to endothelial cells may extend to the renal circulation and result in acute failure.[3] In these cases, clinical signs of the infectious disorder may predominate and biochemical changes reflect renal involvement. Dogs with multisystemic disease should be monitored, as they are at high risk of acute renal failure. Support of the circulating blood volume and of renal perfusion—in addition to specific treatment of the primary disease—are important.

Ongoing investigations into the prevention and treatment of acute renal failure are focused on agents that influence renal hemodynamics and agents that influence cellular repair. Vasodilatory agents under investigation include low-dose norepinephrine, clonidine, propranolol, and endothelin antagonists. The infusion of norepinephrine (a catecholamine) at low dosages appears to selectively vasoconstrict the efferent arteriole and improve glomerular capillary pressure, filtration fraction, and urine output; higher dosages also constrict the afferent arteriole.[5] The effect of low-dose norepinephrine in ischemic acute renal failure may be enhanced by the concurrent infusion of dopamine.[6] Administration of clonidine or propranolol (a beta blocker) may improve renal recovery by improving renal microcirculation.[7] Endothelin is a regulatory peptide secreted from endothelial cells in response to hypoxia. In addition to its multiple effects on renal function, endothelin is a potent vasoconstrictor, and endothelin-neutralizing antibodies have been effective in reversing renal dysfunction in an ischemic model of acute renal failure.[8,9]

Dietary manipulation of eicosanoid production may enhance renal vasodilatory mechanisms by reducing the production of thromboxane A_2. The protective activity of eicosapentaenoic acid and docosahexaenoic acid supplementation was demonstrated in a study in which dogs were treated with fish oils prior to an ischemic insult.[10] The role of dietary lipids in the progression and management of chronic renal disease in dogs and cats is also being studied.

Cellular protectants under investigation include glycine infusions,[11] epidermal growth factor, and insulin-like growth factor. In rats, glycine attenuates the morphologic and functional damage associated with cisplatin administration and hypoxic injury.[12] Epidermal growth factor and insulin-like growth factors helped promote tissue repair in gentamicin-induced and ischemic acute renal failure in rat models.[13,14]

The efficacy of any of these strategies remains purely speculative in clinical practice. In veterinary medicine, efforts have focused on elucidating protocols and strategies for preventing nephrotoxicosis due to commonly used chemotherapeutic agents. Current recommendations for the administration of aminoglycosides, cisplatin, and amphotericin B have been reviewed.[15–17]

REFERENCES

1. Brown SA, Barsanti JA, Finco DR: Effects of vasoactive agents on kidney function, in Kirk RW, Bonagura JD (eds): *Current Veterinary Therapy XI: Small Animal Practice*. Philadelphia, WB Saunders, 1992, pp 832–833.
2. Longhofer SL, Dricsson GF, Cifelli S, Benitz AM: Renal function in heart failure dogs receiving furosemide and enalapril maleate. *Proceedings of 11th ACVIM Forum*, 1993, p 936 (abstract).
3. Forrester SD, Lees GE: Acute renal failure associated with systemic infectious disease, in Kirk RW, Bonagura JD (eds): *Current Veterinary Therapy XI: Small Animal Practice*. Philadelphia, WB Saunders, 1992, pp 829–831.
4. Taboada J, Palmer GH: Renal failure associated with bacterial endocarditis in the dog. *JAAHA* 25:243–251, 1989.
5. Cesare JF, Ligas JR, Hirvela ER: Enhancement of urine output and glomerular filtration in acutely oliguric patients using low-dose norepinephrine. *Circ Shock* 39:207–210, 1993.
6. Schaer GL, Fink MP, Parrillo JE: Norepinephrine alone versus norepinephrine plus low-dose dopamine: Enhanced renal blood flow with combination pressor therapy. *Crit Care Med* 13:492–496, 1985.
7. Mason J: The pathophysiology of ischaemic acute renal failure: A new hypothesis about the initiation phase. *Renal Physiol* 9:129–147, 1986.
8. Simonson MS: Endothelins: Multifunctional renal peptides. *Physiol Rev* 73:375–411, 1993.
9. Kon V, Yoshioka T, Fogo A, Ichikawa: Glomerular actions of endothelin in vivo. *J Clin Invest* 83:1762–1767, 1989.
10. Neumayer HH, Heinrich M, Schmissas M, et al: Amelioration of ischemic acute renal failure by dietary fish oil administration in conscious dogs. *J Am Soc Nephrol* 3:1312–1320, 1992.
11. Heyman SN, Rosen S, Silva P, et al: Protective action of glycine in cisplatin nephrotoxicity. *Kidney Int* 40:273–279, 1991.
12. Weinberg JM, Davis JA, Abarzua M, Raja T: Cytoprotective effects of glycine and glutathione against hypoxic injury to rat tubules. *J Clin Invest* 80:1446–1454, 1987.
13. Morin NJ, Laurent G, Nonclercq D, et al: Epidermal growth factor accelerates renal tissue repair in a model of gentamicin nephrotoxicity in rats. *Am J Physiol* 263:F806–F811, 1992.
14. Ding H, Kopple JD, Cohen A, Hirschberg R: Recombinant human insulin-like growth factor I accelerates recovery and reduces catabolism in rats with ischemic acute renal failure. *J Clin Invest* 91:2281–2287, 1993.
15. Forrester SD: Preventing nephrotoxic acute renal failure. *Proceedings of 10th ACVIM Forum*, 1992, pp 30–132.
16. Forrester SD, Jacobson JD, Fallin EA: Taking measures to prevent acute renal failure. *Vet Med* 89:231–236, 1994.
17. Ogilvie GK, Straw RC, Powers BE, et al: Prevalence of nephrotoxicosis associated with a short-term saline solution diuresis protocol for the administration of cisplatin to dogs with malignant tumors: 61 cases. *JAVMA* 199:613–616, 1991.

Acute Renal Failure. Part II. Diagnosis, Management, and Prognosis*

University of Prince Edward Island
India F. Lane, DVM, MS

Colorado State University
Gregory F. Grauer, DVM, MS
Martin J. Fettman, DVM, MS, PhD

KEY FACTS

❏ Sudden onset of azotemia and clinical signs associated with uremia may result from prerenal or postrenal influences or acute intrinsic renal failure.

❏ To eliminate prerenal influences, initial fluid therapy should be designed to rapidly replace volume deficits.

❏ Hyperkalemia and metabolic acidosis associated with acute renal failure are often reversed with appropriate fluid therapy.

❏ Oliguric acute renal failure may be converted to polyuric acute renal failure by treatment with diuretics or vasodilators.

❏ In cases of acute renal failure, histologic assessment of renal tissue obtained by renal biopsy is important in establishing a definitive diagnosis and prognosis for recovery.

Acute renal failure (ARF) is a sudden, severe reduction in renal function. The condition is often life threatening. In some cases, however, renal lesions associated with acute renal failure are reversible; adequate renal function can be regained with appropriate supportive care.

Part I of this presentation reviewed the pathophysiology of acute renal failure, identification of patients at risk for the development of acute renal failure, and potential strategies for prevention and treatment of the condition.

In Part II, diagnosis and management of acute renal failure are reviewed. Acute versus chronic renal failure, prerenal azotemia, and postrenal azotemia are emphasized; fluid therapy as a general consideration of management is also discussed.

DIAGNOSIS
Acute Versus Chronic Renal Failure

Prerenal azotemia, postrenal azotemia, and both acute and chronic renal failure can lead to such clinical signs as lethargy, depression, anorexia, vomiting, diarrhea, and dehydration. The more severe signs of uremia (including stupor; coma; hemorrhage; oral ulcerations; and, occasionally, seizures) are usually not observed in cases of prerenal azotemia. Such signs may, however, be associated with postrenal azotemia and acute and chronic renal failure.[1]

Diagnosis of renal failure (Figure 1) is made when azotemia is accompanied by isosthenuria (urine specific gravity 1.008 to 1.012) or minimally concentrated urine (urine specific gravity 1.013 to 1.029 in dogs, 1.013 to 1.034 in cats). Other clinicopathologic abnormalities found in cases of renal failure include anemia, electrolyte imbalances, and metabolic acidosis.

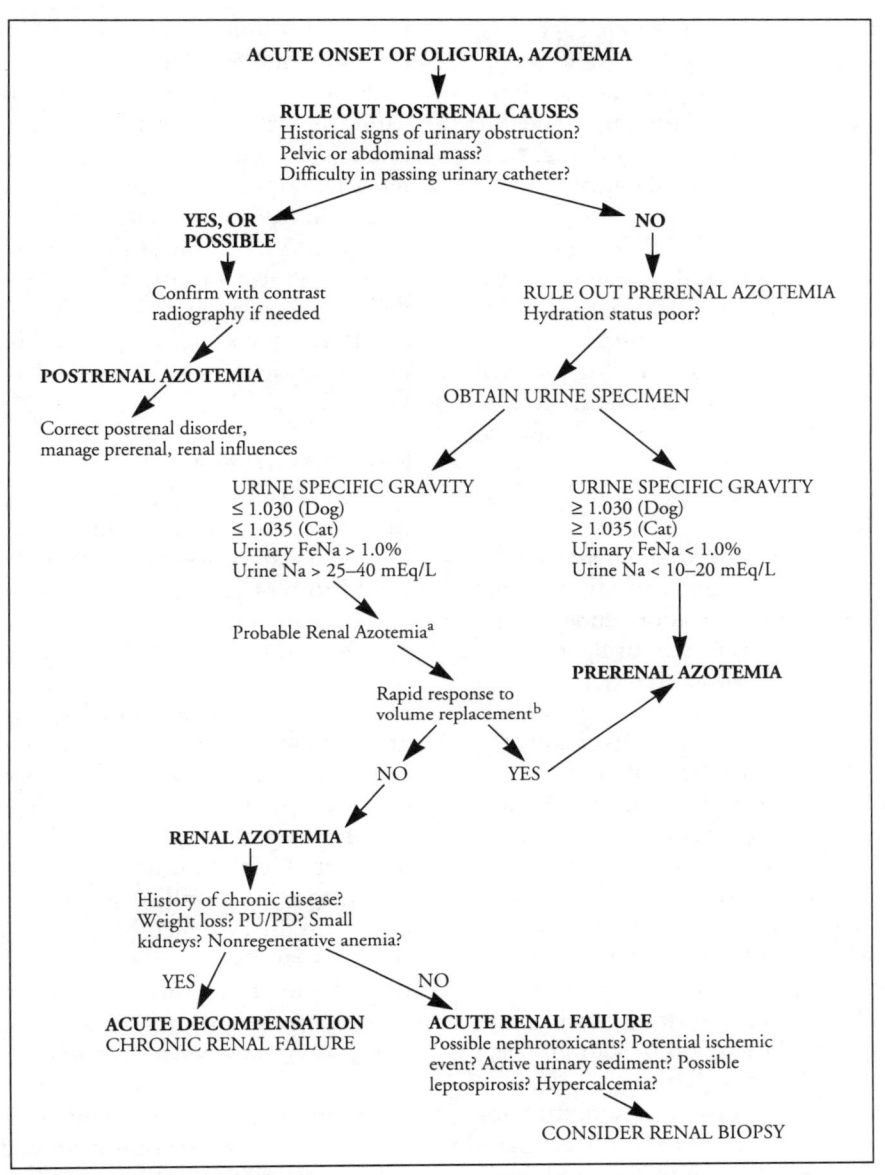

```
                    ACUTE ONSET OF OLIGURIA, AZOTEMIA
                                    │
                         RULE OUT POSTRENAL CAUSES
                         Historical signs of urinary obstruction?
                         Pelvic or abdominal mass?
                         Difficulty in passing urinary catheter?
                    ┌───────────────┴───────────────┐
              YES, OR                              NO
              POSSIBLE                              │
                │                        RULE OUT PRERENAL AZOTEMIA
         Confirm with contrast            Hydration status poor?
         radiography if needed                      │
                │                         OBTAIN URINE SPECIMEN
         POSTRENAL AZOTEMIA              ┌──────────┴──────────┐
         Correct postrenal disorder,  URINE SPECIFIC GRAVITY   URINE SPECIFIC GRAVITY
         manage prerenal, renal        ≤ 1.030 (Dog)            ≥ 1.030 (Dog)
         influences                    ≤ 1.035 (Cat)            ≥ 1.035 (Cat)
                                       Urinary FeNa > 1.0%      Urinary FeNa < 1.0%
                                       Urine Na > 25–40 mEq/L   Urine Na < 10–20 mEq/L
                                              │                        │
                                    Probable Renal Azotemia[a]         │
                                              │                        │
                                    Rapid response to          PRERENAL AZOTEMIA
                                    volume replacement[b]
                                       ┌──────┴──────┐
                                      NO            YES
                                       │
                                 RENAL AZOTEMIA
                                 History of chronic disease?
                                 Weight loss? PU/PD? Small
                                 kidneys? Nonregenerative anemia?
                              ┌──────────┴──────────┐
                             YES                   NO
                              │                     │
                    ACUTE DECOMPENSATION     ACUTE RENAL FAILURE
                    CHRONIC RENAL FAILURE    Possible nephrotoxicants? Potential ischemic
                                             event? Active urinary sediment? Possible
                                             leptospirosis? Hypercalcemia?
                                                     │
                                             CONSIDER RENAL BIOPSY
```

Figure 1—Diagnostic algorithm for the assessment of animals with suspected acute renal failure. (*a*) Impaired concentrating ability exists and is most likely caused by renal parenchymal lesions; however, other causes of impaired tubular concentrating ability (e.g., diuretic administration, hypoadrenocorticism, hypercalcemia, pyometra, and renal medullary washout) must be considered. (*b*) Entails a marked increase in urine production and rapid resolution of azotemia. FE_{Na} = Excreted fraction of filtered sodium, Na = sodium, *PU/PD* = polyuria/polydipsia.

Such findings as previous weight loss or episodes of illness; polyuria; polydipsia; pale mucous membranes; and small, irregular kidneys may be indicative of chronic renal failure.[2,3] A young animal in good body condition without a history of illness that exhibits clinical signs is more likely to have acute rather than chronic renal failure, unless the breed is known to have a high incidence of juvenile renal disease. A history of nephrotoxic drug use, toxicant exposure, trauma, or potential ischemic insult (as discussed in Part I) may indicate that acute renal failure is involved.

In cases of acute renal failure, the kidneys may be painful or enlarged. Clinical signs are often more severe than they are in a patient with chronic renal failure at the same level of dysfunction.

Hyperkalemia and severe metabolic acidosis are most likely to occur in cases of acute renal failure, whereas nonregenerative anemia, normokalemia, hypokalemia, and mild metabolic acidosis are suggestive of chronic renal failure.[2,4] Hyperkalemia and severe azotemia are less likely to occur in animals with nonoliguric acute renal failure.[5] Proteinuria and the presence of granular casts and renal epithelial cells and debris are indicative of acute renal damage.[2,4]

Dogs and cats with chronic renal failure may exhibit an apparently acute onset of clinical signs or an acute exacerbation of the disease (sometimes called *acute-on-chronic* renal failure). In such cases, the distinction between acute and chronic disease may require renal biopsy. Initial management for prerenal azotemia, acute renal failure, and acute-on-chronic disease is similar; the long-term prognoses, however, may differ significantly.

Prerenal Azotemia

Many extrarenal disorders can cause hypovolemia or hypotension and thereby result in reduced renal perfusion, reduced glomerular filtration, and prerenal azotemia. In such cases, urine concentrating ability is usually maintained (urine specific gravity >1.030 in dogs, >1.035 in cats). If urine concentrating ability is impaired by other influences, such as hyperadrenocorticism or hypoadrenocorticism, pyometra, liver disease, hypotonic dehydration, and diuretics, distinguishing between prerenal and renal azotemia can be difficult.[6,7] Under such circumstances, other assessments of urine composition may facilitate diagnosis.

Urinary sodium concentration can be measured; it is generally less than 10 to 20 mEq/L in cases of prerenal azotemia, because sodium retaining ability remains. Urinary sodium concentrations can be variable in dogs; the fractional excretion of sodium (FE_{Na} = [$Urine_{Na}$/$Plasma_{Na}$ × $Plasma_{Cr}$/$Urine_{Cr}$ × 100]) is therefore a more accurate reflection of sodium conservation. In cases of prerenal disorders with adequate tubular function, fractional excretion of sodium is generally less than 1%. Urinary sodium concentrations greater than 25 mEq/L and fractional excretion of sodium values greater than 1% are indicative of renal failure.[3,8,9]

Interpretation of the fractional excretion of sodium may be invalid in cases with such conditions as congestive heart failure, hepatic failure, or nephrotic syndrome. In such cases, excretion of sodium is impaired, and retention of sodium may persist despite renal dysfunction.[9] Other urinary indexes supporting a diagnosis of prerenal azotemia include urine osmolality significantly greater than plasma osmolality (ratio >5 to 6:1) and high urine-to-plasma creatinine ratio (>20:1).[8]

In humans, urinary sodium excretion and urine-to-plasma creatinine values are combined to give a renal failure index (RFI). The renal failure index is determined by the formula $urine_{Na}$/$urine_{Cr}$/$plasma_{Cr}$.[8] Renal failure index values greater than 1.0 are consistent with oliguric acute renal failure; renal failure index values less that 1.0 are indicative of prerenal azotemia.[3,8] In one group of human patients, however, renal failure index values were not found to be reliable indicators of acute renal failure.[10]

Azotemia and clinical signs of prerenal dysfunction should resolve rapidly with correction of volume deficits and restoration of renal perfusion. Initial fluid therapy for azotemic patients is thus designed to rapidly replace fluid deficits and reduce prerenal influences.

Postrenal Azotemia

Trigonal or urethral obstruction and upper or lower urinary tract rupture lead to postrenal azotemia. Lower urinary tract obstruction should be suspected if a history of strangury, dysuria, or complete anuria is reported.[3] Obstruction of the urethra or bladder neck can usually be ruled out by the passage of a urinary catheter. Passage of a catheter also provides an opportunity to obtain urine specimens for specific-gravity determination and other analyses.

Although unilateral obstruction of the renal pelvis or ureter generally does not result in azotemia, upper urinary tract obstruction should be suspected when demonstrable abdominal pain, abdominal masses, or a history of nephroliths is present. Urine sediment may contain evidence of crystals or inflammatory cells. Survey radiographs can be used to assess renal size, shape, and symmetry, as well as to rule out radiodense calculi and mass lesions. Renal ultrasonography may reveal hydronephrosis, hydroureter, nephroliths, or renal masses. Excretory urography or computed tomography might be necessary to completely rule out upper urinary tract disease.[2,4]

The possibility of urinary tract rupture should be considered in cases involving abdominal or pelvic trauma. Hematuria, swelling of the inguinal or perineal area, and abdominal distension are signs suggestive of urine leakage. Peritoneal fluid with a creatinine concentration greater than serum creatinine concentration is supportive of urine leakage, but a contrast radiograph is the best tool for confirming and localizing the rupture site.

MANAGEMENT
General Considerations

When acute renal failure is suspected (Figure 2), use of potentially nephrotoxic drugs should be discontinued. If a toxicant is the suspected cause of acute renal failure, nonspecific therapy to reduce further absorption of the agent should be instituted, including gastric lavage and/or administration of acti-

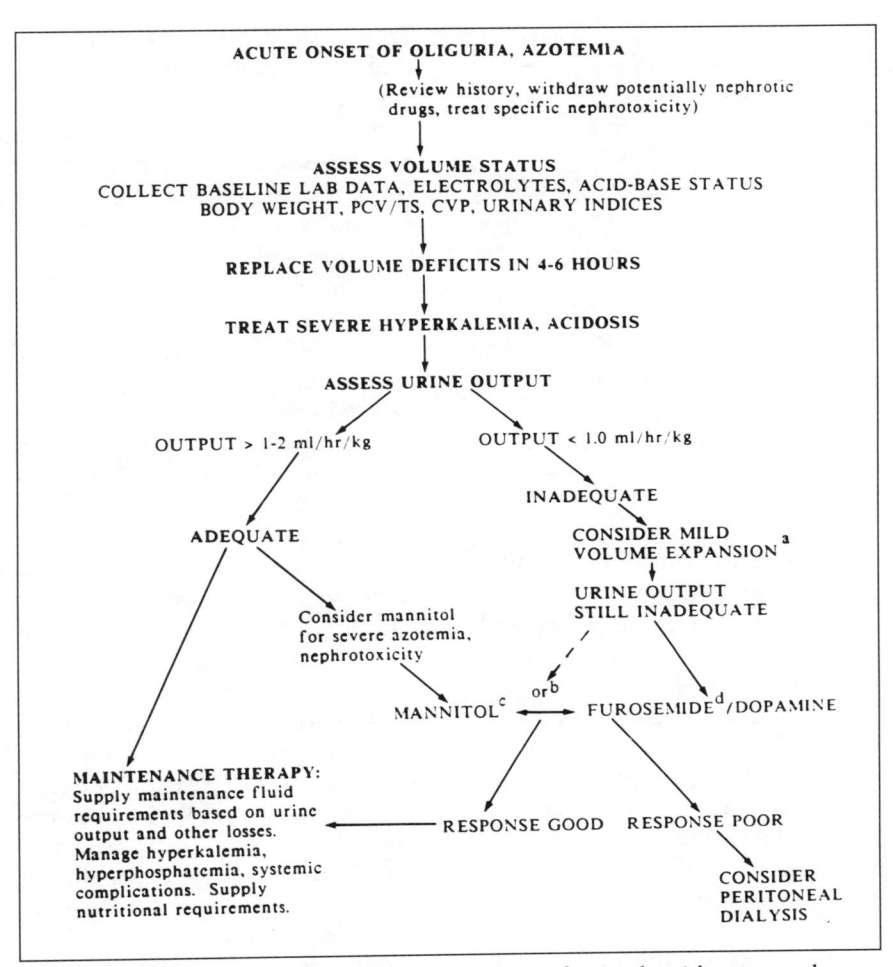

Figure 2—Therapeutic algorithm for management of animals with suspected acute renal failure. (*a*) If no evidence of overhydration exists, there is no increase in central venous pressure. (*b*) If one regimen is unsuccessful, the other may be attempted. (*c*) Avoid in cases with evidence of overhydration. (*d*) Avoid in cases of gentamicin nephrotoxicity. *PCV* = packed cell volume, *TS* = total solids, *CVP* = central venous pressure.

vated charcoal and cathartics. Specific antidotes should be administered if the toxicant is known (e.g., ethylene glycol).

If possible, underlying diseases, such as hypoadrenocorticism, pyometra, and hepatic disease, should be managed specifically. Treatable intrinsic renal disorders, such as leptospirosis and pyelonephritis, should be identified and appropriate management initiated. Obstructions to urine flow should be removed. Supportive therapy is designed to provide time for nephron repair, regeneration, and compensation.[2-4]

Fluid Therapy

Fluid therapy remains the mainstay of treatment for acute renal failure. The goals of fluid therapy are to correct fluid and electrolyte imbalances, improve renal hemodynamics, increase tubular flow, and initiate diuresis. Fluid needs in cases of acute renal failure are such that intravenous infusion is required. Jugular catheters allow administration of fluid loads, facilitate frequent blood sampling, and supply access for central venous pressure (CVP) measurement.

Fluid deficits should be replaced intravenously during the first four to six hours of treatment.[2,4] A 0.45% saline and 2.5% dextrose solution or 0.9% saline solution can be used initially. The amount of fluid required to restore extracellular fluid deficits can be calculated by multiplying the estimated percentage of dehydration by the patient's body weight in kilograms (e.g., for a dog that weighs 10 kilograms and is 5% dehydrated: 0.05 × 10 kg = 0.5 kg = 0.5 liters, or 500 ml).[11] The fluid rate should be reduced in animals with known or suspected cardiovascular dysfunction.

TABLE I
Potassium Supplementation in the Management of Renal Failure

Measured Serum Potassium Concentration	Amount of Potassium Chloride to be Added to Each Liter of Fluid Administered[a] (mEq)
3.5–4.0	20
3.0–3.5	30
2.5–3.0	40
2.0–2.5	60
<2.0	80

[a]Do not exceed an administration rate of 0.5 mEq/kg/hr.

During the rehydration phase, the animal should be carefully monitored for urine output and overhydration. Frequent monitoring of body weight, central venous pressure, packed cell volume, and plasma total solids helps to detect early overhydration.[12] Physical manifestations of overhydration include increased bronchovesicular sounds, tachycardia, restlessness, chemosis, and serous nasal discharge. Auscultation of overt crackles and wheezes is usually a late sign of overhydration with established pulmonary edema.

If overhydration is not apparent after rehydration, a moderate fluid challenge may help to improve urine flow. Because remaining deficits may be difficult to detect clinically, volume expansion with fluids equivalent to an additional 3% to 5% body weight can be administered to facilitate rehydration and improve renal perfusion.[4] If volume expansion is attempted, however, close observation for signs of overhydration is necessary.

Once diuresis has been established (urine output of 1 to 2 ml/kg/hr), and in cases of nonoliguric acute renal failure, fluid therapy should be tailored to match urine volume and other losses. Such losses include insensible losses (e.g., water loss resulting from respiration) and continuing losses (e.g., fluid loss resulting from vomiting, diarrhea, or hemorrhage). Insensible losses are estimated at 20 ml/kg/day. Urine output is quantitated for six- to eight-hour intervals; the amount is replaced during an equivalent time period. Ongoing gastrointestinal losses are also replaced. If hyperkalemia is not present and diuresis has ensued, polyionic maintenance fluids (e.g., lactated Ringer's solution) can be used.

In the recovery phase of acute renal failure, urine volume and electrolyte losses can be great. Maintenance potassium requirements should be administered in fluids based on serum potassium measurements as given in Table I.

Treatment of Hyperkalemia and Metabolic Acidosis

In cases of oliguric acute renal failure, hyperkalemia and metabolic acidosis often develop. Mild to moderate imbalances are often resolved with appropriate fluid therapy; however, hyperkalemia and severe metabolic acidosis can be life threatening and should be treated specifically.

Serum potassium concentrations greater than 6.5 to 7 mEq/L can cause cardiac conduction disturbances and electrocardiographic changes, including peaked T waves, bradycardia, prolonged P–R intervals, widened QRS complexes, and loss of P waves. Severe hyperkalemia can also precipitate atrial standstill, idioventricular rhythms, ventricular tachycardia, fibrillation, and asystole.[13,14]

Moderate hyperkalemia is largely resolved by administration of potassium-free fluids (dilution) and improvement of urine flow (increased excretion). Severe hyperkalemia (K^+ >7 to 8 mEq/L) or hyperkalemia resulting in cardiotoxicity should be treated by administering 10% calcium gluconate (0.5 to 1.0 ml/kg given intravenously during a period of 10 to 15 minutes)[2,14,15] or sodium bicarbonate (0.5 to 2 mEq/kg given intravenously during a period of 20 to 30 minutes, or as calculated to correct metabolic acidosis).[14,15]

Calcium ions counteract the cardiotoxic effects of excess potassium without lowering serum potassium; therefore, calcium treatment is reserved for cases in which immediate treatment of cardiac disturbances is required. Treatment of acidosis with bicarbonate facilitates the entry of potassium into cells. Glucose and insulin can also be used in emergency situations to increase intracellular shifting of potassium. Insulin is administered at a dose of 0.1 to 0.25 U/kg followed by a glucose bolus of 1 to 2 grams per unit of insulin given.[12] Blood glucose monitoring should be maintained for several hours after administration of insulin because hypoglycemia can occur. The effects of a calcium, bicarbonate, or glucose and insulin regimen are, however, short-lived; maintenance therapy, such as fluid diuresis or dialysis, must be initiated to ultimately maintain potassium excretion.[11]

Mild to moderate metabolic acidosis also commonly resolves with fluid therapy; specific treatment is rarely necessary unless blood pH is less than 7.10 to 7.15 or total carbon dioxide measures less than 10 to 12 mEq/L.[2,4] Bicarbonate requirements can be calculated using the base deficit determined from arterial blood or an estimated base deficit (body weight [kg] × 0.5 × base deficit or $[20 - T\ CO_2]$ = mEq bicarbonate required).[12] Optimally, one half of the calculated bicarbonate dose should be administered slowly during a period of 15 to 30 minutes, after which

TABLE II
Pharmacologic Agents and Dose Regimens Used in Treatment of Acute Renal Failure[2,12,21,28]

Drug	Action	Dose Regimen	Comments	Contraindications, Possible Complications
Furosemide	Loop diuretic	D, C: 2–6 mg/kg every 6–8 hours IV	Incrementally increase dose every 1 hour up to 6 mg/kg if urine output remains poor; efficacy improved with concurrent administration of dopamine	Dehydration, hypokalemia, aminoglycoside nephrotoxicity
Mannitol	Osmotic diuretic	D, C: 0.25–1.0 g/kg (10%–25% solution)	Administer as slow bolus over 15–20 minutes; can be repeated every 4–6 hours or administered as infusion (8%–10% solution) if effective	Dehydration, cardiopulmonary insufficiency, overhydration, elevated central venous pressure, intracranial hemorrhage
Dextrose	Osmotic diuretic	D, C: 25–50 ml/kg over 1–2 hours IV (10%–20% solution); repeat every 8–12 hours	Test initial urine for glucose and continue to monitor urine output; adjust maintenance fluid therapy administered between boluses to supply total daily calculated requirements	Discontinue infusion if glucosuria is not present or if adequate urine output does not occur after approximately half the recommended dose is administered
Dopamine	Renal vasodilator	D, C: 1–3 µg/kg/min CRI	Dilute in normal saline, 5% dextrose or lactated Ringer's solution; avoid dilution in alkaline solution; avoid additional additives in solution; efficacy improved if combined with furosemide	Hyperkalemia; may be arrhythmogenic
Sucralfate	Gastrointestinal protectant	D: 0.5–1.0 g every 6–8 hours PO C: 0.25–0.5 g every 8–12 hours PO	Separate administration from concurrent dosing of antacids by 30 minutes to 1 hour	Constipation is a possible side effect
Cimetidine	H_2-receptor antagonist	D: 5–10 mg/kg every 6–8 hours IV or PO C: 2.5–5 mg/kg every 12 hours IV or PO	Administer slowly when given IV	Reduce dose in cases involving hepatic disease
Ranitidine	H_2-receptor antagonist	D: 2 mg/kg every 8–12 hours IV or PO C: Not established	Same as for cimetidine	Reduce dose in cases involving renal disease
Metoclopromide	Antiemetic (antidopaminergic)	D, C: 0.2–0.5 mg/kg every 8 hours PO, SQ, or IV, or 1–2 mg/kg 24 hours CRI	Acts at CRTZ. Enhances gastric emptying	Avoid in epileptics; high doses may cause mental disturbances
Trimethobenzamide	Antiemetic (antihistamine-like)	D: 3 mg/kg every 8 hours IM C: Not established	Acts at CRTZ	

D = dog, C = cat, CRI = constant rate infusion, IV = intravenously, IM = intramuscularly, PO = orally, SQ = subcutaneously, CRTZ = chemoreceptor trigger zone.

acid–base parameters should be reassessed.[12] Overzealous bicarbonate administration can result in ionized calcium deficits, paradoxic cerebrospinal fluid acidosis, and cerebral edema.[4,12]

Treatment of Oliguria

Oliguria is defined as urine output less than 0.27 ml/kg body weight/hr[16]; however, after rehydration, urine output less than 1 to 2 ml/kg/hr is inadequate. If oliguria persists, additional pharmacologic manipulation with diuretics or vasodilators is necessary. Furosemide given in increasing doses (2 to 6 mg/kg; see Table II) has been advocated as an initial treatment for oliguria. Single, high-dose regimens (200 to 500 mg)[8,17] are used in humans to initiate urine flow. Apparently, however, mannitol[18] or dopamine in combination with furosemide[19] is a better choice than furosemide alone to initiate diuresis and possibly increase glomerular filtration rate.

Mannitol (10% or 20% solution) is administered at 0.5 to 1.0 g/kg as a slow bolus during a period of 15 to 20 minutes[2,4,12] (Table II). Urine output should improve within one hour of administration if the agent is effective. A second bolus may be administered, but doing so considerably increases the potential for volume overexpansion and complications, such as pulmonary and tissue edema.

As an osmotic agent, mannitol acts to increase tubular flow and help prevent tubular obstruction or collapse.[8,18] It is also a weak renal vasodilator, in which capacity its effect may be mediated by prostaglandins or atrial natriuretic peptide.[20] Mannitol acts as a scavenger of oxygen-derived free radicals that sometimes form after ischemia and reperfusion (see Part I).[8] Thus, mannitol should increase urine output and perhaps have a mild positive effect on glomerular filtration rate.

Hypertonic (10% to 20%) glucose, another osmotic agent, has been suggested as an alternative therapy to mannitol.[21] Its effects in initiating tubular flow and urine output are similar to those of mannitol. Solutions of 10% or 20% dextrose are easily formulated and supply metabolizable energy. Hypertonic dextrose is administered as an intermittent slow bolus of 25 to 50 ml/kg (see Table II), given during the course of one to two hours, two to three times daily.[21] A potential advantage of administration of hypertonic glucose is that urine can be monitored early after the start of therapy and the infusion can be stopped before the risk of overhydration is incurred. The detection of glucose in the urine should not preclude monitoring urine output; glucosuria can occur without a significant increase in urine production.

Hypertonic glucose lacks certain beneficial effects of mannitol, including vasodilation and oxygen-derived–free radical scavenging.[8] Mannitol may also be a better osmotic agent, because it is not metabolized or resorbed by renal tubules.

Dopamine (Table II) combined with furosemide should be used in overhydrated patients instead of osmotic agents; it may be effective when osmotic diuresis fails. Low-dose dopamine infusion (1 to 3 µg/kg/min) causes renal vasodilation and preserves renal and splanchnic blood flow.[22] Increases in glomerular filtration and sodium excretion may also occur.[8] Although when given in low doses dopamine has minimal systemic effects, it can be arrhythmogenic; electrocardiographic monitoring is therefore advised when dopamine is administered. The half-life of dopamine is extremely short; if arrhythmia is observed, discontinuing dopamine infusion should result in rapid resolution of the arrhythmia.

When furosemide therapy is combined with dopamine infusion, the likelihood of inducing diuresis is increased.[19] Furosemide has been shown to exacerbate gentamicin toxicity[23]; its use should probably be avoided in cases of acute renal failure caused by aminoglycoside use.

Initiation of diuresis facilitates the management of acute renal failure by lowering serum urea nitrogen and potassium concentrations and reducing the risk of overhydration. The increase in urine production, however, is usually the result of decreased tubular reabsorption of water with no real increase in glomerular filtration rate.[2]

Systemic Complications

In cases of acute uremia, gastrointestinal signs occur most frequently. Nausea, anorexia, vomiting, hematemesis, diarrhea, and oral ulcerations are common.[24–26] Intussusceptions occasionally develop in uremic patients.[24] Uremic stomatitis, characterized by oral ulcerations, discoloration or sloughing of the tip of the tongue, and fetid breath, is seen most frequently with chronic disease but may also develop with severe acute uremia. The oral lesions may be a result of the caustic effects of ammonia produced locally by the action of bacterial ureases. It is also possible that mucosal damage is simply a manifestation of a more generalized disruption of gastrointestinal mucosa.[24,26]

In humans, oral lesions are aggravated by periodontal disease; good oral hygiene may reduce the severity of oral ulceration.[24] Severe pain from oral ulceration can be relieved by topical administration of compounds containing lidocaine.

Hemorrhagic or ulcerative gastritis that leads to anorexia and vomiting is commonly induced by uremia. Lesions may be caused by local irritation from high levels of ammonia or an altered gastric mucosal barrier. Increased urea concentrations may also alter the gastric mucosal barrier.[24,25] Renal failure results in decreased clearance of gastrin, which may precipitate hypergastrinemia and increased gastric acid production, two conditions that can exacerbate gastric lesions.[25] Pathologic findings include edema, mastocytosis, fibroplasia and mineralization in the lamina propria, and arteriolar lesions in the submucosa.[27]

Vomiting caused by gastritis can be controlled to a certain extent by administration of histamine (H_2 receptor) blockers, cimetidine (5 to 10 mg/kg given orally every 6 to 8 hours), or ranitidine (2 mg/kg given orally every 8 to 12 hours; see Table II), agents which reduce gastric hydrochloric acid production. Sucralfate (0.5 to 1.0 gram given orally every 6 to 8 hours; see Table II), a gastrointestinal protectant, is administered to coat existing gastric and intestinal mucosal ulcerations. Sucralfate dissociates in the stomach to aluminum hydroxide and sucrose octasulfate, a viscous substance that forms a complex with gastrointestinal mucosa and preferentially adheres to ulcerated areas. Sucralfate also protects the mucosa from gastric acid penetration, inactivates pepsin, and adsorbs damaging bile acids.[28]

In cases of uremia, the large and small bowel are affected by increased serum urea concentrations. Diarrhea results from enterocolitis, partial malabsorption of proteins and carbohydrates, altered bile salt metabolism, and bacterial overgrowth.[1,24-26] Finally, vasculitis and coagulation abnormalities induced by uremia can create severe generalized gastrointestinal hemorrhage.[24,25]

Vomiting can also result from direct stimulation of the chemoreceptor trigger zone (CRTZ) by uremic toxins, such as guanidines.[24] Effects of these toxins can be reduced by administration of centrally acting antiemetics, such as metoclopramide or trimethobenzamide (Table II), which act at the chemoreceptor trigger zone. Because α-adrenergic blockade can result in significant vasodilation and hypotension, phenothiazine compounds (e.g., chlorpromazine) that act at both the emetic center and the chemoreceptor trigger zone should be avoided unless adequate hydration and blood pressure have been restored.

Critically ill uremic patients are highly susceptible to infection; septicemia or other infections are major causes of death in humans with renal failure.[3] Depressed leukocyte function and depressed cellular immunity have been documented.[1,29,30] In cases of uremia, production of chemotactic factors as well as polymorphonuclear chemotactic responses are depressed. Lymphocyte numbers and activity are also depressed.[29,30] Recently, defects in macrophage receptor functions[31] and monocyte responsiveness[32] have been documented in humans with end-stage renal failure. Metabolic acidosis, altered mucosal barriers, and malnutrition can contribute to weakened host defenses.[1] Humoral immunity appears to be less significantly affected by uremia.[29,30]

Prevention of infection is essential in uremic patients; strict aseptic techniques should be used when placing vascular and urinary catheters, administering parenteral medications, and caring for wounds. If urine output is in question, the use of metabolic cages or intermittent catheterization is preferred over placement of indwelling urinary catheters. If peritoneal dialysis is used, infection becomes an even greater concern; peritonitis can be a serious complication.[33,34] Careful attention should therefore be paid to protocol and asepsis when peritoneal dialysis is used.

Other complications in cases of acute renal failure include hemorrhage and neurologic dysfunction. The bleeding tendency in uremic humans is still not completely understood, but it is characterized by an increased bleeding time and altered platelet function. Undetermined uremic compounds produce defects in platelet aggregation, platelet adhesiveness, and platelet factor 3 release in humans; such conditions are reversed by dialytic therapy.[29,30] Limited studies have found whole-blood platelet aggregation in uremic dogs to be normal, however.[35]

Hemorrhage is best managed by decreasing the severity of uremia, although some animals may require transfusions if significant blood loss occurs. Administration of cryoprecipitate,[36] desmopressin (DDAVP),[37] and other vascular factors[38] has recently been shown to alleviate the bleeding tendency in some humans with uremia.

Neurologic abnormalities associated with uremia include encephalopathic signs and peripheral neuropathy.[1,39,40] Uremic encephalopathy occurs in humans when the glomerular filtration rate (GFR) falls below 10% of the normal rate.[40] Clinical signs in such cases include sluggishness; confusion; disorientation; hallucinations; vertigo; ataxia; clonus; and centrally mediated anorexia, nausea, and vomiting.[40] In dogs, tremors, head bobbing, and seizures are reported.[41]

Alterations in calcium levels in the brain have been documented in humans and dogs, and it is speculated that increased calcium entry is facilitated by parathyroid hormone (PTH).[40] In rats, alterations in brain metabolism and energy use have also been observed; other uremic toxins may play a role in the cause.[40] A peripheral neuropathy associated with uremia is also seen in humans and is more likely to be clinically evident in chronic end-stage renal disease. This distal polyneuropathy is characterized clinically by sensory changes in distal limbs and depressed distal reflexes. Motor-nerve conduction velocities are variably reduced. Although similar electrophysiologic changes can be documented in humans with acute renal failure, clinical signs are usually not apparent.[40] Control of uremia is the best method of management of neurologic dysfunction. Seizures may be managed with low-dose diazepam.

Nutritional support must be maintained in animals with acute renal failure. Many such animals cannot tolerate oral intake or cannot consume enough calories to compensate for severe illness. Ongoing catabolic processes then increase the burden of nitrogenous wastes presented to the kidneys.[42] Enteral or parenteral feeding can be considered for these patients. The goal of nutritional therapy in uremic patients is to supply caloric requirements using adequate carbohydrate sources and to supply amino acids or protein sources in an amount that can maintain nitrogen balance but avoid excessive protein load on the damaged kidneys.[42] Ideally, protein should be supplied as amino acids; essential amino acid supplementation has been shown to improve survival in anephric dogs.[43]

Suggested protein requirements for uremic dogs are 0.3 g/kg/day of a basic amino acid solution[42] or 2.2 g/kg/day total protein. Diets should be moderately restricted in phosphorus; intestinal phosphate binders may be needed to control hyperphosphatemia.[4] Methods of enteral and parenteral feeding in dogs and cats have been described.[44,45]

Renal Biopsy

Histologic evaluation of renal tissue is often important in cases of acute renal failure to establish an accurate diagnosis and prognosis for return of renal function. Renal biopsy should be considered in cases in which a definitive diagnosis is required, heavy proteinuria is present, diffuse systemic disease is suspected, or when the type of renal failure (acute or chronic) cannot be established.[4] Biopsy is also indicated when conservative methods of treatment have failed, when oliguria cannot be corrected after one to two days of therapy, or when severe uremia or hyperkalemia persist for long periods.[2,13]

Histologic evidence of tubular regeneration and intact tubular basement membranes are considered good prognostic indicators of reversibility; extensive tubular necrosis and interstitial mineralization with disrupted basement membranes are poor prognostic signs.[2,46] In one group of humans with acute renal failure, renal biopsy results altered the diagnosis in 44% of cases for which a biopsy was obtained.[47] Specific therapy was altered in 37% of such cases, particularly when glomerular disease or interstitial nephritis was identified.[47]

Biopsies are most helpful when performed early in the course of treatment and should always be performed if intensive therapeutics, such as dialysis, are considered. Surgical; laparoscopic; and blind, keyhole, or percutaneous approaches guided by ultrasonography have been described.[48-51] Various percutaneous and laparascopic techniques apparently produce similarly adequate tissue samples.[51]

Serious complications of biopsies are rare. Transient hematuria and occasional incidences of hydronephrosis are reported with needle biopsies.[52] More severe complications, including perirenal hemorrhage or urine leakage, are possible. An open wedge biopsy can be obtained if a dialysis catheter is placed surgically for initiation of peritoneal dialysis. Coagulation parameters, including the platelet count, mucosal bleeding time, and such tests of coagulation as activated clotting time, activated partial thromboplastin time (APTT), and/or one-stage prothrombin time (OSPT) should be performed before renal biopsy.

Peritoneal Dialysis

Dialytic therapy should be considered when initial fluid and diuretic therapy have not been successful in relieving oliguria or uremia. Dialysis can also be used to manage overhydrated patients and to hasten elimination of certain toxicants.[53]

Dialysis must be undertaken early in the course of acute renal failure if it is to be helpful. Hemodialysis is costly and technically demanding, requiring specialized equipment and trained personnel. Peritoneal dialysis can be equally effective and does not require a great deal of specialized equipment or training. The procedure is still expensive and labor intensive,[33] however, and it should not be undertaken without serious consideration of the financial and time commitments involved. The procedure for peritoneal dialysis has been described in the literature[53] and can be accomplished at an experienced 24-hour treatment center or at referral teaching hospitals.

PROGNOSIS

Once acute renal failure is established, treatment is intensive and costly, particularly if dialytic therapy is considered. Because high mortality is associated with acute renal failure, it is helpful to have an accurate prognosis before aggressive therapy is considered.

In general, nonoliguric acute renal failure has a better prognosis than oliguric acute renal failure because hyperkalemia is less likely to be present and the tendency for overhydration to occur is minimized. Nephrotoxicant-induced acute renal failure may have a better prognosis than acute renal failure resulting from ischemia and other causes because tubular basement membranes frequently remain intact following nephrotoxicant-induced damage. Certainly, exceptions to these generalities occur, depending on the degree of damage and dysfunction.

Many prognostic factors have been investigated in humans with acute renal failure. Univariate and multivariate discrimination score systems exist to give a prognosis for survival in individual cases.[54-57] Significant variables contributing to a poor prognosis include preexisting cardiac disease, renal disease, neoplasia, pancreatitis, acute trauma, and such complications as oliguria, respiratory failure, coma, and sepsis.[54-56] The number of complications and number of organ systems failing also correlates with outcome.[54,55,57,58] Mortality is highest in surgical patients (>80%), primarily because of complications and multiple organ-system failure.[54,57,59] The severity of azotemia and the interval before the start of dialysis in surgical patients have been shown to be important,[54] a finding that emphasizes the need for early recognition and treatment.

Age of the patient was a significant factor in several studies, with mortality increasing progressively in human patients over 50 years of age.[54,59] Overall, the conditions most frequently associated with mortality in several studies were hypotension, neurologic coma, and respiratory failure.[57,58] Death, however, is often caused by the initial disease or secondary complications of the condition other than uremia.

Variables affecting humans can be applied to veterinary medical patients. In general, prognosis in cases of acute renal failure is affected by the severity of renal dysfunction, the extent of histologic damage, and the response to treatment. Awareness of the severity of underlying disease, mental status, significant complications, and status of other organ systems should help the clinician to formulate an early prognosis in individual cases. Histologic assessment of renal tissue and the effectiveness of early management may provide a better prognosis for survival as time progresses. In dogs and cats that survive to reach the recovery phase, adequate (although subnormal) renal function is usually recovered.

About the Authors

Dr. Lane is affiliated with the Department of Companion Animals, Atlantic Veterinary College, University of Prince Edward Island, Charlottetown, Prince Edward Island, Canada. Dr. Grauer is affiliated with the Department of Clinical Science and Dr. Fettman is affiliated with the Department of Pathology at the College of Veterinary Medicine and Biomedical Sciences, Colorado State University, Fort Collins, Colorado.

REFERENCES

1. Bovee KC: Metabolic disturbances of uremia, in Bovee KC (ed): *Canine Nephrology*. Media, PA, Harwal Publishing Co, 1984, pp 555–612.
2. Grauer GF: Acute renal failure, in Allen DG (ed): *Small Animal Medicine*. Philadelphia, JB Lippincott Co, 1991, pp 595–604.
3. Brezis M, Rosen S, Epstein FH: Acute renal failure, in Brenner BM, Rector FC (eds): *The Kidney*, ed 3. Philadelphia, WB Saunders Co, 1986, pp 735–799.
4. Polzin D, Osborne C, O'Brien T: Diseases of the kidney and ureters, in Ettinger SJ (ed): *Textbook of Veterinary Internal Medicine*, ed 3. Philadelphia, WB Saunders Co, 1989, pp 1963–2046.
5. Anderson RJ, Linas SC, Berns AS, et al: Nonoliguric acute renal failure. *N Engl J Med* 296:1134–1138, 1977.
6. Feldman EC, Nelson RW: *Canine and Feline Endocrinology and Reproduction*. Philadelphia, WB Saunders Co, 1987, pp 1–28.
7. Tyler RD, Qualls CW, Heald RD: Renal concentrating ability in dehydrated hyponatremia dogs. *JAVMA* 191:1095–1100, 1987.
8. Finn WF: Diagnosis and management of acute tubular necrosis. *Med Clin North Am* 74:873–892, 1990.
9. Zarich SZ, Fang LST, Diamond JR: Fractional excretion of sodium; exceptions to its diagnostic value. *Arch Intern Med* 145:108–112, 1985.
10. Durakovic Z, Durakovic A, Durokovic S: The lack of clinical value of laboratory parameters in predicting outcome in acute renal failure. *Ren Fail* 11:213–219, 1989–1990.
11. Muir WM, DiBartola SP: Fluid therapy, in Kirk RW (ed): *Current Veterinary Therapy. VIII. Small Animal Practice*. Philadelphia, WB Saunders Co, 1983, pp 28–40.
12. Kirby R: Acute renal failure as a complication in the critically ill animal. *Vet Clin North Am Small Anim Pract* 19:1189–1208, 1989.
13. Tilley LP: *Essentials of Canine and Feline Electrocardiography*, ed 2. Philadelphia: Lea & Febiger, 1985, pp 232–233.
14. Willard MD: Treatment of hyperkalemia, in Kirk RW (ed): *Current Veterinary Therapy. IX. Small Animal Practice*. Philadelphia, WB Saunders Co, 1987, pp 94–101.
15. Cowgill LD: Acute renal failure, in Bovee KC (ed): *Canine Nephrology*. Media, PA, Harwal Publishing Co, 1984, pp 405–438.
16. English PB: Acute renal failure in the dog and cat. *Aust Vet J* 50:384–392, 1974.
17. Rose BD: Diuretics. *Kidney Int* 39:336–352, 1991.
18. Burnier M, Schrier RW: Protection from acute renal failure. *Adv Exp Med Biol* 212:275–283, 1986.
19. Lindner A: Synergism of dopamine and furosemide in diuretic-resistant, oliguric acute renal failure. *Nephron* 33:121–126, 1983.
20. Kurnik BR, Weisberg LS, Cuttler IM, Kurnik PB: Effects of atrial natriuretic peptide versus mannitol on renal blood flow during radiocontrast infusion in chronic renal failure. *J Lab Clin Med* 116:27–35, 1990.
21. Finco DR, Low DG: Intensive diuresis in polyuric renal failure, in Kirk RW (ed): *Current Veterinary Therapy. VII. Small Animal Practice*. Philadelphia, WB Saunders Co, 1980, pp 1091–1093.
22. Parker S, Carlon GC, Isaacs M, et al: Dopamine administration in oliguria and oliguric renal failure. *Crit Care Med* 9:630–632, 1981.
23. Adelman RD, Spangler WL, Beasom F, et al: Furosemide enhancement of experimental gentamicin nephrotoxicity: Comparison of functional and morphological changes with activities of urinary enzymes. *J Infect Dis* 140:342–352, 1979.
24. Osborne CA, Stevens JB, Polzin DJ: Gastrointestinal manifestations of urinary diseases, in Anderson NV (ed): *Veteri-*

nary *Gastroenterology*. Philadelphia, Lea & Febiger, 1980, pp 681–704.
25. Strombeck DR, Guilford WG: *Small Animal Gastroenterology*, ed 2. Davis, CA, Stonegate Publishing Co, 1990.
26. Chew DJ, DiBartola SP: Diagnosis and pathophysiology of renal disease, in Ettinger SJ (ed): *Textbook of Veterinary Internal Medicine*, ed 3. Philadelphia, WB Saunders Co, 1989, pp 1893–1961.
27. Cheville NF: Uremic gastropathy in the dog. *Vet Pathol* 16:292–309, 1979.
28. Papich MG: Medical therapy for gastrointestinal ulcers, in Kirk RW (ed): *Current Veterinary Therapy. X. Small Animal Practice*. Philadelphia, WB Saunders Co, pp 911–918.
29. Anagnostou A, Kurtzman NA: Hematological consequences of renal failure, in Brenner BM, Rector FC (eds): *The Kidney*, ed 3. Philadelphia, WB Saunders Co, 1986, pp 1631–1656.
30. Fried W: Hematologic complications of chronic renal failure. *Med Clin North Am* 62:1363–1379, 1978.
31. Ruiz P, Gomez F, Schrieber AD: Impaired function of macrophage Fc gamma receptors in end-stage renal disease. *N Engl J Med* 322:717–722, 1990.
32. Gibbons RA, Martinez OM, Garovoy MR: Altered monocyte function in uremia. *Clin Immunol Immunopath* 56:66–80, 1990.
33. Carter LJ, Wingfield WE, Allen TA: Clinical experience with peritoneal dialysis in small animals. *Compend Contin Educ Pract Vet* 11(11):1335–1343, 1989.
34. Thornhill JA: Therapeutic strategies involving antimicrobial treatment of small animals with peritonitis. *JAVMA* 185:1181–1184, 1984.
35. Forsythe LT, Jackson ML, Meric SM: Whole blood platelet aggregation in uremic dogs. *Am J Vet Res* 50:1754–1757, 1989.
36. Triulzi DJ, Blumberg N: Variability in response to cryoprecipitate treatment for hemostatic defects in uremia. *Yale J Biol Med* 63:1–7, 1990.
37. Vigano GL, Mannucci PM, Lattuada A, et al: Subcutaneous desmopressin (DDAVP) shortens bleeding time in uremia. *Am J Hematol* 31:32–35, 1989.
38. DiPaolo N, Capotondo L, Rossi P, et al: Bleeding tendency of chronic uremia improved by vascular factor. *Nephron* 52:268–272, 1989.
39. Raskin NH, Fishman RA: Neurologic disorders in renal failure (part I). *N Engl J Med* 294:143–148, 1976.
40. Arieff AI: Neurologic manifestations of uremia, in Brenner BM, Rector FC (eds): *The Kidney*, ed 3. Philadelphia, WB Saunders Co, 1986, pp 1731–1758.
41. Wolf AM: Canine uremic encephalopathy. *JAAHA* 16:735–738, 1980.
42. Finco DR, Barsanti JA: Parenteral nutrition during a uremic crisis, in Kirk RW (ed): *Current Veterinary Therapy. VIII. Small Animal Practice*. Philadelphia, WB Saunders Co, 1983, pp 994–996.
43. Van Buren CT, Dudrick SJ, Dworkin L, et al: Effects of intravenous essential L-amino acids and hypertonic dextrose on anephric beagles. *Surg Forum* 23:83–84, 1972.
44. Wheeler SL, McGuire BH: Enteral nutrional support, in Kirk RW (ed): *Current Veterinary Therapy. X. Small Animal Practice*. Philadelphia, WB Saunders Co, 1989, pp 30–37.
45. Lippert AC, Armstrong PJ: Parenteral nutritional support, in Kirk RW (ed): *Current Veterinary Therapy. X. Small Animal Practice*. Philadelphia, WB Saunders Co, 1989, pp 25–30.
46. Maxie MG: The urinary system, in Jubb KV, Kennedy PC, Palmer N (eds): *Pathology of Domestic Animals*, ed 3. Orlando, FL, Academic Press, 1985, pp 343–411.
47. Richet G: When should renal biopsy be done in acute uremia? *Kidney Int* 28(Suppl 17):S152–S153, 1985.
48. Hager DA, Nyland TG, Fisher P: Ultrasound-guided biopsy of the canine liver, kidney and prostate. *Vet Radiol* 26:82–88, 1985.
49. Grauer GF, Twedt DC, Mero KN: Evaluation of laparoscopy for obtaining renal biopsy specimens from dogs and cats. *JAVMA* 183:677–679, 1983.
50. Osborne CA, Finco DR, Low DG, et al: Percutaneous renal biopsy in the dog and cat. *JAVMA* 151:1474–1480, 1967.
51. Wise LA, Allen TA, Cartwright M: Comparison of renal biopsy techniques in dogs. *JAVMA* 195:935–939, 1989.
52. Jeraj K, Osborne CA, Stevens JB: Evaluation of renal biopsy in 197 dogs and cats. *JAVMA* 181:367–369, 1982.
53. Parker HR: Peritoneal dialysis and hemofiltration, in Bovee KC (ed): *Canine Nephrology*. Media, PA, Harwal Publishing Co, 1984, pp 723–754.
54. Cioffi WG, Ashikaga T, Gamelli RL: Probability of surviving postoperative acute renal failure; development of a prognostic index. *Ann Surg* 200:205–211, 1984.
55. Rasmussen HH, Pitt EA, Ibels LS, McNeil DR: Prediction of outcome in acute renal failure by discriminant analysis of clinical variables. *Arch Intern Med* 145:2015–2018, 1985.
56. Lien J, Chan V: Risk factors influencing survival in acute renal failure treated by hemodialysis. *Arch Intern Med* 145:2067–2069, 1985.
57. Liano F, Garci-Martin F, Gallego A, et al: Easy and early prognosis in acute tubular necrosis: A forward analysis of 228 cases. *Nephron* 51:307–313, 1989.
58. Smithies MN, Cameron JS: Can we predict outcome in acute renal failure? *Nephron* 51:297–300, 1989.
59. Wilkes BM, Mailloux LU: Acute renal failure; pathogenesis and prevention. *Am J Med* 80:1129–1136, 1986.

UPDATE

The preceding text outlined the principles of early treatment of acute renal failure, emphasizing restoring volume requirements, achieving diuresis, and correcting early metabolic complications. Patients that survive the early phase of dysfunction require long periods of maintenance therapy. In these cases, attention to fluid therapy remains important, as urine volume and metabolic needs can be variable. Monitoring of urine output, acid–base status, and electrolyte status must be continued.

The patient's fluid requirements are based on estimates of the volume required to:

- Replace persistent volume deficits
- Supply maintenance needs for typical sensible and insensible losses
- Replace ongoing losses due to vomiting, diarrhea, bleeding, or polyuria.

In dogs and cats with acute renal failure, losses due to urine output will be most variable. Therefore, fluid requirements in acute renal failure patients are best determined by calculating volumes required to:

- Correct persistent dehydration (see original text)
- Provide for insensible losses (13 to 20 ml/kg/day)
- Replace urinary and gastrointestinal losses.

Some clinicians factor in a 3% to 5% estimate for subclinical dehydration in renal failure patients, regardless of physical examination findings. Urine volume is quantitated in 6 to 8 hour intervals and replaced during an equivalent period, in addition to other calculated amounts. Overhydration of oliguric patients and further dehydration of polyuric patients should be avoided.

Fluid composition during long-term maintenance therapy should be tailored to the individual patient. After the initial rehydration with normal saline, other polyionic fluids designed to provide buffering capacity and electrolyte replacement (e.g., lactated Ringer's solution, Normosol-R, Plasma-Lyte) are often used in the first few days of treatment, particularly when ongoing gastrointestinal losses are great. For longer term therapy, lower-sodium solutions designed to meet maintenance fluid needs (e.g., half-strength lactated Ringer's solution or 0.45% saline in 2.5% dextrose, Normosol-M, or Plasma-Lyte 56 and 5% dextrose injection) may be more appropriate, particularly when ongoing losses consist primarily of free water losses in polyuria.[1] Alternating administration of 5% dextrose solutions with high-sodium replacement solutions may also be effective in preventing hypernatremia in patients requiring long-term fluid therapy. Other acute renal failure patients continue to require balanced isotonic solutions. Potassium supplementation is usually required in excess of amounts supplied in commercial fluids (see Table I, original text), and serial monitoring of serum electrolytes is recommended as the best way to determine maintenance fluid composition.

Recovering renal tissue may require several weeks of fluid support. The best indicators of recovery include reduced blood urea nitrogen, serum creatinine, and serum phosphorous concentrations accompanied by lessened clinical signs of uremia. Biochemical parameters often do not return to normal, but may stabilize at an acceptable level of azotemia. As these positive indicators are observed and oral intake of food and fluid increases, tapering of fluid therapy can begin. Fluid volumes usually can be reduced by 25% to 50% daily for several days. During this process, monitor the patient carefully. If progressive dehydration or azotemia occurs, attempt to taper the fluid volume more slowly.

ADDITIONAL REFERENCE

1. Chew DJ: Fluid therapy during intrinsic renal failure, in DiBartola SF (ed): *Fluid Therapy in Small Animal Practice*. Philadelphia, WB Saunders, 1992, pp 554–572.

Radiology of Acute Abdominal Disorders in the Dog and Cat (Part 1)

Lawrence J. Kleine, DVM, MS
Associate Professor and Head, Radiology
Tufts University
School of Veterinary Medicine
North Grafton, Massachusetts

Acute abdominal disorders are among the most difficult problems to diagnose in small animal practice. Even though the clinical signs are of short duration, the underlying lesion may be either acute or chronic. Since many of these disorders must be treated promptly to prevent rapid deterioration of the patient's condition, a practical approach is urged. It is suggested that an attempt be made to classify the disorder as *inflammatory, hemorrhagic, obstructive*, or *traumatic*. This initial approach may permit management decisions which will reduce morbidity without excluding other diagnoses. An exact diagnosis can often be made only during an exploratory laparotomy or after biopsy or necropsy.

The inevitable question that must be answered is, should surgery be performed? Survey radiography and specific radiographic procedures often provide crucial data which not only categorize the disorder but determine if surgery is needed. Utilization of special techniques in the diagnosis of acute abdominal disorders is limited by the animal's inability to tolerate stress. These individuals must be handled gently because of their painful and often precarious metabolic state. Yet radiographic examinations must be thorough if morbidity and mortality are to be reduced to a minimum.

Clinical Aspects and Physical Examination—First priority in caring for the dog or cat with an acute abdominal disorder is to determine the necessity for support of both the respiratory and circulatory systems. Such intervention is accomplished by administration of oxygen, colloid or crystalloid fluids, and by maintaining body temperature. After emergency care a more thorough physical examination should be carried out to estimate the need for other tests. The importance of repeating the physical examination cannot be overemphasized in reevaluating the dog or cat's condition.

Careful inspection of the animal's conformation gives an indication of the nature and presence of any abnormality. A recumbent posture may indicate weakness, spinal injury, or pain, and if there is a unilateral painful condition, the affected side is generally kept uppermost. Kyphosis may indicate back or kidney pain. Rapid shallow breathing often accompanies abdominal pain regardless of the organ involved, making a short x-ray exposure time essential. Wounds, bruising, or pain should lead to further examination for internal injuries that are not immediately apparent.

Thorough but careful palpation of the external surface of the body and abdomen is essential for adequate diagnosis. However, routine abdominal palpation may be difficult or even impossible in the injured animal because of pain. Therefore, changing the position, such as laying the animal on its back so that it cannot tense its abdominal muscles, or the use of analgesics may aid in this critical part of the examination.[3]

Body temperature and pulse are criteria used in determining the seriousness and location of an injury. A rapid pulse rate, rising rectal temperature, and concomitant radiographic and clinical signs of obstruction are highly suggestive of small bowel infarction. Simple laboratory tests such as packed cell volume and white blood cell count are useful in determining the likely source, and sometimes the seriousness of the condition. Blood gas evaluations are needed, not only for diagnosis, but as aids in deciding the type of fluid to be administered. When peritoneal effusion is suspected, paracentesis with laboratory examination of any fluid thus obtained may be diagnostic.

General Radiographic Technique—The primary considerations in selecting x-ray exposure factors are the thickness and composition of the tissue being examined. A general technique chart will usually suffice for abdominal radiography. However, if the x-ray generator can produce a short exposure time at high milliamperage it may be desirable to produce a second chart utilizing low kilovoltage technique with a high milliampere-second setting in order to enhance patient contrast. A high milliampere-second setting is necessary to compensate for the decreased radiographic density that would otherwise result from lowering the kilovoltage. If the exposure is longer than 1/10th of a second there will be an inherent lack of sharpness due to motion of viscera during the exposure.

The primary x-ray beam should be collimated only to the area of interest. This reduces the secondary radiation exposure to personnel who restrain the animal and also increases detail on the x-ray film by reducing scatter. The most important factor in reducing scatter, and thereby increasing detail, is the use of a grid. Grids should be used when the area being radiographed is thicker than 10 cm. The grid will absorb scattered radiation that would otherwise fall on the x-ray film thereby reducing contrast and image sharpness. Either a stationary or moving (Bucky) grid can be used. The higher the grid ratio[a] the greater the amount of scatter that will be reduced. When a grid is used, the radiation necessary to produce the image must be increased to compensate for primary beam absorption.

With low output equipment compromise is necessary so that increased radiation exposure does not require a length of exposure time that increases the possibility of motion. For lower power equipment a 5 to 1 stationary table-top grid may be the best compromise, whereas with maximum power equipment a 10 to 1 high speed movable grid may be more desirable.

Both ventrodorsal and lateral projections are necessary for evaluation of the abdomen. One view or the other will not usually give a satisfactory evaluation. Gas within the gastrointestinal tract or the abdominal cavity will rise and fluid will fall; therefore, in the left lateral radiograph one would expect air to rise into the pylorus and fluid to fall into the fundus of the stomach. The reverse is true in the right lateral projection. Bearing these facts in mind, one may choose whether the right or left lateral view is more desirable under a particular set of circumstances. In some cases, both projections are needed.

The ventrodorsal view is generally preferred over the dorsoventral view because in the former the animal may be stretched somewhat thus reducing the amount of tissue to be penetrated by the x-ray beam. It is also usually easier to position the animal correctly in the ventrodorsal view because the landmarks for positioning are more readily seen. Oblique views project an image of the structures that lie at the margin of the abdomen but would be otherwise partially obliterated by overlying viscera in the standard ventrodorsal and lateral projections.

Special views such as recumbent lateral or horizontal beam radiographs are useful in determining whether a particular opacity is fluid or solid. Horizontal beam radiography is also used to demonstrate air-fluid levels in the intestine or free gas in the abdominal cavity.

Radiographic Examination of the Gastrointestinal Tract Utilizing Contrast Medium—There are several reasons why barium is the most commonly used contrast medium in the gastrointestinal tract. Not only is barium unexcelled as a coating agent of mucosal surfaces, it is readily obtainable and inexpensive. As long as it remains in the gastrointestinal tract, it is nontoxic and its transit time through the gastrointestinal tract is predictable.[8] On the other hand, the organic iodides intended for gastrointestinal use are hypertonic and have a tendency to draw fluid into the gastrointestinal tract.[11] In the case of a debilitated patient this feature is highly undesirable and may lead to increased morbidity. The use of isosmotic aqueous agents will overcome this risk. In addition, the transit time of organic iodides through the gastrointestinal tract is less predictable than that of barium, they are more expensive, have a bitter taste, and generally do not provide satisfactory mucosal coating.

However, since these agents are much less irritating to peritoneal and pleural surfaces than barium, it would seem that organic iodides have a place in contrast studies of the gastrointestinal tract where perforation is suspected. A caveat to consider is that these contrast agents are generally

---

[a]This is the ratio between the height and distance between the lead strips that form the grid.

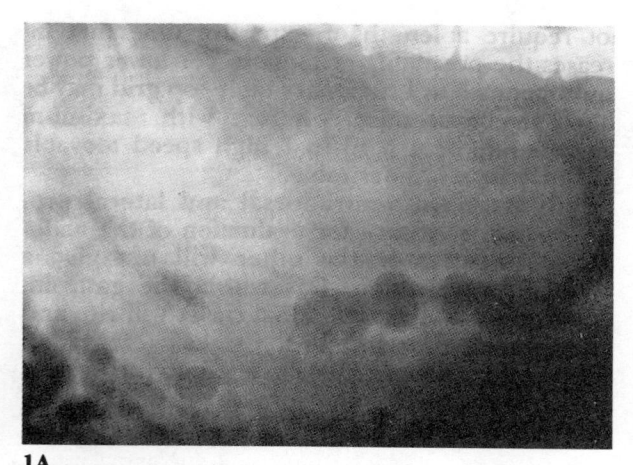

Fig 1—This 13-year-old Beagle had an abdominal mass and pitting rear leg edema. Since only one kidney was seen in the survey radiograph **A** an excretory urogram was performed **B**. Both kidneys were outlined and the mass contains contrast medium. A few hours later the dog suddenly became weak, pale, and died. The mass was a post caval aneurysm.

diluted by fluid that accumulates proximal to the site of obstruction or perforation, and therefore the site of perforation may not be seen radiographically. Moreover, one must recognize that these agents are rapidly absorbed from the peritoneal surface, so that if perforation is present it may not be visualized because of rapid reabsorption of the contrast medium across the peritoneal membrane.

It is *not* true that contrast visualization of the kidneys, ureters, and urinary bladder during organic iodide upper gastrointestinal examination (UGI) indicates gastrointestinal tract perforation. Occasionally the organic iodide is absorbed by the mucosa of the small intestine and excreted by the kidneys.[10] For these reasons organic iodides have a restricted role in gastrointestinal radiography of the dog and cat.

Spilling of barium into the peritoneal cavity as the result of perforation may not be as serious as once thought if lavage of peritoneal surfaces is carried out at exploratory laparotomy immediately upon recognition of such a perforation.[13] Because of the hazards of barium granulomas in the peritoneum and the possibility of not visualizing the perforation when organic iodides are used, it may be desirable to perform exploratory laparotomy based on clinical and survey radiographic findings rather than performing any type of contrast examination when perforation is suspected.

Pure USP barium sulfate is generally an unsatisfactory product for use in an UGI. Commercial barium preparations which are micropulverized and have added suspending agents are much more desirable. Their transit time through the gastrointestinal tract is more predictable and there is much less tendency for these agents to precipitate during the examination.

Barium products may be mixed by the user or may be purchased already mixed. Since the latter are uniform in consistency, they are usually the best and most convenient choice for UGI in the dog and cat. If barium is mixed manually, the manufacturer's instructions should be carefully followed. Vigorous agitation in a blender will produce the most uniform suspension. The contrast medium should be weighed and mixed with the appropriate volume of water.

Before administering any oral contrast agent for the UGI the stomach and small intestine should be free of food and the colon should not contain feces. Without proper preparation, transit of barium through the gastrointestinal tract will be impeded. Furthermore, dense ingesta may overlap and obliterate lesions so that radiographic examination is not only not useful, but possibly misleading.

However, since many patients suffering from acute abdominal conditions cannot receive enemas or laxatives because of the nature of their illness, it may be necessary to perform contrast examination without bowel preparation. Under these circumstances the radiographic study may be limited in its accuracy and if the examination is inconclusive it should be repeated later if the animal's condition will permit.

In general, it is preferable to give a large amount of barium (11 to 15 ml per kg of body weight) for the UGI. Contrast medium is administered by stomach tube to encourage passage through the gastrointestinal tract as a bolus. This permits better evaluation of the gastrointentinal tract than when barium is present in all parts of the GI tract simultaneously. A more accurate judgement of transit time is obtained if the contrast medium is deposited in the stomach quickly.

If the stomach is the primary area of interest, the UGI technique can be modified by administering a small amount of contrast medium (4 to 7 ml per kg of body weight). The animal is then rotated and radiographed in the dorsoventral, ventrodorsal, right, and left lateral projections. Ventrodorsal-oblique views may also be useful if a lesion near the cardia is suspected. After these radiographs are made, the UGI may be continued by administering another 9 to 11 ml per kg of body weight of con-

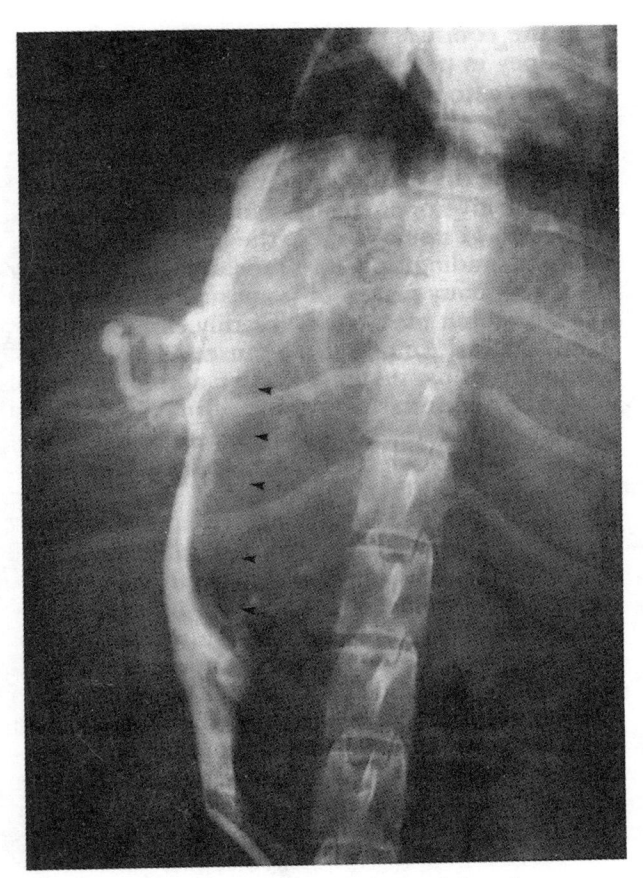

Fig 2—A 7-year-old spayed female Dachshund was examined for ascites and rear leg edema and weakness. The post-vena-cava gram indicates a large filling defect (*arrows*) due to invasion of the vena cava by an adrenal pheochromocytoma. Acute weakness was due to bleeding from the neoplasm.

trast medium by stomach tube and repeating the radiographic procedure. This technique permits evaluation of the stomach in several planes in both the distended and undistended states. Further examination of the stomach can be accomplished by instilling room air or carbon dioxide through the stomach tube or by mixing barium suspension with an effervescent agent.[b]

During the UGI examination, radiographs in both the ventrodorsal and lateral projections are generally made at each of the following times: immediately, 30 minutes, 60 minutes, 3 hours, 6 hours, and 24 hours. However, in each case the examination is tailored to the animal's needs and consideration is given to the expected pathologic change. If the passage of contrast medium is exceptionally rapid, radiographs should be taken more frequently early in the course of the examination. If transit time is slow some of the early films may be eliminated. Both ventrodorsal and lateral radiographs are essential for complete examination of the gastrointestinal tract. Some examiners choose to increase their millampere-seconds by 25% or kilovoltage by 10% to provide penetration of the barium column, permitting better evaluation of the intestinal wall during the UGI.

If the colon is the primary area of interest the best radiographic examination is a barium enema rather than the UGI. The consistency of contrast medium is not uniform when it finally reaches the colon in the UGI, so that its coating characteristics are altered, and there is a longer wait to visualize the colon when barium is given orally rather than by enema.

The barium enema procedure is generally performed under anesthesia and should not be preceded by punch biopsy of the colon or vigorous colonoscopy because the colon can be weakened, increasing the danger of perforation with subsequent spilling of barium into the peritoneum. There is no uniform opinion as to the length of time that should elapse before a barium enema can be given after these procedures, however, a delay of 7 days is preferred.

The most satisfactory barium enema technique is to use a commercially available plastic bag which contains dry barium and has plastic tubing with an attached inflatable cuff.[c] After suspending the barium in water, the tubing is inserted in the rectum so that the cuff lies just beyond the pelvic brim. The cuff is inflated to maintain the position of the tubing and to prevent leakage of barium from the patient during the examination. For small dogs or kittens a bulb syringe inserted into the rectum may serve the same purpose as an inflatable cuff, but air administration is difficult to control when the examination is performed in this manner. The barium is instilled by gravity flow, until the colon and rectum are outlined by contrast. This generally requires 22 to 33 ml of contrast medium per kg of body weight. When the colon has been filled, radiographs are made in the right and left lateral projections and the ventrodorsal and dorsoventral projections.

Barium is drained from the colon by placing the administration bag lower than the level of the dog. Gentle abdominal palpation helps to empty the colon and rectum. Usually 15 to 20 minutes is required to drain most of the contrast medium. After removing the barium, all projections are repeated. Finally the colon is insufflated with carbon dioxide or room air and the four projections are repeated again. This final procedure provides double contrast and distends the colon, providing superior mucosal detail.

Radiographic Examination of the Urogenital Tract Using Contrast Medium—Contrast radiographic examination of the urinary tract is essential in diagnosing many cases of acute abdominal disease. The male canine urethra is most clearly seen when 5 to 10 ml of a sterile aqueous iodine solution, with an iodine concentration of approximately 200 mg per ml, is administered by uri-

---

[b] E-Z Gas, E-Z-EM Company, Inc., Westbury, NY 11590

[c] Barium enema, E-Z-EM Company, Inc., Westbury, NY 11590

nary catheter into the distal urethra while occluding the urethral orifice. X-ray exposure is made at the conclusion of this procedure. The entire urethra and neck of the urinary bladder are outlined to show filling defects or mucosal irregularities.

The urinary bladder is drained and an attempt is made to flush out blood clots or debris with sterile saline. The bladder is then distended with either gas or organic iodine contrast medium until back pressure is exerted on the syringe by the medium, or until the volume of contrast medium administered equals the estimated capacity of the urinary bladder. The potential hazard of fatal air embolism resulting from air insufflation of the urinary bladder, particularly in patients with hematuria, must be considered. Less risk is associated with carbon dioxide insufflation of the bladder. Radiographs are made in the ventrodorsal and lateral projections. Ventrodorsal oblique views are needed if a bladder neck lesion is suspected.

Excretory urography is done to evaluate the kidneys and ureters. For this procedure, aqueous organic iodine contrast medium, at a dose of 250 to 900 mg of iodine per kg body weight, is injected rapidly intravenously. The lower dosage is suggested in giant breeds of dogs and when the pyelographic phase of the urogram is the area of primary interest. The upper dose range is utilized when working with small dogs and cats, when hypotension or uremia are present, or when the nephrographic phase of the urogram is of greatest importance.

The contrast medium can be administered through an indwelling venous catheter rather than a needle to facilitate visualization of the vascular phase of the urogram in the immediate radiographs. Ordinarily, compression techniques are not used because of the diminished visibility which results when there is overlapping of small bowel silhouettes on the kidneys, and because tranquilization is usually necessary for effective compression.

In the conventional intravenous urogram both ventrodorsal and lateral radiographs are obtained at the following times after injection of the contrast medium: immediately, 10 minutes, 30 minutes and 60 minutes. If a lesion is suspected in the trigone area, ventrodorsal oblique radiographs which include the pelvic canal should be taken in addition to the standard lateral and ventrodorsal views. The nephrographic phase is best seen in the immediate radiographs while the pyelographic phase is best seen at 10 and 30 minutes. The one hour radiograph is used to evaluate the renal silhouettes for the presence of a pyelographic phase and prolonged distortion of pelvic diverticula.

In cases of a prolonged nephrogram or pyelogram, additional radiographs are generally taken at 2 and 4 hours. A crude measure of renal function is given by the quantity and density of contrast medium in the kidneys and urinary bladder. The ureters are seldom visualized completely in a single exposure regardless of its timing because the contrast medium is carried away from the kidney in peristaltic waves.

Cholecystography—Where ultrasound is available, it has largely replaced cholecystography in gallbladder evaluation. The oral cholecystogram is generally used to evaluate dogs and cats for cholecystitis. For performing oral cholecystography, 200 mg of iopanic acid tablets[d] per kg of body weight are given per os, and radiographs are then made 10 to 14 hours later. If the gallbladder is not visualized, radiographs are repeated in 24 hours. There are many causes of nonvisualization of the gallbladder, but most can be readily eliminated on a clinical basis. Among these causes are: drug not administered, drug vomited after administration, proximal duodenal obstruction, malabsorption syndrome, insufficient liver excretion of drug, obstruction of cystic duct, absence of gallbladder, and cholecystitis.

When the gallbladder is not visualized by the oral technique, an intravenous cholecystogram using meglumine iodipapide[e] may then be performed. The contrast medium is administered intravenously at a dose rate of 0.5 ml per kg of body weight over a period of ten minutes. Radiographs are made 30, 60 and 180 minutes after injection. This procedure outlines the intrahepatic bile ducts, and may permit the examiner to determine whether or not intrahepatic bile duct obstruction is present.

Angiography—Angiography is used extensively in man to evaluate abdominal trauma.[9] However, this technique has not found wide acceptance in small animal practice because of the need for special equipment and expertise not generally available to the private practitioner. In renal infarction or rupture of the renal pedicle angiography is the preferred method of diagnosis. There are other vascular lesions that may require angiography for ante mortem diagnosis (Figs 1 and 2).

When aortic embolism is suspected the most accurate radiographic approach to the problem is to catheterize the aorta through a carotid artery approach. However, a simpler and usually satisfactory technique is to use a venous catheter inserted by means of the cephalic or jugular vein, making a rapid injection of approximately 2 ml of contrast medium per kg of body weight. Radiographs are made between 7 and 20 seconds following the administration of the medium, which will not be as dense as with the aortic approach, but usually will outline any major obstruction of the abdominal aorta.

ACKNOWLEDGMENT

The author gratefully acknowledges the help of Paula Ruel, BSN, RN, in the preparation of the manuscript.

---

[d]Telepaque, Winthrop Laboratories, New York, NY 10016

[e]Cholegraffin, Squibb & Sons, Princeton, NJ 08540

REFERENCES

1. Dixon JA, et al: Intestinal motility following vascular occlusion of small intestine. *Gastroenterology* 58: 673-678, 1970
2. Donahue JK, Hunter C and Balch HH: Significance of fluid levels in x-ray films of the abdomen. *New Eng J Med* 259: 13-15, 1958.
3. Hornbuckle WE, Kleine LJ: Obstruction of the small intestine, in *Current Veterinary Therapy VI*, Kirk R(ed): Philadelphia, WB Saunders Co, 1977, pp 952-958.
4. Kleine LJ, Hornbuckle WE: Acute pancreatitis: radiographic findings in 182 dogs. *J Am Vet Rad Soc* 19: 102-106, 1978.
5. Kleine LJ: Radiographic Diagnosis of urinary tract trauma in the dog and cat. *Sm An Vet Med Update Series* 7:2-6, 1978.
6. Kleine LJ: Radiography in the diagnosis of intestinal obstruction in dogs and cats. *Compen Contin Educ for Sm An Pract*, 1: 44-51, 1979.
7. Laufman H; Intestinal strangulation. *Surg Gynec and Obst* 135: 271-272, 1972
8. Miller RE, Skucas J: *Radiographic Contrast Agents*. Baltimore, University Park Press, 1977.
9. Osborn D, et al: Role of Angiography in abdominal nonrenal trauma. *Rad Clin N Amer* 11: 579-592, 1973.
10. Poole CA, Rowe MI: Clinical evidence of intestinal absorption of gastrograffin. *Radiology* 118: 151-153, 1976.
11. Rowe MI, et al: Gastrograffin induced hypertonicity: the pathogenesis of neonatal hazard. *Am J Surg* 125: 185-188, 1973.
12. Wolfe DA, Meyer WC: Obstructing intestinal abscess in a dog. *JAVMA* 166: 518-519, 1975.
13. Zhuetlin N, Lasser EC, Rigler LG: Clinical studies on effect of barium in the peritoneal cavity following rupture of the colon. *Surg* 32: 967-979, 1952.

Radiology of Acute Abdominal Disorders in the Dog and Cat (Part II)

Lawrence J. Kleine, DVM, MS
Associate Professor and Head, Radiology
Tufts University
School of Veterinary Medicine
North Grafton, Massachusetts

In acute abdominal disorders survey film findings are exceptionally important because contrast examinations may be impossible to perform due to the animal's poor condition or the need for a rapid diagnosis. When the radiographic findings are correlated with physical and laboratory tests a decision whether a contrast examination should be performed can be made. Survey radiographs also indicate whether the initial radiographic technique was correct and whether factors are present that will preclude a contrast examination or will prevent adequate visualization of the various abdominal structures during the contrast examination. These factors include the presence of feces or excessive gas in the intestine and the presence of gas in the intraperitoneal space.

Each examiner should develop a method of evaluating radiographs to determine whether they are of adequate technical quality and also to evaluate the films so that no abnormality will be overlooked. Clinical judgement is used to assign proper significance to any abnormalities that are found.

When examining the radiograph one should first visualize those structures external to the abdomen, including the bony portion of the spinal column, the ribs and the ilia. Next, the abdominal wall should be evaluated for any break in its integrity, changes in opacity (Fig 1) or the presence of a foreign body. The diaphragmatic silhouette should be examined and the general abdominal configuration evaluated. A search should be made for evidence of free gas or fluid within the peritoneal cavity. Free gas tends to accumulate in the subdiaphragmatic area between the liver and the diaphragm in both the ventrodorsal and lateral projections. Horizontal beam radiography in a recumbent lateral or standing position may be useful in further delineating small amounts of gas. Another manifestation of free intraperitoneal gas is the formation of small bubbles due to gas becoming trapped within the mesentery. These bubbles will tend to occupy a central position in the abdomen, may have the same stippled appearance as hemorrhage of the omentum and be difficult for the inexperienced observer to discern.

Next, the appearance of the retroperitoneum and kidneys should be evaluated for masses or uneven opacity which generally indicates extravasation of fluid. The uneven appearance does not reveal the

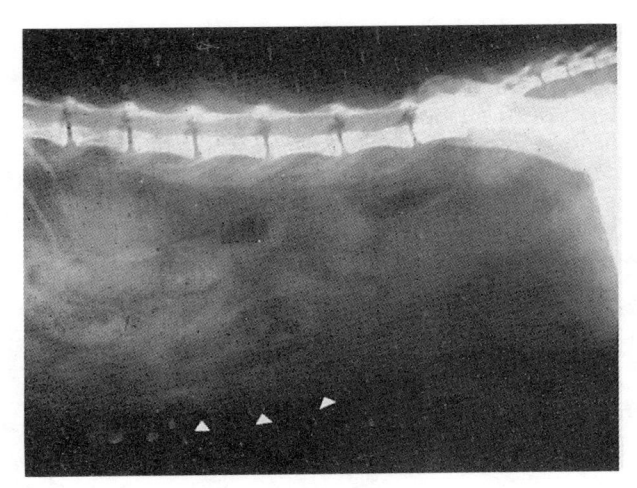

Fig 1—A one-and-a-half-year old cat experienced pain when its abdomen was touched. In abdominal radiographs an irregular opacity was present in the ventral subcutaneous soft tissues (arrows). The microscopic diagnosis was pansteatitis.

nature of the fluid but merely its presence. It may be hemorrhage, an exudate or a transudate. After the evaluation of the skeletal structures of the abdomen, the abdominal wall, the abdominal cavity and retroperitoneum, each abdominal viscus in turn should be examined. The entire gastrointestinal tract including the stomach, small intestine and colon should be evaluated. In addition, special attention should be paid to the liver, spleen and pancreas.

Stomach

The normal gastric silhouette lies parallel to the arch of the rib in the lateral radiograph, except in deep-chested dogs, where it is nearly perpendicular to the sternum. Hepatomegaly displaces the pyloric antrum in a dorsocaudomedial direction causing the fundic-pyloric axis to lie more parallel to the spine than usual. When gastric thickening or edema of mucosal folds is suggested, no specific conclusions can be drawn with respect to the cause. This finding is often associated with vomiting, regardless of whether the vomiting is due to pyloric or intestinal obstruction, irritation of the gastrointestinal tract, or secondary to metabolic upset such as uremia. In chronic uremia, gastric mineralization may occur.

Direct trauma to the stomach is seldom easily evaluated radiographically. Granular material within the stomach is sometimes the result of gastric hemorrhage which may be secondary to trauma, inflammatory disease or a neoplasm. In gastric perforation free air is usually released into the abdominal cavity. Volvulus of the stomach results because of rotation of the stomach around the mesenteric axis. The pylorus comes to lie in a more dorsal and cranial position than normal on the left of the midline. When this occurs neither air nor fluid can easily leave the stomach and further distension leads to toxemia and strangulation. There is reduced venous blood flow to the heart due to compression of the caudal vena cava. Gastric volvulus can be recognized by the displacement of the pylorus and by a dense line along the cranial aspect of the gastric silhouette, resulting from the folding of the pylorus upon the body of the stomach.

Diaphragmatic hernia is a very common acute abdominal injury. It is most often recognized radiographically by the presence of abdominal viscera within the thoracic cavity or by the absence of viscera which would normally be present in the abdomen. These displaced viscera usually partially obliterate the cardiac silhouette. Transudation of fluid into the pleural or intraperitoneal space occurs if there is incarceration of a viscus within the thoracic cavity. A gastric diaphragmatic hernia must be recognized as a surgical emergency because it can be rapidly fatal, leading to strangulation, toxemia, interference with lung expansion, and reduced cardiac filling.

Vomiting is the most frequent clinical sign associated with a gastric foreign body, pyloric obstruction, or mucosal irritation.

Intussusception of the stomach into the esophagus is a rare condition that can be rapidly fatal if not recognized early.

Any time shock or difficult breathing is present, the gastric silhouette may be greatly distended with air.

While neoplasms are not generally considered the cause of acute abdominal disease, if they cause obstruction, massive blood loss, or perforation, clinical signs will be acute.

The stomach may be indirectly involved in either pancreatic or hepatic masses or pancreatitis.[4] In these situations gastric displacement is a prominent finding. With a pancreatic mass or pancreatitis the pylorus may be displaced to the left. Other findings that may be associated with pancreatitis include spreading of the angle between the descending duodenum and the greater curvature of the stomach and lack of definition in the cranial abdominal quadrant due to inflammatory response of the tissues in that region[4] (Fig 2).

Small Intestine

Injury to the small intestine due to blunt trauma is not common because of its ability to be displaced. With a large perforation of the intestine free gas is found in the intraperitoneal space, whereas when small tears occur the free gas may be confined to small bubbles trapped in the mesentery and omentum.

Weeks or months following trauma, an abdominal mass may develop due to adhesions between the lacerated portion of intestine, mesentery, and omentum. Obstruction can occur because of narrowing of the lumen due to fibrosis. Bruising of the intestine may not produce any immediate radiographic abnormality except for a slight loss of contrast due to hemorrhage. An organizing intramural hematoma is capable of producing small bowel obstruction after a period of several hours.

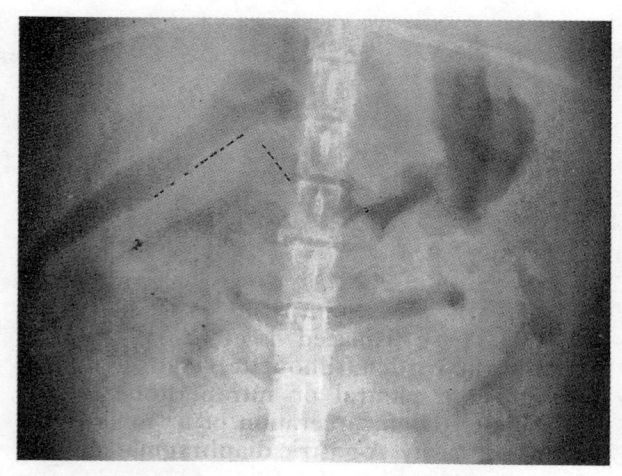

Fig 2—This 6-year-old male miniature poodle had an acute episode of hematemesis. The duodenum and stomach were both displaced caudally by the enlarged liver. In addition, the duodenal-gastric angle was widened (dotted line). The microscopic diagnosis was acute, necrotizing pancreatitis.

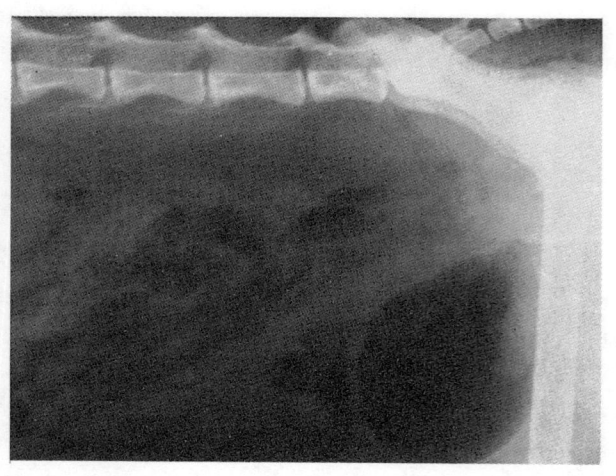

Fig 4—This 3-year-old cat presented with stranguria and ventral-caudal abdominal swelling after an automobile accident. The small intestine was displaced into a ventral hernia. A pneumocystogram demonstrated herniation of the urinary bladder also. There was rupture of the prepubic tendon.

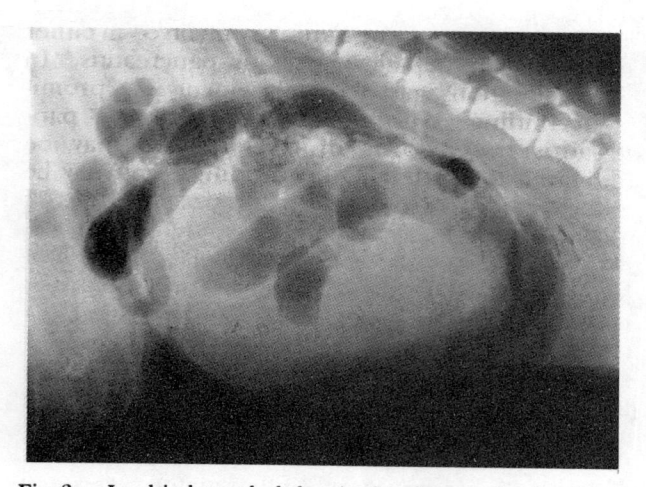

Fig 3—In this lateral abdominal radiograph of a four-year-old male miniature poodle, a large oval midabdominal mass is apparent. There is also gaseous distension of the small intestine. These findings, in the presence of clinical signs of intestinal obstruction, are highly suggestive of small bowel infarction. Surgical examination revealed an 18 cm segment of infarcted jejunum.

If massive infarction of the intestine occurs one expects to find both gas and fluid distending the small intestine due to paralysis and diminished absorption of material from the infarcted segment (Fig 3).[1] Small areas of infarction may not produce any radiographic findings initially but fibrosis can cause obstruction in the subsequent days and weeks.

Small Bowel Herniation

Small bowel herniation through an opening in the diaphragm is one of the most common results of blunt abdominal trauma. Paracostal, abdominal and inguinal herniae containing small intestine are less common but the importance of finding such lesions cannot be overemphasized (Fig 6). Incarceration with or without volvulus in the hernia may result in obstruction and vascular compromise with subsequent toxemia.

Foreign Bodies and Intussusceptions

Foreign bodies and intussusceptions are also considered under the broad definition of trauma. Foreign bodies are the most common cause of intestinal obstruction in the dog and cat, and the size and nature of ingested objects defy the imagination. The most common complication of foreign body ingestion is obstruction of the intestinal lumen. The radiographic signs are those of distension with delayed transit of material through the gastrointestinal tract (Fig 5). When a linear foreign body such as a string is ingested, the small intestine becomes hyperactive and becomes *bunched* as peristalsis causes the bowel to move along the string (Fig 6). Perforation may occur soon after such hyperperistalsis is initiated.

In early intussusception, obstruction may not be complete but vascular compromise can produce infarction and necrosis. Usually a tubular structure of fluid opacity is visualized in mid abdomen, with gas accumulation proximal to the point of obstruction. A barium enema should be diagnostic in cases of cecocolic or ileocolic intussusception (Fig 7). In intussusceptions confined to the small intestine, an UGI may be necessary to reach a definitive diagnosis.

Tumors

Tumors of the small intestine cause acute or chronic clinical signs by obstruction or blood loss from an ulcerated surface. Intestinal adenocarcinoma and lymphoma are the most common

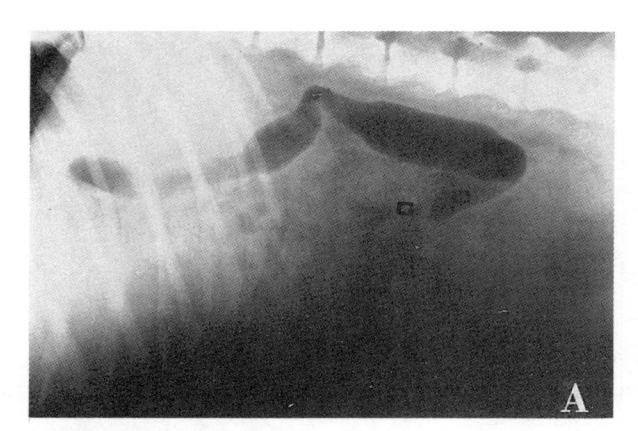

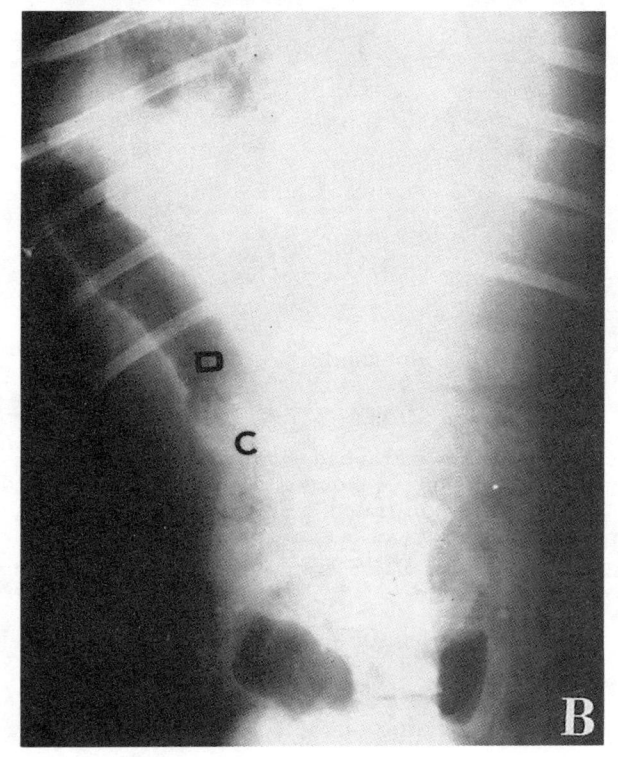

Fig 5 A and B—This 11-year-old terrier dog had an acute onset of vomiting. The gas distended duodenum (D) and the obstructing foreign body (C, corn cob) are clearly seen.

gastrointestinal neoplasms seen in this practice.

Adynamic (Paralytic) Ileus

Adynamic (paralytic) ileus occurs from peritonitis, shock, intestinal obstruction and administration of anticholinergic drugs. In paralytic ileus it may be difficult to determine whether dilated loops of intestine that contain gas are small bowel or colon. As a general rule, small bowel occupies a more central position in the abdomen while the laterally located loops are more likely to be colon.

Simple and Strangulated Obstruction

Intestinal obstruction regardless of its cause may be either simple or strangulated. In simple obstruction there is closure of a loop at a single site, whereas in strangulation there is closure of a loop at two sites resulting in interference with intestinal blood supply. When the ischemic area becomes infarcted, perforation rapidly follows.[1,7] Horizontal beam radiography may demonstrate intralumenal air-fluid levels at different heights in the same loop and can be an invaluable technique in the diagnosis of strangulation obstruction (Fig 8).[2]

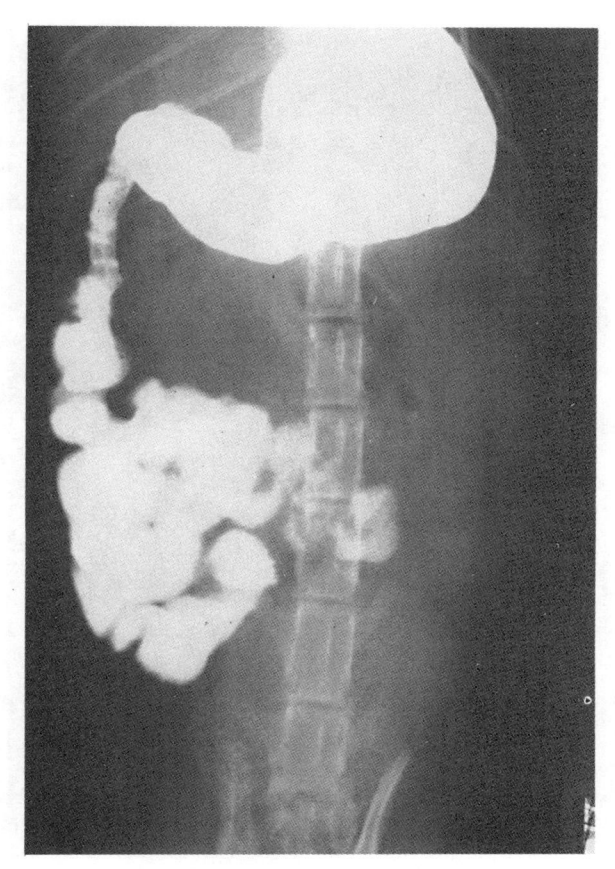

Fig 6—Acute abdominal pain and vomiting were prominent signs in a 9-month-old female cat. A 30-minute radiograph in the UGI shows convolutional plication of the proximal small intestine, highly suggestive of a linear foreign body. An 8-inch string was removed surgically.

Inflammatory Disease

Inflammatory disease of the small intestine is common in dogs and cats but does not always produce radiographic signs. The expected signs include thickening of intestinal walls and evidence of hyperperistalsis during contrast examination (Figs 9 and 10). Abscesses of the small intestine may protrude into the lumen and become large enough to cause obstruction.[12] Often there is resolution before obstruction develops, but fibrosis and occasionally stenosis are possible sequelae to this condition. Adhesions secondary to surgical procedures, previous inflammatory diseases, or external trauma will occasionally produce obstruction of the small intestine. Dogs can develop obstruction due to adhesions as long as three months after a traumatic incident.

Pancreatitis is capable of producing secondary changes in the intestinal tract and this assists in making the diagnosis. The duodenum may be somewhat thickened and distended and displaced to the right. An uneven granular opacity may be

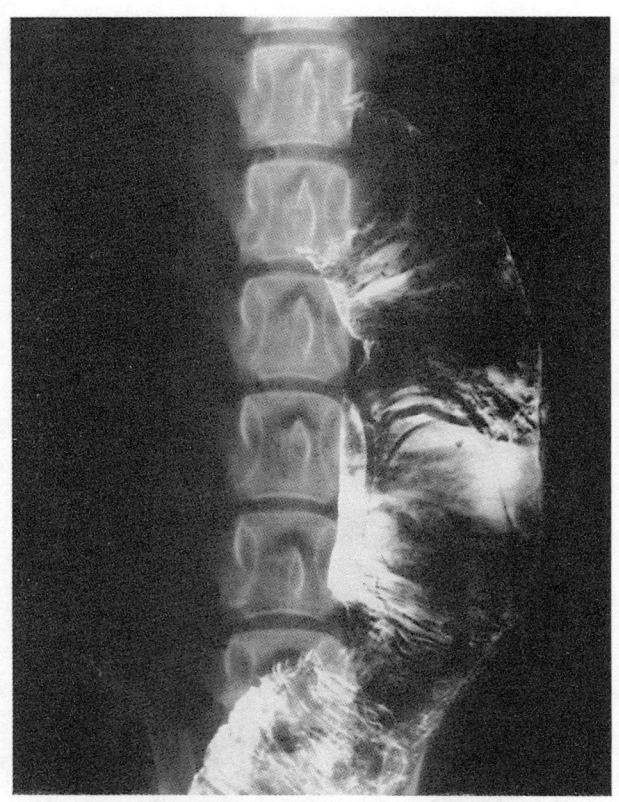

Fig 7—This 4-month-old Golden Retriever had several bouts of vomiting and diarrhea. An abdominal mass was palpated and a barium enema was performed. The multiple circumferential filling defects in the colon were caused by invagination of the small intestine into the lumen of the colon. A large percentage of the small intestine was involved in the intussusception.

present in the left cranial quadrant of the abdomen due to inflammatory disease within the peripancreatic tissues.[4]

Cecum and Colon

Blunt abdominal trauma seldom produces any radiographic changes in the cecum or colon. Penetrating foreign bodies may perforate either of these structures and produce pneumoperitoneum with associated bacterial contamination of the peritoneal cavity. Foreign bodies causing clinical signs in the cecum and colon are much less common than those in the stomach or small intestine.

Volvulus and Intussusception

Volvulus of the cecum associated with neoplasm initiates dramatic distension. Cecocolic intussusception may be a chronic disease with vague signs such as vomiting, intermittent abdominal pain and diarrhea. Cecocolic intussusception is therefore a difficult condition to diagnose clinically, but is easily recognized with a barium enema by noting a coiled filling defect in the ascending and transverse colon. Occasionally the diagnosis can be strongly suspected based on survey film findings of a soft tissue mass (invaginated cecum) in a gas filled ascending or tranverse colon (Fig 11).

Inflammatory Lesions and Tumors

Inflammatory lesions of the cecum are most

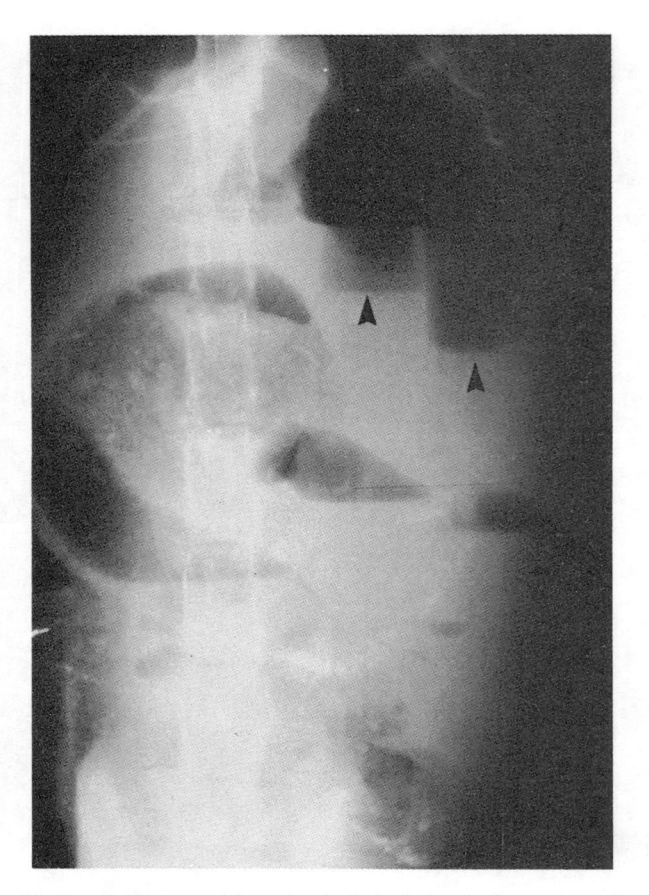

Fig 8—A 13-year-old cat had clinical signs of acute small bowel obstruction. A horizontal beam dorsoventral radiograph demonstrated multiple intralumenal air-fluid levels (*arrows*) in a loop of intestine in the left cranial abdomen. There was strangulating obstruction of the midjejunum.

often due to parasitic infestation or extension of enterocolitis.

Histiocytic colitis is expected to produce ulceration and thickening of the colon and this may be detected by barium enema. Tumors in the cecum

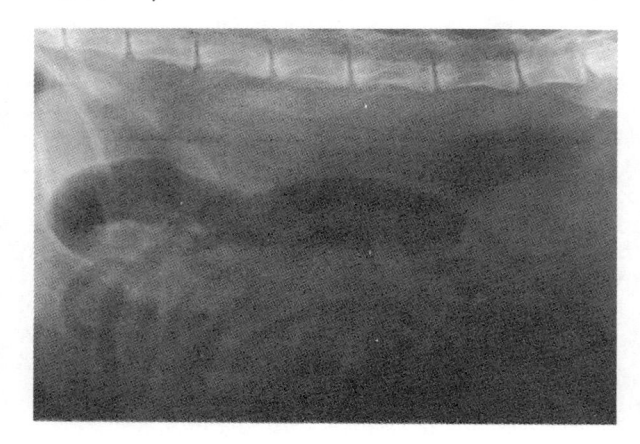

Fig 9—There was thickening of the wall of the entire small intestine with gas accumulation but no evidence of distension in this three-year-old castrated male cat. The cat had a sudden onset of vomiting and anorexia. The clinical and radiographic diagnosis was nonspecific enteritis.

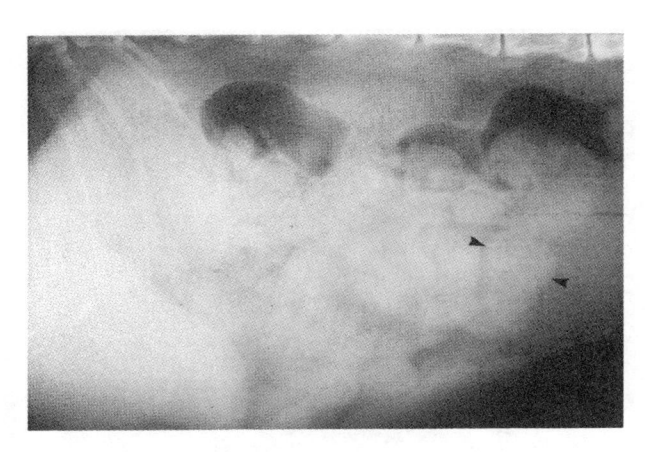

Fig 10—An 11-year-old castrated male cat was presented because of acute blood-stained diarrhea. The major radiographic abnormalities were an enlarged liver and spleen and a turgid small intestine (*arrows*). The biopsy diagnosis was eosinophilic enteritis.

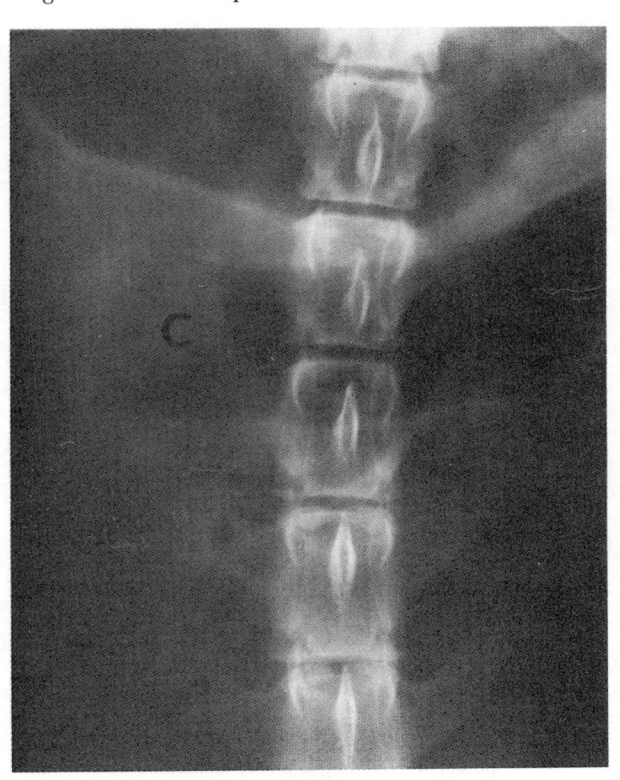

Fig 11—This 4-year-old male Labrador Retriever had several episodes of vomiting and acute abdominal pain. The filling defect (*c*) in the transverse colon (*T*) is the invaginated cecum (cecocolic intussusception).

and colon may produce acute signs of obstruction. Shock may occur due to massive bleeding secondary to ulceration of the free surface of the tumor.

Supporting Structures and Retroperitoneum

Trauma to the abdominal wall is a frequent occurrence in the dog and cat but radiographic findings are usually limited to the recognition of soft tissue swelling due to bruising, or gas accumulation secondary to laceration of the skin and subcutaneous tissue. External hernias or opaque foreign bodies are easily recognized. Increased opacity of the subcutaneous tissue may be caused by inflammatory soft tissue disease, which simulates an acute abdominal disorder (Fig 1). Fractures of the last few ribs or transverse processes of lumbar vertebrae may be associated with lacerations of the liver, spleen, or kidneys. Bleeding into the abdominal cavity has no distinct diagnostic appearance to differentiate blood from a transudate or exudate. Peritoneal effusion can be due to many abdominal disorders such as pancreatitis; rupture of prostatic abscess; mesenteric abscess; rupture of bile ducts, intestine, or uterus (Fig 12); infectious feline peritonitis; penetrating abdominal wounds; and intestinal obstruction with strangulation. Tumors and abscesses involving the omentum and mesentery are recognized by formation of a mass and stippled opacities in the mid ventral abdomen due to breakdown of fat planes which usually provide contrast between the abdominal viscera. Mesenteric and cecal node enlargement can be the cause of acute abdominal pain (Fig 13).

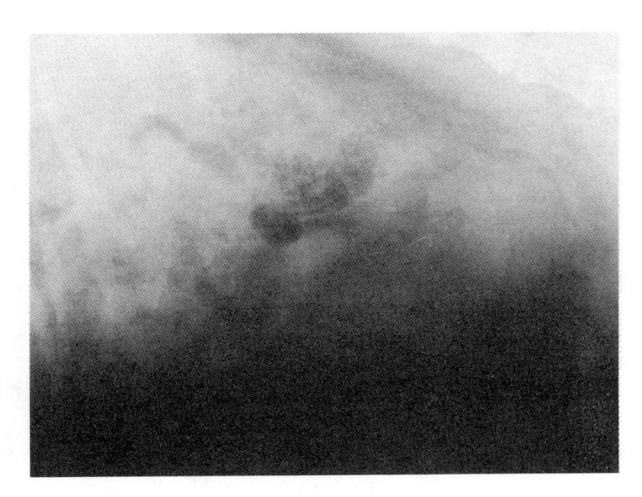

Fig 12—This 13-year-old female, shepherd-cross dog had a persistent purulent vaginal discharge for several weeks, then suddenly developed a distended abdomen and weakness. The abdomen lacked normal definition and there was a tubular, fluid-filled density in the caudal abdomen. The surgical findings were peritonitis secondary to ruptured pyometra.

Trauma to the kidneys and ureters is recognized by increased size and an uneven opacity of the retroperitoneal space. Retroperitoneal hemorrhage, without urinary tract pathology, may produce this same radiographic appearance. Such trauma is often accompanied by fractures of dorsal spinous processes or transverse processes of lumbar vertebrae and fractures of the last few ribs.[5] Retroperitoneal abscesses produce radiographic signs similar to those seen with retroperitoneal hemorrhage or tumor.

Urethra

Perineal swelling, following trauma or associated with anuria, should lead to investigation of the integrity of the urethra by means of positive con-

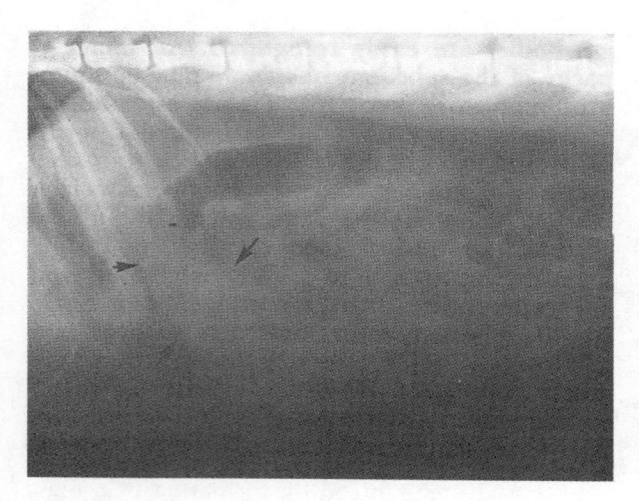

Fig 13—The arrows outline an oval abdominal mass in a 2-year-old male cat that had fever and leucocytosis. The mass was an abscessed ileocecal lymph node.

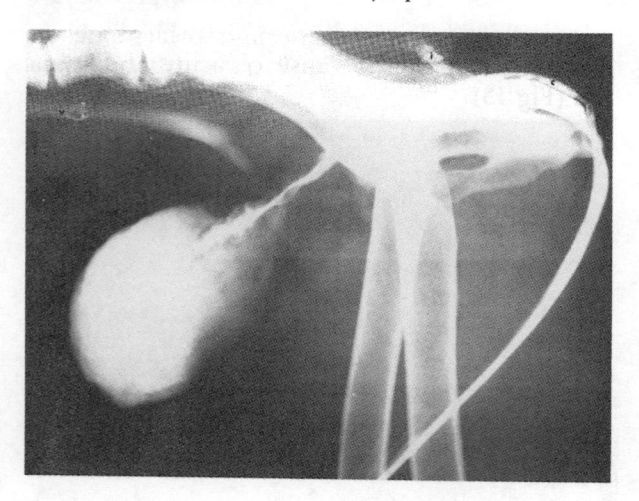

Fig 14—This 6-year-old male retriever has extravasation of contrast medium into the corpus spongiosum penis (*c*). The internal pudendal vein (*i*), and the caudal vena cava (*v*) are outlined. The radiographic findings are due to an injury of the urethra in the region of the ischium. Gas can also escape into the venous system when vascular areas are injured, leading to fatal air embolism.

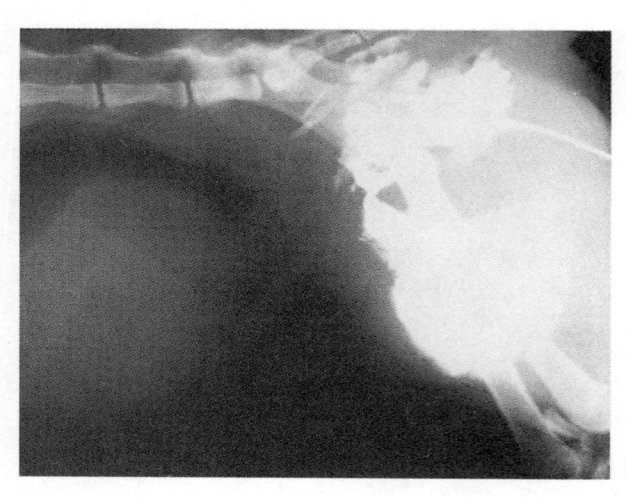

Fig 15—A 2-year-old cat was unable to urinate following an automobile accident. The right ilium and pelvic floor were fractured. The urinary bladder was distended. There was extravasation of contrast medium into an inguinal hernia because of a ruptured urethra.

trast urethrography (Figs 14 and 15). Negative contrast urethrography may also be useful but it carries with it the hazard of air embolism unless carbon dioxide or a soluble gas other than room air is used. In addition to trauma, acute signs may be due to obstructing calculus, urethritis, or post-operative or post-traumatic stricture. Iatrogenic injury may occur with catheters that are too large or inflexible, and occasionally results in tearing of the mucosa with subsequent stricture formation.

Prostate Gland

The prostate gland is generally well-protected by the bony pelvis and is seldom seriously injured by external force. Occasionally, however, a prostatic cyst may be ruptured by external trauma or by passage of a urinary catheter into a cyst which communicates with the prostatic urethra. When a cyst ruptures, hemorrhage, hematoma formation and necrosis occur. Prostatitis and abscess formation may also cause acute abdominal signs due to pain, dysuria, obstruction, infection or sepsis.

The various types of prostatic enlargement can usually not be distinguished from one another by radiographic means alone. Prostatic enlargement is best recognized by abdominal survey radiography and retrograde cystourethrography. Cysts communicating with the prostatic urethra do not mean that the primary prostatic disease is cystic hyperplasia. Communicating cysts may also be present with prostatitis, abscesses or prostatic tumors. Prostatic neoplasms metastasize to the lumbar spine and pelvis and may produce acute lameness and pain.

Urinary Bladder

Blunt trauma to the urinary bladder in an automobile accident is relatively common.[5] Such lesions include lacerations, contusions, hernias and volvulus of the urinary bladder. When an inflexible catheter is inserted too deeply it can penetrate the wall of the bladder. If a flexible catheter is inserted too deeply it can be knotted. Overinflation during pneumocystography can cause local tears in the mucosa or even complete rupture of the bladder wall. The urinary bladder may be traumatized when the uterine stump is litgated during an ovariohysterectomy.

Volvulus of the urinary bladder may occur following removal of its median ligament in abdominal surgery. In acute cystitis the urinary bladder may be only minimally thickened and the signs of cystitis may be functional (straining and spasm) rather than anatomical changes of thickening and irregularity which are most often seen with chronic cystitis. Granulomas sometimes occur at the bladder neck secondary to an infected uterine stump. Tumors of the urinary bladder may cause obstruc-

Kidneys and Ureters

In trauma to the kidneys and ureters the primary survey radiographic signs are accumulation of fluid in the abdominal cavity or retroperitoneal space or renal enlargement or displacement. These lesions are best evaluated by survey radiography and intravenous urography (Fig 16).

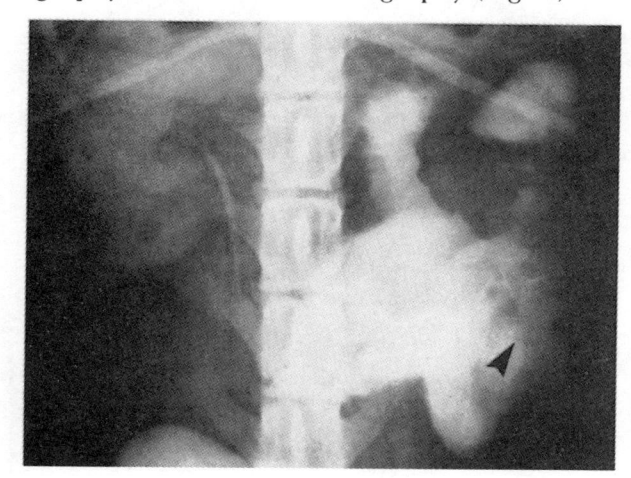

Fig 16—This 5-year-old Cocker Spaniel had been struck by a car several hours before radiographs were made, dislocating its left hip. The black arrow shows the point of rupture of the left renal pelvis in a 30-minute intravenous urogram.

Acute Inflammatory Diseases

Acute inflammatory diseases of the kidneys include pyelitis, pyelonephritis and nephritis. While pyelitis and pyelonephritis are ordinarily caused by infection, nephritis may be either infectious or toxic. The radiographic signs are usually subtle, early and are best recognized by means of intravenous urography. Later in the disease one expects to find distortion of the renal pelvis, a prolonged pyelogram, a variable degree of hydronephrosis, and blunting of the pelvic diverticula. In nephritis there may be enlargement of the parenchymal portion of the kidney with or without hydronephrosis. In some cases of acute nephritis the kidneys may appear more dense than usual.

Calculi Formation

While formation of calculi is not an acute phenomenon, the clinical signs may have a sudden onset due to passage of a renal calculus into a ureter causing obstruction and extreme abdominal pain. Nonradiopaque renal stones cannot be visualized without the aid of intravenous urography.

Tumors

If tumors of the kidneys and ureters rupture, they may cause massive bleeding and the clinical signs will be acute.

Genital Organs

Volvulus of Ovary or Testicle

Volvulus of an ovary or a retained testicle causes

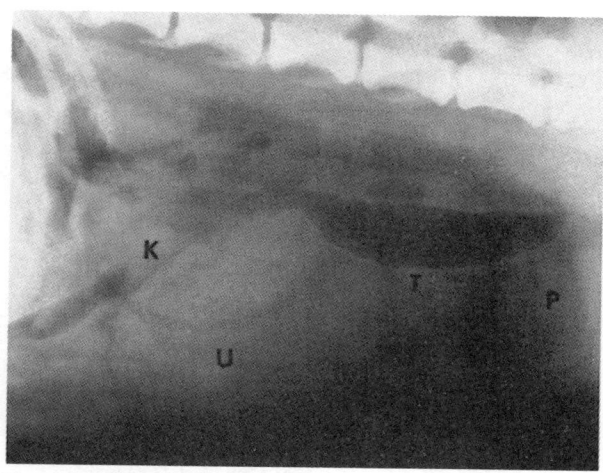

Fig 17—This 6-year-old male dog was presented in acute abdominal pain. The abdominal densities were left kidney (*K*), urinary bladder (*U*), abdominal testicle (*T*), and prostate glad (*P*). There was torsion of the testicle.

abdominal pain due to vascular compromise and swelling of the parenchyma of the organ (Fig 17). A retained testicle or ovary can be recognized radiographically as an oval abdominal mass in the caudal or mid abdomen.

Uterus

The uterus may be traumatized directly by a blunt force such as an automobile accident, causing laceration accompanied by peritoneal bleeding with loss of abdominal contrast. Volvulus of a gravid uterus may occur with vascular compromise, particularly when it enters an inguinal or abdominal hernia. Inflammatory lesions of the uterus are common in both dogs and cats. In endometritis the uterus has a turgid, nodular appearance and is usually two to three times normal size. With pyometra, the uterus is usually not lobulated but instead has a smooth configuration, may be five to eight times its normal diameter and filled with fluid. Both conditions may cause either acute or chronic abdominal signs. Occasionally the infected uterus may rupture, producing radiographic signs of peritoneal effusion and peritonitis (Fig 12).

Dystocia

Dystocia caused by fetal head, maternal pelvis incompatibility, is easily diagnosed radiographically. Fetal death can be recognized by the presence of air within the fetus or uterus or fetal skull fractures (Fig 18).

Other Abdominal Viscera

Liver and Biliary System

Ultrasound examination of the liver and associated viscera is highly effective in evaluation of the acute abdomen. The liver, bile ducts, and gallbladder can be involved in blunt abdominal trauma although they are protected by the rib cage. Laceration and bruising of the liver is usually not clinically significant. Massive laceration with hemorrhage and rupture of the bile ducts or gallbladder results in bile peritonitis. Occasionally

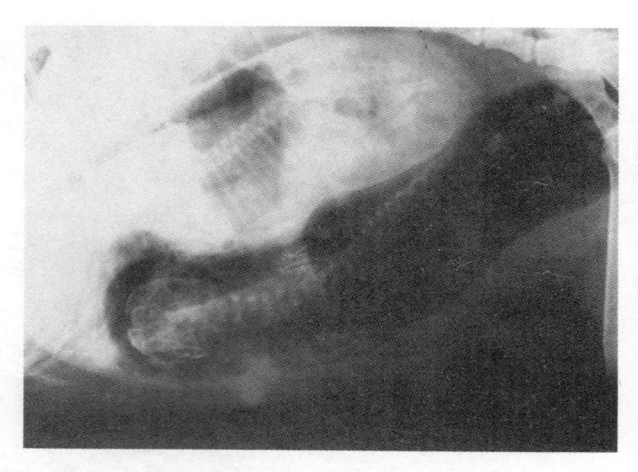

Fig 18—There were clinical signs of septicemia in this 3-year-old female Fox Terrier that had been in labor for 12 hours. Gas surrounds the fetus that is engaged in the pelvic canal in a caudal presentation. The radiographic and clinical findings are those of emphysematous metritis.

traumatic portal vein thrombosis is the cause of an acute abnormality. Tumors of the liver, bile ducts, and gallbladder may cause acute abdominal disease by bleeding. Gallstones with bile duct obstruction produce acute abdominal pain and icterus (Fig 19). Emphysematous cholecystitis can be seen as an accompanying lesion of pancreatitis (Fig 20).

Pancreas

The pancreas is afforded protection by the ribs and associated viscera, but when traumatic pancreatitis occurs, the abdominal findings are similar to those described for acute pancreatitis.[4] Pancreatic neoplasms may produce upper gastrointestinal obstruction when they reach sufficient size or invade the duodenum. Ultrasound examination of the pancreas is often more useful than radiography.

Spleen

The spleen is often involved in abdominal trauma. Lesions that can cause acute abdominal signs include volvulus, infarction, and laceration. Splenic volvulus may be recognized radiographically by emphysema in the organ, usually consisting of many small bubbles. Volvulus of the spleen may produce toxemia due to vascular compromise, while lacerations produce either an abdominal mass when a hematoma forms, or free fluid in the peritoneal cavity in the case of hemorrhage. Infectious disorders of the spleen (splenitis) are an infrequent cause of abdominal pain. Tumors of the spleen may cause acute abdominal signs due to bleeding, especially following vigorous abdominal palpation.

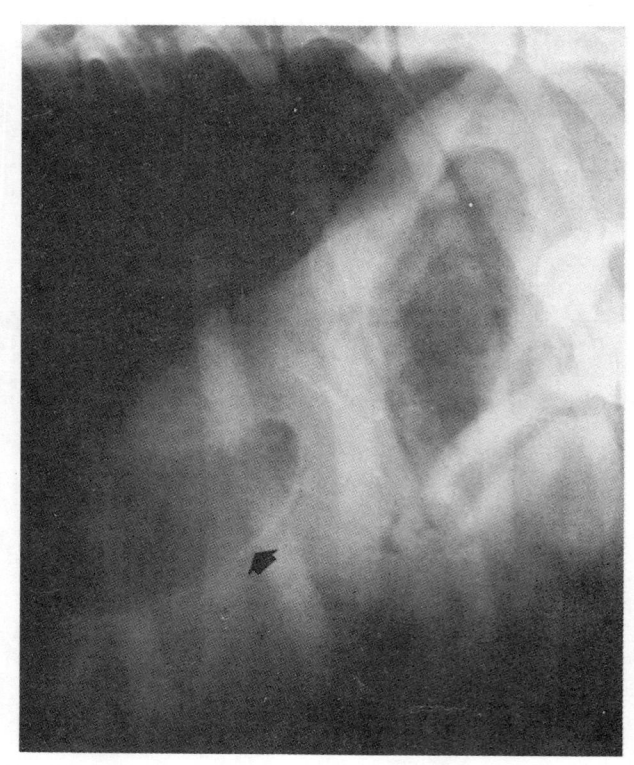

Fig 20—The arrow points to air in the wall of the gallbladder. Intralumenal air was also present in this case of emphysematous cholecystitis in a 6-year-old, male Shepherd-cross dog.

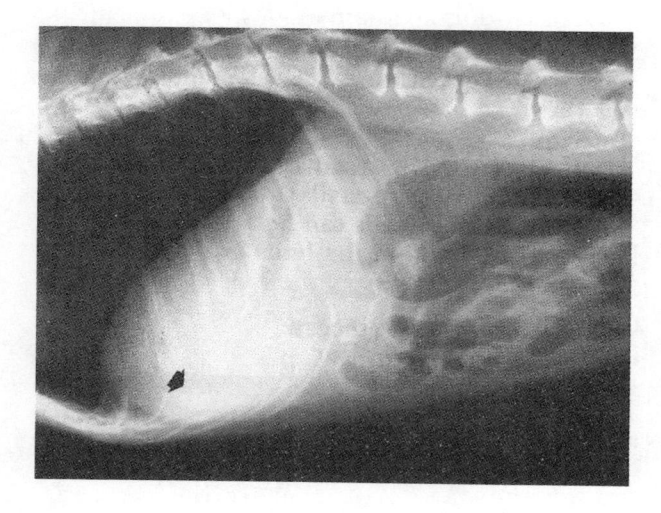

Fig 19—Choleliths are capable of causing cystic duct obstruction and signs of acute pain and jaundice. The arrow points to gallstones in this 7-year-old spayed female cat.

ACKNOWLEDGEMENT

The author gratefully acknowledges the help of Paula Ruel, BSN, RN in the preparation of the manuscript

REFERENCES

1. Dixon JA, et al: Intestinal motility following luminal and vascular occlusion of the small intestine. *Gastroenterology*, 58: 673-678, 1970
2. Donahue JK, Hunter C, Balch HH: Significance of fluid levels in x-ray films of the abdomen. *New Eng J Med* 259: 13-15, 1958
3. Hornbuckle WE, Kleine LL: Obstruction of the small intes-

tine, in Kirk RW, (ed): *Current Veterinary Therapy* VI. Philadelphia, WB Saunders Co., 1977, pp. 952-958.
4. Kleine LJ, Hornbuckle WE: Acute pancreatitis: Radiographic findings in 182 dogs. *J Am Vet Rad Soc* 19: 102-106, 1978.
5. Kleine LJ: Radiographic diagnosis of urinary tract trauma in the dog and cat. *Small Animal Vet Med Update* 7: 1-6, 1978.
6. Kleine LJ: The role of radiography in the diagnosis of intestinal obstruction in dogs and cats. *Compen Contin Educ for Sm An Pract* 1: 44-51, 1979.
7. Laufman H.: Intestinal strangulation fever. *Surg Gynec Obstet* 135: 271-272, 1972.
8. Miller RE, Skucas J.(eds): *Radiographic Contrast Agents*. Baltimore University Park Press, 1977.
9. Osborn D, et al.: The role of angiography in abdominal nonrenal trauma. *Rad Clin No Am* 11: 579-592, 1973.
10. Poole CA, Rowe MI: Clinical evidence of intestinal absorption of gastrografin. *Radiology* 118: 151-153, 1976.
11. Rowe MI, et al. Gastrografin induced hypertonicity: The pathogenesis of neonatal hazard. *Am J Surg* 125: 185-188, 1973.
12. Wolfe DA, Meyer WC: Obstructing intestinal abscess in a dog. *JAVMA* 166: 518-519, 1975.
13. Zheutlin N, Lasser EC, Rigler LG: Clinical studies on effect of barium in the peritoneal cavity following rupture of the colon. *Surg* 32: 967-979, 1952.

Radiologic Aspects of Thoracic Trauma in the Dog and Cat (Part I)

Lawrence J. Kleine, DVM, MS
Associate Professor and Head, Radiology
Tufts University
School of Veterinary Medicine
North Grafton, Massachusetts

Radiology is an important diagnostic tool in the evaluation of thoracic trauma in dogs and cats. It is rapid, nontraumatic and usually easily interpreted. Furthermore, the radiographs form a permanent record which may be used as a basis for checking progress.

Each year about 400 cases of thoracic trauma (1% of all admissions) are seen in our urban practice. Ten percent of these cases die or are euthanatized because of their injuries. Often other major injuries, such as fractures, accompany thoracic trauma. The relative importance of each of the multiple injuries of each individual is determined by an intelligent clinical appraisal, solving the most urgent problem first, followed by the others in a logical sequence. Treatment of life-threatening conditions must take precedence over any diagnostic test. However, treatment can often be undertaken simultaneously with radiography, physical examination and laboratory tests. Gentleness and efficiency are essential in making an accurate and rapid diagnosis.

The basic roentgen signs of thoracic trauma are alterations in density, size, location, shape, and the margin of structures normally located in the thorax, as well as the presence of structures in the thorax which are normally located elsewhere. Decreased radiographic opacity occurs secondary to the presence of air in the subcutaneous tissues or in the pleural, pericardial, or mediastinal spaces. Abnormal soft tissue opacity may occur in the subcutaneous tissues, pleural cavity, or mediastinum due to fluid accumulation.

Atelectasis, edema, or hemorrhage causes increased lung opacity. Intrapericardial fluid will produce a large cardiac silhouette, while the size of the heart may be smaller when there is reduced circulating blood volume. Pulmonary arteries may increase in size proximal to an area of arterial embolism or thrombosis but are generally less prominent in shock.

Technique—Conventional survey radiographs made in the lateral and ventrodorsal or dorsoventral positions are frequently the most accurate and useful diagnostic procedures in thoracic trauma. The standard KVP and MAS x-ray settings for thoracic radiography are used in the initial examination. If a small amount of fluid is present in the lung or pleural cavity, a second radiograph at twice the usual MAS will provide better visualization of thoracic morphology. If a significant amount of the pleural cavity is obliterated by fluid, thoracocentesis should be performed before repeating the radiographs. Better visualization of pneumothorax can be achieved by reducing the MAS to half its usual value. The exposure time of thoracic radiographs should not exceed 1/30th of a second to eliminate unsharpness resulting from cardiac and respiratory motion. Ventrodorsal oblique radiographs demonstrate some rib fractures and esophageal perforations better than conventionally positioned films (Fig 1).

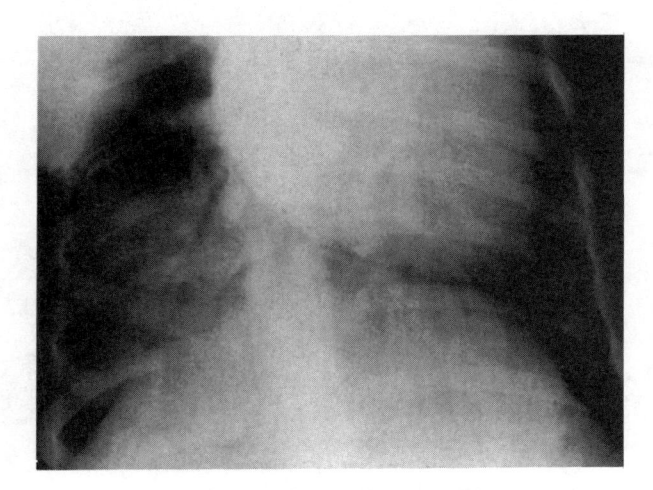

Fig 1—Ventrodorsal oblique radiographs are useful in demonstrating rib fractures because the fractures are displayed over the less dense peripheral lung fields. Fractures of the 7th through 10th right ribs are seen in this dog.

In addition to survey radiographs made with a vertical x-ray beam, certain radiographic aids are available. These include horizontal beam radiography, pleurography and fistulography. Horizontal beam radiography with changes in the animal's posture may be useful in demonstrating whether a density is liquid or solid. For instance, a dog or cat might be placed in sternal, then dorsal recumbency position using a horizontal x-ray beam to make radiographs in each position. Fluid in the pleural cavity is seen in the ventral portion of the thorax in the sternal position and in the dorsal thorax in dorsal recumbency. This technique can also be used to detect small amounts of gas in the pleural cavity. Free gas will always rise to the highest part of the cavity and free fluid will fall to the lowest part. When effusion fills more than about 25% of the pleural cavity, horizontal beam radiography, following withdrawal of fluid, will usually permit better visualization of thoracic viscera.

Contrast Pleurography—Contrast pleurography is not often needed but may occasionally be helpful in delineating pleural and diaphragmatic silhouettes when a diaphragmatic hernia is suspected but cannot be confirmed by noncontrast radiography. A local anesthetic is instilled into the dorsal part of the 7th or 8th interspace, and a short needle is used to enter the pleural space. The needle is aspirated to be sure lung parenchyma has not been punctured. (This test is difficult to evaluate if pneumothorax is present, as air can be aspirated from the pleural space as well as from lung parenchyma.) About one ml of aqueous contrast medium per kg of body weight is instilled (a concentration of about 300 mg of iodine per ml of solution is satisfactory). The animal is then rotated 360° several times to distribute the contrast medium throughout the pleural space. Conventional ventrodorsal and lateral radiographs are made. The coating produced by the procedure outlines the pleural space, defining the otherwise homogenous abdominal viscera which may have herniated into the thoracic cavity. In some cases the contrast medium also enters the abdominal cavity through the diaphragmatic opening.

Fistulography—Fistulography is performed to locate the origin of sinus tracts and to visualize nonopaque foreign bodies which have produced fistulae to the skin. A flexible end-hole catheter whose diameter is large enough to occlude the external opening of the fistula is selected. The catheter is inserted deeply into the tract and viscous contrast medium is injected.[a] Ventrodorsal and lateral radiographs are made as soon as backflow of contrast medium out of the tract is seen. The procedure is not generally useful if there are multiple, large skin openings which cannot be occluded, but discrete tracts which lead to a definitive focus can be effectively outlined.

Esophagram—If an esophagram is needed to evaluate potential perforation, an oily contrast medium intended for bronchographic use is preferred. This medium is considered safer than either barium or the water soluble organic iodides intended for gastrointestinal use, in the event that an esophageal pulmonary fistula is present.[1,4] Water soluble organic iodides are not used because they do not provide satisfactory mucosal coating. Recognition of erosions and ulcerations of the mucosa is important in rendering an accurate prognosis when an esophageal foreign body or other type of perforation is present.

Thoracic Cage—Lesions of the bone and soft tissue of the thoracic cage are usually easily seen and interpreted. However, attention may be drawn to the intrathoracic injury, and damage to the supporting structure may be overlooked. A careful, systematic observation is needed in every case to avoid this common error (Fig 2).

Fractures and dislocations of ribs, and fractures of dorsal spinous processes and scapulae without displacement, can often be treated conservatively, however they should be recognized as significant injuries and a source of pain to the animal. Rib fracture fragments sometimes penetrate either the lung or subcutaneous tissues and skin of the

---

[a]Author's note: Aqueous iodide media can be mixed with KY jelly. However, preferred products are Hypaque 90 (Winthrop Laboratories, New York, NY) or Dionosil (Glaxo).

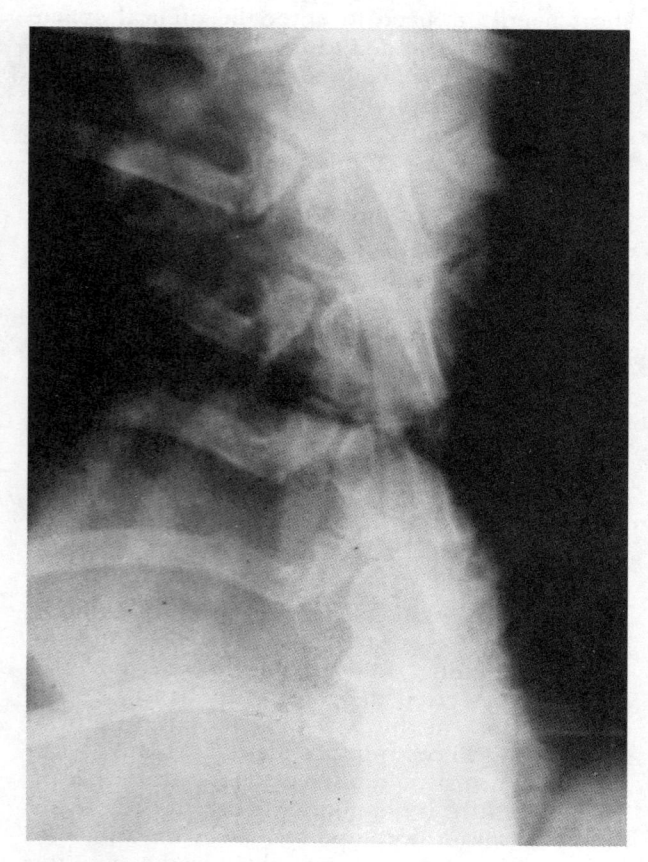

Fig 2—A ventrodorsal radiograph was taken of this dog because the clinician suspected spinal trauma. Fractures of the 7th through 11th right ribs are seen near the costo-vertebral articulation.

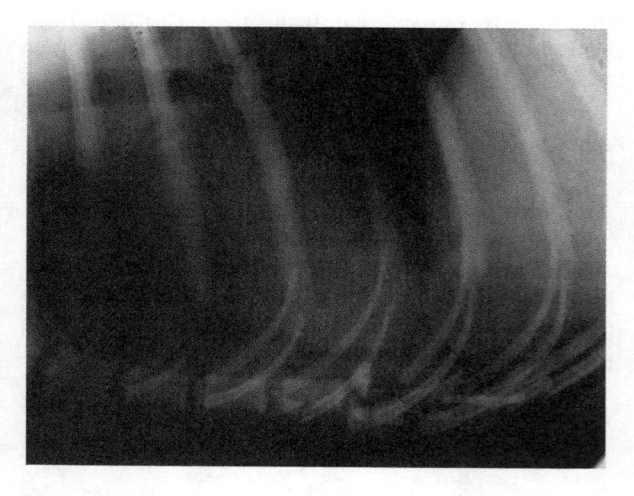

Fig 3—This dog had sternal pain after a fall of 15 feet. There is ventral displacement and fragmentation of the 7th sternebra. Density in the ventral caudal thorax is due to pleural hemorrhage.

thorax resulting in hemo-pneumothorax which must be treated surgically.

When there are multiple segmental rib fractures, a flail chest may develop.[b] This injury is usually a surgical emergency because of the serious degree of pulmonary insufficiency which results. Fractures of the scapulae are seldom seen clearly in thoracic radiographs but are easily diagnosed by a combination of palpation and radiography of the specific area. Sternebrae and vertebral bodies can be dislocated as well as fractured. Pain and swelling are usually the only clinical signs associated with sternebral dislocation; however, sternebral fractures or dislocations may be displaced with enough violence to rupture the internal thoracic vessels causing substantial hemorrhage (Fig 3).

Fractures and dislocations of the thoracic vertebrae are significant findings indicating the need for thorough and sometimes repeated neurologic examination. An accurate prognosis can seldom be based on the radiographic findings alone. Neurological data are generally much more valuable.

---

[b]Editor's note: A flail chest develops when the chest wall is so mobile because of rib fractures, that it moves in a paradoxical fashion on respiration, i.e. the mobile segment moves in on inspiration.

The subcutaneous tissues of the thorax should be scrutinized for evidence of changes in opacity. In the case of breaks in the skin, air may be seen at the site of the puncture, and small amounts of air are often inadvertently introduced by subcutaneous fluid administration. When the cervical trachea is perforated or a large penetrating wound is created in the loose cervical soft tissues, dissecting emphysema may extend into the mediastinum and over the entire body (Fig 4).

Subcutaneous hemorrhage is recognizable as a swelling which has the radiographic opacity of soft tissue, and is most often associated with rib fractures. Teeth, knife fragments, and shotgun pellets are some of the opaque foreign bodies which can be seen in the thoracic cavity or soft tissues surrounding the thorax. Foreign bodies such as wood splinters or plastic which are usually radiolucent can sometimes be seen if they are surrounded by air. More often, however, fistulography is needed.

Intercostal hernia often appears as a uniform soft tissue density outside of and parallel to the rib cage, because the herniated viscus is usually omental or mesenteric fat. If the hernia contains small intestine or colon gas shadows should be seen.

Thoracic Cavity—Radiographic signs of thoracic trauma may be reflected in the pleural cavity by air or fluid accumulation in the pleural or mediastinal spaces. Pneumothorax is commonly seen following thoracic trauma and is often accompanied by pulmonary and pleural hemorrhage. Radiographic recognition of pneumothorax is easiest in the conventional lateral view. When the dog or cat lies on its side, air in the thoracic cavity rises to the highest point. In so doing, the heart and unexpanded lungs are displaced downward. This phenomenon separates the heart from the sternum so that air is seen ventral to the cardiac silhouette.

In the ventrodorsal view small amounts of air will rise to occupy the retrosternal area without

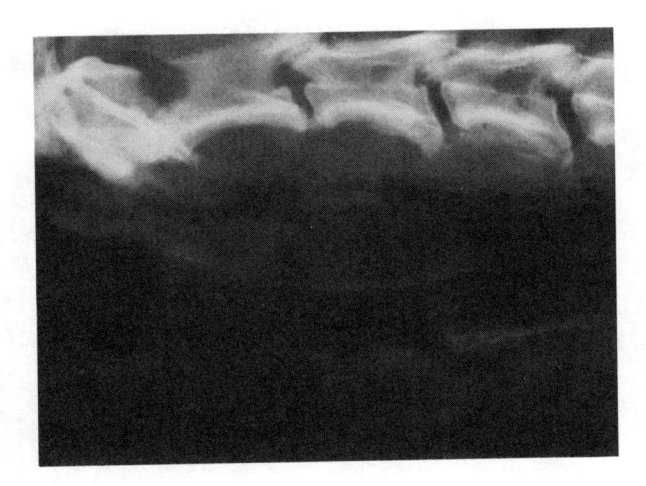

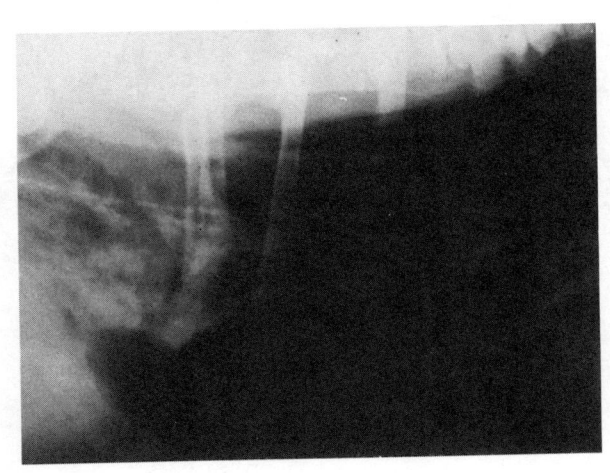

Fig 4A, B—The ventral trachea was torn by a bite wound resulting in separation of the tracheal rings and extensive subcutaneous and mediastinal emphysema in this dog.

being seen in the peripheral lung fields. In the horizontal beam lateral view air rises to the dorsal part of the thoracic cavity depressing the dorsal portion of the lungs. When a small amount of pneumothorax is suspected, a high intensity light may be useful to examine the areas of the lung for peripheral pulmonary vessels. If vessels can be identified in the peripheral lung fields, and the lungs are normally expanded, pneumothorax is probably not present. When the lungs are atelectatic because of elevated intrathoracic pressure, the visceral pleural surfaces are often seen more clearly than usual because of the air surrounding the lung and the outlining of the pleura which results.

Generally pneumothorax is a self-limiting process. The elevated intrathoracic pressure produces a tamponade effect. When the air leak has sealed, pneumothorax is dramatically reduced within 72 hours. The source of pneumothorax is seldom identifiable at the time of injury. Ordinarily the mediastinum in the dog and cat does not prevent the free passage of air from one side of the thorax to the other; therefore, unilateral pneumothorax is rarely seen.

Pneumomediastinum—Pneumomediastinum can occur secondary to a penetrating wound at the thoracic inlet, tracheal penetration due to trauma, (Fig 5) or instrumentation or dissection of air through the anatomical openings in the diaphragm, when extensive pneumoretroperitoneum is present'. Pneumomediastinum is recognized radiographically by clear outlining of mediastinal structures which are not usually seen, such as the esophagus, brachiocephalic, left subclavian and azygos vessels. Pneumomediastinum is seldom associated with any clinical signs and when the air leak is eliminated, the lesion usually resolves in 48 to 72 hours.

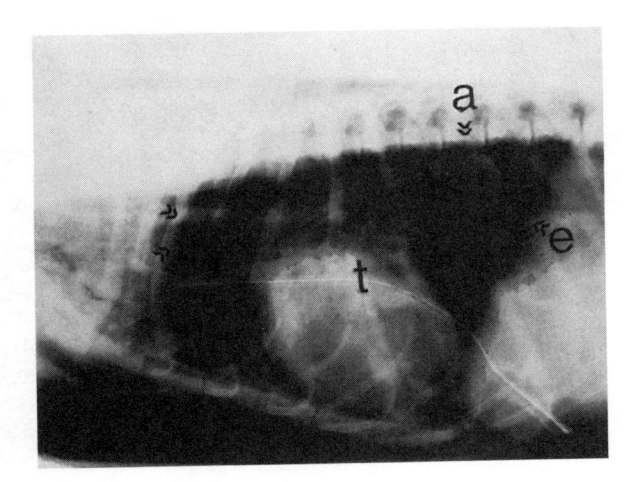

Fig 5—The recognition of pneumomediastinum depends upon visualization of both walls of the trachea (arrows), the aorta (A), and the esophagus (E). Occasionally the azygos vein is also seen. A thoracic drain tube (T) has been used to remove pleural hemorrhage.

Pleural effusion, regardless of its cause, is recognized radiographically by increased opacity and widening of the pleural space. When the effusion is slight, the only radiographic signs may be increased visualization of interlobar fissures and the rounding of the lung margin in the costophrenic angle in the ventrodorsal view. These minor changes are best seen when the radiograph is exposed on expiration. In the conventional lateral thoracic radiograph, fluid will flow to the lowest part of the thorax, obscuring the lung fields in this area.

The fluid will generally be seen dorsal to the caudal lung lobes in this view. When an x-ray film is exposed with the horizontal beam, the dorsal margin of the fluid level generally has a scalloped appearance unless pneumothorax is also present, in which case the fluid level will be horizontal and even. Plueral blood, bile, transudate and exudate can usually not be distinguished from one another on the basis of their radiographic appearance.

Cranial mediastinal hemorrhage often occurs

'Editor's note: Two additional causes of pneumomediastinum are perforation of the esophagus and the escape of intrapulmonary air dissecting along bronchi into the mediastinum.

along with pulmonary and pleural hemorrhage. Occasionally, however, hemorrhage or effusion is the only indication of thoracic injury and may be due to either blunt trauma or penetration of the esophagus near the heart base. Radiographic findings in either case are widening and increased density in the cranial mediastinum, blending with and obsuring the cranial aspect of the cardiac silhouette. Both pleural and mediastinal hemorrhage may mimic masses and other effusions. Therefore, thoracocentesis is often needed for definitive diagnosis.

REFERENCES

1. Chiu, C.L. and Gambach, R.R.: Hypaque Pulmonary Edema: A case report. Radiology, 111 (1974); 91-92.
2. Genereux, G.P.: The End-Stage Lung. Radiology, 116 (1975): 279-289.
3. Lord, P.F., Greiner, T.P., Greene, R.W. and DeHoff, W.D.: Lung Lobe Torsion in the Dog. JAAHA, 9 (1973): 473-482.
4. Reich, S.B.: Production of Pulmonary Edema by Aspiration of Water-Soluble Nonabsorbable Contrast Media. Radiology, 92 (1969): 367-370.

Radiologic Aspects of Thoracic Trauma in the Dog and Cat (Part II)

Lawrence J. Kleine, DVM, MS
Associate Professor and Head, Radiology
Tufts University
School of Veterinary Medicine
North Grafton, Massachusetts

Upper Airway—Occasionally, respiratory distress is associated with upper airway trauma. The degree of respiratory difficulty associated with tracheal or bronchial obstruction is directly related to the degree and level of obstruction. Complete obstruction of the trachea will result in death within minutes while partial bronchial obstruction may produce no clinical or radiographic signs.

Radiographic evidence of obstruction is primarily interruption of the air density in the trachea or major bronchi. Foreign bodies (Fig 6) and blood are common causes of airway obstruction. Foreign bodies such as plastic, which are normally radiolucent, may be seen because of the contrast provided by the surrounding air. Tracheal stenosis following tracheal injury is an infrequent cause of airway obstruction (Fig 7). Traumatic tracheal stenosis can result from overinflation of the cuff of an endotracheal tube with secondary vascular compromise, necrosis and scar tissue formation.

Lung—Some pulmonary abnormalities associated with trauma are intrapulmonary hemorrhage, pulmonary collapse, lung lobe torsion, electric shock and formation of tracheoesophageal fistulae. Trauma to the lung can range from a small localized contusion without clinical signs to massive laceration which produces rapid atelectasis and exsanguination due to pneumothorax and hemorrhage.

Pulmonary Hemorrhage—Pulmonary hemorrhage is the most common radiologic diagnosis following thoracic trauma. Radiographically, it appears as a focal increase in opacity of lung parenchyma with the presence of air bronchograms.

Since the radiographic changes are due to fluid accumulation within the air spaces, they cannot be radiographically distinguished from inflammatory lung disease. In single acute episodes of hemorrhage, the radiographic abnormalities usually resolve in 48 to 72 hours. Persistence of the radiographic changes for a longer period of time indicates continued bleeding or superimposition of inflammatory lung disease.

Lobar Collapse—Lobar collapse most often occurs as the result of the presence of space occupying material (air, fluid, mass) in the pleural space, but may also result from bronchial obstruction due to blood accumulation or foreign material within a bronchus, or lung torsion.

Lobar Torsion—Lung lobe torsion usually occurs in deep-chested dogs, but can occur in any dog or cat.[3] The left cranial and right middle lobes are most frequently involved. There is often a history of trauma or a long-standing pleural effusion. The clinical signs are ambiguous and may not be severe enough to cause the owner to seek veterinary aid until the lesion has been present for several days or weeks. Lung torsion is nearly always accompanied by trapped clotted blood in the pleural space. The twisted lung lobe is usually totally consolidated and increased in size. Air bronchograms are usually not seen within the affected lobe.

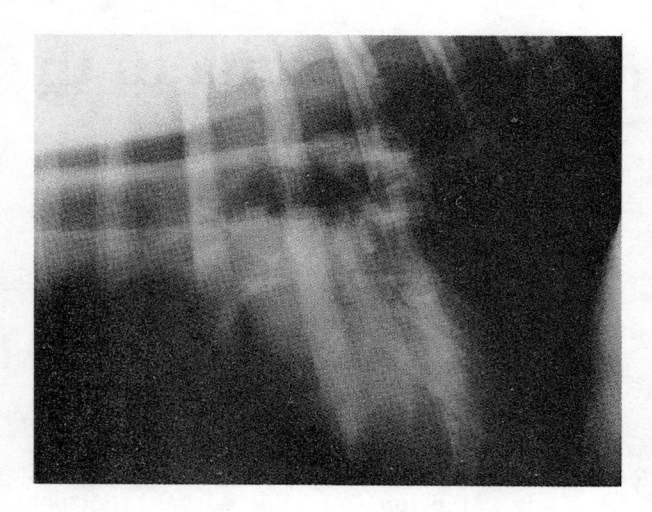

Fig 6—An oval density lies dorsal to the left atrium interrupting the air pattern of the distal trachea. Moderate dyspnea and coughing were prominent clinical signs in this dog. The oval density was an acorn.

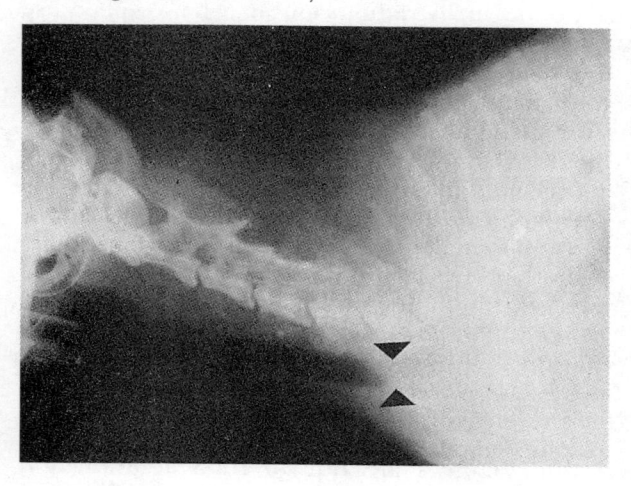

Fig 7—This radiograph was made two weeks following an episode of pneumomediastinum which had resolved. At the time of this radiograph the cat was mildly dyspneic. The arrows outline a stenotic area of the trachea which was presumed to be the site of the previous tracheal rupture which had lead to pneumomediastinum.

Electric Shock—Severe electric shock produces pulmonary edema which is frequently confined to the caudal lung lobes. Within 48 to 72 hours the lungs will become normal unless secondary infection occurs.

Tracheo-esophageal Fistulae—Tracheo-esophageal fistulae are rare. They may be congenital or acquired. Acquired trancheo-esophageal fistulae may be associated with external trauma, or more likely, chronic esophageal inflammation secondary to penetration by an esophageal foreign body. Contrast esophagraphy is necessary to confirm the diagnosis. In doing so, one must be aware that both the barium and aqueous iodide contrast agents can produce serious lung damage. Therefore a medium which is intended for bronchographic use should be employed.

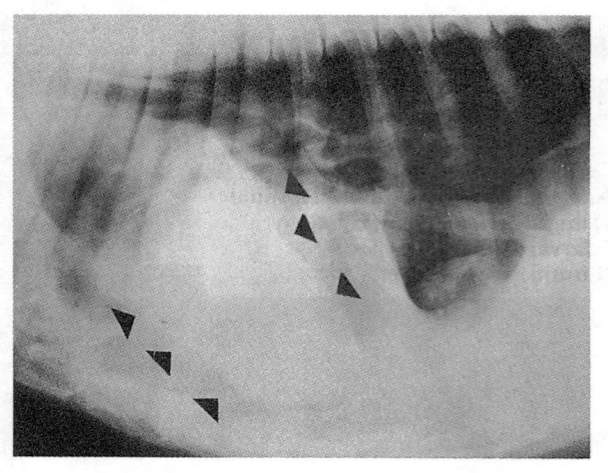

Fig 8—Lung lobe torsion usually produces pleural effusion and consolidation of the affected lobe. In this case, the left cranial middle lobe was involved. (arrows)

Inhalation Injuries—In addition to external trauma, the lung can be injured by inhalation of noxious gases or aspiration of foreign material. The quantity of material inhaled or aspirated, its irritative properties, and the presence of concomitant disease determine the severity of the radiographic signs (Fig 9). Both the physical character and the force of inhalation determine the location of the inhaled substance in the airways. Generally the dependent portions of the caudal and middle lung lobes are most severely affected.

While inhalation of solid or liquid can occur secondary to vomiting or regurgitation due to any cause, it is most often associated with esophageal paralysis, cricopharyngeal achalasia, or a persistent vascular ring at the heart base causing esophageal dilation. Occasionally solid or liquid medication or food is inhaled because of struggling during misguided efforts to force feed a dog or cat.

Smoke or hydrocarbon inhalation may not produce any radiographic signs in spite of clinical evidence of moderate dyspnea. Early radiographic changes are usually confined to the bronchial tree. Later, interstitial opacities may be prominent and, in severe cases, pulmonary edema may follow.

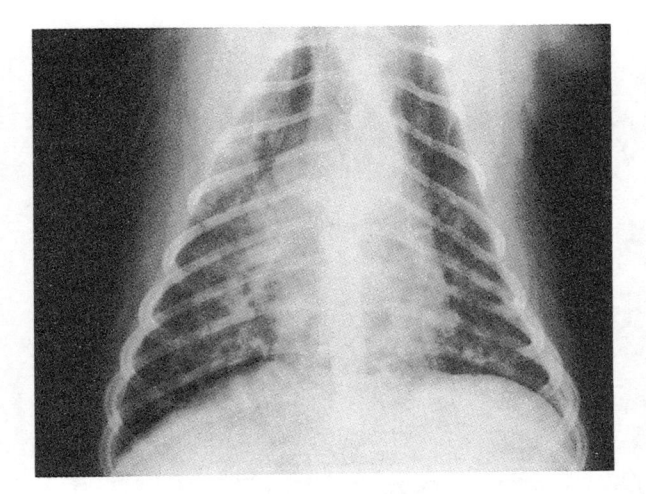

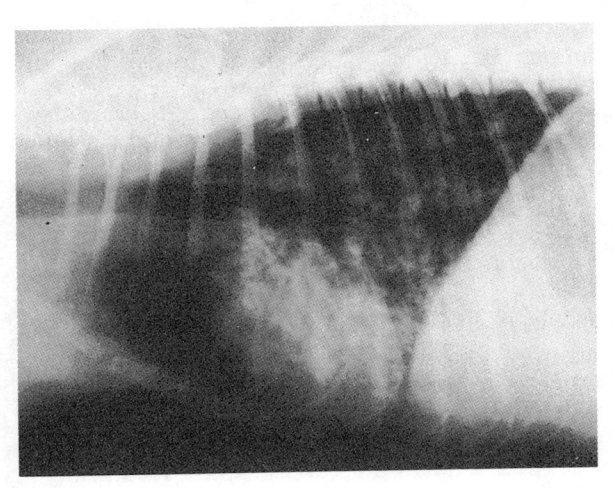

Fig 9A and B—Uniform linear densities producing pulmonary consolidation were seen in this four-year-old dog after it inhaled a saturated salt solution. The owner administered the solution to induce vomiting in the dog because of possible toxin ingestion.

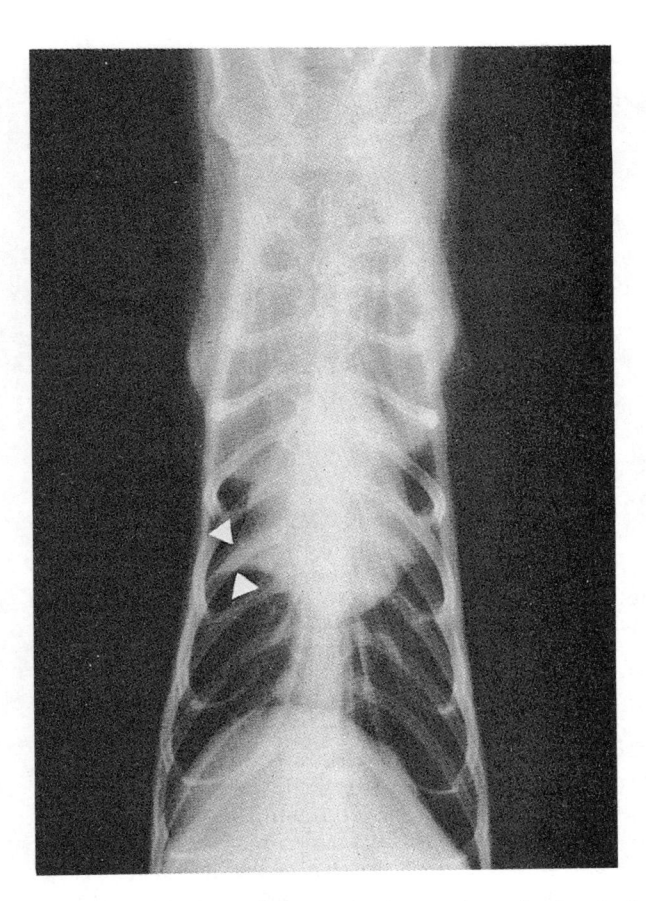

Fig 10—The triangular opacity (arrows) at the level of the right middle lung lobe is the result of atelectasis and pleural adhesions. These lesions were secondary to pleural and pulmonary hemorrhage three weeks earlier. (Editor's note: Without confirming evidence, this radiographic appearance is consistent with collapse of the right middle lung lobe, as well as the diagnosis of pleural adhesions.)

Esophagus—Blunt thoracic trauma rarely causes esophageal injury. The most common type of esophageal trauma is secondary to foreign body ingestion. Foreign bodies which are radiolucent may be seen if they are surrounded by intra-esophageal air. Esophageal foreign bodies usually cause the clinical signs of salivation, dysphagia, and regurgitation, but occasionally the only clinical sign is anorexia, and the clinician does not suspect the foreign body which is found incidentally by thoracic radiography.

Esophageal perforation results in esophageal contents entering the mediastinum or pleural space. Fluid in the pleural space leads to opacification of the interlobar fissures and blunting of the costophrenic angles.

Both of these phenomena are best seen in the ventrodorsal projection. Mediastinitis, pyothorax, and septicemia may occur soon after esophageal perforation. Esophageal scarring with subsequent stenosis may occur after esophageal surgery or endoscopic removal of a foreign body.

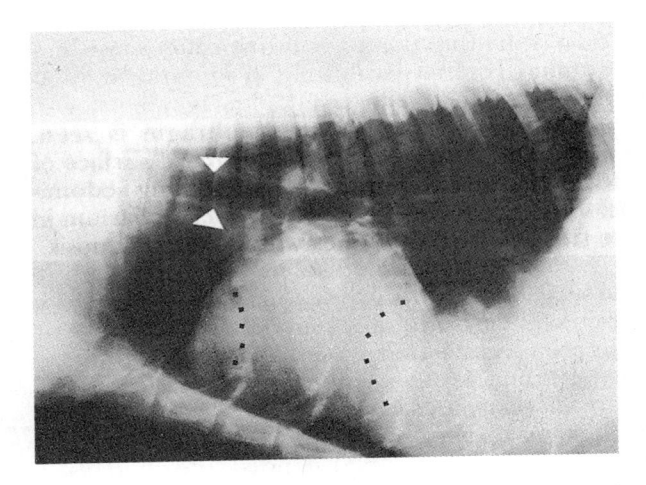

Fig. 11—Pneumomediastinum (arrows) and a wide, lobular ventral cardiac silhouette were the radiographic abnormalities in this seven-year-old spayed German Shepherd dog. The lobular appearance was due to the spleen which had passed through a diaphragmatic rupture and enveloped the heart (dotted lines).

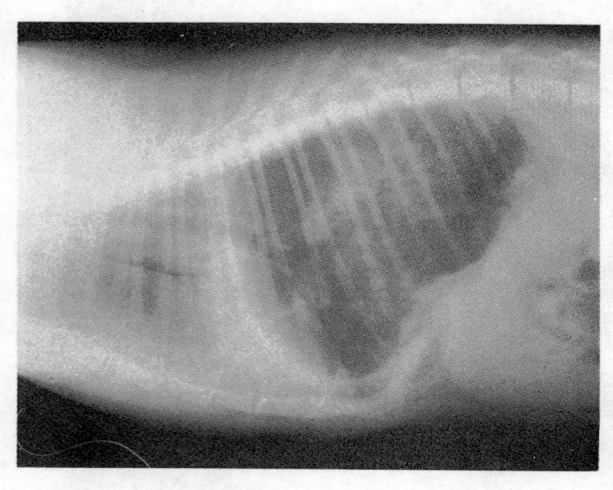

Fig 12—A large gas shadow cranial to the level of the diaphragm obliterates the heart in this five-month-old female cat. The gas is contained in a distended stomach which has passed through a ruptured diaphragm. The degree of distension suggests obstruction of the pylorus or proximal small intestine.

Diaphragm—Diaphragmatic hernia is probably the most common thoracic injury which requires surgical correction. The tear in the diaphragm may be so small as to be an incidental finding at necropsy, or so large as to permit passage of nearly all the freely movable abdominal viscera into the thoracic cavity.

Diagnosis of a diaphragmatic hernia may be easily made radiographically due to the presence of abdominal viscera in the pleural space. However, if incarceration of an organ such as omentum or liver occurs, secondary pleural effusion may obliterate the herniated organs. For this reason, repeat radiography of the thorax after thoracocentesis may be helpful if pleural effusion is significant. If sufficient fluid cannot be withdrawn to permit visualization of the caudal mediastinum and ventral diaphragm, horizontal beam radiography with the patient in dorsal recumbency may allow better visualization of the area in question. In instances where effusion is not present, but an irregularity of the diaphragm is seen, pleurography may outline the thoracic surface of the diaphragm along with any protruding abdominal viscera. Barium in the stomach and intestines will aid the diagnosis if they are herniated.

Identification of the displaced organs may give the surgeon an estimate of the size of the diaphragmatic tear (Fig 11). Also, some diaphragmatic hernias are surgical emergencies (Fig 12). For instance, if the stomach or intestine is incarcerated in the thoracic cavity and greatly distended, the abdominal viscus may become infarcted and perforate. Also the distended stomach or intestine may produce pulmonary insufficiency due to encroachment upon the lung.

Heart and Thoracic Vessels—Myocardial contusions, infarctions and a small volume of in-

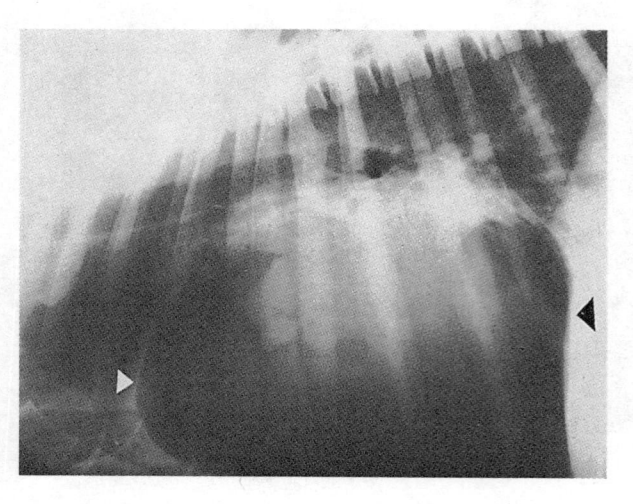

Fig 13—This three-year-old male Beagle developed severe cough with hemoptysis after a day of hunting. Hemorrhagic pericardial effusion was withdrawn and these radiographs were made. The arrows point to the margins of the air distended pericardium. A stick had been inhaled, penetrated the left mainstem bronchus and the left auricular appendage producing the hemorrhagic pericardial effusion. The hole in the left auricular appendage had sealed but when the effusion was relieved, air filled the pericardium through the bronchial-pericardial fistula.

trapericardial fluid do not result in detectable radiographic changes. Except in extreme instances, cardiac and great vessel trauma is difficult to recognize on survey radiographs. Exceptions include large volume pericardial effusion, pneumopericardium, rupture of a cardiac chamber, and aneurysm.

Hemopericardium can result from rupture of a cardiac chamber due to blunt trauma, instrumentation, chronic mitral regurgitation, or rupture of blood vessels in the epicardium or pericardium. The heart generally assumes a spherical configuration in these cases. If there is a single episode of bleeding which is arrested, considerable reduction in the size of the cardiac silhouette occurs in 48 to 72 hours. Massive hemopericardium can result in cardiac failure and death due to tamponade.

Pneumopericardium is the result of communication between the pericardium and a positive pressure air source, such as a bronchial-pericardial fistula or introduction of air during pericardiocentesis (Fig 13) or traumatic air passage from a hilar bronchus into the pericardium.

REFERENCES

1. Chiu, C.L. and Gambach, R.R.: Hypaque Pulmonary Edema: A case report. Radiology, 111, (1974):91-92.
2. Genereux, G.P.: The End-Stage Lung. Radiology, 116, (1975):225-289.
3. Lord, P.F., Greiner, T.P., Greene, R.W. and DeHoff, W.D.: Lung Lobe Torsion in the Dog. JAAHA, 9, (1973):473-482.
4. Reich, S.B.: Production of Pulmonary Edema by Aspiration of Water-Soluble Nonabsorable Contrast Media. Radiology, 92, (1969):367-370.

Acute Gastroenteritis *(continued from page 310)*

rospective investigation were Great Dane, Weimaraner, Saint Bernard, Gordon Setter, and Irish Setter.

ACUTE PANCREATITIS

This disorder is notoriously difficult to diagnose in both dogs and cats. Recently, a sensitive and specific immunoassay for trypsin-like immunoreactivity (TLI) has been developed and appears to be a useful serologic marker for acute pancreatitis in the cat.[4] In one clinical study,[5] cats with acute pancreatitis had significantly elevated serum TLI when compared to healthy cats or to cats ill with other diseases. Also of interest, none of the 12 cats with pancreatitis in this study had elevations in serum amylase or lipase concentrations.

Other investigators[6] are evaluating the clinical utility of urine trypsin activation peptide (TAP) by ELISA in diagnosing canine pancreatitis.

REFERENCES

1. Murtaugh RJ, Herring DS, Jacobs RM, et al: Pancreatic ultrasonography in dogs with experimentally induced acute pancreatitis. *Vet Radiol* 26:27-32, 1985.
2. Glickman LT, Glickman NW, Perez CM, et al: Analysis of risk factors for gastric dilatation and dilatation-volvulus in dogs. *JAVMA* 204:1465-1471, 1994.
3. Hall JA, Willer RL, Seim HB, et al: Gross and histologic evaluation of hepatogastric ligaments in clinically normal dogs and dogs with gastric dilatation-volvulus. *Am J Vet Res* 56:1611-1614, 1995.
4. Medlinger TL, Burchfield T, Williams DA: Assay of trypsin-like immunoreactivity (TLI) in feline serum. *J Vet Intern Med* 7:133, 1993.
5. Parent C, Washabau RJ, Williams DA, et al: Serum trypsin-like immunoreactivity, amylase, and lipase in the diagnosis of feline acute pancreatitis. *Am J Vet Intern Med* 9:144, 1995.
6. Williams DA, Melgarejo T, Henderson J, et al: Serum trypsin-like immunoreactivity (TLI), trypsinogen activation peptides (TAP), amylase, and lipase in canine experimental pancreatitis. *J Vet Intern Med* 10:159, 1996.

INDEX

A

Abdominal
  disorders, acute, 336–351
  trauma, 58–59
Acute renal failure (ARF), 261, 311–335
  drugs used, 329
  ischemic, 312–313
  nephrotoxic, 313–314
  protective agents used, 317
Adenosine nucleotides, 319–320
Afterdrop, temperature, 268
Airway obstruction, 227–232
Allopurinol, 77, 144, 319
Analgesia, 95, 185, 253, 280, 282–288
  guidelines for administration, 286–287
Anaphylaxis, 122, 182–183
Anesthesia, 78
Angiography, 340
Angiotensin converting enzyme (ACE) inhibitors, 28, 322
Anthropomorphism, 279
Antibiotic drugs, 116, 125, 185, 294, 301–302, 308
Antibodies, venom, 181
Anticoagulant intoxication, 133
Antiemetics, 309
Antifreeze consumption, 159–162
Antimicrobial agents. See Antibiotic drugs
Antioxidant drugs, 77
Antiplatelet drugs, 35
Antivenin, 182–183
Aortic thromboembolism, 29–36
Apnea, 68
Apneustic respiration, 68, 80
Arginine supplementation, 8
Arterial blood gas analysis, 50, 53–54, 59, 73, 97, 337
Arteriotomy, 33
Aspirin, 19, 35–36, 38
Ataxia, 159, 204
Ataxic respiration, 68, 80
Atrial natriuretic peptide (ANP), 318
Azotemia, 164, 326

B

Bacterial infection, life-threatening. See Systemic inflammatory response syndrome (SIDS)
β-adrenergic-blocking drugs (BABD), 18, 115, 320
Barbiturates, 76–77
Barium enemas, 338–339
Bicarbonate. See Sodium bicarbonate
Biopsies, 332
Bladder
  rupture, 58, 94, 97, 105
  tube graft, 107
Blood
  coagulation pathways, 170
  culture samples, 294
  gas analysis, arterial, 50, 53–54, 59, 73, 97, 337
  pressure, 117, 258
  transfusions, 114, 132–137, 182
    determining need for, 133
Borborygmi, 95
Brachycephalic airway syndrome, 228–229
Bradykinin activity of venoms, 169
Brain injury, 63–83
  drugs used, 72
  therapeutic flowchart, 71
Bronchodilators, 239

C

Calcium channel blockers, 13, 18, 28, 35, 38, 43–45, 77–78, 319
Capnography, 73
Captopril, 18, 322
Carbon monoxide poisoning, 234
Cardiac
  activity of venoms, 170–172
  arrhythmia, 15, 28, 95, 116–117, 164
Cardiogenic shock, 110–111, 120
Cardiomyopathy, 10, 29–31
  dilated, 30–31
  with excessive moderator bands, 31–32
  hypertrophic (HCM), 10, 12–20, 30–31
  restrictive, 31–32
Cardiopulmonary resuscitation (CPR), 269
Cardiovascular support, 294–297, 302
Catheterization, posttrauma, 103, 105–107
Central venous pressure monitoring, 117–118, 123–124
Cerebellar trauma, 64
Cerebral
  edema, 64–65, 157
  hemispheric damage, focal, 63
  hemorrhage, 64–65
Cerebrospinal fluid analysis, 195, 204
Cheyne-Stokes respiration, 68
Cholecalciferol intoxication, 163–166
Cholecystography, 340
Chylothorax, 242
Circulatory
  failure, 121
  stasis, 31
Clotting abnormalities, 297
Coagulative properties of venoms, 172–173
Coagulopathies, 132–133
Coma, 80
Coma scale, 72
Computed tomography (CT), 69, 83, 99–101, 195, 209, 326
Congestive heart failure (CHF), 8–9, 22–28
Consciousness, level of, 66–67, 80, 266
Convulsions, 157
Core temperature, 259, 262
  rewarming options, 269–270
Corneal
  laceration, 214–217
  ulcer, deep, 215
Corticosteroid drugs, 41–43, 52–53, 74, 83, 115, 125–129, 165, 183–185, 234–239, 253
Coxofemoral luxations, 84–91
Crackles, 15
Craniotomy, 79
Crystalloid administration, 114, 123–124, 128–129, 296
Cystoscopy, 99
Cystostomy, 103–104, 107
Cystourethrography, positive-contrast retrograde, 98

D

Decerebrate rigidity, 68, 80
Decompression of spinal cord, 40
Deferoxamine, 77, 144
DeVita pin, 86–87
Dexamethasone, 41
Dialysis, 311, 332
Diarrhea, 303–304, 330–331
Diazepam, 157, 199, 207, 209, 286
Dietary
  indiscretion, 304
  protein, 318

Diltiazem, 18, 38
Dimethyl sulfoxide (DMSO), 43, 76, 144
Distributive shock, 110–111
Diuresis, osmotic, 43, 159, 252–253, 318
Dobutamine, 296–297
Dopamine, 45, 115, 297, 330
Dyspnea, 52, 95
    acute, 15
    expiratory, 228

E

Echinocytosis, 188
Echocardiography, 34, 117
Ectoparasitic control, 154–157
Edema, 23
    cerebral, 64–65, 157
    pulmonary, 15, 34, 53
Electrical shock, 237, 358
Electrocardiography (ECG), 25, 28, 34, 52, 99, 268
    abnormalities seen in, 266
    continuous, 258
Electroencephalography (EEG), 179, 203
Electrolyte imbalance, 164, 315
Electromyography, 99
ELISA kit for venom identification, 188
Embolectomy, 33, 38
Encephalopathy, 195
Endocardial damage, 31
Endophthalmitis, 216
Endoscopy, 229
Endothelium-derived relaxing factor (EDRF), 7–10
    nonendothelial agents mimicking EDRF effects, 8–9
Enteral feeding, 298–299
Epileptiform seizures, 66. *See also* Seizure disorders
Epinephrine, 239
Epistaxis, 132, 134, 229
Esophageal foreign bodies, 359
Esophagraphy, 353
Ethanol administration, 160–161
Ethical responsibility, 278–279
Ethylene glycol consumption, 159–162, 314, 327
Evaporative cooling technique, 262

F

Facial trauma, 56–57
Fasting, 304
Fecal cytology, 305
Feline asthma, 239
    drugs used, 240
Fentanyl, 53, 284–285
Fetal death, 349
Fibrinolytic-producing pathways in snakebite, 171
Fibrosis
    interstitial, 13
    pulmonary, 50
Fistulography, 353
Flail chest, 245, 248–258
Fluid replacement therapy, 52, 73, 83, 114–115, 122–123, 181–182, 252, 296, 306–308, 327–335
    cautions regarding, 263
    hypertonic saline solutions, 114, 124, 127–129
    intraosseous infusion, 147–153
Fly biting, 203
Focal seizures, 194, 202
Foreign bodies
    esophageal, 359
    tracheal, 228
Furosemide, 17, 27–28, 76, 165, 252, 330

G

Gastric lavage, 326
Gastroenteritis, acute, 303–309
    common causes, 304
    drugs used, 307
Gastrointestinal hemorrhage, 132, 134
Glaucoma, acute, 217–218
Glucocorticoid drugs. *See* Corticosteroid drugs
Glutathione peroxidase, 143–144

H

Head trauma, 63–83
Healing, 103, 105, 109
Heart failure
    congestive (CHF), 8–9, 22–28
    noncongestive, 24
Heat syncope, 275
Heatstroke. *See* Hyperthermia
Hematuria, 97, 105, 326
Hemiparesis, 63
Hemolytic activity of venoms, 171
Hemopericardium, 360
Hemoptysis, 235
Hemorrhage, 128, 131–137
    cerebral, 64–65
    gastrointestinal, 132, 134
    pulmonary, 357
Hemothorax, 242
Heparin, 10, 297
Hepatic
    damage, heatstroke-induced, 261
    encephalopathy, 195
Hepatotoxicity, 197
Hernia
    diaphragmatic, 242, 254, 343, 360
    small bowel, 344
Hetastarch administration, 83, 114, 124, 129, 252, 258, 296
High-rise syndrome, 56–61
Hindlimb paralysis, 15–16, 30
Hip luxations, 84–91
Histamine activity of venoms, 169
Hydrochlorothiazide, 18
Hypercalcemia, 163–164, 177
Hyperemia, 213
Hyperkalemia, 38, 177, 272, 325–326, 328
Hyperoxygenation, 72
Hyperphosphatemia, 163–164
Hypertension, 7
Hyperthermia, 259–263, 272–276
Hypertonic solution administration
    glucose, 330
    sodium, 114, 124, 127–129, 132
Hypertrophic cardiomyopathy (HCM), 10, 12–20, 30–31
Hyperventilation, 68
Hyphema, 219
Hypocalcemia, 274
Hypokalemia, 274–275
Hypoplasia, tracheal, 228
Hypoproteinemia, 168
Hypotension, 297
Hypothermia, 265–270
Hypoventilation, 49, 72
Hypovolemic shock, 72, 110–111, 120–132, 149, 181, 275
Hypoxemia, 49, 51–52, 227–232
Hypoxia, 72, 140, 143, 229, 234

I

Inflammatory disease. *See* Systemic inflammatory response syndrome (SIDS)

Insecticides, 154–157
International Association of the Study of Pain, 279
Intoxicants
    anticoagulant rodenticides, 133
    cholecalciferol rodenticides, 163–166
    ethylene glycol, 159–162, 314, 327
    mushrooms, 190–192
    pyrethrin/pyrethroid insecticides, 154–157
Intracranial
    neoplasias, 204
    pressure, elevated, 65, 79, 270
Intraosseous infusion, 147–153, 293
    catheter placement, 152
Intubation, 53
Intussusception, 344–346
Iridocyclitis, acute, 218–219
Ischemia, 139–146
Ischemic
    neuromyopathy, 34
    neuropathy, 33
Isoproterenol, 239

J

Jacksonian seizure, 202–203
Jejunal feeding, 297, 299

K

Keratitis, ulcerative, 216
Kinin-producing pathways in snakebite, 171

L

Laparoscopy, 99, 101
Laparotomy, 103
Laryngeal paralysis, 228
Lazaroids, 144
Left ventricular dysfunction, 14
Lens luxation, 216
Level of consciousness, 66–67, 80, 266
Lidocaine, 116
Lipids, dietary, 322–323
Lobular collapse, 357
Low-recording thermometer, 268
Lung sounds, abnormal, 15
Luxations, 57–61
    hip, 84–91
    lens, 216
Lymphosarcoma, 228

M

Magnetic resonance imaging (MRI), 69, 101, 195, 209
Mannitol, 75–76
Mechanical ventilation, 53
Methocarbamol, 157
Methylprednisolone, 41, 44–45, 74–75
4-methylpyrazole, 161–162
Mitral
    regurgitation, 14
    valvular insufficiency, 24
Morphine sulfate, 34, 36, 53, 283–284
Muscle tissue effects of snakebite, 176–177
Musculoskeletal injuries, 57–58
Mushroom consumption, 190–192
Mycetismus, 190–192
Myocardial
    contusions, 52
    hypertrophy, 13–14

N

Naloxone hydrochloride, 43, 77, 116, 285
Neoplasias, intracranial, 204
Nephrography, 340
Neurogenic shock, 111
Neuromyopathy, ischemic, 29, 33–34
Neuropathy, 155–156
    ischemic, 33
Neurotoxic effects of snakebite, 175–176
Nitrate therapy, 7–10
Nitrovasodilators, 8–10
Noncongestive heart failure, 24
Nonglucocorticoid aminosteroids, 144
Nonsteroidal antiinflammatory drugs (NSAIDs), 285–286, 315
Nutritional support, 299, 307–308, 332

O

Obstructive shock, 120
Old dog cough, 10
Oliguria, 330
Ophthalmic emergencies, 210–224
    adnexal injuries, 212–214, 220–221
    injuries to the globe, 214–219, 222–224
Ophthalmoscopy, indirect, 224
Opioids, 53, 282–285, 308
Opisthotonos, 194
Optic neuritis, 224
Oral trauma, 56–57
Osmotic diuresis, 43, 159, 252–253, 318
Oximetry, pulse, 52, 258
Oxygen
    free-radical-induced brain injury, 65–66, 77
    supplementation, 72–73, 233–239, 268, 297–298

P

Pain, 281
    management, 278–289
Panting response, 259, 261
Paracentesis, needle, 98, 337
Paradoxic motion, 245–246, 253
Parenchymal disease, 232–241
    drugs used, 238
Pelvic fractures, 93–101
    soft tissue injuries, 94, 96
Pentastarch administration, 124, 129
Peripheral nerve damage, 94–96
Peritoneal
    fluid analysis, 99
    lavage, 98, 297
Peritonitis, 301
Phenobarbital, 196–197, 206, 209
Phospholipase A_2 activity of venoms, 169
Pin selection, 86–89
Pinning, 58
Plasma transfusions, 115, 124, 135, 182, 302
Platelet
    disorders, 132–133
    hyperreactivity, 31
Pleural cavity disease, 93, 241–244
Pleurography, contrast, 353
Pneumomediastinum, 355
Pneumonia, 232–235
    aspiration, 234
Pneumothorax, 48, 51, 93, 241–242, 354–355
Positive-contrast retrograde
    cystourethrography, 98
    urethrography, 106, 108
Postrenal azotemia, 326

Potassium bromide, 209
Prednisolone, 41
Prerenal azotemia, 326
Propranolol, 38
Proptosis, reduction of, 213–215
Prostaglandin activity of venoms, 169, 186
Prostatic enlargement, 348
Pulmonary
    contusion, 48–54, 93, 234–235, 250
    edema, 15, 34, 53, 235–239, 275, 358
    hemorrhage, 357
    thromboembolism, 239–241
Pulse
    femoral, 15, 34
    oximetry, 52, 258
Pupillary size and reactivity, 67
Pyelography, 340

R

Radiography, 50, 69, 97, 106, 195, 204–205, 229, 241
    abdominal, 336–351
    contrast, 326, 337–340, 360
    interpretation of, 342–351
    thoracic, 16, 34, 236–237, 352–360
Radioisotope brain scans, 205
Rales, 15, 50
Reduction, 86–88, 91
Renal failure. *See* Acute renal failure (ARF)
Renal failure index, 326
Reperfusion injury, 139–146. *See also* Oxygen free-radical-induced brain injury
    postischemic, 65
Respiratory
    emergencies, 227–258
    failure, 113, 245–246
Resuscitation
    cardiopulmonary (CPR), 269
    recommended procedure, 296–297
Reticulosis, 224
Retinal detachment, 224
Rhabdomyolysis, 181, 270
Rodenticide consumption, 133

S

Scintigraphy, ventilation-perfusion, 240
Secondary autolytic brain tissue destruction, 71
Sedation, 185–186, 237
Seizure disorders, 164, 193–210
    antiepileptic drugs, 195–196, 199, 206–209
    causes, 194, 203–204
    realistic therapy goals, 195, 205–206
    refractory cases, 197–198
Septic shock. *See* Systemic inflammatory response syndrome (SIDS)
Shock, 59, 110–130
    monitoring of, 117–118
    pathophysiology of, 112
Skull fractures, 78
    basilar, 66
Small airway disease, chronic, 229
Small Animal Coma Scale (SACS), 67, 80
Smoke-inhalation injury, 234, 358
Snakes
    envenomization by, 167–189
    genera and species, 168
Sodium bicarbonate, 116, 125, 160, 165, 328
Sodium loading, 317–318
Spinal cord
    decompression, 40
    trauma, 40–45, 58, 61
Splenic rupture, 132, 134
Stabilization of vertebral column, 40
Status asthmaticus, 239
Status epilepticus, 198, 207–208
Steinmann pin, 88–89
Stenosis, subaortic, 28
Steroid drugs. *See* Corticosteroid drugs
Stoicism in animals, 280
Superoxide dismutase, 77, 143, 319
Systemic inflammatory response syndrome (SIDS), 110–111, 146, 290–302, 345–346, 349
    drugs used, 295–296
    monitoring variables, 293
    specific bacterial infections, 291, 322

T

Tachypnea, 235
Taurine in commercial cat foods, 12, 28
Thermometer, low-recording, 268
Thermoregulation, 259–260, 265
Thoracentesis, 58, 243–244
Thoracic trauma, 48–54, 56, 59
Thoracocentesis, 241–242
Thrombocytopenic activity of venoms, 172
Thromboembolism, aortic, 29–36
Thrombosis, 7, 10, 31
Tirilazad mesylate, 44–45
Tissue plasminogen activator (TPA), 38
Tonometry, 217
Toxicoses, general treatment, 156–157, 191
Tracheal
    foreign bodies, 228
    obstruction, 228–229
    stenosis, 228
Tracheostomy, 230–232, 234, 251–252
Transfusion reactions, 135–137
Tromethamine, 77
Tumors, 344–347, 350

U

Ultrasonography, 28, 99, 101, 326
Urethral trauma, 102–109
Urethrography, positive-contrast retrograde, 106, 108
Urethrostomy, 109
Urethrotomy, 109
Urinary system effects of snakebite, 177–178
Urinary tract trauma, 93–94
Urography, 340
    excretory, 326
    intravenous, 98

V

Valvular insufficiency, mitral, 24
Vascular permeability of snakebite, 169–170
Vasoactive drugs, 8–10, 115, 125, 318–319, 322
Vasoconstriction, 49, 112
    renal, 312
Vasogenic shock, 120
Venodilators, 185–186, 237
Venom identification, 188
Venomous snake genera and species, 168
Ventilation-perfusion scintigraphy, 240
Ventilatory compromise, 51
Ventricular dysfunction, 14
Vertebral column stabilization, 40
Vestibular system lesions, 64
Vomiting, 303–305, 330–331, 343

W

Warfarin, 38
Whole blood clotting test (WBCT20), 188
Wiring, 58, 88–89, 253